The Sepsis Codex

The Sepsis Codex

Edited by

MARCIO BORGES SA
Multidisciplinary Sepsis Unit Intensive Care Department
Son Llatzer University Hospital

Associate Professor of Infectious Diseases in the Balearic Islands
University (UIB) Palma de Mallorca, Spain

Principal Investigator of Sepsis Group of the Balearic Islands
Health Research Institute (IDISBA) Palma de Mallorca, Spain

Director of Sepsis Committee of the Iberian and Pan-american
Intensive Care Federation (FEPIMCTI) Mexico, Mexico

Sepsis Code Foundation, Palma de Mallorca, Spain

JORGE HIDALGO
Head of the Intensive Care Unit and COVID-19 Unit Belize Healthcare Partners,
Belize, Central America
President-Elect World Federation of Intensive and Critical Care

JAVIER PEREZ-FERNANDEZ
Intensive Care Solutions, Baptist Hospital of Miami,
Miami, FL, United States

ELSEVIER

The Sepsis Codex

ISBN: 978-0-323-88271-2

Copyright © 2023 Elsevier Inc. All rights reserved.

Publisher: Dolores Meloni
Acquisitions Editor: Charlotta Kryhl
Editorial Project Manager: Pat Gonzalez
Production Project Manager: Omer Mukthar
Cover Designer: Greg Harris

3251 Riverport Lane
St. Louis, Missouri 63043

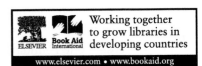

Working together to grow libraries in developing countries

www.elsevier.com • www.bookaid.org

Dedicated to the healthcare professionals, fearless, generous, and compromised with their patients. For you all, in the frontline of the fight against illnesses.
Javier, Jorge, and Marcio.

Picture Inflammation. An original Watercolor Painting from:
Dra. Gerhaldine Morazan. Clinico-Pathologist: inflammation

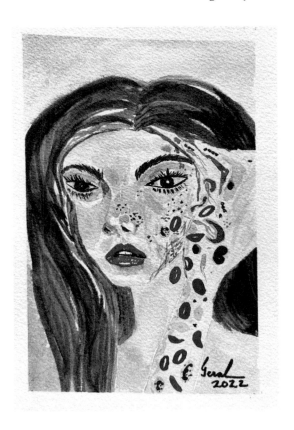

List of Contributors

Ahsan Ahmed
Critical Care Medicine, M H Samorita Hospital, Dhaka, Bangladesh
Assistant Professor and ICU In charge, KPC Medical College and Hospital, Kolkata, India

Tharawt Aisa
Critical Care Department, Manchester University Hospitals, Manchester Foundation Trust, Manchester, United Kingdom

Maria Jimena Aleman
School of Medicine, Universidad Francisco Marroquin, Guatemala

Gabriela Alvarado
Head of the General ICU at Hospital Regional de Occidente
Quetzaltenango, Guatemala

Javier Gil Anton
Department of Pediatric, Pediatric Intensive Care Unit, Biocruces, Bizkaia Health Research Institute, Cruces University Hospital, University of Basque Country, UPV/EHU, Barakaldo, Bizkaia, Spain

Zulmi Aranda
Department of Medicine
Pacific University
North University and South-America University
Chief Division of Critical Care
Regional Hospital
Pedro Juan Caballero, Paraguay

Pietro Arina
Bloomsbury Institute of Intensive Care Medicine
University College London
London, United Kingdom

Kazuaki Atagi
Division of Critical Care Medicine
Nara Prefecture General Medical Center
Shichijo Nishimachi
Nara City, Japan

Josep Maria Badia
Department of Surgery, Hospital General de Granollers, Universitat Internacional de Catalunya, Barcelona, Spain

Marie Baldisseri
Professor of Critical Care Medicine and Neurocritical Care
Critical Care Medicine
University of Pittsburgh Medical Center
Pittsburgh, PA, United States

Helena Barrasa
Intensive Care Medicine, Araba University Hospital, Vitoria, Alava, Spain

Juan Carlos de Carlos
Pediatric Intensive Care Unit
Univeristy Hospital Son Espases
Palma de Mallorca, Spain

Clara Centeno
Department of Urology, Parc Tauli, Hospital Universitari, Sabadell, Spain

Rajesh Chandra Mishra
Honorary Consultant Intensivist & Internist
Critical Care and Internal Medicine
Shaibya Comprehensive Care Clinic
Ahmedabad, Gujarat, India

Luis Chiscano-Camón
Intensive Care Department
Vall d'Hebron University Hospital
Vall d'Hebron Barcelona Hospital Campus
Barcelona, Spain
Shock, Organ Dysfunction and Resuscitation Research Group
Vall d'Hebron Research Institute (VHIR)
Vall d'Hebron University Hospital
Vall d'Hebron Barcelona Hospital Campus
Barcelona, Spain
Departament de Medicina, Universitat Autònoma de Barcelona, Barcelona, Spain

Craig Coopersmith
Professor Surgery
  Emory University
  Atlanta, GA, United States

Rafael Zaragoza Crespo
Sepsis Code Foundation
  Palma de Mallorca, Spain
Chief-head of Intensive Care Unit
  University Hospital Dr Peset
  Valencia, Spain

Luisa Cruz
School of Medicine, Universidad Francisco Marroquin,
  Guatemala

Jeanette Zúñiga Escorza
Adult, Intensive Care Unit, Hospital Juárez de México,
  Mexico City, Mexico

Elisabeth Esteban
Pediatric Intensive Care Unit
  Pediatric Transport Team
  University Hospital Sant Joan de Déu
  Barcelona, Spain

Ricard Ferrer
Intensive Care Department
  Vall d'Hebron University Hospital
  Vall d'Hebron Barcelona Hospital Campus
  Barcelona, Spain
Shock, Organ Dysfunction and Resuscitation Research
  Group
  Vall d'Hebron Research Institute (VHIR)
  Vall d'Hebron University Hospital
  Vall d'Hebron Barcelona Hospital Campus
  Barcelona, Spain
Departament de Medicina, Universitat Autònoma de
  Barcelona, Barcelona, Spain
Ciber Enfermedades Respiratorias (Ciberes), Instituto
  de Salud Carlos III, Madrid, Spain

Vanessa Fonseca-Ferrer
Pulmonary Disease and Critical Care Fellowship
  Program, Caribbean Healthcare System, San Juan,
  Puerto Rico, VA, United States

Fernando Fonseca
Chief, Intensive Care
  Hospital Universitario Araba
  Vitoria, Spain

Luis Gerena-Montano
Pulmonary Disease and Critical Care Fellowship
  Program, Caribbean Healthcare System, San Juan,
  Puerto Rico, VA, United States

Luis Antonio Gorordo-Delsol
Care Support Division, Hospital Juárez de México,
  Mexico City, Mexico

Deepa Gotur
Department of Medicine, Houston Methodist Hospital,
  Houston, TX, United States

Xavier Guirao
Unit of Endocrine Head/Neck Surgery. Department of
  Surgery, Unit of Surgical Site Prevention, Parc Tauli,
  Hospital Universitari, Sabadell, Spain

Jamila Hedjal
France Sepsis Association
  Ile de France
  Maisons Alfort, France

Ahmed F. Hegazy
Associate Professor of Anesthesiology and Critical Care
  Medicine, University of Western Ontario, London,
  ON, Canada

Allyson Hidalgo
Biochemistry, Arizona State University
  Phoenix, AZ, United States

Jorge Hidalgo
Head of the Intensive Care Unit and COVID-19 Unit
  Belize Healthcare Partners
  Belize City, Belize
President-Elect, World Federation of Intensive and
  Critical Care

Judith Jacobi
Critical Care Pharmacy Specialist
Sr. Consultant Visante, LLC.
Lebanon, IN, United States

Laura S. Johnson
Associate Professor of Surgery, Department of Surgery,
Emory University School of Medicine, Burn Medical
Director, Grady Memorial Hospital, Atlanta, GA,
United States

Montserrat Juvany
Department of Surgery, Hospital General de
Granollers, Granollers, Spain

Ryoung-Eun Ko
Department of Critical Medicine, Samsung Medical
Center, Sungkyunkwan University School of
Medicine, Seoul, South Korea

Christopher Lai
Medical Intensive Care Unit, Bicêtre Hospital, Paris-
Saclay University, AP-HP, Le Kremlin-Bicêtre, France

Ahsina Jahan Lopa
Critical Care Medicine
M H Samorita Hospital
Dhaka, Bangladesh

Consultant and Incharge ICU and Emergency, Shaha-
buddin Medical College, Dhaka, Bangladesh

John Lyons
Assistant Professor of Surgery
Department of Surgery
Emory University
Atlanta, GA, United States

Saad Mahdy
Consultant Anaesthesiology, University Hospital
Limerick, Dooradoyle, Limerick, Ireland

Adjunct Senior Clinical Lecturer, University of
Limerick, Limerick, Ireland

Manu L.N.G. Malbrain
First Department of Anaesthesiology and Intensive
Therapy, Medical University of Lublin, Lublin,
Poland

Medical Data Management, Medaman, Geel, Belgium

International Fluid Academy
Lovenjoel, Belgium

Alex Martin
Intensive Care, Araba University Hospital,
Vitoria, Spain

Javier Maynar
Clinical Chief
Intensive Care Medicine
Araba University Hospital
Vitoria, Alava, Spain

Michael Mazzei
Critical Care Fellow, University of Pittsburg, Pittsburg,
PA, United States

Michaël Mekeirele
Department of Critical Care
Vrije Universiteit Brussel (VUB)
Universitair Ziekenhuis Brussel (UZB)
Jette, Belgium

Graciela Merinos-Sánchez
Adult Emergency Department, General Hospital "Dr.
Eduardo Liceaga", Mexico City, Mexico

Sulimar Morales-Colón
Pulmonary Disease and Critical Care Fellowship
Program, Caribbean Healthcare System, San Juan,
Puerto Rico, VA, United States

Gerhaldine Morazan
AFI Medical Surveillance, Baylor College of Medicine
Houston, TX, United States

Prabath W.B. Nanayakkara
Amsterdam UMC location Vrije Universiteit Amsterdam, Department of Internal Medicine, Amsterdam,
the Netherlands

Amsterdam Public Health, Amsterdam, the
Netherlands

Victor Manuel Sanchez Nava
Chairman, Critical Care & Internal Medicine Hospital,
San Jose y Zambrano Hellion TEC Salud, Tecnolo-
gico de Monterrey, Monterrey, N.L., Mexico

Hector Alejandro Ramirez Garcia
Chairman, Critical Care & Internal Medicine Hospital,
San Jose y Zambrano Hellion TEC Salud, Tecnolo-
gico de Monterrey, Monterrey, N.L., Mexico

Lucila Nieves-Torres
Gynecology and Obstetrics Service, Hospital Juárez de
México, Mexico City, Mexico

Lorenzo Olivero
Faculty of Medicine
University of Panama, Transístmica, Panamá,
Panama

Carlos Enrique A. Orellana Jimenez
Critical Care Unit
General Hospital
Salvadoran Social Security Institute (ISSS)
San Salvador, El Salvador

José-Artur Paiva
Centro Hospitalar Universitario Sao Joao
Porto, Portugal

Faculty of Medicine
University of Porto
Porto, Portugal

Ketan Paranjape
Amsterdam UMC location Vrije Universiteit Amsterdam, Department of Internal Medicine, Amsterdam,
the Netherlands

Amsterdam Public Health, Amsterdam, the
Netherlands

Javier Perez-Fernandez
Intensive Care Solutions, Baptist Hospital of Miami,
Miami, FL, United States

Orlando Pérez-Nieto
Emergency and Critical Care
Hospital General San Juan del Río
Querétaro, Mexico

Paola Perez
School of Medicine, University of Virginia,
Charlottesville, VA, United States

Erika-Paola Plata Menchaca
Intensive Care Department
Vall d'Hebron University Hospital
Vall d'Hebron Barcelona Hospital Campus
Barcelona, Spain

Shock, Organ Dysfunction and Resuscitation Research
Group
Vall d'Hebron Research Institute (VHIR)
Vall d'Hebron University Hospital

Vall d'Hebron Barcelona Hospital Campus
Barcelona, Spain

Mary Jane Reed
Medical Director Biocontainment Unit
Department of Critical Care Medicine and Trauma
Surgery
Geisinger Medical Center
Danville, PA, United States

Jordi Rello
Vall d'Hebron Campus Hospital
Barcelona, Spain

William Rodríguez-Cintrón
Pulmonary Disease and Critical Care Fellowship Pro-
gram, Caribbean Healthcare System, San Juan,
Puerto Rico, VA, United States

Gloria M. Rodríguez-Vega
Department of Critical Care Medicine, HIMA-San
Pablo Caguas, Puerto Rico, United States

Jose Alfonso Rubio Mateo-Sidron
Cardiothoracic ICU
Hospital Universitario
Madrid, Spain

Juan Carlos Ruiz-Rodríguez
Intensive Care Department
Vall d'Hebron University Hospital
Vall d'Hebron Barcelona Hospital Campus
Barcelona, Spain

Shock, Organ Dysfunction and Resuscitation Research
Group
Vall d'Hebron Research Institute (VHIR)
Vall d'Hebron University Hospital
Vall d'Hebron Barcelona Hospital Campus
Barcelona, Spain

Departament de Medicina. Universitat Autònoma de
Barcelona, Barcelona, Spain

Carlos Sánchez
Head of Critical Care Services
Critical Care Services
Hospital General IESS Quevedo, Quevedo,
Ecuador

Juan Ignacio Sánchez
Pediatric Intensive Care Unit and Pediatric Emergency
Department

University Hospital
Madrid, Spain

Associate Professor, Faculty of Medicine, UCM,
Madrid, Spain

Marcio Borges Sa
Multidisciplinary Sepsis Unit
Intensive Care Department
Son Llatzer University Hospital
Associate Professor of Infectious Diseases in the
Balearic Islands University (UIB)
Palma de Mallorca, Spain

Principal Investigator of Sepsis Group of the Balearic
Islands Health Research Institute (IDISBA)
Palma de Mallorca, Spain

Director of Sepsis Committee of the Iberian and Pan-
american Intensive Care Federation (FEPIMCTI)
Mexico, Mexico

Sepsis Code Foundation
Palma de Mallorca, Spain

Michiel Schinkel
Amsterdam UMC location University of Amsterdam,
Center for Experimental and Molecular Medicine
(CEMM), Amsterdam, the Netherlands

Amsterdam UMC location Vrije Universiteit Amsterdam, Department of Internal Medicine, Amsterdam,
the Netherlands

Amsterdam Institute for Infection and Immunity (AII),
Amsterdam, the Netherlands

Reena Shah
Internal Medicine
Aga Khan University Hospital Nairobi
Nairobi, Kenya

Jorge E. Sinclair De Frías
Department of Physiology
Faculty of Medicine
University of Panama, Transístmica, Panamá,
Panama

Jorge E. Sinclair Avila
Punta Pacific Hospital/Johns Hopkins Medicine Panama, Pacífica, Panamá, Panama

Mervyn Singer
Bloomsbury Institute of Intensive Care Medicine
University College London
London, United Kingdom

Sharmili Sinha
Critical Care
Apollo Hospitals
Bhubaneswar, Odisha, India

Gee Young Suh
Department of Critical Medicine, Samsung Medical
Center, Sungkyunkwan University School of
Medicine, Seoul, South Korea

Ahmed Taha
Assistant Clinical Professor - Cleveland Clinic Learner
collage of Medicine, Case Western Reserve University, Cleveland, OH, United States

Critical Care Institute, Cleveland Clinic, Abu Dhabi,
United Arab Emirates

Jean-Louis Teboul
Medical Intensive Care Unit, Bicêtre Hospital, Paris-
Saclay University, AP-HP, Le Kremlin-Bicêtre, France

Arlene C. Torres
Intensive Care Solutions (ICS)
Baptist Hospital of Miami
Miami, FL, United States

Elena Usón
Intensive Care Medicine, Can Missees Hospital. Eivissa,
Spain

Domien Vanhonacker
Department of Critical Care
Vrije Universiteit Brussel (VUB),
Universitair Ziekenhuis Brussel (UZB),
Jette, Belgium

Department of Anesthesiology,
Vrije Universiteit Brussel (VUB),
Universitair Ziekenhuis Brussel (UZB),
Jette, Belgium

W. Joost Wiersinga
Amsterdam UMC location University of Amsterdam,
Center for Experimental and Molecular Medicine
(CEMM), Amsterdam, the Netherlands

Amsterdam UMC University of Amsterdam, Department of Internal Medicine, Amsterdam, the
Netherlands

Amsterdam Institute for Infection and Immunity (AII),
Amsterdam, the Netherlands

Eder Zamarrón
Emergency and Critical Care
    Hospital Regional #6 IMSS
    Madero City, Tamaulipas, Mexico

Janice L. Zimmerman
Adjunct Professor of Medicine
    Medicine
    Baylor College of Medicine
    Houston, TX, United States

Preface

While in medical school, we spend many hours understanding the complexity of the disease and the several diagnostic tests and therapeutic options for a patient. Countless clinical and theoretical sessions cover differential diagnosis, complicated organ interactions, and the constantly changing world of evidence.

A precise definition of diseases is important as they allow accurate diagnosis, which is essential to enable appropriate therapeutic interventions to be given and hence outcome to be maximized. Much has been written over the last decade about Sepsis. Some medical conditions have fairly clear-cut pathophysiology, which is relatively simple to define and diagnose and can be made in the presence of comparatively specific clinical symptoms and supported by images and laboratory testing. However, in Sepsis, the situation is more complex. Sepsis can be caused by various microorganisms in individuals of different ages, predisposing factors, and genetic traits, among others, resulting in varying degrees of the immune response.

The "one-size-fits-all" approach in a patient with Sepsis is insufficient to meet individual patients' needs.

Advances in medical knowledge in genetics, biomarkers, and other features, with subsequent acknowledgment of the heterogeneity of patients and treatments effects in clinical trials, have required clinicians to be ever more cognizant of the need to approach therapeutic endeavors by patient subgroups.

Working with an exceptional group of physicians and researchers worldwide, we have led an effort to present *The Sepsis Codex*, a 35-chapter book to summarize the cutting edge of science regarding Sepsis. We want to thank all the authors for their excellent contributions. We hope all the readers will have a good time reading the book.

Jorge Hidalgo, MD, MACP, MCCM, FCCP
Belize City, Belize

Marcio Borges Sa, MD
Palma de Mallorca, Spain

Javier Perez-Fernandez, MD, FCCM, FCCP
Miami, Florida

Acknowledgments

The preparation of this project required the effort of many individuals. We want to thank the authors or collaborators for coming on board on this endeavor, being able to support the pressure of a timeline, taking a moment to satisfy the call for expertise and help, and keeping aside multiple other tasks and, indeed, personal time.

We sincerely appreciate the talent and accomplishments of the Elsevier professionals, Charlotta Kryhl and, in particular, Ms. Patricia Gonzalez, who partnered with us all along and took our manuscript and produced it into this book.

Finally, many thanks to our patients, the ultimate motive of our existence, to whom we must express our gratitude. They trust us with their life and impulse our learning and actions to make us always keep the utmost attention to details. We welcome all comments, pros, cons, and suggested revisions.

Contents

CHAPTER 1

Sepsis: Past, Present, and Future—Lessons Learned from COVID-19

JOSÉ-ARTUR PAIVA • JORDI RELLO

COVID-19, in its most severe forms, is a model of sepsis [1]. It is caused by a microorganism, characterized by a thrombotic endotheliopathy involving the entire body, which has been called the cornerstone of organ dysfunction in COVID-19 [2]. The initial phase of viral replication may be followed by inadequate host response, leading to generalized disease, although blood cytokine levels are not always very high in COVID-19 [3]. They are still raised, both Th1 and Th2, compared with healthy individuals and can reach levels similar to those in patients with sepsis due to other causes [4,5]. It is associated with increased neutrophil extracellular trap release that may be involved in the thrombotic endotheliopathy, endotoxin levels, probably endogenously released from Gram-negative bacteria in the gut, are often increased in severe COVID-19, and are directly related to the severity of the disease [6], suggesting the possibility of inadequate blood flow to the various organs [7] and in the subpopulation of COVID-10 patients admitted to an intensive care medicine (ICM) service, multiple organ dysfunction syndrome (MODS) accounts for most of the deaths.

Even characteristics usually presented as disparities between COVID-19 and sepsis may be better viewed as similarities. There is more marked hypercoagulable state and more frequent pulmonary vascular injury in severe COVID-19, but similar features may exist in subsets of patients with sepsis due to other individual pathogens that have not been subject to the same intense investigation [1]. Children are mostly spared, but childhood deaths from sepsis occur mainly in low- and middle-income countries, particularly in sub-Saharan Africa, and many are due to sepsis related to respiratory infections and diarrheal diseases [8]. Around 10% of the COVID-19 cases develop "long COVID", but it is demonstrated that up to 50% of sepsis survivors suffer from a postsepsis syndrome with persisting physical, cognitive, and psychological sequelae [9].

Therefore, severe COVID-19 is a disease that respects the criteria for sepsis and for which we do not yet have an effective standardized management. Yet, in spite of this formidable handicap, several studies have shown that there was a substantial improvement in survival among people admitted to critical care with COVID-19 from March to June 2020, during the first wave of the pandemic, and that this improvement was not due to temporal changes in age, sex, ethnicity, or major comorbidity burden of admitted patients, as the reduction persisted after adjusting for illness severity and changes in patient case mix [10,11]. In fact, in spite of the inexistence of an etiotropic therapy of COVID-19, hospital mortality from critical COVID-19 at end of the first wave was around 20%−25%, in Europe, similar to those observed in other forms of sepsis.

What were the potential reasons for this fall in mortality along the first wave and for a sustained good response thereafter? In our opinion, much of it was due to a combination of factors that are listed in Table 1.1.

When we reflect on the huge and intense effort put up to overcome the COVID-19 challenge, we may end up thinking that we may have been taking severe infection and sepsis too lightly. And this may be partially true. Indeed, it advisable to leverage sepsis response

TABLE 1.1
Factors Associated With Reduction in Critical COVID-19 Mortality

1. Patient and society awareness: patient presented earlier to hospital when feeling unwell

2. Focus on prevention
   2.1 Vaccine development
   2.2 Mass vaccination
   2.3 Infection control practices at health units and at societal levels

3. Better and easier access to intensive care
   3.1 Expansion of intensive care unit (ICU) facilities
   3.2 Fast track assessment and specific flows with fast ICU admission
   3.3 Fast diagnostic methodologies

4. Advances in clinical management
   4.1. Pharmacological and respiratory support strategies reducing iatrogeny

5. New research paradigm
   5.1 Adaptive platform trials
   5.2 Shortened Clinical Research Form (CRFs) and/or automated data collection
   5.3 Preference for pragmatic versus explanatory studies.
   5.4 Development of international registries with harmonized data collection
   5.5 Encouragement of collaboration between investigators and research groups with similar interests

on the COVID-19 challenge. COVID-19 may be a game changer for sepsis research and clinical practice.

The new game laws coming up and changing sepsis management scenario are summarized in Table 1.2.

The pace for COVID-19 research has been much faster, and the process of implementation of new knowledge into clinical practice is more consequential. The investigation of corticosteroids to treat non-COVID sepsis lasts for five decades and at least 40 clinical trials have resulted in equivocal evidence of their effectiveness [12], while it took less than one year to show a clear benefit of dexamethasone in COVID-19 [13,14] and to apply it in clinical practice. On the same line, there is no immunomodulatory therapy approved for non-COVID sepsis, while interleukin-6 inhibitors—tocilizumab (or sarilumab)—and Janus kinase inhibitors—baricitinib (or tofacitinib)—are already used for severe COVID-19. This means that a new model for biomedical research was attained, understanding that clinical research is not complete prior to implementation and that research and practice can

and should coexist. The wheel that converges Implementation Science with Precision Medicine and with Learning Health Care System [15] was put to move much faster and therefore new knowledge was achieved and implemented more efficiently. Transforming ongoing data on ongoing learning, understanding clinical patterns, optimizing the use of behavior data and genomics to drive clinical and patient decision-making are key features of a modern intensive care department.

For decades, ICM lumped different diseases into syndromes and developed guidelines for a common framework of treatment of these syndromes. Adult respiratory distress syndrome (ARDS) and sepsis are two very good examples of this strategy.

The diversity of ARDS has long been perceived. Factors used to identify ARDS subphenotypes may be clinical—pulmonary versus nonpulmonary, medical versus trauma, focal versus diffuse—physiological—PaO_2/FiO_2, dead space fraction, ventilator ratio, driving pressure—or, more recently, biological—genomic,

TABLE 1.2
New Perspectives That are Changing Sepsis Management Scenario

1. Link research to change of clinical practice

2. Avoid lumping the unlumpable

3. Recognize phenotypes and subphenotypes

4. Move toward personalized medicine

transcriptomic, proteomic, or metabolomic. ARDS patients can be stratified according to markers of inflammation for prognostic enrichment [16]. Using latent class analysis, two distinct subphenotypes of ARDS were identified based on combined clinical and biologic data from patients enrolled in two large clinical trial cohorts [17]: the "hyperinflammatory" subphenotype, characterized by enhanced inflammation, fewer ventilator-free days, and increased mortality, compared to the "hypoinflammatory" subphenotype. These two subphenotypes have been found in subsequent independent analyses of multiple other ARDS trial cohorts, and the poor prognosis associated with the hyper inflammatory phenotype persists [18–20]. In spite of no trials have yet used biologic phenotyping prerandomization, due to unavailability of bedside biomarkers testing, there is mounting evidence that biologic phenotype predicts treatment response to several different interventions, namely positive end-expiratory pressure (PEEP) [17], fluid management strategies [19], and simvastatin [21]. High PEEP, liberal fluid management, and simvastatin were associated to better outcome in the "hyperinflammatory" subphenotype, and this benefit did not occur in the "hypoinflammatory" subphenotype. Using hierarchical clustering, two similar subphenotypes—the "uninflamed" and the "reactive" subphenotypes—were identified, based on plasma protein biomarkers [22]. It was shown later that there were differences in blood leukocyte gene expression between groups: approximately one-third of genes were differentially expressed, with upregulation of oxidative phosphorylation genes in the "reactive" subphenotype [23].

Studies have shown that COVID-19, itself, had different subphenotypes. Vasquez et al. performed a study to investigate the existence of distinct subphenotypes of COVID-19 in a large, geographically and demographically diverse population of critically ill patients and to replicate the results in a second independent population. Latent class analysis identified four subphenotypes with consistent characteristics across the discovery (45 centers; $n = 2188$) and replication (22 centers; $n = 1112$) cohorts, leading to different clinical outcomes and to diverse mortality, 17% in the least severe and 37% in the most severe subphenotype [24]. In another study, Bos et al. showed that there was no statistical evidence for respiratory subphenotypes using static data at any time during the first four days of mechanical ventilation, but time-dependent analysis showed that two subphenotypes were developed within the first days of mechanical ventilation. Patients with an upward trajectory of

ventilatory ratio, a marker of dead space ventilation, had a higher risk of venous thrombotic events, more frequently developed acute kidney injury, required longer invasive mechanical ventilation, and had higher mortality [25].

Sepsis is another heterogeneous syndrome that has historically been treated with a protocolized approach. A recent study on the global burden of sepsis [8] showed that, in 2017, an estimated 48.9 million incident cases of sepsis were recorded worldwide and 11.0 million sepsis-related deaths were reported, representing 19.7% of all global deaths. Age-standardized sepsis incidence fell by 37.0% and mortality decreased by 52.8% from 1990 to 2017. However, this estimated burden of sepsis is twice that thought previously, which is largely attributable to the far higher burden among people living in areas with a lower sociodemographic index, for whom data had previously been lacking. There are substantial differences between regions, in total number of sepsis deaths, age distribution of sepsis deaths, and case fatality, with the highest burden in sub-Saharan Africa, Oceania, south Asia, east Asia, and southeast Asia. These differences by location are alarming and deserve urgent attention from the global health, research, and policy communities. Antimicrobial resistance (AMR) poses an additional challenge to sepsis treatment, and the combination of high incidence of sepsis and high incidence of AMR is a cradle to the vicious circle of broad-spectrum antibiotic use and AMR selection. The use of a protocolized approach for sepsis, namely the surviving sepsis campaign guidelines [26] or their local adaptations, has significantly contributed to the decrease in sepsis mortality in the last two decades. In spite of the protocolized approach, the existence of different subphenotypes has long been acknowledged. Wong et al. have developed a biomarker-based mortality risk model for pediatric sepsis, as well as gene expression-based subphenotypes of pediatric septic shock. They found that among intermediate- and high-risk patients, corticosteroids were associated with a more than tenfold reduction in the risk of a complicated course in one subphenotype but not in the other [27]. Gårdlund et al. used latent class analysis to identify six distinct subphenotypes of septic shock in adults using clinical data from PROWESS Shock study, each with a typical profile: (a) "Uncomplicated Septic Shock," (b) "Pneumonia with ARDS," (c) "Postoperative Abdominal," (d) "Severe Septic Shock," (e) "Pneumonia with ARDS and MODS," and (f) "Late Septic Shock" [28]. The six-class showed high entropy approaching 1 (i.e., 0.92), indicating there was excellent separation between classes. Seymour et al. used machine learning applied to electronic health record data, limited to 29 variables, mostly vital signs and laboratory tests collected within the initial 6 h following hospital presentation, and identified four subphenotypes with different genetic and inflammatory markers and markedly different mortality rates [29]. The α phenotype was the most common (33%) and included patients with the lowest need of a vasopressor; in the β phenotype (27%), patients were older and had more chronic illness and renal dysfunction; in the γ phenotype (27%), patients had more inflammation and pulmonary dysfunction; patients of the δ phenotype (13%) had more liver dysfunction and septic shock. Simulation models showed that varying the phenotype frequencies within a randomized control trial of early goal-directed therapy changed the results from more than 33% chance of benefit to more than 60% chance of harm, suggesting that these phenotypes may help in understanding heterogeneity of treatment effects and that different phenotypes deserve different therapeutic approaches.

This raising awareness of the existence of subphenotypes among critical care syndromes, potentially targetable with different therapeutic approaches, led to the proposal of a new lexicon. Gattinoni and Marini [30] defended that, while rearranging and rethink these broad ultra-lumped definitions would be acceptable, they would prefer and support a delumping scenario, labeling diseases on the basis of their etiology. This would certainly push toward personalized medicine, admitting that not only the etiological treatment but also the appropriate respiratory support approach might be different in different situations and at different stages of the disease process.

In our opinion, we absolutely need to reform the lexicon but not to abandon it. In spite of all the reasons stated above, these umbrella concepts, such as sepsis and ARDS, are useful and fundamental to promote public awareness and societal lobby, to potentiate public and professional education, to facilitate early recognition and implementation of specific patient care pathways, to support research, and finally to gain and maintain political and policymaker focus. Being able to grab citizen's and policymakers' attention to sepsis as a public health threat is a prerequisite for a maximized strategy. However, to improve results, acknowledgment of subphenotypes to tailor therapy and support and to test therapeutics in clinical trials is necessary. Anchored in consensus guidelines, a quantum leap of personalized approach is an unmet clinical need.

CONCLUSIONS

Sepsis is defined as an aberrant and dysfunctional response to an infection. Past studies have been characterized by many efforts to improve diagnostic tools and unsuccessful efforts to reduce mortality based on adjunctive therapies.

The present epidemic of COVID has provided a good sepsis paradigm originated from a viral trigger. It emphasizes the importance on individualization on different clinical phenotypes and the importance of time in therapeutic management. Whereas measures effective in reducing the viral burden can be effective if started very early, they are useless if delayed. Lack of success of convalescent plasma is a clear evidence on the need to individualize management based on time after disease onset. Moreover, the effectiveness of some monoclonal antibodies used very early opens an opportunity to expand therapy in other viral or bacterial infections, particularly in solid organ transplant recipients or other immunocompromised subjects. Lastly, the success in reducing mortality by the use of steroids in patients requiring additional oxygen is a new paradigm to be expanded through the use of different immunomodulatory agents in a precision therapy approach.

All together, these observations represent an opportunity for further research development to cover management gaps. It is paradoxical that being the immune response the key of the evolution from infection to sepsis, rapid tests for monitoring the immune response at bedside have not been developed and successfully implemented. With the experience learned from COVID-19 disease, next steps for sepsis management improvement with potential impact on outcomes should focus on: (a) identification of subclinical phenotypes at the bedside, using clinical and biological markers; (b) implementation of a precision medicine strategy, balancing the use of therapy targeted to reduce the organism burden at the onset and of immunomodulatory agents in a second time window; (c) development of immune response assessment at the bedside, early after the diagnosis of serious infections, to anticipate individual infected patients at high risk of developing sepsis and to customize specific preemptive therapies based on the risk.

REFERENCES

[1] Vincent JL. COVID-19: it's all about sepsis. Future Microbiol 2021;16(3):131–3.
[2] Pons S, Fodil S, Azoulay E, Zafrani L. The vascular endothelium: the cornerstone of organ dysfunction in severe SARS-CoV-2 infection. Crit Care 2020;24(1):353.

[3] Sinha P, Matthay MA, Calfee CS. Is a "cytokine storm" relevant to COVID-19? JAMA Intern Med 2020;180(9): 1152−4.

[4] Kox M, Waalders N, Kooistra E, et al. Cytokine levels in critically ill patients with COVID-19 and other conditions. JAMA 2020;324(15):1565−7.

[5] McElvaney OJ, McEvoy N, McElvaney O, Carroll T, Murphy M, Dunlea D, Choileain O, et al. Characterization of the inflammatory response to severe COVID-19 illness. Am J Respir Crit Care Med 2020;202(6):812−21.

[6] Arunachalam PS, Wimmers F, Mok CKP, Perera R, Scott M, Hagan T, Sigal N, et al. Systems biological assessment of immunity to mild versus severe COVID-19 infections in humans. Science 2020;369(6508):1210−20.

[7] Zuo Y, Yalavarthi S, Shi H, Gockman K, Zuo M, Madison J, Blair C, et al. JCI Insight 2020;5(11):e138999.

[8] Ruud KE, Johnson SC, Agesa KM, Shackelford KA, Tsoi D, Kieylan DR, Colombara DV, et al. Global, regional, and national sepsis incidence and mortality, 1990-2017: analysis for the global burden of disease study. Lancet 2020; 395(10219):200−11.

[9] Prescott HC, Iwashyna TJ, Blackwood B, Calandra T, Chlan LL, Choong K, Connolly B, et al. Understanding and enhancing sepsis survivorship. Priorities for research and practice. Am J Respir Crit Care Med 2019;200(8): 972−81.

[10] Docherty AB, Mulholland RH, Lone NI, Cheyne CP, De Angelis D, Diaz-Ordaz K, Donegan C, et al. Changes in in-hospital mortality in the first wave of COVID-19: a multicentre prospective observational cohort study using the WHO Clinical Characterisation Protocol UK. Lancet Respir Med 2021;9(7):773−85.

[11] Dennis JM, McGovern AP, Vollmer SJ, Mateen BA. Improving survival of critical care patients with coronavirus disease 2019 in England: a national cohort study, March to June 2020. Crit Care Med 2021;49(2):209−14.

[12] Rygard SL, Butler E, Granholm A, Hylander Moller M, Cohen J, Finfer S, et al. Low-dose corticosteroids for adult patients with septic shock: a systematic review with meta-analysis and trial sequential analysis. Intensive Care Med 2018;44(7):1003−16.

[13] The RECOVERY Collaborative Group. Dexamethasone in hospitalized patients with covid-19. N Engl J Med 2021; 384:693−704.

[14] Sterne JA, for the The WHO Rapid Evidence Appraisal for COVID-19 Therapies (REACT) Working Group. Association between administration of systemic corticosteroids and mortality among critically ill patients with COVID-19: a meta-analysis. JAMA 2020;324(13):1330−41.

[15] Chambers D, Feero WG, Khoury MJ. Convergence of implementation science, precision medicine, and the learning health care System: a new model for biomedical research. JAMA 2016;315(18):1941−2.

[16] Wilson JG, Calfee CS. ARDS subphenotypes: understanding a heterogeneous syndrome. Crit Care 2020;24:102.

[17] Calfee CS, Delucchi K, Parsons PE, Thompson BT, Ware LB, Matthay MA. Subphenotypes in acute respiratory distress syndrome: latent class analysis of data from two randomised controlled trials. Lancet Respir Med 2014;2:611−20.

[18] Delucchi K, Famous KR, Ware LB, Parsons PE, Thompson BT, Calfee CS, ARDS Network. Stability of ARDS subphenotypes over time in two randomized controlled trials. Thorax 2018;73:439−45.

[19] Famous KR, Delucchi K, Ware LB, Kangelaris KN, Liu KD, Thompson BT, Calfee CS, ARDS Network. Acute respiratory distress syndrome sub-phenotypes respond differently to randomized fluid management strategy. Am J Respir Crit Care Med 2017;195:331−8.

[20] Sinha P, Delucchi KL, Thompson BT, McAuley DF, Matthay MA, Calfee CS, NHLBI ARDS Network. Latent class analysis of ARDS sub-phenotypes: a secondary analysis of the statins for acutely injured lungs from sepsis (SAILS) study. Intensive Care Med 2018;44:1859−69.

[21] Calfee CS, Delucchi KL, Sinha P, Matthay MA, Hackett J, Shankar-Hari M, NcDowell C, et al. Acute respiratory distress syndrome subphenotypes and differential response to simvastatin: secondary analysis of a randomised controlled trial. Lancet Respir Med 2018;6:691−8.

[22] Bos LD, Schouten LR, van Vught LA, Wiewel MA, Ong DSY, Cremer O, Artigas A, et al. Identification and validation of distinct biological phenotypes in patients with acute respiratory distress syndrome by cluster analysis. Thorax 2017;72:876−83.

[23] Bos LDJ, Scicluna BP, Ong DSY, Cremer O, van der Poll T, Schultz MJ. Understanding heterogeneity in biological phenotypes of acute respiratory distress syndrome by leukocyte expression profiles. Am J Respir Crit Care Med 2019;200:42−50.

[24] Vasquez CR, Gupta S, Miano TA, Roche M, Hsu J, Yang W, Holena DN, , et alfor the STOP-COVID investigators. Identification of distinct clinical subphenotypes in critically ill patients with COVID-19. Chest 2021;160(3): 929−43.

[25] Bos LDJ, Sjoding M, Sinha P, Bhavani SV, Lyons PG, Bewley AF, Botta M, et al. Longitudinal respiratory subphenotypes in patients with COVID-19-related acute respiratory distress syndrome: results from three observational cohorts. Lancet Respir Med 2021;9(12): 1377−86.

[26] Evans L, Rhodes A, Alhazzani W, Antonelli M, Coopersmith CM, French C, Machado F, et al. Surviving sepsis campaign: international guidelines for management of sepsis and septic shock 2021. Intensive Care Med 2021;47(11):1181−247.

[27] Wong HR, Atkinson S, Cvijanovich N, Anas N, Allen G, Thomas N, Bigham M, et al. Combining prognostic and predictive enrichment strategies to identify children with septic shock responsive to corticosteroids. Crit Care Med 2016;44. e1000−3.

[28] Gårdlund B, Dmitrieva N, Pieper C, Finfer S, Marshall J, Thompson BT. Six subphenotypes in septic shock: latent class analysis of the PROWESS Shock study. J Crit Care 2018;47:70–9.

[29] Seymour CW, Kennedy JN, Wang S, Chang CCH, et al. Derivation, validation, and potential treatment implications of novel clinical phenotypes for sepsis. JAMA 2019;321:2003–17.

[30] Gattinoni L, Marini J. Isn't it time to abandon ARDS? The COVID-19 lesson. Crit Care 2021;25:326.

CHAPTER 2

Sepsis Definitions: A Historical Perspective

JAVIER PEREZ-FERNANDEZ • ARLENE C. TORRES • PAOLA PEREZ

The definitions of sepsis have been the subject of statements, consensus conferences, and controversy for the last four decades. Since the 1980s when several multicenter trials failed to consistently demonstrate improved outcomes in patients with sepsis, many explained those suboptimal results by the different patient populations in the trials and the lack of consistent inclusion criteria. It was clear then that there was a need for standard definitions. The multifaceted nature of sepsis and its clinical manifestations, crossing several specialties, have also been part of the heterogenicity in the definitions and the pathophysiologic explanations. Requirements to define sepsis have included microbiologic samples, inflammatory markers, and physiologic variations of vital signs. For the last four decades, multiple consensus conferences and publications have covered the topic of sepsis definition aiming to create standard criteria and to enhance our ability to early diagnose sepsis [1].

According to the World Health Organization, sepsis is responsible for one in five deaths globally. In the United States, the Centers for Disease Control and Prevention report that sepsis affects over 1.7 million adults accounting for nearly 270,000 deaths [2]. Despite the burden of disease and the importance of prompt identification to provide better outcomes, a major disparity still exists regarding the definition of sepsis and its effects.

The COVID-19 pandemic has brought this topic to an even more relevant position. Throughout the pandemic, COVID-19 complications have been considered a secondary insult or consequence of the virus itself. Sepsis, a frequent complication of the COVID-19 infection, has many times been overseen, not being addressed, or diagnosed in patients with COVID-19 infection [3]. This might have highlighted the lack of clinical meaningfulness of the actual definitions expressed by some.

When reviewing the actual definitions, some aspects will need to be considered. The purpose of the chapter is to review the current scenario regarding the definitions and to determine the wish list for any updated ones. The need for standardization of the criteria is evident, and it will help us to better tackle this impacting disease.

WHAT IS SEPSIS?

Even classical definitions are broad and varied. From simple dictionary statements to more complicated ones, the literature is full of different subjects defining sepsis-related conditions. During many years, to define sepsis, it was required the presence of a source of infection. As our knowledge in sepsis expanded, there was a move to consider sepsis as an intrinsic body response to an infectious insult and hence the focus of the definitions was placed in the inflammatory cascade [4,5].

Regardless of the conceptual definition used, the consensus is that sepsis is a medical emergency requiring a timely response [2]. Despite significant advancements in the understanding and management of the pathophysiology of this clinical syndrome, including hemodynamic monitoring tools, resuscitation measures, etc., sepsis remains one of the major causes of morbidity and mortality in critically ill patients [6]. For that reason alone, defining sepsis and more specifically, diagnosing sepsis at an early stage, is of utmost importance.

SEPSIS THROUGH THE YEARS

As previously discussed, for decades, the presence of bacteremia was required to define sepsis. Both terms were frequently interchanged in the literature [7,8]. The trials conducted included a great variety of patients with sepsis, and the inclusion criteria were obscured by frequently using a disparity of definitions. It was not

The Sepsis Codex. https://doi.org/10.1016/B978-0-323-88271-2.00004-3

surprising for many that the results from those trials showed varied outcomes, many times failed to prove impact, and sometimes lacked replicability [9,10]. Additionally, the diverse number of definitions used made the comparison among trials difficult at least, and the term "tower of Babel" was introduced to explain the heterogenicity found in those definitions [11,12].

The Consensus Conferences

The first consensus conference occurred in August 1991 [13]. The members of the taskforce from the Society of Critical Care Medicine (SCCM) and the American College of Chest Physicians (ACCP) had the goal to define sepsis and to create uniformity and standardization. The first consensus introduced the term systemic inflammatory response syndrome (SIRS), a subject of ulterior discussion and controversy [5,8,14]. Other nomenclature coined were the definitions of severe sepsis (sepsis with the presence of an associated organ failure), septic shock, and multiple organ dysfunction syndrome. The conference brought fresh air to a congested world of names and subjects and paved the wave for multicenter trials and further advances in our knowledge of sepsis. The controversial point of the definitions was the term SIRS, its concepts, and its clinical meaningfulness. For most, SIRS criteria were highly sensitive and its application to define sepsis would include most patients in the intensive care unit lacking then, from clinical value [15–17]. This controversy remained for years.

In 2001, the Sepsis-2 Consensus definitions further clarified the concepts of sepsis and septic shock to include threshold values for organ damage [18]. The consensus was a joined effort from the European Society of Intensive and Critical Care Medicine, the ACCP, the SCCM, the American Thoracic Society, and the Surgical Infection Society. The taskforce introduced suspected infection-specific definitions and those were categorized as inflammatory, hemodynamic, general, organ dysfunction, and tissue perfusion variations. Biochemical indicators in the early detection of sepsis were also emphasized. Although new terminology was used, a critique to Sepsis-2 was the no modification of the diagnostic criteria from 1991 [19,20].

More recently published, in 2016, Sepsis-3 Consensus definitions deviated from SIRS criteria and defined sepsis as a "life-threatening organ dysfunction caused by a dysregulated host response to infection" [21]. The concept of organ dysfunction was emphasized. These Sepsis-3 definitions updated sepsis and septic shock and introduced the use of the quick Sequential Organ Failure

Assessment (qSOFA) scoring system, created for the early identification of simultaneous organ dysfunction in sepsis. The latest guidelines highlighted the requirement of early diagnosis in conjunction with speedy interventions during the ongoing sepsis process. One of the caveats of the Sepsis-3 was the unfortunate misrepresentation of the use of qSOFA by the medical community. Sepsis-3 did not propose the use of qSOFA as a screening tool to identify sepsis [22]. Rather, its use is meant to be a warning or prognosticator of an increased risk of deterioration for patients with a suspected infection.

Surviving Sepsis Campaign

At the beginning of the century, in parallel with the effort of defining sepsis, and with the goal to reduce sepsis mortality by 25% by 2009, the Institute for Healthcare Improvement in collaboration with a group of experts launched the Surviving Sepsis Campaign [23]. This initiative has had great acceptance in the medical community and has become a worldwide reference in the management of sepsis. The guidelines were updated in 2016 and most recently in 2021 [24,25].

Other Initiatives

For the last two decades, additional initiatives have been created internationally to reduce the global burden of sepsis, to enhance our knowledge of the disease and to promote education. Some of these have a local or regional scope, whereas others have transcended borders introducing new tools for the fight against sepsis. The Sepsis Alliance, the Global Sepsis Alliance, the International Sepsis Forum, or Code Sepsis Foundation are some examples of those. Albeit these initiatives seem to favor the expansion of our knowledge and the recognition of sepsis, a concern brought by several is that the number of different organizations, in parallel with the need to compete for the limited funding sources available, is creating an atmosphere of heterogenicity and competency and driving us afar from standardization.

FUTURE DIRECTIONS

Perhaps the lack of standardization in many sepsis trials has been an obstacle to reach a better understanding of the diagnosis and has created a limitation to achieve improved outcomes. It is for that reason that it becomes even more essential to evolve the definitions according to our increasing knowledge of the disease. Both clinical requirements and technologic advancements need to be included in our definitions to better serve the purpose of a timely diagnosis.

Clinical Needs

For definitions to work, they need to be easy to understand, simple to apply, and clear to interpret. Basically, the application of definitions in clinical practice is surrogated to the simplicity of these definitions. The present definitions are overly sensitive, and far from being specific, they introduce significant diagnostic challenges at the bedside. Many patients present with characteristics include in the defining criteria for sepsis. The introduction of the "sepsis alert" in many US institutions is an example of that. An increasingly number of false-positive alerts are deviating care and resources motivated by the nonspecific and highly sensitive criteria used [26,27]. Moreover, their lack of specificity is also manifested by the limitation of the diagnostic techniques, heavily resting into microbiologic tests complemented with radiologic images and clinical data.

Big data and possibly the use of artificial intelligence might be in the horizon to better formulate screening tools. Promising results with early warning systems, some of them in place nowadays, open a door for a hope in our fight against sepsis and might be helpful tools to better define sepsis [28,29]. The possibilities offered by big data analytics seem to be endless. The opportunities can go from classifying patients in different groups for prognostic purposes, based on historical cohorts of millions of patients, to the opportunity to cross-link references and physiologic variables to observe otherwise imperceptible meaningful details. The future will give us more answers in this direction, but the opportunities are certainly exciting.

Biomarkers

The introduction of biomarkers into sepsis definitions becomes a challenge itself. As the lack of a universally accepted biomarker remains and as the sensitivity and specificity of those are less than optimal in most cases, using a biomarker as a surrogate of the presence of sepsis is more than questionable.

Sepsis biomarkers have been commercialized over the last decades. Among them, the most popular included interleukin-6, C-reactive protein, presepsine, or procalcitonin. Although their role in the identification of sepsis has certainly deviated from the optimal, some (like procalcitonin) have demonstrated a role in the antibiotic de-escalation or stewardship [30,31].

Genetics and Phenotyping

Some more research is needed in advanced genetic techniques such as nucleic acid amplification, aiming to obtain detectable levels of the pathogen involved in the sepsis cascade [32]. Other efforts have been placed into predicting sepsis at an early phase with the combination of genetic information and artificial intelligence [33]. Up to date, those techniques have failed to demonstrate reasonable cost-value benefit and further investigation and refinement is needed to consider a broader use.

In the absence of clearly demonstrated biomarkers, our refinement in the sepsis definition must rest into a multistep approach including clinical pretest probability and diagnostic algorithms that will help us refine the presence of sepsis.

CONCLUSIONS

Albeit our knowledge of sepsis and its pathophysiology has evolved over the last decades, our definitions are yet to evolve at the same pace. Thirty years after the first consensus conference, the early identification of sepsis rests in physiologic parameters, nonspecific and overly sensitive. Medicine is evolving into personalization and phenotyping. Big data and artificial intelligence are being applied to diagnostic and treatment processes. We need to turn our eyes to these resources and consider our next step in defining not only sepsis but also its myriad of repercussions. As it is universally agreed that sepsis management is time-sensitive and that early diagnosis of the condition is ulteriorly determinant of the outcomes, we need to develop definitions that can be applied to screening tools, simple and at the same time sophisticated with high sensitivity and specificity.

REFERENCES

[1] Perez J, Dellinger RP. Sepsis definitions. In: Eichacker PQ, Pugin J, editors. Evolving concepts in sepsis and septic shock. Netherlands: Kluwer Publishers; 2001.

[2] Sepsis (nih.gov). Content source: Centers for disease Control and prevention, National Center for Emerging and Zoonotic Infectious Diseases (NCEZID), Division of Healthcare Quality Promotion DHQP August 17, 2021.

[3] Zhou F, Yu T, Du R, et al. Clinical course and risk factors for mortality of adult inpatients with COVID-19 in Wuhan, China: a retrospective cohort study. Lancet 2020;395:1054−62.

[4] Stedman's medical dictionary. 26th ed. Baltimore: Williams and Wilkins; 1995.

[5] Sibbald WJ, Marshall J. Christou N and the Canadian multiple organ failure study group. "Sepsis": clarity of existing terminology… or more confusion? Crit Care Med 1991;19:996−8.

[6] Kaukonen K, Bailey M, Suzuki S, et al. Mortality related to severe sepsis and septic shock among critically ill patients in Australia and New Zealand. 2000-2012. JAMA 2014; 311(13):1308−16.

[7] Bone RC, Fisher CJ, Clemmer TP, et al. Sepsis syndrome: a valid clinical entity. Methylprednisolone severe sepsis study group. Crit Care Med 1989;17:389−93.

[8] Sprung CL. Definitions of sepsis-Have we reached a consensus? Crit Care Med 1991;19:849−51.

[9] The Veterans Administration Systemic Sepsis Cooperative Study Group. Effect of high-dose glucocorticoid therapy on mortality in patients with clinical signs of sepsis. N Engl J Med 1987;317:659−65.

[10] Zeni F, Freeman B, Natanson C. Anti-inflammatory therapies to treat sepsis and septic shock: a reassessment. Crit Care Med 1997;25:1095−100.

[11] Bone RC. Let's agree on terminology: definitions of sepsis. Crit Care Med 1991;19:973−6.

[12] Dellinger RP, Bone RC. To SIRS with love. Crit Care Med 1998;26:178−9.

[13] Members of the American College of Chest Physicians/ Society of Critical Care Medicine Consensus Conference Committee. Definitions for sepsis and organ failure and guidelines for the use of innovative therapies in sepsis. Crit Care Med 1992;20:864−74.

[14] Levy MM, Dellinger RP, Townsend SR, et al. The Surviving Sepsis Campaign: results of an international guideline-based performance improvement program targeting severe sepsis. Intensive Care Med 2010;38:367−74.

[15] Rangel Frausto MS, Pittet D, Cortigan M, et al. The natural history of the Systemic Inflammatory Response Syndrome (SIRS). A prospective study. JAMA 1995;273: 117−23.

[16] Salvo I, De Cian W, Mussico M, et al. The Italian SEPSIS study: preliminary results on the incidence and evolution of SIRS, sepsis, severe sepsis and septic shock. Intensive Care Med 1995;21:S244−9.

[17] Opal SM. The uncertain value of the definition for SIRS. Chest 1998;113:1442−3.

[18] Levy MM, Fink MP, Marshall JC, et al. SCCM/ESICM/ ACCP/ATS/SIS international sepsis definitions conference. Crit Care Med 2003;31:1250−6.

[19] Kaukonen KM, et al. Systemic inflammatory response syndrome criteria in defining severe sepsis. N Engl J Med 2015;372(17):1629−38.

[20] Vincent JL. Dear SIRS, I'm sorry to say that I don't like you. Crit Care Med 1997;25(2):372−4.

[21] Singer M, Deutschman CS, Seymour CW, et al. The third international consensus definitions for sepsis and septic shock (Sepsis-3). JAMA 2016;315(8):801−10.

[22] Abraham E. New definitions for sepsis and septic shock: continuing evolution but with much still to be done. JAMA 2016;315(8):757−9.

[23] Dellinger RP, Levy MM, Carlet JM, et al. Surviving sepsis campaign: international guidelines for management of severe sepsis and septic shock: 2008. Intensive Care Med 2008;34(1):17−60.

[24] Rhodes A, Evans LE, Alhazzani W, et al. Surviving sepsis campaign: international guidelines for management of sepsis and septic shock: 2016. Intensive Care Med 2017; 43(3):304−77.

[25] Evans L, Rhodes A, Alhazzani W, et al. Surviving sepsis campaign: international guidelines for management of sepsis and septic shock 2021. Crit Care Med 2021; 49(11):e1063−143.

[26] Nguyen SQ, Mwakalindile E, Booth JS, et al. Automated electronic medical record sepsis detection in the emergency department. PeerJ 2014;2:e343.

[27] Parks Taylor S, Rozario N, Kowalkowski M, et al. Trends in false-positive code sepsis activation in the emergency department. Ann Am Thorac Soc 2020;17(4):520−2.

[28] Goh KH, Wang L, Yeow AYK, et al. Artificial intelligence in sepsis early prediction and diagnosis using unstructured data in healthcare. Nat Commun 2021;12:711.

[29] Zargoush M, Sameh A, Javadi M, et al. The impact of recency and adequacy of historical information on sepsis predictions using machine learning. Sci Rep 2021;11: 20869. https://doi.org/10.1038/s41598-021-00220-x.

[30] Lippi G, Montagnana M, Balboni F, et al. Academy of emergency medicine and care-society of clinical biochemistry and clinical molecular biology consensus recommendations for clinical use of sepsis biomarkers in the emergency department. Emerg Care J 2017;13:68.

[31] Schuetz P, Beishuizen A, Broyles M, Ferrer R, Gavazzi G, Gluck EH, et al. Procalcitonin (PCT)-guided antibiotic stewardship: an international experts' consensus on optimized clinical use. Clin Chem Lab Med 2019;57: 1308−18.

[32] Sinha M, Jupe J, Mack H, Coleman TP, Lawrence SM, Fraley SI. Emerging technologies for molecular diagnosis of sepsis. Clin Microbiol Rev 2018;31. https://doi.org/ 10.1128/CMR.00089-17.

[33] El-Rashidy N, Abuhmed T, Alarabi L, et al. Sepsis prediction in intensive care unit based on genetic feature optimization and stacked deep ensemble learning. Neural Comput Appl 2022;34:3603−32.

FURTHER READING

[1] Dellinger RP, Levy MM, Rhodes A, et al. Surviving sepsis campaign: international guidelines for management of severe sepsis and septic shock, 2012. Intensive Care Med February 2013;39(2):165−228. https://doi.org/10.1007/ s00134-012-2769-8. Epub 2013 Jan 30. PMID:23361625.

CHAPTER 3

The Epidemiology of Sepsis

JAMILA HEDJAL

INTRODUCTION

I found myself committed to actively fighting sepsis following the death of my thirteen-year-old son Farès from septic shock on appendicular peritonitis. In order to create awareness among both health professionals and the general public, I created the first French association for the fight against sepsis by surrounding myself with health professionals but also families of patients.

As a result, I have been contacted by several international, European, and national scholarly societies to help combat this unknown scourge.

That's why, I find myself sharing my experience by writing this chapter reporting my research.

I did not fail to train with the renowned French Universities of Medicine, the Sorbonne University, and University of Lorraine.

My goal is to popularize sepsis so that the general public can identify and thus learn to recognize its symptoms.

I will first address the definition of sepsis and its impact, its historical overview, and in a second step, we will focus on the microbial etiology, the need for rapid and optimal management, how to recognize symptoms, and we will conclude with prospects for improvement and directions for the future.

Definition of Sepsis and Its Impact

Sepsis is the most serious form of infection and causes an average of 11 million deaths each year according to the World Health Organization (WHO), and for its survivors, it leaves room for serious sequelae (more than 50% of survivors will have serious sequelae).

This is a global public health priority and emergency. One death by sepsis occurs every 2.8 s in the world.

At its World Assembly on May 29, 2017, the WHO called on all states to take action to combat sepsis, through actions in the fields of education, information, prevention, diagnosis, care, and research. The world figures are:
- 50 million people affected by sepsis worldwide.
- Nearly 700,000 deaths in Europe.
- In France, 57,000 deaths.
- The average cost of hospitalization is 16,000 euros.
- 40% of deaths in resuscitation (first cause of death).

Sepsis is defined by European and American learned societies as: an acute state of dysregulation of the body's response to infection (bacterial, viral, fungal, or parasitic) resulting in loss of organ function and life-threatening risk to the patient and therefore death.

In short, an excessive and abnormal response of the body to bacteria, viruses, fungi, or parasites destroying its own tissues and loss of vital organ functions one or more.

It is a general infection from an initial outbreak that discharges into the bloodstream. Most often, it formed by an untreated or poorly treated infection.

Its sources can come from lung infection, abdominal infections, skin and soft tissue infections, meningeal infections, urinary tract infections, care-related infections.

More than 80% of infections occur outside the hospital.

A global public health priority and emergency.

Sepsis can affect all of us. However, people with a weakened immune system are particularly at risk: people over 60 years of age, infants under one year of age, people with chronic diseases, immunodepressed people, people infected with acquired immunodeficiency syndrome (AIDS), and people who have had their spleen removed.

The severity of sepsis is not related to the infection but rather to the delay of diagnosis and therefore of its management because there is ignorance of the symptoms and recognition of its signs by the general public and health professionals.

Yet the scientific community has established international recommendations [1].

Faced with this unknown scourge, the WHO, at its World Assembly on May 29, 2017, drew the attention of all member countries to respond to the fight against sepsis, through actions in the fields of education, information, prevention, diagnosis, care, and research in each respective country.

The Sepsis Codex. https://doi.org/10.1016/B978-0-323-88271-2.00027-4

In addition, the scientific community has also established an alert indicator, simple to collect, in order to detect early in case of infection the risk of developing sepsis.

This alert indicator is called quick SOFA (qSOFA).

It is composed of three items: Sepsis = Infection + SOFA = or >2

(1) Systolic blood pressure <100 mmHg
(2) Respiratory rate >22 cycles/min
(3) Obnubilation or confusion

When at least two of these three criteria are present in a patient with an infection, then the patient is considered at very high risk of developing sepsis [2].

History of Sepsis

Sepsis has always cohabited with man; its origin can be found in ancient Greek which means putrefaction. For a better historical and precise understanding, I will remember here the concise summary of the Pasteur Institute: We can even go back to ancient Egypt. *After several theories in the 19th century, sepsis is defined as the diffusion of a pathogenic organism into the bloodstream.*

But the realization of severe septic states despite the development of effective antimicrobial treatments gradually leads to an awareness of the interaction between the responsible germ and the host response, leading to the concept of systemic inflammatory response syndrome.

Previously, for example, we used to refer to "hospital (or nosocomial) gangrene (or rot)." It often affected soldiers, following war wounds, which were frequently infected. The most famous of these cases is undoubtedly Richard Lionheart, who died in 1199 after the infection that followed his wound by an arrow. Puerperal fever has also been used to describe an infection that occurs in women after childbirth. This is how Lucretius Borgia died in 1519 giving birth to his seventh child. It was the French doctor Armand Trousseau who first suggested that nosocomial gangrene and puerperal fever corresponded to similar pathologies.

Ignaz Semmelweis, a Hungarian doctor who demonstrated in Vienna in 1847 the importance of hand hygiene in order to avoid the contagion of women in childbirth. But the contagiousness had been suspected by the late 18th century Scottish doctor Alexander Gordon.

It was two Alsatian doctors, Victor Feltz (1835–93) and Léon Coze (1819–96), who first demonstrated the presence of bacteria in the blood of a patient with puerperal fever, a deadly infection secondarily attributed to streptococci. Louis Pasteur, in collaboration with the maternity wards of Port-Royal, Cochin, and Lariboisière, confirmed these observations in 1879–80 and advocated hygiene during childbirth.

Sepsis is the result of a serious infection that usually begins locally (peritonitis, pneumonia, urinary tract infection, catheter infection, etc.). It often affects patients with weakened immune systems. When it occurs after surgery or other procedures, it can be called nosocomial infection. [3].

Epidemiology of Sepsis Worldwide

The overall incidence of sepsis and septic shock appears to be increasing, mainly due to the increasing prevalence of vulnerable populations (aging of the population, increased chronic failure, and immunocompromised patients) and improved detection. In most western registries, septic shock accounts for 10%–15% of ICU admissions. The incidence of sepsis and septic shock in resuscitation is estimated at 75,000 cases per year in France, 750,000 in the United States, and probably more than 19 million worldwide [4].

Alarming figures!

50 million patients affected per year worldwide.

11 million deaths a year worldwide.

40% of deaths in resuscitation (first cause of death).

350,000 newborns die worldwide each year.

2.9 million children die from sepsis each year.

49% of patients with sepsis in intensive care units contracted the infection in hospital.

25% of patients who survive sepsis have cognitive impairment.

Pediatric and Neonatal Sepsis are Distinguished

Of the 50 million cases of sepsis recorded worldwide each year, 20 million are among children under five. Newborns are particularly affected since sepsis is the cause of about 15% (2018 figure) of infant deaths (with an increased risk for preterm or low-weight babies).

Maternal Sepsis

Maternal sepsis results from infection during pregnancy, childbirth, following abortion or during the postpartum period. Obstetric infections are the third leading cause of maternal death (about 10%), most in low- and middle-income countries.

Sepsis Acquired in Hospital

Sepsis contracted directly in a hospital represents one in four cases of sepsis. It results from a complication of care and results in longer hospital stays and increased risks of antimicrobial resistance.

The available global epidemiological data on sepsis are insufficient, and even more so in low- and middle-income countries, where sepsis mortality is highest. 85% of sepsis cases and 84.8% of sepsis-related deaths occur in countries with low, low-medium, or medium sociodemographic indices, especially in sub-Saharan Africa and Southeast Asia.

Often, mortality from sepsis depends on the quality of care, health infrastructure, preventive measures, diagnosis, and management. There is an urgent need to improve infection prevention and control (for example, access to vaccines), sanitation (water, hygiene, and health), and the fight against antimicrobial resistance.

In industrialized countries, sepsis accounts for as many deaths as myocardial infarction: there are 95 cases of sepsis per 100,000 population for those under 65, and 1220 cases for those over 65. In developing countries, sepsis puerperal remains a major cause of death for women after childbirth (18,000 deaths per year). Neonatal sepsis is estimated to cause more than 350,000 newborn deaths worldwide.

In France
Mortality of sepsis patients is 30%, but mortality of the most serious form (septic shock) can reach 50%. It is estimated that 30,000 people die from sepsis in France. Projections for the future suggest a doubling of the number of cases in the next 50 years due, in particular, to the aging of the population. Despite these impressive figures, sepsis remains far behind other diseases in terms of research priority: while in industrialized countries, sepsis affects 1.8 times more people than heart disease, The funds invested in sepsis research are 13 times less than those invested in heart disease and 32 times less than those invested in AIDS research.

According to the researchers, 85% of sepsis cases in 2017 occurred in low- and middle-income countries, including sub-Saharan Africa, the South Pacific Islands near Australia, and South, East, and Southeast Asia.

In Africa
A significant proportion of sepsis can be attributed to the consequences of weak health systems, including poor sanitation and hygiene, and poor health care.

In fact, it is estimated that at least 2 million people die from sepsis in Africa.

In the United States
The epidemiology of severe sepsis in children has been particularly well studied in the United States of America. Of the 1,586,253 hospitalizations in 1995 among children (0−18 years) in seven states representing 24% of the American population, 9675 were sepsis according to the 9th International Classification of Diseases (ICD) [5].

LIMITATIONS AND CHALLENGES
Managing sepsis remains a challenge:
- Golden hours (6 h to save life: an emergency for its management) [6].
- Constantly changing area of research and therefore not enough investment in research compared to other diseases.
- The misuse of antibiotics in uninfected patients poses the problem of side effects and thus the development of microbial resistance.
- Increased demand from health professionals for biomarkers that improve their ability to distinguish patients under antiinfective treatment, that is, to differentiate patients with sepsis (microbial aggression) from those showing sterile aggression.

It is clear that currently, no biomarker, among the multitude of molecules evaluated, does not allow this distinction with certainty.
- Lack of awareness of sepsis by city health professionals, attending physicians, and specialists out of resuscitation leading to delays in management with sometimes a misorientation of the patient in an inappropriate department.
- Blood culture wait time to administer effective antibiotic to germ.
- Exposure to the risk of nosocomial infections for the already very fragile patient.

Epidemiology by Microbial Etiology
40% of sepsis and septic shock are linked to bacteremia.

The most common sources of sepsis input are:

Streptococcus, *Streptococcus pneumonia*, *Streptococcus pyogenes*, Staphylococcus, *Escherichia coli*, Enterobacteria, Candida.

The patient must be identified and treated quickly and referred to the appropriate care services upon arrival in the emergency department (cf Golden hours):
- Importance of clinical signs, close reassessment of patients in the emergency department septic.
- Benefits of a biomarker to quickly estimate the severity of sepsis.
- The predominant place of lactate (venous or arterial) at present: Tool very relevant prognosis.
- Determination of procalcitonin (PCT).

Interest in systematic initial dosing on entry into USC or resuscitation.

Proven role in reassessment of indication and duration of antibiotic therapy.

Blood culture, not to be neglected to appropriate antibiotic therapy [7].

Prospects for Improvement

Often, mortality due to sepsis depends on the quality of care, health infrastructure, preventive measures, hygiene measures, vaccination, diagnosis, and management. There is an urgent need to work to improve infection prevention and control and to combat antimicrobial resistance.

Prospects for Future Orientation

Several recommendations can be put in place to fight effectively against sepsis.

We can here refer to recommendations already made in France by learned societies of resuscitation and requested by the Directorate General of Health in a report where 10 recommendations were elaborated:

- Assessing the place of new molecular tools for microbiological diagnosis;
- Develop innovative biological and microbiological diagnostic tools for early patient, organizational and technical management (place of lactate, new molecular diagnostic tools for infections, quality of blood cultures and other diagnostic tests, relevance and risk of overuse, biomarkers of severity, imaging, etc.);
- Assessment of the place of existing biomarkers (C-reactive protein, PCT, lactate, etc.) in primary care pending international harmonization of ICD. Codification of sepsis by the ICD should be a tool for epidemiological monitoring of this condition.

In terms of translational research, it is proposed:

- develop new experimental models of sepsis by promoting cross-research between physicians and veterinarians;
- develop "digital-3D" organ models;
- promote interactions with cancer research, given the commonalities in terms of physiopathology between cancer and sepsis; this mission could be entrusted to multiagency thematic institutes;
- allow one or two CICs to develop the endotoxin model in healthy volunteers.

In terms of clinical research, it is proposed to:

- develop relevant criteria of judgment; mission entrusted to the learned societies involved in this mission in connection with users and under the aegis of the Ministry of Solidarity and Health;
- encourage the inclusion of all patients in cohorts or therapeutic trials—especially in the context of medical projects of hospital groups in the territory, since there is currently no reference treatment for sepsis;
- promote the development of research after sepsis both in the hospital and after discharge from the

hospital, in medical and social settings, and in the city;

- organize a national population epidemiological study under the auspices of the Ministry of Solidarity and Health [8];
- organize the epidemiological study for the child based on the Premature Newborn Cohort as a reference for epidemiological study on a pediatric cohort—the assessment of the role of qSOFA by primary care professionals [2].

CONCLUSIONS

The sooner sepsis is detected and its quality management assured, the greater the chances of survival.

Deaths from sepsis can be prevented if symptoms are recognized and quality management is assured.

Is It Still Necessary to Recognize the Signs?

For this, an awareness of health professionals and the general public with an education and training program is essential. Many international learned societies, associations, and organizations are mobilizing around the world to fight against sepsis: Global Sepsis Alliance, European Sepsis Alliance, Sepsis Trust, France Sepsis Association, etc. It is by working together that we could reduce this mortality.

At first in France, the association France Sepsis www. francesepsisassociation.com was created following a tragedy in a hospital setting, a death of a child by septic shock on appendicular peritonitis and whose mission is to raise awareness among health professionals and the general public in France and around the world.

How to Recognize Sepsis in Adults and Children Over 12 Years?

Symptoms in adults and children over 12 years of age:

- Drowsiness or confusion, difficulty speaking
- Extreme muscle pain
- Fever or chills (fever greater than 38 degrees or less than 36 degrees)
- Sense of impending death
- No urine for an entire day
- Shortness of breath and tachycardia
- Pale or mottled, cold extremities

How to Recognize Sepsis in Infant and Child—12 Years Old?

Symptoms in infants and children—12 years old:

- Fever (greater than 38 degrees or less than 36 degrees)
- Does not feed
- Vomit several times
- No urine all day

- Rapid breathing
- Seizure or convulsion
- Skin eruption (purpura)
- Lethargic and having trouble waking up

How to Avoid Sepsis?

Sepsis can be avoided through:
- vaccination;
- basic hygiene measures: hand washing;
- collective awareness by the general public and health professionals [9].

If an infection develops sepsis, the gateway to infection must be quickly identified and antibiotic treatment implemented. Identifying sepsis and treating it early saves lives (see Golden hours, the golden six hours).

Through my militant approach, I hope that the awareness of the fight against sepsis is generalized because the cases of sepsis will increase with the aging of the population plus antimicrobial resistance.

I warmly thank all the international and national learned societies that have accompanied me to educate me on sepsis, the Universities of Medicine, the Ministry of Health in France, my faithful professors Djillali Annane, Jean Carlet, and Jean Marc Cavaillon as well as my co-editors, professors Jorge Hidalgo, Marcio Borges, and Javier Perez.

REFERENCES

[1] Rhodes A. Surviving Sepsis Campaign: international guidelines for management of sepsis and septic shock: 2016. Intensive Care Med 2017;43:304–77.

[2] Singer M, Deutschman CS, Seymour C, Shankar-Hari M, Annane D, Bauer M, et al. The third international consensus definitions for sepsis and septic shock (Sepsis-3). JAMA 2016;315(8):801–10 (Le score qSOFA (pour quick SOFA)).

[3] Reference website Institut Pasteur.

[4] Septic shock J. Lemarié, S. Gibot (Chapter 167 of the full Treaty).

[5] WHO World Health Assembly. Improving the prevention, diagnosis and clinical management of sepsis, agenda item 12.2, AMS70.7. World Health Assembly Resolution. NHS England; 2017 (17 July 2017). Information on specifications of CQUIN indicators for CQUIN models 2017/18–2018/19 (Annex). Retrieved January 16, 2019 from NHS England website).

[6] Dellinger RP, Carlet JM, Masur H, Gerlach H, Calandra T, Cohen J, et al. Surviving Sepsis Campaign guidelines for a management of severe sepsis and septic shock. Soins Intensifs Méd 2004;30:536–55.

[7] Surviving sepsis Campaign: an international guide to managing sepsis and septic shock: 2016.

[8] Report 2019 "all united against an unknown scourge" professor Djillali Annane.

[9] Site de l'Association France Sepsis. www.francesepsisassociation.com.

CHAPTER 4

Pathophysiology of Sepsis

MARIA JIMENA ALEMAN • LUISA CRUZ • JORGE HIDALGO • ALLYSON HIDALGO

INTRODUCTION

The term sepsis originated from the ancient Greek term of "decomposition" and "putrefaction" [1,2]; however, it wasn't until 1914 when Hugo Schottmüller provided the first definition of sepsis as: a "state caused by microbial invasion from a local infectious source into the bloodstream which leads to signs of systemic illness in remote organs" [3]. Although an infection is required to diagnose sepsis, we now know that the catastrophic clinical picture is caused by the host's response to the invading pathogen more than the pathogen itself. Over the past decades, there has been a dramatic increase in the evidence behind the origin and pathophysiology of sepsis; however, sepsis remains as one of the most common causes of death in hospitalized patients [1]. In this chapter, we will dilucidate some of the mysteries behind the immunology, vascular, neuroendocrine, and metabolic response in sepsis.

IMMUNOLOGY

Sepsis refers to a dysregulated multisystem response to an infection [4]. Although the immune system begins with a compartmentalized microbial recognition, unknown triggers amplify the immune response leading to systemic inflammation and homeostatic unbalance. This complex process involves different cells, receptors, secreted proteins, enzymes, structural and chemical elements of defense which together protect the host from infection [5]. The immune system is able to recognize danger and pathogen signals, respond to them through different effector functions, regulate the inflammation, and generate an immunological memory (Fig. 4.1). However, this immune response widely varies across individuals, and even in the same individual at different times [5–7]. The reasons for the dysregulation and

maladaptive responses of the immune system in sepsis are still unanswered [3].

Immune Phenotypes

In most individuals, the immune response in sepsis will generate two distinct response patterns [8]. The first pattern has been the most traditionally recognizable phenotype. The majority of patients will have a phenotype pattern with both pro- and antiinflammatory responses present at the start of the infectious illness mounted by both innate and adaptive immune systems. These individuals eventually recover with restoration of homeostasis in both immune systems with a full disappearance of inflammation and recovery of immune cell paresis. These individuals initially have excessive innate immune system inflammation leading to early death and later have adaptive immune system impairment leading to long-term immunosuppression and late deaths [3,5] (Fig. 4.2).

In a second group of individuals, the same pattern of pro- and antiinflammatory response is activated with the onset of sepsis; however, instead of restoring homeostasis, they experience incontrollable inflammation and secondary organ injury. In this phenotype, both early and late deaths are caused by an intractable and excessive immune response. Eventually, the immune system does recede leading to immunosuppression and further deaths in the long term [3,5,9,10]. This pattern has been observed in a cohort of pneumonia patients who had subclinical inflammation beyond the acute phase; an exaggerated immune response assed with interleukin (IL)-6 and IL-10 profiling was associated with worse survival characteristics [11].

Other less common phenotypes include patients with a more severe and aggressive course, like patients with Waterhouse–Friderichsen syndrome, in which

The Sepsis Codex. https://doi.org/10.1016/B978-0-323-88271-2.00003-1

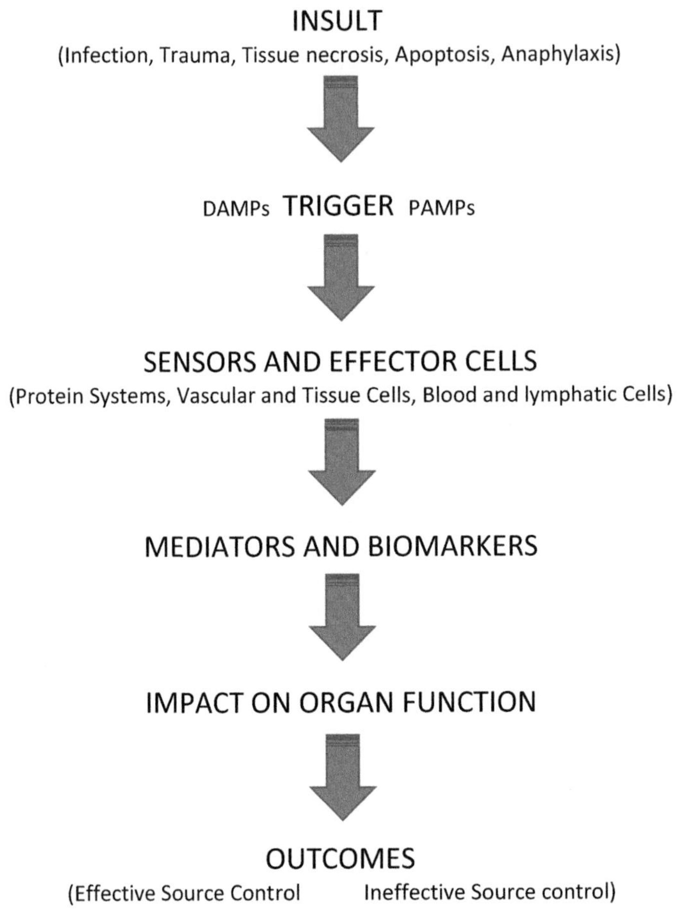

INSULT
(Infection, Trauma, Tissue necrosis, Apoptosis, Anaphylaxis)

DAMPs TRIGGER PAMPs

SENSORS AND EFFECTOR CELLS
(Protein Systems, Vascular and Tissue Cells, Blood and lymphatic Cells)

MEDIATORS AND BIOMARKERS

IMPACT ON ORGAN FUNCTION

OUTCOMES
(Effective Source Control   Ineffective Source control)

FIG. 4.1 The inflammatory response. This simplified overview shows the course of the inflammatory response. An insult triggers the release of PAMPs (pathogen-associated molecular patterns) and/or DAMPs (danger-associated molecular patterns), which are sensed by pattern recognition mechanisms such as receptors (pattern recognition receptors (PRRs) on the cell surface or within the cytosol or nucleus of sensor cells as well as by pattern-recognizing complex systems such as the complement system and others. Therefore, sensors can be different types of cells, tissues/organs, or proteins/other molecules, which themselves may function as effectors to modulate the immune response through various different pro- or anti-inflammatory mediators or biomarkers. As a result, the underlying insult can be cleared or not, and organ function may be temporarily or permanently impaired. *aPPT*, activated partial thromboplastin time; *AT*, antithrombin; *CD64 and CD48*, integral membrane glycoproteins; *C5a and C3a*, complement components 5a and 3a; *C5aR*, C5a receptor protein; *C5b-9*, terminal complement complex; *CRP*, C-reactive protein; *DIC*, disseminated intravascular coagulation; *ELAM-1*, endothelial leukocyte adhesion molecule 1; *HMGB1*, high-mobility-group protein B1; *ICAM-1*, intercellular adhesion molecule 1; *IL-6*, interleukin-6; *LBP*, LPS-binding protein; *LPS*, lipopolysaccharide (part of the membrane of Gram-negative bacteria); *LTA*, lipoteichoic acid (part of the cell wall of Gram-positive bacteria); *mHLA-DR*, monocytic human leukocyte antigen DR; *MIF*, macrophage migration inhibitory factor; *PT*, prothrombin time; *PCT*, procalcitonin; *sTNF*, soluble tumor necrosis factor; *sTREM-1*, soluble triggering receptor expressed on myeloid cells 1; *suPAR*, soluble urokinase-type plasminogen activator receptor. (https://doi.org/10.1128/CMR.00016-12.)

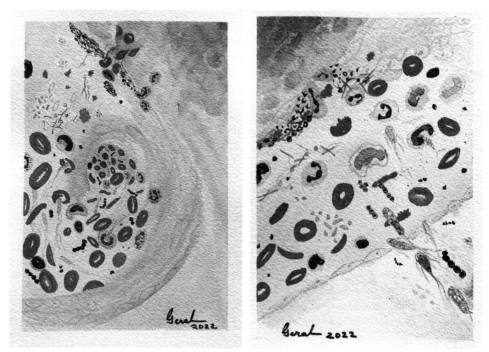

FIG. 4.2 Water color of the inflammation mediators. *With permission of Dra. Gerhaldine Morazan.*

death occurs before any immunosuppression is seen [3]. Contrarily, individuals with a preexisting severe immunosuppression may not display any proinflammatory response at all, such as transplant patients on immunosuppressive therapy [3,12,13]. Lastly, to highlight the importance of surgical source control, patients in whom no source control can be established display multiple proinflammatory courses of sepsis followed by more and more pronounced immunosuppression [3,14,15].

As most phenotypes overlap at different points, with varying levels of proinflammatory and immunosuppressive responses, it is difficult to analyze the course a patient might experience with a single snapshot in time of their clinical immune response [3,6,8].

Immune Activation

The innate immune system is the primary defense line against infections, working on surveillance, identification, and clearance of foreign bodies. The innate immune system includes myeloid cells, the complement system, and epithelial and mucosal structural and chemical defense mechanisms. Sepsis begins with the detection of the presence of pathogens in a normally sterile tissue. Diverse triggers release pathogen-associated molecular patterns (PAMPs) and/or danger-associated molecular patterns (DAMPs) that can be sensed by the immune system through receptors of sensor cells and through pattern-recognizing complex systems like the complement system. Microorganisms express a range of molecules that work like PAMPS such as lipopolysaccharide, peptidoglycan, flagellin, and double-stranded RNA that can activate leukocytes directly. While damaged tissue sends signals to communicate an established infection and activate the immune system indirectly through DAMPs. The tissue can express heat shock proteins, cathelicidins, uric acid, fibrinogen, free cellular and mitochondrial DNA, and high-mobility group box-1 that are sensed by different receptors such as RAGE, Toll-like receptors (TLRs), and specific receptors such as IL-1R [1,16,17]. After pattern-recognition receptors sense PAMPs and DAMPs, the signal activates the inflammasome protein complex which induces the transcription of inflammatory genes via nuclear factor kappa-B (NF-kappaB). This multimeric inflammasome protein complex cleaves and activates cytokines involved in the elimination of pathogens. As the NF-kappaB increases the transcription of precedent proteins (e.g., pro-IL-1beta), this provides more substrate for the inflammasome to cleave and activate. Together they induce NF-kappaB in neighboring cells, sustaining and amplifying the inflammatory response [18,19].

DAMPs are not limited to sepsis, which may explain why noninfectious conditions, like pancreatitis and trauma, cause sepsis-like clinical pictures. Cellular necrosis from any major physical injury or trauma can trigger the release of mitochondrial DNA causing inflammatory signals mimicking PAMPs released during infection [20].

The link between the innate immune system and the adaptive immune system occurs through antigen-presenting cells (APCs). APCs are immune cells with the ability to process and deliver antigens to adaptive immune cells in secondary lymphoid organs, such as the spleen, lymph nodes, and mucosal-associated lymphoid tissues. Through the communication between APCs and B and T lymphocytes, a specific immune response against the inciting pathogen is triggered [5].

Coagulation Cascade and Complement System

The pathogens also activate different protein systems such as the complement system, the coagulation cascade, and fibrinolytic system. The complement system proteins are a group of soluble proteins that are produced in the liver and circulate inactively that enhance the immune response. They can be activated by: antibody-coated pathogens (classical pathway), by the pathogen alone (alternative pathway), or by carbohydrate-binding proteins (e.g., mannose-binding lectin, ficolins) that coat the pathogens (lectin pathway). These three mechanisms converge on a C4 convertase enzyme that cleaves the complement protein C3 into the subunits C3a and C3b. C3b acts as an opsonin improving phagocytes while C3a and C5a act as anaphylotoxins, which are released into circulation and act as proinflammatory agents that gather phagocytes to the infection site [5,21].

The deposition of fibrin and formation of microthrombi in the microcirculation is the result of the systemic activation of the coagulation and fibrinolytic systems which seems to contribute to the impaired microcirculation seen in sepsis. This is triggered by proinflammatory cytokines, for example, IL-6 and tumour necrosis factor-alpha (TNF-α). Thrombocyte counts, antithrombin, protein C and S, activated partial thromboplastin time, D-dimers, fibrin, plasminogen activator inhibitor, and thrombomodulin are considered to be markers that measure the severity of the host response and following these can be used for prognostic purposes [5].

The complement system, part of the innate immune system, intersects with the extrinsic pathway of the coagulation system through C5a, an activated complement product that activates endothelial tissue factor. The coagulation system also interacts with the complement system as thrombin cleaves C5 into the active C5a and C5b. These positive feedback loops between both systems can worsen tissue damage and organ dysfunction [22].

Immunosuppression

After the initial exaggerated hyperinflammatory state, the immune response evolves to a subsequent antiinflammatory response leading to significant immunosuppression. This phenomenon is known as immunoparalysis. Profound acquired immunosuppression develops a few days after patients develop septic shock [1,23,24].

This immunosuppression is seen in multiple components of the immune system. Neutrophils lose their antiinfectious properties and change to an immature and immunosuppressive state. Monocytes and dendritic cells lose their ability to present antigens due to a diminished expression of major histocompatibility complex class II. A majority of effector lymphocytes suffer from apoptosis, while the remaining lymphocytes present an exhausted phenotype [25]. These exhausted lymphocytes lose their effector functions and reduce their proliferation, cytokine production, and increase their coinhibitory receptor expression. On the other hand, regulatory T and B cells subpopulations expand increasing the immunosuppression [23,24].

This immunosuppression reflects clinically with a loss of delayed-type hypersensitivity reactions, failure to clear the original infection regardless of antibiotic treatment and consequently secondary infections [3,9]. The magnitude and persistence of sepsis-induced immunosuppression increases the susceptibility to reactivation of viruses (Cytomegalovirus or Herpes Simplex Virus), nosocomial infections, fungal infection and increases the mortality rate [23,26–28]. This concept has been observed in deceased patients whose biochemical, flow cytometric, and immunohistochemical findings are associated with immunosuppression [29]. Late-phase immunosuppression has also been supported by postmortem findings of patients who died during the late stage of sepsis and had evidence of extensive depletion of splenic CD4, CD8, HLA-DR cells, and the expression of ligands for inhibitory receptors on lung epithelial cells. This immunosuppression can be long-lasting, possibly explaining the excess mortality rate seen in septic patients over weeks and years after the initial disease [24,29].

Acquired immunosuppression is not specific to septic patients. Different clinical conditions create a similar inflammatory response, although the magnitude of this immune dysfunction may vary depending on the clinical condition [30]. Immune alterations and secondary infections have been reported in patients with burns, trauma, major surgery, pancreatitis, and other infectious diseases such as Ebola [31−35].

The immune response in sepsis is still a biological and clinical challenge. Different genetic, physiologic, and microbiological factors may explain the differences seen across individuals and provide an exciting opportunity for future research and therapeutic targets.

ENDOTHELIUM

The glycocalyx lays on the apical side of endothelial cells on the inner side of the heart, blood vessels, and lymphatic vessels and is a key agent in microvascular and endothelial physiology. It regulates microvascular tone and endothelial permeability, maintains oncotic gradients across the endothelial barrier, regulates the adhesion/migration of leukocytes, and inhibits intravascular thrombosis [36−38]. During inflammation, there are characteristic changes to the glycocalyx which include loss of vascular tone with local blood pooling, degradation of heparan sulfate leading to a shift to a procoagulant state with consequent microthrombosis, enhanced expression of adhesion molecules with increased leukocyte trafficking, and loss of antioxidative properties with progressive oxidative injury to the endothelium [36,37,39].

The glycocalyx regulates vasomotor tone through changes in its shape that results in the release of nitric oxide. With the regulation of vascular tone, the glycocalyx is involved in the peripheral distribution of blood flow and oxygen to tissues [40]. The glycocalyx also regulates endothelial permeability by maintaining an oncotic gradient between intravascular and interstitial spaces. The glycocalyx involves cell-bound proteoglycans, glycosaminoglycan (GAG) side chains, and sialoproteins, which guard the endothelial cells on their luminal side and inside endothelial clefts (the space between two contiguous endothelial cells). Due to the high density of negative electric charges of its GAG side chains, the glycocalyx retains a high reflection capacity for albumin [41]. On the luminal portion of the glycocalyx, soluble components such as albumin, free hyaluronic acid molecules, thrombomodulin, and various serum proteins (i.e., superoxide dismutase, antithrombin III, and cell adhesion molecules) are bound [42].

The intracapillar hydrostatic pressure (PIV) and the interstitial colloid oncotic pressure ($\pi$is) have been emphasized as the driving forces of flow in the traditional Starling model; however, the subglycocalyx colloid oncotic pressure has been recently proposed as a major determinant of transcapillary flow. This space is normally free of protein, and thus the only determinant of transcapillary flow is the PIV. The $\pi$is opposes the flux caused by the PIV, but it is not enough to reverse filtration through the endothelial barrier. In regular conditions, only small amounts of fluid are filtered, which is mostly reabsorbed by the lymphatic system. In sepsis, the inflammatory injury to the glycocalyx increases the porosity of endothelium allowing albumin and other proteins to be present in the extravascular space. As a consequence, the PIS rises increasing the flow of fluid [36,43].

The πiv also increases which further opposes back filtration of fluid and drives edema formation [43]. Despite colloid infusion showing a relatively better volemic effect, it cannot resolve the interstitial edema in patients with sepsis. Infusion of albumin or synthetic colloids cannot reverse the process of edema formation since the PIC opposes the fluid transcapillary flux but cannot reverse it. Furthermore, the use of colloids accumulates colloidal molecules in the interstitial space of injured endothelium which worsens edema [36,44]. This has been associated with increased need for renal replacement therapy and mortality in septic patients [45].The interstitial edema secondary to endothelial/glycocalyx damage is directly associated with sepsis-induced organ failure [36,39]. This is commonly observed in the lung which will be discussed later in this chapter.

The glycocalyx's geometry normally prevents the interaction between the circulating leukocytes and adhesion molecules or selectins inhibiting leukocyte adhesion to the endothelium, and preventing the migration of neutrophils in noninflamed tissues [39]. When shedding occurs on this layer, adhesion molecules become exposed which results in further endothelial-cellular interactions [40]. Endothelial activation and a significant increase in glycocalyx expression of endothelial leukocyte adhesion molecule 1, intercellular adhesion molecule 1 (ICAM-1), and vascular cell adhesion molecule 1 (VCAM-1) result from exposure to proinflammatory mediators (IL-1, IL-2, IL-6, TNF-α, and other molecules released during acute inflammation such as bradykinin, thrombin, vascular endothelial growth factor [VEGF], and histamine). These proteins promote leukocyte rolling, adherence, and migration to initiate the inflammatory damage to endothelium and tissues [36,46].

With shedding of the glycocalyx, there is also release of syndecans which downregulates the inflammatory damage caused by TNF-α. This is a maladaptive behavior as it reduces inflammation but also causes the endothelial cells to rearrange and loosens its intercellular junctions. This rearrangement increases the paracellular permeability allowing more passage of fluids, albumin, and solutes [36,43,47]. Circulating components of the glycocalyx (endocan, syndecan, and cadherins) can be potentially used as a biomarker in sepsis [48].

Other important mediators in endothelial physiology includes heparan sulfate and VEGF. Heparan sulfate binds to endothelial superoxide dismutase and xanthine oxidoreductase protecting endothelial cells from oxidative stress and promoting an anticoagulant state [36]. VEGF induces angiogenesis and increases significantly the endothelial permeability [49]. Gram-negative lipopolysaccharides can induce VEGF-mRNA expression and trigger leukocytes and platelets to release VEGF [50]. The increased vascular permeability by VEGF involves the stimulation of collagenase production and proteolytic disruption of the endothelial basement membrane [51,52]. The main source of VEGF are the kidneys which have been suggested to play an important role in the regulation of glomerular permeability to protein. Urinary microalbuminuria has been observed to be a reliable marker of sepsis-induced alterations of endothelial barrier and changes in paracellular permeability [53]. Furthermore, renal release of VEGF in septic acute kidney injury (AKI) contributes to distal organ endothelial damage [54].

SHOCK AND ORGAN FAILURE

Sepsis with hypotension is referred as septic shock, regardless of the response to fluid resuscitation. Sepsis causes a distributive shock secondary to inflammatory mediators causing arterial and venous distribution [55]. This is further worsened by leakage of intravascular fluid into the interstitial space secondary to endothelial damage covered previously in this chapter [36]. Along with shock, concomitant organ dysfunction or perfusion abnormalities (e.g., lactic acidosis, oliguria, or coma) are present, with sepsis the most common cause of multiple organ failure [3,56]. This clinical picture began to develop only after intensive care units

(ICUs) were available. Before the ICU life-saving organ support, most patients with septic shock ultimately died from irreversible shock within a few days without time to develop progressive multiple organ failure [3].

Septicemic organ dysfunction involves endothelial, vascular, and immune dysfunction, and changes in cellular metabolism [57]. Organ dysfunction, which directly correlates with mortality and morbidity, is the most important clinical event in sepsis. Two main changes have occurred to our understanding of septic shock: organ dysfunction can develop in the absence of hypoperfusion and in the absence of significant cell death [56]. The study of these mechanisms has allowed us to reframe and redefine organ dysfunction in the setting of critical illnesses.

Microvascular dysfunction is caused primarily by endothelium and glycocalyx injury, secondary loss of autoregulation, and altered cell–cell communication [36,58]. Other mechanisms such as the deformation of red blood cells [59], increased blood viscosity [60], activation of the coagulation and complement systems [61], and increased nitric oxide levels are also involved. During septic shock, there is an increase in overall NO production throughout the body albeit with a heterogeneous pattern due to the distribution of inducible NO synthase [62]. The inhibition of inducible NO synthase has been associated with improvement in renal circulation. Endothelial NO synthase, on the other hand, normally has a protective role in the endothelium as it inhibits cell aggregation and promotes vasodilation. During sepsis, there are reduced levels of NO synthase further contributing to a circulation collapse [37,62,63].

Microvascular dysfunction causes hypoperfusion leading to a decreased delivery of oxygen to cells and ultimately tissue and organ dysfunction. Tissue perfusion is determined by diffusion and convection. Diffusion depends on vessel density: as this increases, the distance for oxygen to diffuse into cells decreases. Diffusion-related hypoxia occurs due to capillary dropout (a decrease in vessel density). Convection depends on the velocity of red blood cells and hemoglobin saturation. Convection-related hypoxia occurs due to a reduced proportion of vessels with adequate flow as there is an increase in the proportion of vessels with intermittent flow or stopped flow altogether [64]. These changes increase the heterogeneity of blood flow distribution seen in sepsis. Although normally, different organs metabolically demand different levels of supply of nutrients and oxygen (and thus blood flow); in sepsis, the oxygen delivered is uncoupled to its demand. These causes some cells to have excess supply of oxygen (luxury flow), while others are underperfused.

Sustained uptake of oxygen is seen by the low capillary oxygen saturation of perfused vessels adequately matching the tissue's metabolic demand. However, the tissues with overperfusion will have a reduced extraction of oxygen and thus these luxury flow capillaries will have increased levels of capillary oxygen saturation and contribute to an overall increase in venous oxygen saturation (SvO_2). The contradictory presence of both low capillary oxygen saturation and an increase SvO_2 is termed the oxygen partial pressure gap. The oxygen partial pressure gap indicates the simultaneous occurrence of regional deficiencies in oxygen supply and functional shunting. The deficient blood flow supply uncoupled to local tissue metabolic demands also causes an increase in venous PCO_2 levels. An increase in PCO_2 gap (venoarterial difference of PCO_2) suggests areas of stagnant flow to tissues with increased hypoxia risk [56,65].

There is evidence in septic patients, in which organs can become dysfunctional without any decrease in oxygen delivery, suggesting that hypoxia of tissues is not an isolated phenomenon. Therefore, perfusion-based therapeutic efforts may only be partially effective or may have no effect at all. In addition, organ dysfunction can occur when no significant cell death occurs, which suggests that a loss of organ function may be an adaptation to a more severe, inflammatory injury [66].

In the heart, septic cardiomyopathy is characterized by an acute onset and reversible behavior. The left ventricular ejection fraction is low with a normal or low ventricular filling pressure and an increased left ventricular compliance [67].

In the lungs, a disruption of the alveolar endothelial glycocalyx causes pulmonary edema and sepsis-induced lung injury. The alveolar—endothelial barrier is disrupted by the accumulation of protein-rich fluid in the interstitial lung spaces and alveoli. The consequences of this event are ventilation—perfusion mismatch, hypoxia, and decreased lung compliance producing acute respiratory distress syndrome in extreme situations [1,68,69].

In the kidneys, sepsis can lead to reduced renal perfusion, acute tubular necrosis, and minimal defects in the microvasculature and tubules [1,70].

In the gastrointestinal tract, sepsis can lead to increased permeability of the mucosal lining. This causes bacterial translocation across the bowel and autodigestion of the bowl by luminal enzymes. The liver can undergo endothelial architecture alteration causing hepatocellular injury and cholestasis [1,56].

In the nervous system, changes in endothelial cells weaken the blood—brain barrier allowing the entry of toxins, inflammatory cells, and cytokines. Damage, such as changes of cerebral edema, neurotransmitter disruption, oxidative stress, and white matter injury lead to an increase risk of septic encephalopathy. These can range from mild confusion to delirium and coma [1].

Organ cross talk is a complicated and poorly understood biological communication process in which malfunctioning organs can affect other organs. Lung—brain cross talk happens in patients who have a lung injury and afterward present with brain impairment, who previously had normal neurologic function [56]. Inflammatory interaction between the kidney and the lungs via systemic cytokines has been found in preclinical and clinical research, with ventilator-induced lung damage linked with high tidal volume mechanical ventilation leading to AKI development. In kidney—lung cross talk, there appears to be a distinct pattern of renal inflammation [56,71].

In the event of sepsis, the coagulation and complement systems influence each other through connected pathways, despite the fact that they are not solid organs. Early sepsis potentially links the powerful complement activation and disseminated intravascular coagulation. Complement end products make the blood more thrombogenic, cause procoagulant and antifibrinolytic proteins to be produced, and block anticoagulant pathways. Mammals with bacteria-induced sepsis and inhibition of C3 convertase avoided complement activation, diminished levels of thrombocytopenia and coagulopathy, and conserved endothelium anticoagulant properties [56,72].

THE NEUROENDOCRINE RESPONSE

The neuroendocrine response to any form of stress, even sepsis, follows a particular biphasic pattern. An acute neuroendocrine response is characterized by an activated hypothalamopituitary profile with downregulation of peripheral anabolic pathways.

This response is adaptive as it shuts down anabolic processes temporarily in order to provide the body with metabolic substrates for essential functions. The acute neuroendocrine changes might be adaptive in trying to limit unnecessary energy expenditure and target the restoration of homeostasis. However, as these changes become prolonged, they become maladaptive ultimately causing a central suppression of the neuroendocrine axes contributing to an increase morbidity and mortality in critical illness and sepsis [73—75].

The Hypothalamic—Pituitary—Adrenal Axis

The hypothalamic—pituitary—adrenal (HPA) axis, in acute critical illness, is activated by neural circuits and a massive release of inflammatory cytokines (particularly IL-6, TNF-α, and IL-1). These cytokines stimulate corticotropin-releasing hormone (CRH) and adrenocorticotropic hormone (ACTH) secretion [73].

Macrophage-inhibiting factor secretion is triggered by excessive inflammation and can also modulate the HPA in septic shock. Once the HPA is activated, it increases levels of ACTH, total and free cortisol. Additionally, impaired glucocorticoid clearance and suppressed levels of corticosteroid-binding globulin contribute to the very high cortisol levels seen in critical illness. The number and binding affinity of glucocorticoid receptors is reduced due to an excess or inappropriate cytokine production. Poor suppressibility by the administration of exogenous steroids is observed during enhanced cortisol availability in acute stress [76].

In the chronic stage, the circulating cortisol levels increase by corticotropin-mediated independent mechanisms as ACTH remains low. Cytokines, ANF, endothelin, and substance P are elements that drive cortisol secretion besides from CRH.

Persisting hypercortisolism may provide advantages in protracted critical illness such as providing energy from gluconeogenesis, minimizing excessive inflammation, and preserving vascular tone. However, it also mediates harmful complications such as hyperglycemia, myopathy, and increased susceptibility to infection [73,77].

The Hypothalamic–Pituitary–Thyroid Axis

Thyroid hormones are responsible for the regulation of energy metabolism in all tissues and is a key factor in physiologic processes of cell differentiation, growth, and metabolism. Immediately after a stressful event, the circulating levels of T3 decrease, while the levels of rT3 increase. Both thyrotropin and T4 momentarily increase but quickly return to normal. The phenomenon of a persisting low T3 with an inappropriately normal TSH is known as low T3 syndrome, sick euthyroid syndrome, or nonthyroidal illness (NTI). NTI is an attempt to protect the organism by reducing energy consumption and catabolism [78].

The Somatotropic Axis

The regular pattern of growth hormone (GH) secretion changes as a response to acute stress with higher pulse frequency, amplitude, and interpulse levels observed. This occurs in the presence of peripheral GH resistance, such as in the liver, ultimately causing a decrease in IGF-1, IGFBP-3, and the acid labile subunit.

Enhanced GH secretion promotes lipolysis and antagonizes insulin's actions, thus providing essential fatty acids and glucose for energy. Simultaneously, the indirect anabolic effects of IGF-1 are supressed, as they are considered nonessential for the body's survival in the acute setting.

In a prolonged course, there is a dramatic reduction in the pulsatile GH secretion with a more profound reduction in IGF-1 and IGFEBP-3. The existence of these contributes to hypercatabolism, an inability to rebuild tissues, and wasting syndrome [73,79].

The Male Gonadal Axis and Prolactin

Men in the acute phase of critical illness have been observed to have low testosterone concentrations even with high levels of circulating LH. In the chronic phase, LH secretion is reduced further contributing to low circulating levels of testosterone. Testosterone is a strong anabolic hormone; therefore, low levels increases catabolism [73,80].

Prolactin levels are high after the onset of critical illness which represent an attempt to activate the immune system. However, with a prolonged critical course, there is reduced PRL secretion further contributing to immunosuppression [75,80].

METABOLIC RESPONSE TO SEPSIS

Metabolic changes in response to sepsis are consequences of neuroendocrine and inflammatory alterations. Such responses include stress hyperglycemia and anorexia.

Stress hyperglycemia develops from any form of severe physical stress, including sepsis. This metabolic response is induced by stress hormones, such as cortisol, GH, glucagon, and catecholamines. Proinflammatory cytokines also contribute to stress hyperglycemia. Once induced, gluconeogenesis and peripheral insulin resistance occur. The severity of hyperglycemia can increase if drugs, such as catecholamines and corticosteroids, or (parenteral) nutrition are used. It is highly debated whether hyperglycemia is a primary indicator of the severity of illness or a cause for it [81]. The prevention of severe hyperglycemia is recommended for all critically ill patients until more findings are presented [73,82].

As a response to infection, the central and peripheral effects of proinflammatory cytokines regulate anorexia. Long-term underfeeding is linked to ongoing catabolism, higher risk of infections, and mortality [83,84]. Early full enteral nutrition is recommended by the clinical practice guidelines and may require parenteral nutrition. However, the timing to add parenteral nutrition may differ. As low macronutrient intake may be tolerated during the acute phase of sepsis, the use of early parenteral nutrition may not be necessary at this stage [85–87].

Metabolic Reprogramming

It has been proposed that the cellular metabolic down-regulation in sepsis is an adaptive response to reprioritize energy consumption to limit additional injury, maintain energy balance, prevent DNA damage, and preserve cellular composition. In sepsis, a preferential oxidation of glucose occurs regardless of the availability of oxygen (Warburg effect). Although the use of glycolysis for activation roles is less energetically efficient than oxidative phosphorylation, it has two key benefits. First, it facilitates the production of structural components such as fatty acids, amino acids, and nucleotides. These play an important role in producing sufficient energy for cell survival. Second, it involves the shunting of glycolytic intermediaries through the pentose phosphate pathway which increases the levels of nicotinamide adenine dinucleotide phosphate (NADPH). NADPH is a key element in reducing oxidative damage from the production of mitochondrial radical oxygen species [56,88].

Autophagy, the cellular digestion of unnecessary or dysfunctional cell components, is increased during sepsis. This occurs as a response to TLR-4–mediated inflammation, oxidative stress, and mitochondrial damage. Increased autophagy is a proposed mechanism of metabolic reprogramming in response to inflammation, removal of damaged mitochondria, and reduction of radical oxygen species during sepsis. Diminished levels of an autophagic response is associated with prolonged critical illness and poor recovery from organ dysfunction [56].

Mitochondria are also key regulators of the cell cycle that can cause cell cycle arrest during sepsis as a protective strategy. Causing a cell cycle arrest reduces the energetic cost of cells that are not suitable to undergo replication and also prevent cell death in the event of harm [89].

Furthermore, in response to hypoxic insult, there is early inactivation and internalization of sodium and chloride transporters and ATPase-linked transmembrane pumps to prevent the excessive use of energy.

CONCLUSION

Sepsis is an inflammatory condition caused by a tainted immune system response to an infection that can result in shock and death. Although the immune response begins with a compartmentalized recognition of microbes, the response rapidly involves multiple systems

and organs in the body causing varying degrees of inflammation and immunosuppression, homeostatic instability, endothelial damage, organ failure, and diverse neuroendocrine and metabolic responses. Although unanswered questions remain regarding the mechanisms that lead to the dysregulation and erratic immune responses in sepsis, we are hopeful new evidence will emerge in the near future.

REFERENCES

[1] Gyawali B, Ramakrishna K, Dhamoon AS. Sepsis: the evolution in definition, pathophysiology, and management. SAGE Open Med 2019;7. https://doi.org/10.1177/2050312119835043. 2050312119835043.

[2] Gruithuisen VPF, editor. Hippocrates des Zweyten ächte medizinische Schriften, ins Deutsche übersetzt. Munich, Germany: Ignaz Josef Lentner; 1814.

[3] Reinhart K, Bauer M, Riedemann NC, Hartog CS. New approaches to sepsis: molecular diagnostics and biomarkers. Clin Microbiol Rev 2012;25(4):609–34. https://doi.org/10.1128/CMR.00016-12.

[4] Dugar S, Choudhary C, Duggal A. Sepsis and septic shock: guideline-based management. Cleve Clin J Med 2020; 87(1):53–64. https://doi.org/10.3949/ccjm.87a.18143.

[5] Conway-Morris A, Wilson J, Shankar-Hari M. Immune activation in sepsis. Crit Care Clin 2018;34(1):29–42. https://doi.org/10.1016/j.ccc.2017.08.002.

[6] Hotchkiss RS, Moldawer LL, Opal SM, Reinhart K, Turnbull IR, Vincent JL. Sepsis and septic shock. Nat Rev Dis Prim 2016;2:16045. https://doi.org/10.1038/nrdp.2016.45.

[7] Hotchkiss RS, Karl IE. The pathophysiology and treatment of sepsis. N Engl J Med 2003;348(2):138–50. https://doi.org/10.1056/NEJMra021333.

[8] Bone RC. Sir Isaac Newton, sepsis, SIRS, and CARS. Crit Care Med 1996;24(7):1125–8. https://doi.org/10.1097/00003246-199607000-00010.

[9] Hotchkiss RS, Coopersmith CM, McDunn JE, Ferguson TA. The sepsis seesaw: tilting toward immunosuppression. Nat Med 2009;15(5):496–7. https://doi.org/10.1038/nm0509-496.

[10] Steinhagen F, Schmidt SV, Schewe JC, Peukert K, Klinman DM, Bode C. Immunotherapy in sepsis—brake or accelerate? Pharmacol Ther 2020;208:107476. https://doi.org/10.1016/j.pharmthera.2020.107476.

[11] Kellum JA, Kong L, Fink MP, et al. Understanding the inflammatory cytokine response in pneumonia and sepsis: results of the genetic and inflammatory markers of sepsis (GenIMS) study. Arch Intern Med 2007; 167(15):1655–63. https://doi.org/10.1001/archinte.167.15.1655.

[12] Schachtner T, Stein M, Reinke P. Sepsis after renal transplantation: clinical, immunological, and microbiological risk factors. Transpl Infect Dis 2017;19(3). https://doi.org/10.1111/tid.12695.

[13] Bafi AT, Tomotani DY, de Freitas FG. Sepsis in solid-organ transplant patients. Shock 2017;47(1S Suppl. 1):12−6. https://doi.org/10.1097/SHK.0000000000000700.

[14] Marshall JC, al Naqbi A. Principles of source control in the management of sepsis. Crit Care Clin 2009;25(4): 753−68. https://doi.org/10.1016/j.ccc.2009.08.001.

[15] Gentile LF, Cuenca AG, Efron PA, et al. Persistent inflammation and immunosuppression: a common syndrome and new horizon for surgical intensive care. J Trauma Acute Care Surg 2012;72(6):1491−501. https://doi.org/10.1097/TA.0b013e318256e000.

[16] Mogensen TH. Pathogen recognition and inflammatory signaling in innate immune defenses. Clin Microbiol Rev 2009;22(2):240−73. https://doi.org/10.1128/CMR.00046-08.

[17] Takeuchi O, Akira S. Pattern recognition receptors and inflammation. Cell 2010;140(6):805−20. https://doi.org/10.1016/j.cell.2010.01.022.

[18] Guo H, Callaway JB, Ting JP. Inflammasomes: mechanism of action, role in disease, and therapeutics. Nat Med 2015;21(7):677−87. https://doi.org/10.1038/nm.3893.

[19] Kumar V. Inflammasomes: Pandora's box for sepsis. J Inflamm Res 2018;11:477−502. https://doi.org/10.2147/JIR.S178084.

[20] Bianchi ME. DAMPs, PAMPs and alarmins: all we need to know about danger. J Leukoc Biol 2007;81(1):1−5. https://doi.org/10.1189/jlb.0306164.

[21] Ward PA. The harmful role of c5a on innate immunity in sepsis. J Innate Immun 2010;2(5):439−45. https://doi.org/10.1159/000317194.

[22] Amara U, Flierl MA, Rittirsch D, et al. Molecular intercommunication between the complement and coagulation systems. J Immunol 2010;185(9):5628−36. https://doi.org/10.4049/jimmunol.0903678.

[23] Venet F, Rimmelé T, Monneret G. Management of sepsis-induced immunosuppression. Crit Care Clin 2018;34(1): 97−106. https://doi.org/10.1016/j.ccc.2017.08.007.

[24] Hotchkiss RS, Monneret G, Payen D. Sepsis-induced immunosuppression: from cellular dysfunctions to immunotherapy. Nat Rev Immunol 2013;13(12): 862−74. https://doi.org/10.1038/nri3552.

[25] Hotchkiss RS, Swanson PE, Freeman BD, et al. Apoptotic cell death in patients with sepsis, shock, and multiple organ dysfunction. Crit Care Med 1999;27(7):1230−51. https://doi.org/10.1097/00003246-199907000-00002.

[26] Limaye AP, Kirby KA, Rubenfeld GD, et al. Cytomegalovirus reactivation in critically ill immunocompetent patients. JAMA 2008;300(4):413−22. https://doi.org/10.1001/jama.300.4.413.

[27] Walton AH, Muenzer JT, Rasche D, et al. Reactivation of multiple viruses in patients with sepsis. PLoS One 2014;9(2):e98819. https://doi.org/10.1371/journal.pone.0098819.

[28] Otto GP, Sossdorf M, Claus RA, et al. The late phase of sepsis is characterized by an increased microbiological burden and death rate. Crit Care 2011;15(4):R183. https://doi.org/10.1186/cc10332.

[29] Boomer JS, To K, Chang KC, et al. Immunosuppression in patients who die of sepsis and multiple organ failure. JAMA 2011;306(23):2594−605. https://doi.org/10.1001/jama.2011.1829.

[30] Hotchkiss RS, Moldawer LL. Parallels between cancer and infectious disease. N Engl J Med 2014;371(4):380−3. https://doi.org/10.1056/NEJMcibr1404664.

[31] Greenhalgh DG. Sepsis in the burn patient: a different problem than sepsis in the general population. Burns Trauma 2017;5:23. https://doi.org/10.1186/s41038-017-0089-5.

[32] Schlömmer C, Meier J. Inflammatory response in trauma patients: are there ways to decrease the inflammatory reaction? Curr Opin Anaesthesiol 2020;33(2):253−8. https://doi.org/10.1097/ACO.0000000000000842.

[33] Wilson PG, Manji M, Neoptolemos JP. Acute pancreatitis as a model of sepsis. J Antimicrob Chemother 1998; 41(Suppl. A):51−63. https://doi.org/10.1093/jac/41.suppl_1.51.

[34] Ruibal P, Oestereich L, Lüdtke A, et al. Unique human immune signature of Ebola virus disease in Guinea. Nature 2016;533(7601):100−4. https://doi.org/10.1038/nature17949.

[35] Mina MJ, Metcalf CJ, de Swart RL, Osterhaus AD, Grenfell BT. Long-term measles-induced immunomodulation increases overall childhood infectious disease mortality. Science 2015;348(6235):694−9. https://doi.org/10.1126/science.aaa3662.

[36] Chelazzi C, Villa G, Mancinelli P, De Gaudio AR, Adembri C. Glycocalyx and sepsis-induced alterations in vascular permeability. Crit Care 2015;19(1):26. https://doi.org/10.1186/s13054-015-0741-z.

[37] Ince C, Mayeux PR, Nguyen T, et al. The endothelium in sepsis. Shock 2016;45(3):259−70. https://doi.org/10.1097/SHK.0000000000000473.

[38] Frati-Munari AC. Importancia médica del glucocáliz endotelial [Medical significance of endothelial glycocalyx]. Arch Cardiol Mex 2013;83(4):303−12. https://doi.org/10.1016/j.acmx.2013.04.015.

[39] Donati A, Domizi R, Damiani E, Adrario E, Pelaia P, Ince C. From macrohemodynamic to the microcirculation. Crit Care Res Pract 2013;2013: 892710. https://doi.org/10.1155/2013/892710.

[40] Kolářová H, Ambrůzová B, Svihálková Šindlerová L, Klinke A, Kubala L. Modulation of endothelial glycocalyx structure under inflammatory conditions. Mediat Inflamm 2014;2014:694312. https://doi.org/10.1155/2014/694312.

[41] Yuan SY, Rigor RR. Regulation of endothelial barrier function. San Rafael (CA): Morgan & Claypool Life Sciences; 2010.

[42] Paulus P, Jennewein C, Zacharowski K. Biomarkers of endothelial dysfunction: can they help us deciphering systemic inflammation and sepsis? Biomarkers 2011; 16(Suppl. 1):S11−21. https://doi.org/10.3109/1354750X.2011.587893.

[43] Woodcock TE, Woodcock TM. Revised Starling equation and the glycocalyx model of transvascular fluid exchange:

an improved paradigm for prescribing intravenous fluid therapy. Br J Anaesth 2012;108(3):384—94. https://doi.org/10.1093/bja/aer515.

[44] Brown RM, Semler MW. Fluid management in sepsis. J Intensive Care Med 2019;34(5):364—73. https://doi.org/10.1177/0885066618784861.

[45] Serpa Neto A, Veelo DP, Peireira VG, et al. Fluid resuscitation with hydroxyethyl starches in patients with sepsis is associated with an increased incidence of acute kidney injury and use of renal replacement therapy: a systematic review and meta-analysis of the literature. J Crit Care 2014;29(1):185.e1—185.e1857. https://doi.org/10.1016/j.jcrc.2013.09.031.

[46] Karamysheva AF. Mechanisms of angiogenesis. Biochemistry (Mosc) 2008;73(7):751—62. https://doi.org/10.1134/s0006297908070031.

[47] Christaki E, Opal SM. Is the mortality rate for septic shock really decreasing? Curr Opin Crit Care 2008;14(5):580—6. https://doi.org/10.1097/MCC.0b013e32830f1e25.

[48] Piotti A, Novelli D, Meessen JMTA, et al. Endothelial damage in septic shock patients as evidenced by circulating syndecan-1, sphingosine-1-phosphate and soluble VE-cadherin: a substudy of ALBIOS. Crit Care 2021;25(1):113. https://doi.org/10.1186/s13054-021-03545-1.

[49] Pierrakos C, Vincent JL. Sepsis biomarkers: a review. Crit Care 2010;14(1):R15. https://doi.org/10.1186/cc8872.

[50] Nakamura T, Ushiyama C, Suzuki Y, Shoji H, Shimada N, Koide H. Hemoperfusion with polymyxin B immobilized fibers for urinary albumin excretion in septic patients with trauma. Am Soc Artif Intern Organs J 2002;48(3):244—8. https://doi.org/10.1097/00002480-200205000-00008.

[51] Becker BF, Chappell D, Bruegger D, Annecke T, Jacob M. Therapeutic strategies targeting the endothelial glycocalyx: acute deficits, but great potential. Cardiovasc Res 2010;87(2):300—10. https://doi.org/10.1093/cvr/cvq137.

[52] Hu Z, Cano I, D'Amore PA. Update on the role of the endothelial glycocalyx in angiogenesis and vascular inflammation. Front Cell Dev Biol 2021;9:734276. https://doi.org/10.3389/fcell.2021.734276.

[53] Omar W, Elsayed M. Mortality prediction of microalbuminuria in septic patients. Open Access Maced J Med Sci 2019;7(23):4048—52. https://doi.org/10.3889/oamjms.2019.633.

[54] Dubin A, Kanoore Edul VS, Caminos Eguillor JF, Ferrara G. Monitoring microcirculation: utility and barriers—a point-of-view review. Vasc Health Risk Manag 2020;16:577—89. https://doi.org/10.2147/VHRM.S242635.

[55] Thompson K, Venkatesh B, Finfer S. Sepsis and septic shock: current approaches to management. Intern Med J 2019;49(2):160—70. https://doi.org/10.1111/imj.14199.

[56] Pool R, Gomez H, Kellum JA. Mechanisms of organ dysfunction in sepsis. Crit Care Clin 2018;34(1):63—80. https://doi.org/10.1016/j.ccc.2017.08.003.

[57] Singer M, De Santis V, Vitale D, Jeffcoate W. Multiorgan failure is an adaptive, endocrine-mediated, metabolic response to overwhelming systemic inflammation. Lancet 2004;364(9433):545—8. https://doi.org/10.1016/S0140-6736(04)16815-3.

[58] De Backer D, Creteur J, Preiser JC, Dubois MJ, Vincent JL. Microvascular blood flow is altered in patients with sepsis. Am J Respir Crit Care Med 2002;166(1):98—104. https://doi.org/10.1164/rccm.200109-016oc.

[59] Lee HJ, Lee S, Park H, Park Y, Shin J. Three-dimensional shapes and cell deformability of rat red blood cells during and after asphyxial cardiac arrest. Emerg Med Int 2019;2019:6027236. https://doi.org/10.1155/2019/6027236.

[60] Kazune S, Piebalga A, Strike E, Vanags I. Impaired vascular reactivity in sepsis—a systematic review with meta-analysis. Arch Med Sci Atheroscler Dis 2019;4:e151—61. https://doi.org/10.5114/amsad.2019.86754.

[61] De Backer D, Donadello K, Taccone FS, Ospina-Tascon G, Salgado D, Vincent JL. Microcirculatory alterations: potential mechanisms and implications for therapy. Ann Intensive Care 2011;1(1):27. https://doi.org/10.1186/2110-5820-1-27.

[62] Cunha FQ, Assreuy J, Moss DW, et al. Differential induction of nitric oxide synthase in various organs of the mouse during endotoxaemia: role of TNF-alpha and IL-1-beta. Immunology 1994;81(2):211—5.

[63] Tiwari MM, Brock RW, Megyesi JK, Kaushal GP, Mayeux PR. Disruption of renal peritubular blood flow in lipopolysaccharide-induced renal failure: role of nitric oxide and caspases. Am J Physiol Ren Physiol 2005;289(6):F1324—32. https://doi.org/10.1152/ajprenal.00124.2005.

[64] Ince C. The rationale for microcirculatory guided fluid therapy. Curr Opin Crit Care 2014;20(3):301—8. https://doi.org/10.1097/MCC.0000000000000091.

[65] Ellis CG, Bateman RM, Sharpe MD, Sibbald WJ, Gill R. Effect of a maldistribution of microvascular blood flow on capillary O(2) extraction in sepsis. Am J Physiol Heart Circ Physiol 2002;282(1):H156—64. https://doi.org/10.1152/ajpheart.2002.282.1.H156.

[66] ProCESS Investigators, Yealy DM, Kellum JA, et al. A randomized trial of protocol-based care for early septic shock. N Engl J Med 2014;370(18):1683—93. https://doi.org/10.1056/NEJMoa1401602.

[67] Vieillard-Baron A. Septic cardiomyopathy. Ann Intensive Care 2011;1(1):6. https://doi.org/10.1186/2110-5820-1-6.

[68] Schmidt EP, Yang Y, Janssen WJ, et al. The pulmonary endothelial glycocalyx regulates neutrophil adhesion and lung injury during experimental sepsis. Nat Med 2012;18(8):1217—23. https://doi.org/10.1038/nm.2843.

[69] Marchetti M, Gomez-Rosas P, Sanga E, et al. Endothelium activation markers in severe hospitalized COVID-19 patients: role in mortality risk prediction. TH Open 2021;5(3):e253—63. https://doi.org/10.1055/s-0041-1731711.

[70] Russell JA, Rush B, Boyd J. Pathophysiology of septic shock. Crit Care Clin 2018;34(1):43—61. https://doi.org/10.1016/j.ccc.2017.08.005.

[71] Liu M, Liang Y, Chigurupati S, et al. Acute kidney injury leads to inflammation and functional changes in the brain. J Am Soc Nephrol 2008;19(7):1360–70. https://doi.org/10.1681/ASN.2007080901.

[72] Markiewski MM, Nilsson B, Ekdahl KN, Mollnes TE, Lambris JD. Complement and coagulation: strangers or partners in crime? Trends Immunol 2007;28(4):184–92. https://doi.org/10.1016/j.it.2007.02.006.

[73] Ingels C, Gunst J, Van den Berghe G. Endocrine and metabolic alterations in sepsis and implications for treatment. Crit Care Clin 2018;34(1):81–96. https://doi.org/10.1016/j.ccc.2017.08.006.

[74] Gheorghiță V, Barbu AE, Gheorghiu ML, Căruntu FA. Endocrine dysfunction in sepsis: a beneficial or deleterious host response? Germs 2015;5(1):17–25. https://doi.org/10.11599/germs.2015.1067.

[75] Wasyluk W, Wasyluk M, Zwolak A. Sepsis as a pan-endocrine illness-endocrine disorders in septic patients. J Clin Med 2021;10(10):2075. https://doi.org/10.3390/jcm10102075.

[76] Boonen E, Vervenne H, Meersseman P, et al. Reduced cortisol metabolism during critical illness. N Engl J Med 2013;368(16):1477–88. https://doi.org/10.1056/NEJMoa1214969.

[77] Peeters B, Güiza F, Boonen E, Meersseman P, Langouche L, Van den Berghe G. Drug-induced HPA axis alterations during acute critical illness: a multivariable association study. Clin Endocrinol 2017;86(1):26–36. https://doi.org/10.1111/cen.13155.

[78] Mebis L, Debaveye Y, Visser TJ, Van den Berghe G. Changes within the thyroid axis during the course of critical illness. Endocrinol Metab Clin N Am 2006;35(4):807–x. https://doi.org/10.1016/j.ecl.2006.09.009.

[79] Marquardt DJ, Knatz NL, Wetterau LA, Wewers MD, Hall MW. Failure to recover somatotropic axis function is associated with mortality from pediatric sepsis-induced multiple organ dysfunction syndrome. Pediatr Crit Care Med 2010;11(1):18–25. https://doi.org/10.1097/PCC.0b013e3181b06046.

[80] Mechanick JI, Nierman DM. Gonadal steroids in critical illness. Crit Care Clin 2006;22(1):87–vii. https://doi.org/10.1016/j.ccc.2005.08.005.

[81] Ingels C, Vanhorebeek I, Van den Berghe G. Glucose homeostasis, nutrition and infections during critical illness. Clin Microbiol Infect 2018;24(1):10–5. https://doi.org/10.1016/j.cmi.2016.12.033.

[82] Becker CD, Sabang RL, Nogueira Cordeiro MF, Hassan IF, Goldberg MD, Scurlock CS. Hyperglycemia in medically critically ill patients: risk factors and clinical outcomes. Am J Med 2020;133(10):e568–74. https://doi.org/10.1016/j.amjmed.2020.03.012.

[83] Alberda C, Gramlich L, Jones N, et al. The relationship between nutritional intake and clinical outcomes in critically ill patients: results of an international multicenter observational study [published correction appears in Intensive Care Med. 2009 Oct;35(10):1821]. Intensive Care Med 2009;35(10):1728–37. https://doi.org/10.1007/s00134-009-1567-4.

[84] Hajimohammadebrahim-Ketabforoush M, Vahdat Shariatpanahi Z, Vahdat Shariatpanahi M, Shahbazi E, Shahbazi S. Protein and energy intake assessment and their association with in-hospital mortality in critically ill COVID-19 patients: a prospective cohort study. Front Nutr 2021;8:708271. https://doi.org/10.3389/fnut.2021.708271.

[85] Kott M, Hartl WH, Elke G. Enteral vs. parenteral nutrition in septic shock: are they equivalent? Curr Opin Crit Care 2019;25(4):340–8. https://doi.org/10.1097/MCC.0000000000000618.

[86] Wischmeyer PE. Nutrition therapy in sepsis. Crit Care Clin 2018;34(1):107–25. https://doi.org/10.1016/j.ccc.2017.08.008.

[87] Casaer MP, Mesotten D, Schetz MR. Bench-to-bedside review: metabolism and nutrition. Crit Care 2008;12(4):222. https://doi.org/10.1186/cc6945.

[88] Toro J, Manrique-Caballero CL, Gómez H. Metabolic reprogramming and host tolerance: a novel concept to understand sepsis-associated AKI. J Clin Med 2021;10(18):4184. https://doi.org/10.3390/jcm10184184.

[89] Green DR, Galluzzi L, Kroemer G. Mitochondria and the autophagy-inflammation-cell death axis in organismal aging. Science 2011;333(6046):1109–12. https://doi.org/10.1126/science.1201940.

CHAPTER 5

Sepsis and Microcirculation

CARLOS ENRIQUE A. ORELLANA JIMENEZ

INTRODUCTION

Sepsis is considered as a life-threatening condition with organ dysfunction due to a dysregulate host response to infection. Septic shock is defined as a subset of sepsis in which profound circulatory, cellular, and metabolic abnormalities are present, which include a persistent hypotension despite adequate volume resuscitation and that require vasopressors to maintain a mean arterial pressure (MAP) more than 65 mm Hg and serum lactate level, 2 mmol/L (18 mg/dL), in which oxygen delivery to cells is insufficient to maintain cellular activity and support organ function [1].

Sepsis is characterized by macrocirculatory disturbances such as relative hypovolemia, a decrease in vascular tone, myocardial depression, and heterogeneous patterns of blood flow in the microcirculation, as well as the inability of cells to adequately extract and use oxygen [2].

Sepsis is involucred in around 50 million people worldwide each year, with 11 million deaths, and nearly 20% of global deaths [3].

MACROCIRCULATION

The main determinants of macrocirculation are pressure and flow.

The static and dynamic variables of hemodynamic monitoring (MAP, central venous pressure, vena cava collapsibility index, etc.) are considered indicators of macrocirculation. Resuscitation from states of shock is claimed to be achieved by restoration of systemic macrohemodynamic variables using fluids and vasoactive drugs with the goal of promoting tissue perfusion and oxygen transport to the tissues. However, if this goal is actually achieved, it is uncertain. These variables of macrohemodynamics were used to guide the initial resuscitation endpoints, but these parameters do not assess at tissue perfusion level. A MAP of 65 mm Hg do not guarantee a sufficient perfusion; therefore, it is necessary to ensure an adequate perfusion at the macro- and microcirculation level, which is crucial for tissue oxygenation and organ perfusion [4].

In fact, systemic hemodynamic variables indicate the onset of cardiovascular decompensation, but rather do not indicate the onset of shock.

MICROCIRCULATION IN SEPSIS

The microcirculation is the terminal vascular network of the systemic circulation. This network is made up of microvessels with diameters <100 μm. This network consists of arterioles, postcapillary venules, capillaries, and their cellular constituents (Fig. 5.1) [4].

The functions of microcirculation are, among others:
1. Transfer the oxygen from red blood cells (RBCs) in capillaries to parenchymal cells, where oxygen is delivered to carry out metabolic reactions at the cellular level.
2. Regulation of solute exchange between the intravascular and tissular space.
3. The transport of all blood-borne hormones and nutrients to the tissue cells including mediating the functional activity of the immune system and hemostasis [5].

Endothelial cells (ECs) almost entirely line the vessels of the microcirculation. ECs have fenestrations and pores and are held together by various molecules, including cadherins and gap junctions, which allow upstream electrical communication between them. These endothelial structures can vary in density and morphology between different organs and vessels. The regulation of the microvascular blood flow is thanks to the regulation of the vascular tone of the arterioles. The main mechanisms that cause this regulation are: myogenic, metabolic, and neurohumoral control mechanisms [6].

The glycocalyx is one of the most important subcellular structures of the endothelium, and its function is present on the luminal side of the endothelium [7–9].

The glycocalyx is a 0.2–0.5 μm gel-like layer synthesized by ECs. It is composed of three main components, proteoglycans, glycosaminoglycans, and plasma proteins, and contains several substances such as

The Sepsis Codex. https://doi.org/10.1016/B978-0-323-88271-2.00031-6

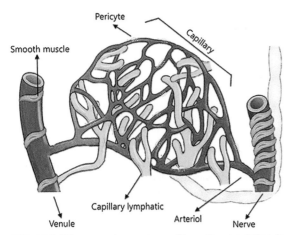

FIG. 5.1 Microvascular anatomy. The microcirculation is the part of the vascular system and consists of the small vessels so-called arterioles, capillaries, and venules. The lymphatic capillaries carry the extravascular fluid into the venous system. The arterioles are surrounded by vascular smooth muscle cells responsible for the regulation of arteriole tone. Taken from Ref. [4].

antithrombin and superoxide dismutase. The glycocalyx is responsible for various physiological processes including homeostasis, solute transport, hemostasis, and immune functions. Until recently, the integrity of the glycocalyx was thought to be the main determinant of the vascular barrier. However, a recent study showed that the glycocalyx can detach under conditions of shock without compromising vascular barrier function [4–6]. Fig. 5.2.

Dependency on macrocirculation, organ-specific autoregulatory mechanisms, and interaction between certain organs make the assessment of microcirculation a complex issue.

The pathophysiology of the microcirculation in shock has been extensively reviewed elsewhere [10].

Sepsis microcirculatory alterations increase the diffusion distance for oxygen and also, due to the heterogeneity of microcirculatory perfusion, can promote the formation of areas of tissue hypoxia in the vicinity of well-oxygenated areas.

Microcirculatory derangements in sepsis are [11]:

1. Reduction in vessel density.
2. Alteration in flow.
3. Heterogeneous distribution of perfusion.

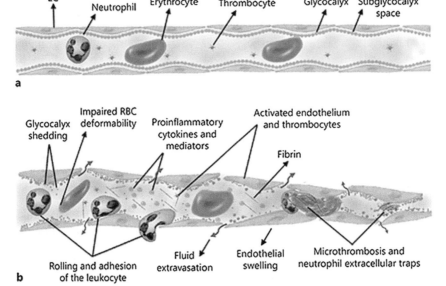

FIG. 5.2 Microvascular dysfunction and vascular endothelial damage. a The structure of a healthy microvessel is shown. EC and glycocalyx cover the lumen of the microvessel. The blood cells (leukocytes, RBC, thrombocytes) flow together with plasma inside the microvessels. b Microcirculatory damage can be caused by ischemia, reperfusion, inflammation, and hypoxia, resulting in endothelial and glycocalyx and RBC damage. Activation of leukocytes induces rolling, adhesion, and ultimately extravasation to the tissue, which further accelerates the inflammation. Decreased vascular permeability causes vascular leakage and edema formation. RBC, red blood cell; EC, endothelial cells. Taken from Ref. [4].

- Intermittently underperfused capillaries in close to well-perfused capillaries.
- Decrease in capillary density.
- Increase in heterogeneity of vessels.

For resuscitation measures to be effective, there must be coherence between the macro- and microcirculation. This coherence should be conceptualized as the normalization of systemic variables in a parallel improvement of microcirculatory perfusion, parenchymal oxygenation cells, and the restoration of normal cell activity. In many shock states, the tissues may remain hypoperfused even after MAP has been restored, as previously mentioned.

Persistence of microcirculatory hypoperfusion after restoration of macrocirculation has been shown in numerous studies and is associated with poor outcomes [12].

Four different types of underlying microcirculatory disorders have been suggested by the loss of hemodynamic coherence [13]:

Type 1 (obstructive): heterogeneous microcirculatory flow in which there are obstructed capillaries next to capillaries with flow of RBCs. The persistence of this type of microcirculatory dysfunction in the presence of normal systemic hemodynamic variables has been associated with adverse outcomes [12]. Increased microcirculatory perfusion during resuscitation is associated with decreased organ failure in septic patients with comparable global hemodynamics [14].

Type 2 (hemodilution/anemic): there is reduced capillary density induced by hemodilution and anemia, in which the dilution of the blood causes the loss of capillaries filled with RBCs and results in increased diffusion distances between oxygen-carrying RBCs and cells in tissues.

Type 3 (hypoperfused): there is reduced microcirculatory flow caused by vasoconstriction or tamponade in which vasoconstriction of arterial vessels causes ischemia or elevated venous pressures that induce microcirculatory tamponade.

Type 4 (distributive): tissue edema caused by capillary leak, resulting in increased diffusion distances between RBCs and tissue cells.

In 2018, a Task Force of the European Society of Intensive Care Medicine published the Second Consensus on the Assessment of Sublingual Microcirculation [15], which proposed a classification system to better characterize microcirculatory disorders other than those associated solely with sepsis.

Types of alterations include:
- Type 1: completely stagnant capillaries (circulatory arrest, excessive use of vasopressors).
- Type 2: reduced number of flowing capillaries (hemodilution).
- Type 3: vessels with stopped flow are seen alongside vessels with flowing cells (sepsis, hemorrhage and hemodilution).
- Type 4: hyperdynamic flow within the capillaries (hemodilution, sepsis).

The early detection of shock is the main objective of microcirculation monitoring.

Microcirculation assessment measurements can be performed according to clinical availability in [11]:
- Clinical assessment.
- Biochemical markers.
- No invasive techniques.

CLINICAL ASSESSMENT

Capillary refill time (CRT) is defined as the time required for return of color after the application of blanching pressure to a distal capillary bed [16], with upper normal values likely ranging 3.5—4.5 s. Confounder as age, temperature, and interrater variability can be difficult their interpretation [17].

A trial found that for a successful resuscitation, CRT and central-to-toe temperature difference (Tc-toe) were more significant predictors compared to metabolic parameters such as central venous oxygen saturation ($ScvO_2$) and central venous arterial CO_2 difference (P [cv-a]CO_2 gap).

SKIN MOTTLING

Skin mottling is defined as a bluish skin discoloration that typically manifest near the elbows or knees and has a distinct patchy pattern [11]. Abnormal skin perfusion is the result of heterogenic small vessel vasoconstriction [18]. At this context, the mottling scoring system, grading from 0 to 5, according to mottling area extension from the knees to the periphery, is a reliable and simple tool (Table 5.1). A trial found that higher skin mottling was predictive of mortality in critical care patients [19].

PERIPHERAL PERFUSION INDEX

The analysis of the pulse oximetry signal is the base of peripheral perfusion index (PPI). PPI is the ratio between the pulsatile blood flow and nonpulsatile static blood flow in peripheral tissues. A trial suggested a cutoff of 1.4 to predict poor peripheral perfusion [20], and a PPI <0.2 predicted mortality in septic patients following resuscitation [21].

TABLE 5.1
Mottling Score System

0	No mottling.
1	Small mottling area localized to the center of the knee.
2	Mottling area not exceeding the superior edge of the kneecap.
3	Mottling does not exceed the middle thigh.
4	Mottling not exceeding the fold of the groin.
5	Mottling that extends beyond the groin

Modified of Ferraris A, Bouisse C, Mottard N et al. Mottling score and skin temperature in septic shock: relation and impact on prognosis in ICU. PLoS One 2018;13(8):e0202329.

The evidence suggests that on-invasive assessment (CRT, Tc-toe, skin mottling, and PPI) may be used as surrogates of peripheral perfusion.

BIOCHEMICAL MARKERS

SvO_2 and $ScvO_2$.

Mixed venous oxygen saturation (SvO_2), vena cava saturation ($ScvO_2$), plasma lactate, and $P[cv-a]CO_2$ gap are used to indicate global perfusion. SvO_2 requires a pulmonary artery catheter; $ScvO_2$, a central venous catheter (CVC).

To calculate the cardiac output, the Fick equation can be used, utilizing the SvO_2 [22]:

$$SvO_2 = SaO_2 - (VO_2 / cardiac\ output \times Hb \times 1.34)$$

where SaO_2 is the arterial oxygen saturation, Hb, hemoglobin concentration, and VO_2, whole O_2 consumption. 70%−75% is the range of normal value of SvO_2.

Decreasing values of cardiac output result in decreases in SvO_2 in the oxygen extraction rate, if SaO_2, VO_2, and hemoglobin remain constant [11].

PLASMA LACTATE

Lactate, in most cases, is a product of anaerobic metabolism and thus indicates inadequate oxygen delivery to or metabolism of tissues. An elevated lactate (>2 mmol/L) is often the result of a mismatch between relative oxygen supply and tissue demand. Epinephrine,

beta-agonists, and metformin can elevate lactate. Lactate clearance as a target of resuscitation has been shown to be noninferior to using $ScvO_2$ monitoring [23].

It is a need to interpret hyperlactatemia with caution due to the complexity of lactate metabolism. Lactate metabolism has been extensively revised elsewhere [24].

Central − Venous − Arterial CO_2 Difference($P[cv − a]CO_2$ gap).

In the assessment of the micro- and macrocirculation, the $P[cv-a]CO_2$ gap can be used. Under physiological conditions, the CO_2 content venous is greater than the arterial, product of the production of CO_2 at peripheral level coupled to oxygen consumption and metabolism in general. In normal ranges, the content has a linear relationship with the pressures, so which the measurement of such pressures has been proposed. In theory, low-flow states and nonanaerobic sources of CO_2 production can increase venous content and thus amplify the normal difference [25].

$P[cv-a]CO_2$ gap can be calculated and used as a surrogate for the cardiac index, and utilizing a CVC, the $ScvO_2$ can be measured and utilized as a surrogate for global tissue hypoxia. A pCO_2 gap >0.8 kPa (6 mm Hg) has been associated with a higher mortality after 24 h of treatment [26].

The pCO_2 delta can be normal in cases of evident hypoperfusion and elevated cardiac output and may also be increased in the absence of hypoperfusion taking into account the Haldane effect [27]. Therefore, the evaluation of the contents has been proposed of CO_2 in relation to those of oxygen as another form to approach the state of tissue perfusion. The $CvaCO_2$/$Da-vO_2$ is a variable that can identify patients with anaerobic metabolism in various critical conditions [27−29].

HANDHELD VITAL MICROSCOPY

Use of handheld vital microscopy (HVM) has permitted direct visualization of the microcirculation for three decades, initially with orthogonal polarization spectral imaging, then with sidestream dark-field imaging, and currently with incident dark-field imaging, which allows a better visualization of capillaries with an optimized resolution [12]. The sublingual circulation is the most common anatomical location imaged.

The assessment of RBC flow though the capillaries (microvascular flow index), the density of the perfuse capillaries (functional capillary density) is achieved by visualization of the sublingual microcirculation.

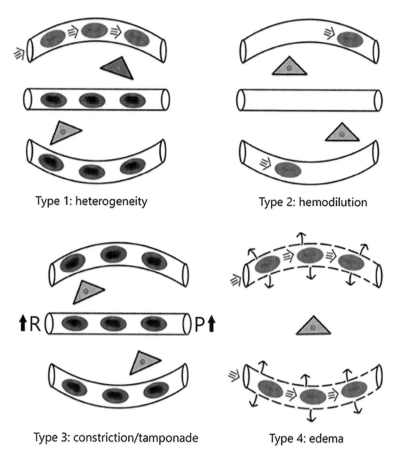

Type 1: heterogeneity

Type 2: hemodilution

Type 3: constriction/tamponade

Type 4: edema

FIG. 5.3 Condition of microcirculatory alterations associated with loss of hemodynamic coherence and reduced oxygen capacity of the tissues. Type 1: Heterogenous RBC flow caused by RBC and endothelial cell injury induced for example by sepsis results in RBC stagnant capillaries next to perfused capillaries resulting in microcirculatory shunts and a reduction of tissue oxygen extraction capacity. Type 2: A decrease in the oxygen-carrying potential of the microcirculation due to hemodilution induced anemia resulting from a low FCD. Type 3: A stasis in the RBC flow due to increased vascular resistance (R) and/or elevated venous pressure (P). Type 4: Increased oxygen diffusion distances due to edema caused by capillary leak syndrome. Taken from Ref. [4].

Some limitations have been pointed out to HVMs [22]:
— Are time consuming.
— The equipment is expensive.
— Require training.
— The measurements need a complex analysis.
— Artifacts induced by compression and saliva.

Despite the use of standardized protocol and support software, the assessment is still slow and limits more widespread use (Fig. 5.3).

REFERENCES

[1] Singer M, Deutschman CS, Seymour C, et al. The Third international consensus definitions for sepsis and septic shock (sepsis-3). JAMA 2016;315(8):801—10.

[2] De Backer D, Durand A, Donadello K. Microcirculation alterations in patients with severe sepsis. Clin Pulm Med 2015;22:31—5.

[3] Mok G, Hendin A, Reardon P, et al. Macrocirculatory and microcirculatory endpoints in sepsis resuscitation. J Intensive Care Med 2020;36:1385—91.

[4] Guven G, Hilty MP, Ince C. Microcirculation: physiology, pathophysiology, and clinical application. Blood Purif 2020;49:143−50.

[5] Bateman RM, Sharpe MD, Ellis CG. Bench-to-bedside review: microvascular dysfunction in sepsis hemodynamics, oxygen transport, and nitric oxide. Crit Care October 2003;7(5):359−73.

[6] Guerci P, Ergin B, Uz Z, et al. Glycocalyx degradation is independent of vascular barrier permeability increase in nontraumatic hemorrhagic shock in rats. Anesth Analg August 2019;129(2):598−607.

[7] Weinbaum S, Tarbell JM, Damiano ER. The structure and function of the endothelial glycocalyx layer. Annu Rev Biomed Eng 2007;9(1):121−67.

[8] Ince C, Mayeux PR, Nguyen T, et al. ADQI XIV Workgroup. The endothelium in sepsis. Shock March 2016;45(3):259−70.

[9] Uchimido R, Schmidt EP, Shapiro NI. The glycocalyx: a novel diagnostic and therapeutic target in sepsis. Crit Care January 2019;23(1):16.

[10] Ince C, De Backer D, Mayeux PR. Microvascular dysfunction in the critically ill. Crit Care Clin April 2020;36(2):323−31.

[11] Cantan B, Martin-Loeches I. Microcirculation in patients with sepsis: from physiology to interventions annual update in intensive care and emergency medicine 2020. Cham: Springer; 2020. p. 245−58.

[12] De Backer D, Donadello K, Sakr Y, et al. Microcirculatory alterations in patients with severe sepsis: impact of time of assessment and relationship with outcome. Crit Care Med 2013;41:791−9.

[13] Ince C. Hemodynamic coherence and the rationale for monitoring the microcirculation. Crit Care 2015;19:S8.

[14] Trzeciak S, McCoy JV, Dellinger RP, et al. Early increases in microcirculatory perfusion during protocol-directed resuscitation are associated with reduced multi-organ failure at 24 h in patients with sepsis. Intensive Care Med 2008;34:2210−7.

[15] Ince C, Boerma EC, Cecconi M, et al. Second consensus on the assessment of sublingual microcirculation in critically ill patients: results from a task force of the European Society of Intensive Care Medicine. Intensive Care Med 2018;44:281−99.

[16] Pandey A, Maj. Capillary refill time. Is it time to fill the gaps? Med J Armed Forces India January 2013;69(1):97−8.

[17] Anderson B, Kelly AM, Kerr D, et al. Impact of patient and environmental factors on capillary refill time in adults. Am J Emerg Med 2008;26:62−5.

[18] Lima A, Bakker J. Clinical assessment of peripheral circulation. Curr Opin Crit Care 2015;21:226−31.

[19] Dumas G, Lavillegrand JR, Joffre J, et al. Mottling score is a strong predictor of 14-day mortality in septic patients whatever vasopressor doses and other tissue perfusion parameters. Crit Care 2019;23:211.

[20] Lima AP, Beelen P, Bakker J. Use of a peripheral perfusion index derived from the pulse oximetry signal as a noninvasive indicator of perfusion. Crit Care Med 2002;17:1210−3.

[21] He HW, Liu DW, Long Y, et al. The peripheral perfusion index and transcutaneous oxygen challenge test are predictive of mortality in septic patients after resuscitation. Crit Care 2013;17:R116.

[22] Huber W, Zanner R, Schneider G, et al. Assessment of regional perfusion and organ function: less and noninvasive techniques. Front Med 2019;6:50.

[23] Jones AE, Shapiro NI, Trzeciak S, et al. Lactate clearance vs central venous oxygen saturation as goals of early sepsis therapy: a randomized clinical trial. JAMA 2010;303:739−46.

[24] Ferguson BS, Rogatzki MJ, Goodwin ML, et al. Lactate metabolism: historical context, prior misinterpretations, and current understanding. Eur J Appl Physiol April 2018;118(4):691−728.

[25] Diaztagle Fernández JJ, Rodríguez Murcia JC, Sprockel Díaz JJ. Venous-to-arterial carbon dioxide difference in the resuscitation of patients with severe sepsis and septic shock: a systematic review. Med Intensiva October 2017;41(7):401−10.

[26] Van Beest PA, Lont MC, Holman ND, et al. Central venous-arterial pCO2 difference as a tool in resuscitation of septic patients. Intensive Care Med 2013;39:1034−9.

[27] Ospina-Tascón GA, Umana M, Bermudez W, et al. Combination of arterial lactate levels and venous-arterial CO_2 to arterial-venous O_2 content difference ratio as markers of resuscitation in patients with septic shock. Intensive Care Med 2015;41:796−805.

[28] Monnet X, Julien F, Ait-Hamou N, et al. Lactate and venoarterial carbon dioxide difference/arterial-venous oxygen difference ratio, but not central venous oxygen saturation, predict increase in oxygen consumption in fluid responders. Crit Care Med 2013;41:1412−20.

[29] Mesquida J, Saludes P, Gruartmoner G, et al. Central venous-to-arterial carbon dioxide difference combined with arterial-to-venous oxygen content difference is associated with lactate evolution in the hemodynamic resuscitation process in early septic shock. Crit Care 2015;19:126.

FURTHER READING

[1] Ferraris A, Bouisse C, Mottard N, et al. Mottling score and skin temperature in septic shock: relation and impact on prognosis in ICU. PLoS One 2018;13(8):e0202329.

CHAPTER 6

Genetics and Sepsis

GABRIELA ALVARADO

GENETICS AND SEPSIS

From Gregor Mendel's first descriptions of inheritance patterns in plants to the decoding of the human genome, genetic engineering has advanced in a very impressive way. The expansion of scientific knowledge about the human genome has a profound impact on humanity, and physicians may be able to use genetic information to dictate immune-based therapies to modulate the response in sepsis patients. Genotyping is likely to become increasingly important in clinical medicine.

SEPSIS RESPONSE

Sepsis is a heterogeneous state associated with significant morbidity and mortality and is a leading cause of mortality worldwide. In addition, the survivors of sepsis frequently have long-term physical, psychological, and cognitive impairments. Despite advances in care, existing epidemiologic studies suggest that sepsis remains a huge burden across all economic regions, and the epidemiologic data for sepsis are scarce to nonexistent for low- and middle-income countries [1].

This syndrome develops as a result of a severe infection by different microorganisms, which explains the diversity of clinical manifestations between patients with sepsis. Each patient with sepsis responds differently, and most likely the responses are modulated by the inflammatory, oxidative, or immune response. The clinical evolution of the characteristics of sepsis makes both diagnosis and treatment difficult because patients proceed through different stages of sepsis, with each stage requiring treatment specifically targeted to counteract these variations. Sepsis patients are still treated as groups rather than individuals, even though there are reported examples of treatments that are proven to be efficacious for some septic patients but not others.

Early recognition of sepsis is one of the principal priorities in the approaches of critical cases, since treatment strategies remain limited and there are no specific treatments for sepsis. Management for patients currently consists mainly of cardiorespiratory resuscitation and treatment of infection. Immunomodulatory therapies in which patients with sepsis are prescribed corticosteroids, antitumor necrosis factor-α (TNF-α) antibodies, antiinterleukin antibodies, platelet-activating factor antagonists, antioxidants, and other new drugs have been accepted as beneficial [2].

However, intensivists continue to be frustrated in their inability to predict the outcome of any one patient with sepsis. Even more frustrating is that despite an explosion of knowledge of the inflammatory response to sepsis and the enormous financial resources invested in randomized controlled trials of antiinflammatory therapies, physicians still lack effective therapies targeting the inflammatory response to sepsis [3].

A high percentage of critical patients with sepsis develop multiple organ failure, making the death rate significantly higher among these patients. This phenomenon is due to the infections as well as the overlapping inflammatory immune events. Analogous sepsis endotypes have been identified in adults with the use of interindividual variations in host response to sepsis; the generated inflammatory responses are different based on the type of tissue, function, and the receptors that trigger the reactions responsible for the biosynthesis of mediators.

While the exact pathophysiology of sepsis remains largely unknown, a variety of factors interfere with the response of the host to an infectious stimulus and this has direct implications both on clinical severity and outcome. The innate immunity responsiveness to an infection is shaped by the genetic differences between individuals, which shows the crucial role of the host defense in the pathophysiology of this complex syndrome [4].

Due to developmental age playing a key role in the host's response to sepsis, pediatric cases differ from adult sepsis cases [5]. The lack of substantial overlap between adults and children likely reflects this developmental difference in host response, so interventions that show promise in adults may not show similar results in pediatric patients.

The Sepsis Codex. https://doi.org/10.1016/B978-0-323-88271-2.00002-X

Some disorders of immune deficiency are detected in childhood due to recurrent serious infections. However, in adults with no known immune deficiency, it is more challenging to determine which genetic polymorphisms lead to an increased risk of acquiring infection. Despite this inherent limitation, some polymorphisms appear to confer increased risk to specific pathogens [6].

Given the underlying heterogeneity, it is conceivable that a subset of the population may benefit from a given therapy and another potentially harmed. There is growing interest in the application of a precision medicine approach to sepsis to identify patients, who are more likely to benefit from targeted therapeutic interventions.

GENETIC VARIABILITY

Sepsis comprises a cascade of pro- and antiinflammatory cytokines and mediators in the systemic circulation, which are found at different stages of sepsis. The most common inflammatory cytokines in sepsis are tumor necrosis factor-α(TNF-α), interleukin-1 (IL-1), and proinflammatory cytokines IL-6 and IL-8. They are released by activating macrophages and CD4 T cells. Antiinflammatory mediators such as IL-10, IL-13, IL-14 and transforming growth factor-β (TGF-β) are present in a later stage [7].

Human host genetics may determine the risk of acquiring an infection. The innate immunity responsiveness to an infection is shaped by the genetic differences between individuals, which emphasizes the crucial role of the host defense in the pathophysiology of sepsis. Studies have reported an increased risk of death from infections when one of their biological parents had died from infections [8]. A genetic basis for interindividual variation in susceptibility to human infectious diseases has been found in twins and adopted persons.

There are many examples of genetic variability that influence physiological activity in sepsis, and there has been great interest in exploring the possibility that a polymorphism in the TNF promoter results in significantly higher TNF levels, which might be associated with a worse outcome from sepsis. Of particular interest was the recent report that mutations in TLR4 are associated with an increased susceptibility to Gram-negative sepsis [9].

HUMAN GENOME

DNA is made up of a wide range of nucleotides that are packaged into chromosomes. Each chromosome contains genes, which are regions that code for specific proteins that allow an organism to function. Genes make up only a small part of an organism's genome, less than 2% of human DNA. The human genome contains approximately three billion nucleotides and about 20,000 protein-coding genes, representing 1% of the total genome length. The remaining 99% are noncoding DNA sequences that do not produce proteins.

Alternative forms of a gene are alleles. An allele is one of two or more versions of a DNA sequence at a given genomic location. People inherit two alleles, one from each parent, for any given genomic location where such variation exists. If the two alleles are the same, the person is homozygous for that allele. If the alleles are different, the person is heterozygous. Alleles can undergo mutations and alter the amino acid sequence of the protein they encode.

A small group of diseases can be predicted by the presence of genetic mutations. In addition to its genome, each cell has an epigenome, which is defined by the gene expression profile in response to environmental stimuli and regulatory mechanisms at the molecular level. Through epigenetics, the causal interactions between genes and their products that give rise to the phenotype are studied [10].

In recent years and with advances in the knowledge of the human genome, great interest has been given to genetic susceptibility to infections, due to the high variability in the human genome. One of the main causes of this variability is what we know as genetic polymorphism. A genetic polymorphism is an allelic variant that exists in at least 1% of the population. They are different from mutations, are much less frequent, and are associated with hereditary diseases. Polymorphisms of the endotoxin-binding protein, CD14 receptor, tumor necrosis factor-beta (TNF-β), TNF-α, interleukin 1 alpha (IL-1α), IL-1β, IL-1ra, IL-6, and IL-10 have been described [11].

FINDING THE GENES

Two types of polymorphisms can be distinguished: variable number of tandem repeats (VNTRs) and single nucleotide polymorphisms (SNPs). When SNP polymorphisms occur within the coding region of the gene, or exon, the probability that the biological function of the protein will be altered is greater, since the base change can result in the substitution of one amino acid for another. SNPs can be genotyped using the restriction fragment length polymorphism technique. Repeat polymorphisms can be genotyped using PCR [11].

Several gene association studies have evaluated SNPs in pediatric sepsis and septic shock. Genome-wide association studies (GWASs) examine a large number of

SNPs simultaneously and identify common variants associated with specific disease states [5].

GWASs are allowed to identify SNPs associated with mortality in septic shock patients. SNPs were associated with early and late mortality, and the genetic variations in different genes alter the activation of immune cells [12]. The early stimulation of inflammation processes appears to be rapidly followed by a downregulation of these processes through dominant antiinflammatory patterns.

Several genetic variants were significantly associated with the risk of sepsis [13]. The association between host genetic variants containing SNPs and VNTRs with genes, which regulate the host's immune response and sepsis susceptibility, has been described. Sequence variants within genes have been considered candidates for the promotion of sepsis pathogenesis.

Increasing evidence has suggested that genetic variants, particularly SNPs, are critical determinants of interindividual differences in both inflammatory responses and clinical outcomes in sepsis patients [13].

SNPs residing on each of the following structures may affect susceptibility and outcome: (I) Pattern recognition receptors (PRRs) on antigen (Ag)-presenting cells, Toll-like receptors (TLRs), and triggering receptor expressed on myeloid cells [14]; (II) Proinflammatory cytokines such as TNFα, IL-1 beta, IL-12, type 1 and 2 interferons, predominately antiinflammatory cytokines such as IL-4, IL-10, and TGF-β; (III) Immunoglobulins (IGs) and their receptor-binding sites found on the crystallizable fragment of immunoglobulin (Fc) of IG bind to receptors expressed on Ag-presenting cells, phagocytes, and natural killer cells [15].

KEY GENES

The genetic basis of susceptibility to major infectious diseases is potentially the most complex area in the genetics of diseases. Sepsis has multiple pathways involving many enzymes, mediators, and proteins coded by genes, making sepsis a polygenic disease.

The sepsis pathophysiology involves highly complex interactions between microorganisms, the host's innate and adaptive immune systems, and multiple organ dysfunction and death [12]. Altered cellular signaling due to circulating cellular mediators contributes to dysregulation of immunity, tissue repair, and cellular stress responses [16].

Polymorphisms in TLRs are a crucial family of pathogen-recognition receptors (PRRs) that provide a major mechanism for innate immune cells to recognize and respond to pathogens. TLR1/2 is responsible for recognizing cell wall components of Gram-positive bacteria. TLR4 is responsible for recognizing the lipopolysaccharide of Gram-negative bacteria. Increasing evidence indicates that polymorphisms of TLR genes influence susceptibility to various infectious diseases, including sepsis [13].

Polygenic diseases have a well-documented interpopulation heterogeneity, and in all cases, require environmental factors in addition to genetic load. Progress is being made in untangling the complex interplay of host genes and microorganisms that results in some striking interindividual variation in susceptibility.

Studies have implicated many genes across a large spectrum of immune and coagulation proteins, including interleukins, receptors, and fibrinogen [17]. Human diseases may be explored using genetic approaches to gain insight into the complex functional pathways that characterize the disease.

Identification of genetic variations in the genes involved in bacterial-induced cellular response and those involved in the pathogenesis of sepsis may allow the development of new diagnostic tools, improved classification of sepsis, and more accurate predictors of patient outcomes [16].

The use of monoclonal antibodies (mAbs) in the treatment of bacterial sepsis targeting the pathogen responsible for inducing sepsis has only recently been investigated. MAbs can now be directed against bacterial infections like *Staphylococcus aureus*, *Staphylococcus epidermidis*, and multidrug-resistant strains of *Pseudomonas aeruginosa*, *Escherichia coli*, and *Klebsiella pneumoniae* [18].

Every patient has a different response to drugs and infections. Individual risks and cellular responses can be related to each patient's unique DNA. Genetics seeks to correlate the variation in DNA sequence with phenotypic differences. The recognition of genetic predisposition to sepsis might facilitate the search for therapeutic targets in patients with an impaired innate immune system [19].

PERSONALIZED AND PRECISION MEDICINE

The evaluation of sepsis-specific genetic polymorphisms can significantly improve the intensive therapy options in critically ill patients with sepsis, and the identification of genetic polymorphisms in critical patients with sepsis can become a revolutionary method for evaluating and monitoring patients.

Personalized medicine is based on the idea that if enough informative risk factors are known, we can come up with a more effective risk stratification models given our limited knowledge of the genes that contribute to shaping the differences in sepsis survival between patients, and the poor predictive utility of the identified genetic variant.

RNA sequencing techniques deliver for log scale greater dynamic range than microarray and can identify even single molecules present in several lectures of genes. Using this new technology to accurately and rapidly identify infecting pathogens and to probe and obtain signatures of the host immune response to infection will likely result in the identification of novel critical regulators of immune function and secondary organ dysfunction, and earlier, more accurate treatment decisions in severe infections.

Technology is now available to rapidly test an individual's numerous polymorphisms using DNA chips (microarrays), a single DNA test done once in a lifetime, could identify the predisposition of a patient to many diseases and the predicted response to therapy. Hundreds of thousands of polymorphisms can be identified and precisely ordered on an SNP map.

Microarrays and other new technologies used to establish an individual's base-line genomic scan could provide useful information about a person's risk profile and expected response to therapy. Knowledge of an individual's polymorphisms that predispose susceptibility to sepsis and predict response to therapy would be invaluable [3].

To increase the power to detect additional risk variants underlying the diversity of sepsis manifestations, further genetic studies should focus on particular infections, rather than on a broadly defined syndrome. The genetic manifestations of some diseases in studies only form a fraction of the real human genetic diversity.

Successful application of precision medicine in clinical practice will require rigorous testing and validation; based on perturbations in shared biological pathways, groups of patients may be subclassified into endotypes and those at risk of poor outcomes identified. Select patients based on their inherent risk may be subject to receive therapeutic interventions in clinical trials.

A lot of research is necessary to identify novel molecular targets and new drugs in sepsis. Rigorous clinical trials in humans are required to test the safety and efficacy of new therapies. Precision medicine approach in sepsis requires simultaneous advancement in three interconnected areas, in preclinical studies, clinical trials, and implementation science [20].

The selection of patients with heterogeneous diseases, such as sepsis, to enrollment in clinical trials remains a major challenge. Strategies and efforts are directed at selecting a study population, in which a drug or intervention is most likely to be effective.

The ongoing search for new therapies for sepsis, new prognostic and diagnostic biomarkers has generated several genome-wide expression studies over the past decade, variously focusing on the diagnosis, prognosis, pathogen response, and underlying sepsis pathophysiology. Despite tremendous efforts to understand gene expression in sepsis, few insights have translated to improvements in clinical practice [2].

The precision medicine in critical patients with sepsis poses unique challenges, for example: the diverse host immune response in sepsis, evolution of gene expression profiles in the same patient, and the limited opportunity between detection and outcome during which an intervention may be applied.

The recent identification of critical illness subtypes points to an emerging need for relating them to precise therapies. Creating these subtypes was done by gene expression analysis, which helped differentiate sepsis from nonseptic states. Despite new advances in this new area of medicine, precision therapies in the ICU are at present, neither clearly defined nor generally accepted.

REFERENCES

[1] Fleischmann C, Schrag A, Adhikari NKJ, Hartog CS, Tsaganos T, Schlattmann P, et al. Assessment of global incidence and mortality of hospital-treated sepsis: current estimates and limitations. Am J Respir Crit Care Med February 1, 2016;193(3):259–72. https://doi.org/10.1164/rccm.201504-0781OC.

[2] Lazăr A, Georgescu AM, Alexander V, Leonard A. Precision medicine and its role in the treatment of sepsis: a personalised view. J Crit Care Med (Targu Mures) July 2019; 5(3):90–6. https://doi.org/10.2478/jccm-2019-0017. Published online 2019 Aug 9.

[3] Holmes CL, et al. Genetic polymorphisms in sepsis and septic shock: role in prognosis and potential for therapy. Chest 2003;124(3):1103–15. https://doi.org/10.1378/chest.124.3.1103.

[4] Flores C. Host genetics shapes adult sepsis survival. Lancet Respir Med 2015;3(1):7–8. https://doi.org/10.1016/S2213-2600(14)70307-8.

[5] Atreya MR, Wong HR. Precision medicine in pediatric sepsis. Curr Opin Pediatr June 2019;31(3):322–7. https://doi.org/10.1097/mop.0000000000000753.

[6] Boyd JH, et al. The meta-genome of sepsis: host genetics, pathogens and the acute immune response. J Innate Immun 2014;6(3):272–83. https://doi.org/10.1159/000358835.

[7] Schulte W, Bernhagen J, Bucala R. Cytokines in sepsis: potent immunoregulators and potential therapeutic targets–an updated view. Mediat Inflamm 2013;2013: 165974. https://doi.org/10.1155/2013/165974.

[8] Petersen L, Andersen PK, Sorensen TI. Genetic influences on incidence and case-fatality of infectious disease. PLoS One 2010;5(5):e10603. https://doi.org/10.1371/journal.pone.0010603. Published 2010 May 14.

[9] Cohen J. The immunopathogenesis of sepsis. Nature December 19–26, 2002;420(6917):885–91. https://doi.org/10.1038/nature01326.

[10] Dupont C, Armant DR, Brenner CA. Epigenetics: definition, mechanisms and clinical perspective. Semin Reprod Med 2009;27(5):351—7. https://doi.org/10.1055/s-0029-1237423.

[11] Garnacho Montero, J.; Garnacho Montero, M. C.; Ortiz Leyba, C.; Aldabó Pallás, T. Genetic polymorphisms in sepsis, Med Intensiva. DOI:10.1016/S0210-5691(05)74226-1

[12] Rosier F, et al. Genetic predisposition to the mortality in septic shock patients: from GWAS to the identification of a regulatory variant modulating the activity of a CISH enhancer. Int J Mol Sci May 29, 2021;22(11):5852. https://doi.org/10.3390/ijms22115852.

[13] Lu H, et al. Host genetic variants in sepsis risk: a field synopsis and meta-analysis. Crit Care January 25, 2019; 23(1):26. https://doi.org/10.1186/s13054-019-2313-0.

[14] Hotchkiss RS, et al. Immunosuppression in sepsis: a novel understanding of the disorder and a new therapeutic approach. Lancet Infect Dis 2013;13(3):260—8. https://doi.org/10.1016/S1473-3099(13)70001-X.

[15] Guilliams M, et al. The function of Fcγ receptors in dendritic cells and macrophages. Nat Rev Immunol 2014; 14(2):94—108. https://doi.org/10.1038/nri3582.

[16] Abu-Maziad A, Schaa K, Bell EF, et al. Role of polymorphic variants as genetic modulators of infection in neonatal sepsis. Pediatr Res 2010;68(4):323—9. https://doi.org/10.1203/PDR.0b013e3181e6a068.

[17] Sutherland AM, Walley KR. Bench-to-bedside review: association of genetic variation with sepsis. Crit Care 2009;13(2):210. https://doi.org/10.1186/cc7702.

[18] Giamarellos-Bourboulis EJ, Opal SM. The role of genetics and antibodies in sepsis. Ann Transl Med 2016;4(17): 328. https://doi.org/10.21037/atm.2016.08.63.

[19] Villar J, et al. Bench-to-bedside review: understanding genetic predisposition to sepsis. Critical care (London).

[20] Seymour CW, Gomez H, Chang C-CH, et al. Precision medicine for all? Challenges and opportunities for a precision medicine approach to critical illness. Crit Care Lond Engl 2017;21(1):257. https://doi.org/10.1186/s13054-017-1836-5.

CHAPTER 7

Screening and early detection of sepsis

MARCIO BORGES SA • RAFAEL ZARAGOZA CRESPO

INTRODUCTION

Sepsis (SE) and septic shock (SS) are a medical emergency, and its rapid and appropriate initial comprehensive diagnostic-therapeutic management will be key to the patient's prognosis. It affects an estimated 30–40 million individuals worldwide each year, although these figures are probably underestimated. And the consequences are also increasingly well known, although they vary greatly according to sources, types of patients, countries, etc. The mortality of SE varies between 10% and 20%, while that of SS between 22% and 57% [1–5]. Mortality has varied in recent years with the introduction of bundles and mainly due to better early management of SE/SS, as described by several groups [1,3–9]. Other consequences of having SE/SS are longer hospital stay, use of resources, and costs compared to other patients. Regarding costs, we have more and more information: it is estimated that a case of SE in Europe consumes about 15,000 euros, while an SS up to 30,000 [3,10,11].

It is important to know in which hospital setting we will have to identify potential septic patients, since the professionals, care experience, human and technical resources are different if it is an emergency department (ED), a hospital ward, or in the intensive care unit (ICU). Therefore, it is important to develop homogeneous mechanisms for such care management to prevent fundamental steps from being missed [1–4,7,8,12–15]. However, for greater complexity, rigid protocols have not been shown to be superior to those adapted to each situation, so we *must always individualize* each case [1–3,12].

The Surviving Sepsis Campaign (SSC) in its various documents, including the latest one, recommends that hospitals have sepsis care programs, strong recommendation with moderate quality of evidence that hospitals have a screening system and programs to improve sepsis detection [16–18].

These programs value a comprehensive view of the process, including screening, educational programs, evaluation of quality indicators, and new diagnostic and therapeutic possibilities. The SSC considers screening programs for the early identification of sepsis with a strong recommendation and with moderate quality of evidence [18].

In our Spanish Consensus Document of Sepsis (SCDS), we recommend to use screening methods with a grade of evidence 1-C for the early detection of potential SE/SS patients in all areas of the hospital [1–3]. And we also recommend with the same degree of evidence comprehensive SE/SS management programs, strongly considering the whole educational process aimed at physicians, nurses, pharmacists, managers, and other health agents.

A key point, in both consensuses, is the need to measure the different actions through balanced but feasible quality indicators. In this case, screening, educational, and bundle evaluation programs are recommended [1,17,18].

LIMITATIONS FOR SEPSIS DETECTION

Sepsis is a complex and heterogeneous clinical syndrome caused by different pathogens (bacteria, viruses, fungi, or parasites) that cause a series of biological consequences in the host. The host in turn presents different forms of physiological response to this aggression. This complex pathogen–host relationship generates different pathophysiological reactions with different phenotypes. These phenotypes of sepsis are

The Sepsis Codex. https://doi.org/10.1016/B978-0-323-88271-2.00026-2

extremely varied and depend, in turn, on other factors such as the immunological situation of the host, its basic treatments, its genotype, etc [3,5,12,19–21].

All this complicates the detection of sepsis itself, since there will be a variability of clinical and analytical criteria that may be related to the sepsis of a given individual against one or more pathogens that have caused the infection (212). And this great phenotypic variability complicates rapid detection, since we do not have clear criteria in the definition of SE/SS [2,12].

Basically, we can detect a septic patient in three ways: the human way we use every day, in an automated electronic alert systems (AEASs) way based on rules or certain scores as Sequential Organ Failure Assessment (SOFA), or through new techniques of big data (BD), artificial intelligence (AI), and machine learning (ML) [2,3].

EARLY DETECTION

In the epidemiology of sepsis, hospital episodes of SE/SS about 60%–75% are identified in the ED, 25%–40% in the wards, and 5%–10% in the critical patient areas [1,3–7,13,18,22,23]. Early detection of a patient with potential sepsis is the most important starting point for adequate care, but fundamental, as it is a time-dependent entity [1–9,13,16–18,21–23].

For this reason, the ED is the main department where we must pay special attention [1,3,12,13,18,22,23]. Most septic patients will pass through the triage area, so organizing a fast and efficient system to identify potential SE/SS patients is a crucial point in proper management. The problem is to generate, in very few minutes, an excellent predictive system based on the clinical history and some signs with sufficient sensitivity to initiate diagnostic-therapeutic measures [1–4,12,23].

In our SCDS, we have developed a simple system of triage in the ED, based on different studies, care protocols, and clinical experiences [1]. In Table 7.1, we highlight the three points in triage: history, clinical examination with signs of systemic inflammatory response syndrome (SIRS) (temperature, heart rate, and respiratory rate), and possible organ dysfunction (OD) (blood pressure, oxygen saturation, neurological, skin lesions). A fundamental point is to recognize the comorbidities and risk factors for an SE/SS of each patient, therefore, and in order not to waste time, we must have simple but effective questions. Referring to

---

TABLE 7.1
The Three Different Criteria of Possible Sepsis in Triage of Emergency Department

1. Comorbidities (CMs) criterion

- Recent hospital admission (<15 days)
- Recent surgery (mainly major interventions)
- HIV or others immunosuppression syndromes
- Recent chemotherapy (<15 days)
- Neutropenic patients
- Bone marrow or solid transplantation
- Immunosuppressive therapies (e.g., steroids)
- Haemodialysis or peritoneal dialysis
- Cirrhosis patient
- Splenectomy
- Worse clinical evolution with antibiotic therapy

2. SRIS criteria (minor criterion)

- Temperature (>38.1 or < 36°C)
- Tachycardia (>90 lpm)
- Tachypnea (>24 rpm) or increased work of breathing

3. Organ dysfunction (OD) (major criterion)

- Arterial hypotension (SABP <90 mmHg or MABP <65 mmHg)
- Desaturation (SatO$_2$ < 90%)
- Altered consciousness
- Skin lesions (compatible with infections)

MABP, median arterial blood pressure; *SABP*, systolic arterial blood pressure.
(Adapted with permission by Borges M, Vidal P, Aranda P. Código sepsis. Capítulo 16. In: Borges Sa M, editor. Manual código sepsis. 2022. ISBN 978-958-5577-48-0. Editorial Distribuna. Bogotá, caracas, Lima, Madrid, Panamá y Pttsbrugh.)

the SRIS criteria in an early phase can guide us, mainly in those patients who have not been on medication (with antipyretics, antiinflammatory drugs, beta-blockers, etc.) that can mask these variables [15−18]. And finally, the presence of potential OD, which can also be recognized in a few minutes and can guide and even accelerate triage times, depending on the severity at this time: blood arterial pressure, oxygen saturation by pulse oximetry, or and level of consciousness [1,2,18].

Based on the combination of variables, we recommend one or another attitude, but as always, we emphasize the need to *individualize* each case, as described in Table 7.2. In Fig. 7.1, we propose, according to the findings and combinations of factors, to activate the sepsis code for this patient to enter as priority and be evaluated by a physician in less than five minutes, and to

initiate the entire diagnostic-therapeutic process adapted to each case. In this section, we can add, depending on availability, the performance of venous/arterial blood gases and obtain pH, $paCO_2$, paO_2, and plasma lactate, which can help us even more in our decision-making [1].

If the process of early detection is complicated in the ED, in hospitalization wards, such suspicion can be much more complicated for several reasons: patients are on different drugs or have undergone different medical or surgical procedures which make it difficult to discern cause-effect, and many clinical and analytical variables are altered by such treatments [1−3,18,22−24].

Currently, several screening programs have been designed with different degrees of sensitivity and specificity for the early detection of sepsis, precisely because

---

TABLE 7.2
Detection and Combination Criteria of Possible Sepsis in Triage of Emergency Department

Consider the different combinations for sepsis detection and activate sepsis code in emergency department based on the three different variables

- 1 major +2 minors
- $>/= 2$ majors
- 1 major +1 minor + CM
- 2 minors + CM
- 1 minor + $>/= 2$ CM
- Consider activate sepsis code in others risk clinical situations
- Always individualize each case

CM, comorbidities; *ED*, emergency department; $>/=$, greater than or equal to.
(Adapted with permission by Borges M, Vidal P, Aranda P. Código sepsis. Capítulo 16. In: Borges Sa M, editor. Manual código sepsis. 2022. ISBN 978-958-5577-48-0. Editorial Distribuna. Bogotá, caracas, Lima, Madrid, Panamá y Pttsbrugh.)

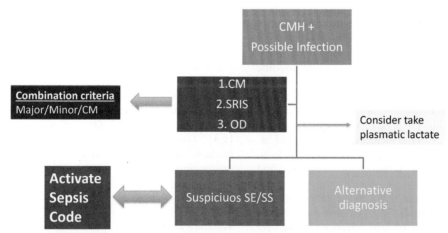

FIG. 7.1 Triage decision-making for SE/SS suspicious in ED. *CM*, comorbidity; *CMH*, clinical medical history; *ED*, emergency department, *OD*, organ disfunction; *SE*, sepsis; *SS*, septic shock. (Adapted with permission by Borges M, Vidal P, Aranda P. Código sepsis. Capítulo 16. In: Borges Sa M, editor. Manual código sepsis. 2022. ISBN 978-958-5577-48-0. Editorial Distribuna. Bogotá, caracas, Lima, Madrid, Panamá y Pttsbrugh.)

of the different diagnostic-therapeutic processes that can influence the early detection of sepsis. Nurses and physicians should be extremely attentive and clinically predisposed to diagnosis so as not to cause delays that often have prognostic consequences in these critically ill patients [1–3,5,8,12,13,22].

An important and possible fact is to train the professionals who are in more direct contact with these potential patients with suspected SE/SS, mainly nurses and physicians of some key specialties, such as ED, intensive care, internal medicine, as well as medical and surgical specialties [1,2,8,22–25]. Only with a continuous educational process, these professionals can maintain the high degree of predisposition for such early identification, which we know is the main key to improve prognostic outcomes and optimize the use of resources [1–4,6,8,12,13,22–25].

DIAGNOSIS

In Table 7.3, we define the different stratified degrees of sepsis, according to Sepsis-2 and Sepsis-3 criteria, but it is a process where it is necessary to *individualize* and evaluate each particular context rather than having rigid criteria (e.g., Two criteria of SIRS plus one of OD to define SE, or use only SOFA criteria). Since many times, even patients with SS and/or multiorgan dysfunction with bacteremia do not have any criteria of SIRS [3,18,26,27].

The diagnosis of sepsis is a dynamic process that requires individualization, since there are no pathognomonic or defining signs or symptoms of sepsis and we need a combination of them to generate a reasonable suspicion. The great variability of etiologies according to focus (e.g., lung or abdominal), pathogen (e.g., bacterial or viral), as well as the different clinical responses (signs/symptoms and analytical findings) makes this diagnostic process difficult [3,18–21,26,27]. Such variability also depends on genetic predisposition and the enormous inter- and intraindividual variability. It is also influenced by the patient's previous situation, e.g., whether he/she is immunosuppressed, concomitant medications, etc. [1–3,12,13,15,17–21,25–27].

The definition of SS has included the presence of tissue hypoperfusion in the setting of an infection, identified in the setting of serum hyperlactatemia and hypotension [1,18,27].

The latest definition of SE/SS, the so-called Sepsis-3, has been extensively studied for its subsequent validation. It has undoubtedly been an advance to categorize patients and try to homogenize the evaluation of trials [26,27]. On the other hand, it has generated many

TABLE 7.3
Sepsis-2 and Sepsis-3 Definitions

Definition	Previous (SEPSIS-2)	Current SEPSIS-3 (Singer et al.)
Sepsis	SRIS + Suspected or documented (Susp/Doc) infection	Infection (Susp/Doc) + 2-3/3 variables qSOFA or increase ≥2 SOFA points
Severe sepsis	Sepsis + Hypotension, Lactate >2 mmol/L Coagulopathy Platelets count <100.000 Bilirubin count >4 mg/L Creatinine increase Urine output <0.5 mL/h (2 hs) Basal $SatO_2$ < 90% Paralytic ilieous, hyperglycemia Other OD as altered consciousness	Disappears this group
Septic shock	Sepsis + Hypotension despite adequate fluid resuscitation	Sepsis + Need for vasopressors (MABP>65) + Lactate >2 mmol/L despite adequate fluid resuscitation

MABP, median arterial blood pressure; *OD*, organ dysfunction.

doubts, as it has been associated with a delay in the detection of patients with SE/SS. In many studies, it has shown a worse sensitivity for the early detection of patients with SE/SS.

It is important to recognize that such classic criteria in the definition of sepsis as fever and leukocytosis are present in about 50%–60% of all cases of SG/SS [1,3]. Many other clinical processes such as, for example, heart failure, severe trauma, some drug or postoperative can cause fever, leukocytosis, tachycardia [3,12,18,28].

Clinical Criteria

We know that a variable percentage of patients with SE or SS (with their OD) may not have SRIS or qSOFA criteria and have a documented infection because of the immense variability of each individual's response to the different pathogens responsible for sepsis [1,3,12,23,26−28]. Although we should not discard the clinical SIRS criteria, since the sum of them increases the risk of having sepsis and also more complications and worse prognosis [3,12].

Although after its publication, the use of qSOFA was recommended to help identify patients potentially with SE/SS, finally the latest SSC document recommends against its use as a single screening tool compared to SRIS, NEWS, or MEWS. And this document described it with a strong recommendation and moderate quality of evidence [18].

Although the Sepsis-3 definition restricted the variables included to those of the SOFA, the authors encourage using other variables, including those of the SRIS to suspect possible sepsis [26].

The biggest problem in the diagnostic process is that both SIRS and OD criteria are not very sensitive and specific, although their combination increases the probability of having sepsis [1−5,12,18]. And in a very early stage, we generally do not have microbiological information to help us support the suspicion of sepsis. Therefore, we must combine different variables, such as risk factors (e.g., immunosuppression, recent admission or surgery, use of Antibiotic (ATB)), medical history (signs and symptoms), and clinical variables (fever, tachycardia, tachypnea, hypotension, desaturation, etc.) [2,3,18].

One problem is that the different types, foci of infection and intra- and interpersonal variability may generate different degrees of clinical response, so that generalization and homogenization of criteria for diagnosing sepsis are impossible [1−4,14−21].

In our SDCS, we recommend the use of severity stratification and prognostic assessment scales such as the APACHE II and mainly the SOFA generalizing to all patients with suspected SE/SS and not only restricted to patients in ICU, with a level of evidence 2-A [1]. And we also suggest incorporating general scales adapted (customized) to the septic patient and scales designed specifically for them (for example, the predisposition, insult, response, organ dysfunction (PIRO) for septic or pneumonia patients) with a level of evidence 2-B [1,3,29−31].

Biomarkers

One of the objectives of the use of biomarker (BM) is to aid in the early detection and diagnosis of different clinical syndromes [12,19,20]. Classically BMs such as leukocyte count or C-reactive protein (CRP) have

helped us in the suspicion of different infections since many years [2].

An important field, in recent years, has been the introduction of new BM of inflammation and infection to try to help in the diagnosis, as well as in the monitoring of response, support in the use of therapies such as antibiotics, and prognosis of septic patients [3,12,17,18]. While classic BM of infection such as the number of leukocytosis has shown poor results, with low specificity for diagnosis, others such as CRP and procalcitonin (PCT), the two most widely used at present, have presented much more encouraging results [1−4]. In the SDCS, we recommend the determination of these two BMs in plasma as they are a tool that improves the diagnosis of sepsis, 1-A [1].

CRP may still be the most widely used BM (after the classics, of course), but in recent years, its limitations and worse sensitivity, specificity, and AUC when compared to PCT have also been described in multiple studies and metaanalyses [2,3,12,13,32−37]. PCT is the BM with the most scientific evidence, at this time, for the diagnosis of sepsis, although, of course, like all BM, it is necessary to contextualize in each case and *always* associated with the clinic [1−3,32−34]. And of course, there are other clinical processes that can have elevated BM (e.g., CRP and PCT) where there is no infection and these BM are elevated, such as severe trauma, major burns, complicates surgeries, or oncological patients [1−3,18,32].

In recent years, other new BMs have been introduced, such as STREM-1, suPAR, presepsin, which are still being studied, although they are already being marketed. More studies are needed, but in Table 7.4, we describe and compare the different BMs and their role in the diagnosis of sepsis [2,3,12].

Despite all this, the SSC does not recommend the use of BM for the diagnosis of sepsis [17,18]. In its latest document, the SSC suggests with a low level of recommendation and a very low level of evidence, the use of PCT plus clinical evaluation to decide when to initiate antibiotic treatment compared to clinical evaluation alone. On the contrary, it does consider stopping antibiotic treatment when PCT is lowered or normalized [18].

The BMs provide us with different aspects of the septic process. And undoubtedly, a fundamental one is that referring to tissue perfusion (shock). Therefore, in the SDCS, we describe that the alteration of a BM of tissue perfusion (such as plasma lactate or venous/central oxygen-oxygen saturation—SvO/SvcO$_2$) will define shock in a suggestive clinical situation, whether or not

TABLE 7.4
Role of Biomarkers to Diagnosis and Prognosis of SE/SS

BM	DIAG	SENSIB-DIAGN	AUC-diagn	PROGN	Syndrome
CRP	+/−	0.75	0.77	NO	Sepsis
PCT	YES++	0.82	0.89	YES	Sepsis, LRTI, bact, ABD
IL-6	YES−−	0.76	0.79	+/−	Sepsis
sTREM1	YES+	0.79	0.89	YES	Pneumonia, meningitis
suPAR	+/−	0.78	0.68	YES	Sepsis, TBC
Pro-ADM	NO	0.53	0.72	YES	Pneumonia, Sepsis
Presepsin	YES+	0.79	0.82	YES	Sepsis

ABD, abdominal infection; *Bact*, bacteremia; *DIAG*, diagnosis; *LRTI*, lower respiratory tract infection; *PROGN*, prognosis; *Pro-ADM*, pro-adrenomedullin; *SENSIB*, sensitivity; *TBC*, tuberculosis.
+, effect positive; −, effect negative.

accompanied by arterial hypotension, which some authors define as occult shock, with a level of evidence of 1-B [1,18,37]. Undoubtedly, the use of plasma lactate has provided valuable information when considering the initiation and intensity of fluid resuscitation and the rapid initiation of vasoactive support [2,7,8,16,18,37]. In the SDCS, with a level 1-A, we recommend that initial SS resuscitation will seek correction of tissue hypoxia, defined by restoration of normal global BMs: $SvcO_2 > 70\%$ or $SvO_2 > 65\%$ and/or normalization of plasma lactate [1]. And guidance of resuscitation of septic patients by monitoring lactate clearance (>15%) has not been shown to be inferior to $SavcO_2$ and is even more reproducible and easier to obtain, 1-B [1].

And its monitoring, since an increase independently means a worse prognosis and the need to increase therapeutic measures to try to reverse tissue hypoperfusion [2,12,16,21,27].

BUNDLE OF THE EARLY DETECTION
In the SDCS, we evaluate four different bundles that address the entire septic process from its early detection to its completion, considering the different phases that the septic patient goes through in the hospital [1,3]. Specifically, we designed the early detection bundle as described below.
- *Definition*: this is the crucial phase for the identification of potential patients with suspected SG/SS, mainly according to clinical criteria (signs and symptoms), sometimes with analytical or even radiological support.
- *Objective*: to detect all patients with suspected sepsis, mainly those with at least one OD, and to activate the Sepsis Code (SC).
- *Place*: at any point in the hospital, from triage, ED area, medical-surgical hospitalization floors, and ICU or semicritical. Maintain an active early detection system in the areas of greater complexity and risk of septic patients, such as emergency, surgery, immunosuppressed, and critical care wards. Assess daily visits to the areas with the highest incidence/prevalence of cases.
- *Structural needs*: minimal, adapted place to perform an adequate anamnesis and physical examination; possibility of portable noninvasive monitoring such as pulse oximetry. Possibility of having a computer system that can automatically record and activate alarm systems.
- *Human resources*: nursing professionals and physicians trained in the recognition of patients with suspected sepsis.
- *Measures (quality indicators)*:
  - Identification of signs and symptoms compatible with sepsis and its possible associated ODs.
  - Activation of the in-hospital CS: paper or computerized record adapted to the resources of each hospital.
  - In hospitals with integrated computer systems, alert alarms can be developed to detect patients with suspected SG/SS for early evaluation.

- *Evaluation*: measure activated cases in total and in each area (e.g., ED or ICU).

EXPERIENCE AND IMPACT OF THE EARLY SEPSIS DETECTION

A study involving 20% of USA hospitals using ICD-9-CM coding to identify SE/SS cases showed an increase from 25.6% in 1993 to 43.8% in 2003 [38]. They also identified that the age-adjusted hospitalization rate for OS had increased from 66.8 to 132.3 cases per 100,000 population ($P < .001$) and also an annual hospitalization increase of 8.2%. Age-adjusted mortality rates for OS continue to increase, from 30.3 in 1993 to 49.7 per 100,000 population in 2003, an increase of 5.6% ($P < .001$).

In Spain, a study conducted in three hospitals in Madrid identified a cumulative incidence of 367 cases per 100,000 inhabitants/year (SG 104 cases and SS 31 cases per 100,000 inhabitants, respectively) and a cumulative incidence rate of hospital admissions of 4.4% [23]. And it has been described with an overall hospital mortality of 20.7% and SS of 45.7%.

The study by Bouza et al. evaluating a six-year period (2006−11), using cases registered with the ICD-9CM identified 240,936 cases of OS, with an incidence of 87 cases per 100,000 population. But this incidence changed according to the years: from 63.7 per 100,000 in 2006 to 105.5 per 100,000 in 2011. Fifty-eight percent of cases were male and 66% were older than 65 years. The overall mortality of septic patients was 43%, with 37.1 cases per 100,000 during the study period. Although cases were increasing, the severity-adjusted mortality decreased significantly from 2006 (45.4%) to 2001 (40.2%), an indirect sign that the recommendations and the change in the management of sepsis in recent years have had positive consequences. Such a trend is corroborated in different international studies, such as those based on the SSC database [4,7,9]. Logically, an important factor is to modulate such mortality according to the severity of the clinical presentation of sepsis.

In Spain, the Edusepsis project [8], in which 23 Spanish ICUs participated, studied the impact of a training program based on training medical and nursing staff in the identification and management of SG/SS in the ED, hospital wards, and ICU. As in the SSC, two bundles were established, the resuscitation bundle (six measures to be completed in the first 6 h) and the management bundle (four measures to be completed in the first 24 h). After the educational intervention, the degree of compliance with the bundles increased significantly, with overall compliance with the resuscitation bundle increasing from 5.3% to 10.0% ($P < .001$) and with the management bundle from 10.9% to 15.7% ($P = .001$). This greater adherence to the treatments proposed by the SSC was associated with a reduction in hospital mortality (44.0% vs. 39.7%; $P = .04$). Despite the results obtained, and the fact that higher levels of compliance were achieved in certain measures included in the bundles, in general, the degree of adherence to both bundles remained low after the intervention, lower than that described by the SSC [7,8]. Moreover, the increase in the degree of compliance achieved, especially with regard to the resuscitation bundle, disappeared in the long term (one year). But these improvements diminished when analyzing a subsequent period of consolidation after the first intervention, indicating the need to maintain an educational process on an ongoing basis. And this is an aspect that requires an enormous training and follow-up effort [8].

A similar training strategy was carried out at the Marqués de Valdecilla Hospital in Santander, Spain [39]. Castellanos et al. reduced in-hospital mortality in patients with SS from 57.3% to 37.5% ($P = .001$) with the implementation of a training program. They also observed that the more bundle measures were fulfilled, the greater the survival rate.

OTHER POSSIBILITIES FOR EARLY SEPSIS DETECTION/SCREENING

One problem with sepsis detection is the immense variability of sepsis presentation. And then there is the human variability of the physician who will perform it. For example, a resident on his first day in the ED does not have the same capacity and knowledge as a specialist with more than 25 years of experience. The probability of rapid detection between one and the other is notorious. And also among physicians with more experience due to their specialty, knowledge, and the variability in the interpretation and identification of the variables associated with sepsis. Undoubtedly, we must have a predisposition to think and include sepsis in the differential diagnosis of a patient with severity criteria. Sometimes the case will be very clear, but many other times, mainly in patients at the extremes of life, immunosuppressed, with recent interventions, it is usually more complicated.

The use of only clinical criteria (such as the presence of fever or arterial hypotension) and analytical criteria (such as leukocyte count or CRP), considered as classic, is not very sensitive and even less specific for detection.

The SIRS criteria and SOFA scores are based on rules derived from the knowledge and experience of clinical experts [2,3,12]. Moreover, the use of the new BM does not dispel doubts and still does not unequivocally discriminate patients with sepsis from those who do not have it [2,3,12,18]. All this suggests that there are considerable limitations in the complex diagnostic process. In recent years, different studies using different scales with BM exclusively or combined with clinical criteria have increased the sensitivity and specificity of sepsis detection, mainly in patients located in the ED and ICU [2,18,33−35].

This reinforces the importance of incorporating other factors and systems in this study that can improve the models.

Automated Electronic Alert Systems

For this reason, in recent years, the application of computer tools for the automation of sepsis detection has been applied in many centers. Their aim is to try to improve the identification of possible cases of sepsis [22,24,40−51].

In recent years, there is growing evidence that automated sepsis detection using different computer tools could improve sepsis diagnosis and consequently increase survival and optimize the use of resources [2,43,44]. The first automated approaches developed in relation to sepsis are defined by systems based on static rules such as the SIRS and SOFA criteria [9,42,44,50]. Due to their characteristics, these systems provide a high false-positive rate and low positive predictive values (PPVs) (around 20%−40%) generating a high number of false alerts with the risk that this entails: excessive misdiagnosis, increased use of resources, excessive diagnostic tests and treatments, fatigue, and lack of confidence of the personnel receiving the alerts, among others [3,22,42−51].

In accordance with the recommendations of, among others, the SSC in the event of a patient with a severe infection, empirical antibiotic treatment must be appropriate and administered as early as possible due to the fact that sepsis mortality decreases with early recognition and treatment. Therefore, sepsis screening and early, aggressive care are vital to increasing the chance of survival. As all we know, implementation of SSC guidelines, an international effort promoting widespread early recognition and implementation of treatment bundles have been associated with mortality reduction in sepsis [18].

In this setting, in one hand, electronic systems that are designed to connect information sources together, and automatically collate, analyze, and continuously monitor the information, as well as alerting healthcare staff when predetermined diagnostic thresholds are met, may offer benefits by facilitating earlier recognition of sepsis and faster initiation of treatment, such as antimicrobial therapy, fluid resuscitation, inotropes, and vasopressors if appropriate [44].

However, on the other hand, there is the possibility that electronic, automated systems do not offer benefits or even cause harm as shows a recent interventional review published recently by Cochrane Library [44] that compared automated sepsis-monitoring systems to standard care in participants admitted to intensive or critical care units for critical illness. They included three RCTs in this review involving 1199 participants in total. Their objective was to evaluate whether automated systems for the early detection of sepsis can reduce the time to appropriate treatment (such as initiation of antibiotics, fluids, inotropes, and vasopressors) and improve clinical outcomes in critically ill patients in the ICU. The study failed to demonstrate any advantage or positive effect in favor or electronic alerts. No benefit also was found in terms of length of stay (LOS) or quality of life. This might happen if the systems are unable to correctly detect sepsis (meaning that treatment is not started when it should be, or it is started when it shouldn't be), or healthcare staff may not respond to alerts quickly enough, or get "alarm fatigue" especially if the alarms go off frequently or give too many false alarms.

However, as reported by Hwang et al. [45] in a systematic review studying sepsis alerts in EDs, noted that all systems used different criteria based on SIRS to define sepsis, ranging sensitivities from 10% to 100% and specificities from 78% to 99%. Negative predictive value was consistently high at 99%−100%, but PPV was low. Then automated sepsis alerts derived from electronic health data may improve care processes but tend to have poor PPV and do not clearly improve mortality or LOS [46]. Moreover, the high rate of solicited consultations and acceptance of recommended prescription changes described by De dios et al. [22] suggest could be perceived to be useful and convenient to use, as it is the main source of referral.

In this way, two studies have reported some benefits in sepsis outcome based on the use of electronic alerts [47,48]. The first one is a unicenter study performed in Florida with before-after design which included 3917 sepsis admissions: 1929 admissions before and 1988 in the after phase. Patients with a discharge ICD-9 code for sepsis, severe sepsis, or SS were identified electronically via their electronic system. Patients were also required to meet clinical criteria for sepsis including two of four SIRS criteria as well as a documented source of infection. Only patients 18 years of age and older were included in the retrospective study. Mean age (57.3 vs. 57.1, $P = .94$) and Charlson comorbidity scores (2.52 vs. 2.47, $P = .35$) were similar between groups. Multivariable analyses identified significant reductions in the after phase for odds of death (OR 0.62, 95% CI 0.39−0.99, $P = .046$), mean ICU LOS (2.12 days before, 95%CI 1.97, 2.34; 1.95 days after, 95%CI 1.75, 2.06; $P < .001$), mean overall hospital LOS (11.7 days before, 95% CI 10.9, 12.7 days; 9.9 days after, 95% CI 9.3, 10.6 days, $P < .001$), odds of mechanical ventilation use (OR 0.62, 95% CI 0.39, 0.99, $P = .007$), and total charges with a savings of $7159 per sepsis admission ($P = .036$). There was no reduction in vasopressor use (OR 0.89, 95% CI 0.75, 0.1.06, $P = .18$) [47].

The second study published by Arabi et al. [48] was a prepost two-phased implementation study that consisted of a preintervention phase (21 months), intervention phase I (multifaceted intervention including e-alert, six months), and intervention phase II when sepsis response team (SRT) was added (six months). The objective of this study was to describe the results of implementing a multifaceted intervention including an electronic alert (e-alert) with an SRT on the outcome of patients with sepsis and SS presenting to the ED.

The primary outcome measures were hospital mortality. Secondary outcomes were the need for mechanical ventilation and LOS in the intensive unit and in the hospital. After implementing the multifaceted intervention including e-alert and SRT, cases were identified with less severe clinical and laboratory abnormalities and the processes of care improved. When adjusted to propensity score, the interventions were associated with reduction in hospital mortality (for intervention phase II compared to preintervention: adjusted odds ratio [aOR] 0.71, 95% CI 0.58−0.85, $P = .003$), reduction in the need for mechanical ventilation (aOR 0.45, 95% CI 0.37−0.55, $P < .0001$), and reduction in ICU LOS and hospital LOS for all patients as well as ICU LOS for survivors.

This same group is currently ongoing a trial [49] to evaluate the effect of screening for sepsis using an electronic sepsis alert versus no alert in hospitalized ward patients on 90-day in-hospital mortality. The intervention includes the implementation of an electronic alert system developed in the hospital electronic medical records based on the quick SOFA (qSOFA). The alert system sends notifications of "possible sepsis alert" to the bedside nurse, charge nurse, and primary medical team and requires an acknowledgment in the health information system from the bedside nurse and physician. The calculated sample size is 65,250. The primary endpoint is in-hospital mortality by 90 days.

There are many published experiences, some with excellent results, but in most of them, there is a common denominator: variability and a large number of false-positive cases. This causes fatigue on the part of the clinicians who receive these alerts, where the majority are positive cases [22,50,51].

Gatewood et al. designed a project of progressive implementation of several measures to improve sepsis care over two years in the ED of their hospital. They started with a baseline resuscitation bundle completion rate of 28% and by the end of the period had reached 71%. And the initiation of antibiotic treatment in less than 3 h had risen from 46% to 82%. During this quality program, they included briefings, automatic alerts, and computerized orders to assist clinicians [51].

But Makam in a systematized review of the literature objectified a poor predictive value for sepsis detection using AEASs derived from electronic health data. And these automated alerts do not improve mortality or LOS [42].

And the most recent systematized review of 2022, the authors conclude the enormous variability of the studies and their results with very different qualities and biases. Therefore, the risk of reporting false-positive cases is very high [5].

Big Data, Artificial Intelligence, and Machine Learning

Recently, however, the use of new technological tools is changing healthcare. Undoubtedly, the application of BD, AI, and ML techniques is being, progressively, more used in medical practice. Mainly in areas such as chronic patient management such as oncology, epidemiology, genetics, pharmacology and, to a much lesser extent, in acute diseases such as sepsis [52].

In recent years, a number of studies, systematic reviews, and metaanalyses have been published using these techniques for the prediction and detection of sepsis. Indeed, the results are extremely positive, compared to human capacity or automated alerts. They have much higher AUC, sensitivities, specialties, with very low false-positive rates compared with classical tools [2,3,12,52−58].

The new definitions of sepsis (Sepsis-3) were developed under BD-AI-ML techniques [26,27].

Studies such as that of Nemati et al. describe the ability of using AI-ML to predict sepsis in the ICU. They generated an algorithm that had an AUC of 0.85 for the detection of sepsis. But another significant fact was that said algorithm detected the case of sepsis between 4 and 12 h before the clinical ones [56].

In a recent retrospective study, the authors developed algorithm demonstrated a sensitivity of 26% and specificity of 98%, with a positive predictive value of 29% and positive likelihood ratio of 13. The alert resulted in a small statistically significant increase in lactate testing and intravenous fluid (IV) administration. However, there was no significant difference in mortality, discharge disposition, or transfer to ICU, although there was a reduction in time-to-ICU transfer [59].

The ability to be able to detect different phenotypes of patients is a potential advantage of using BD-AI-ML. Recent studies have identified different phenotypes of patients with their distinct clinical, analytical, resource use, or prognostic characteristics. An example is the excellent retrospective study by Seymour and colleagues who identified four different types of genotypes in septic ICU patients with AI-ML [60]. These groups had different demographic, clinical, inflammatory, and OD characteristics and had different resource use (such as need for ICU admission or vasopressors) as well as outcomes such as mortality and mortality.

The excellent systematized review and metaanalysis by Lucas Fleuren and colleagues on the ability of AI-ML techniques to predict SE/SS included different studies with more than 3,500,000. They describe that the different algorithms predicted SE/SS with high accuracy, an AUC between 0.75 and 0.90. Of course, there are many limitations: most of the studies are retrospective, were performed in the USA, 30% are from one database, from the MIMMIC group and were performed

in the ICU setting. And they were also studies with moderate to high risk of bias [54].

Of course, the use of different omics (genomics, transcriptomics) exponentially multiplies the variables to be analyzed. This is impossible to do without including automated resources with the capacity to analyze huge amounts of data. And this is only possible with BD-AI-ML techniques [2,3,12,53−58].

To sum up, implementing a multifaceted intervention including sepsis e-alert with SRT or BD-AI-ML techniques may be associated with earlier identification of sepsis, increase in compliance with sepsis resuscitation bundle, and reduction in the need for mechanical ventilation and reduction in hospital mortality and LOS. The role of new algorithms based on Sepsis-3 definitions and/or ML must be defined although seem to offer great advantages.

SUMMARY

We must consider that improving early and adequate detection, with minimal cases of false positives, will have repercussions on the outcome of patients with SE/SS.

Without a doubt, we are facing a new challenge in the history of sepsis. It is about trying to improve its early detection and for this, we must generate paradigm changes. These are to improve screening, educational, monitoring, and quality control programs. To do this, we need to include new technologies to increase diagnosis. These are the use of new laboratory tests with new BMs (and their combination), microbiological molecular tests, and of course the BD-AL-ML techniques (Figs. 7.2 and 7.3).

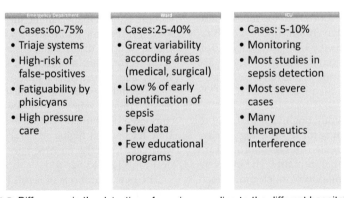

FIG. 7.2 Differences in the detection of sepsis according to the different hospital areas.

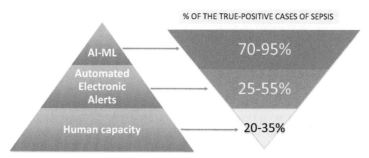

% OF THE TRUE-POSITIVE CASES OF SEPSIS

AI-ML — 70-95%

Automated Electronic Alerts — 25-55%

Human capacity — 20-35%

FIG. 7.3 Sepsis detection methods and true-positive cases. *AI*, Artifitial Intelligence; *ML*, Machine Learning.

REFERENCES

[1] Borges M, Candel FJ, Ferrer R, et al. Documento de Consenso : código sepsis [internet]. Madrid, España: IMC; 2015. Disponible en: https://www.seguridaddelpaciente.es/resources/documentos/2016/SEPSIS-DOCUMENTO-DE-CONSENSO.pdf.

[2] Candel FJ, Borges Sá M, Belda S, et al. Current aspects in sepsis approach. Turning things around. Rev Española Quimioter 2018;31(4):298−315.

[3] Borges M, Vidal P, Aranda P. Código sepsis. Capítulo 16. In: Borges Sa M, editor. Manual código sepsis. 2022. ISBN 978-958-5577-48-0. Editorial Distribuna. Bogotá, caracas, Lima, Madrid, Panamá y Pttsbrugh.

[4] Fleischmann C, Thomas-Rueddel DO, Hartmann M, et al. Hospital incidence and mortality rates of sepsis. Dtsch Arztebl Int 2016;113(10):159−66.

[5] Reinhart K, Daniels R, Kissoon N, et al. Recognizing sepsis as a global health priority - a WHO resolution. N Engl J Med 2017;377(5):414−7.

[6] Fleischmann C, Scherag A, Adhikari NK, et al. Assessment of global incidence and mortality of hospital-treated sepsis. Current estimates and limitations. Am J Respir Crit Care Med 2016;193(3):259−72.

[7] Levy MM, Dellinger RP, Townsend SR, et al. The Surviving Sepsis Campaign: results of an international guideline-based performance improvement program targeting severe sepsis. Intensive Care Med 2010;36(2):222−31.

[8] Ferrer R, Artigas A, Levy MM, et al. Improvement in process of care and outcome after a multicenter severe sepsis educational program in Spain. JAMA 2008;299(19):2294−303.

[9] Ferrer R, Artigas A, Suarez D, et al. Effectiveness of treatments for severe sepsis: a prospective, multicenter, observational study. Am J Respir Crit Care Med 2009;180(9):861−6.

[10] Suarez D, Ferrer R, Artigas A, et al. Cost-effectiveness of the Surviving Sepsis Campaign protocol for severe sepsis: a prospective nation-wide study in Spain. Intensive Care Med 2011;37(3):444−52.

[11] Shorr AF, Micek ST, Jackson Jr WL, et al. Economic implications of an evidence-based sepsis protocol: can we improve outcomes and lower costs? Crit Care Med 2007;35(5):1257−62.

[12] Marti-Loeches I, Levy MM, Artigas A. Management of severe sepsis: advances, challanges, and current status. Drug Des Dev Ther 2015;9:2079−88.

[13] León Gil C, García-Castrillo Riesgo L, Moya Mir M, Artigas Raventós A, Borges SM, Candel González FJ, et al. [Consensus document (SEMES-SEMICYUC). Recommendations for the initial and multidisciplinary diagnostic management of severe sepsis in the hospital Emergency Departments]. Med Intensiva 2007;31(7):375−87.

[14] Yealy DM, Kellum JA, Huang DT, Barnato AE, Weissfeld LA, Pike F, et al. PROCESS Trial. A randomized trial of protocol-based care for early septic shock. N Engl J Med 2014;370(18):1683−93.

[15] Moreno RP, Metnitz B, Adler L, Hoechtl A, Bauer P, Metnitz PG, et al. Sepsis mortality prediction based on predisposition, infection and response. Intensive Care Med 2008;34(3):496−504.

[16] Levy MM, Evans LE, Rhodes A. The surviving sepsis campaign bundle: 2018 update. Intensive Care Med 2018;44(6):925−8.

[17] Rhodes A, Evans LE, Alhazzani W, et al. Surviving sepsis campaign: international guidelines for management of sepsis and septic shock: 2016. Intensive Care Med 2017; 43(3):304−77.

[18] Evans L, Rhodes A, Alhazzani W, Antonelli M, Coopersmith CM, French C, et al. Surviving sepsis campaign: international guidelines for management of sepsis and septic shock 2021. Intensive Care Med November 2021;47(11):1181−247. https://doi.org/10.1007/s00134-021-06506-y. Epub 2021 Oct 2.

[19] Angus DC, van der Poll T. Severe sepsis and septic shock. N Engl J Med 2013;369(21):2063.

[20] Vincent JL, Moreno R, Takala J, Willatts S, De Mendonça A, Bruining H, et al. The SOFA (Sepsis-related organ failure assessment) score to describe organ

dysfunction/failure. On behalf of the working group on sepsis-related problems of the European society of intensive care medicine. Intensive Care Med 1996;22(7):707–10.

[21] Seymor C, Resongart M. Septic shock: advances in diagnosis and treatment. JAMA 2015;18:708–17.

[22] de Dios B, Borges M, Smith TD, et al. Computerised sepsis protocol management. Description of an early warning system. Enferm Infecc Microbiol Clín 2018;36(2):84–90.

[23] Esteban A, Frutos-Vivar F, Ferguson ND, et al. Sepsis incidence and outcome: contrasting the intensive care unit with the hospital ward. Crit Care Med 2007;35(5):1284–9.

[24] Ramasco F, Figuerola A, Mendez R, et al. Initial clinical outcomes and prognostic variables in the implementation of a Code Sepsis in a high complexity University Hospital. Rev Española Quimioter 2019;32(3):238–45.

[25] Yébenes JC, Lorencio C, Esteban E, et al. Interhospital Sepsis Code in Catalonia (Spain): territorial model for initial care of patients with sepsis. Med Intensiva 2020;44(1):36–45.

[26] Singer M, Deutschman CS, Seymour CW, et al. The third international consensus definitions for sepsis and septic shock (Sepsis-3). JAMA 2016;315(8):801–10.

[27] Shankar-Hari M, Phillips GS, Levy ML, et al. Developing a new definition and assessing new clinical criteria for septic shock: for the third international consensus definitions for sepsis and septic shock (Sepsis-3). JAMA 2016;315(8):775–87.

[28] Vincent JL, Sakr Y, Sprung CL, et al. Sepsis in European intensive care units: results of the SOAP study. Crit Care Med 2006;34(2):344–53.

[29] Rello J, Rodriguez A, Lisboa T, Gallego M, Lujan M, Wunderink R. PIRO score for community-acquired pneumonia: a new prediction rule for assessment of severity in intensive care unit patients with community-acquired pneumonia. Crit Care Med 2009;37(2):456–62.

[30] Granja C, Póvoa P, Lobo C, Teixeira-Pinto A, Carneiro A, Costa-Pereira A. The predisposition, infection, response and organ failure (Piro) sepsis classification system: results of hospital mortality using a novel concept and methodological approach. PLoS One 2013;8(1):e53885.

[31] Lisboa T, Diaz E, Sa-Borges M, Socias A, Sole-Violan J, Rodríguez A, et al. The ventilator-associated pneumonia PIRO score: a tool for predicting ICU mortality and health-care resources use in ventilator-associated pneumonia. Chest 2008;134(6):1208–16.

[32] Harbarth S, Holeckova K, Froidevaux C, Pittet D, Ricou B, Grau GE, et al. Diagnostic value of procalcitonin, interleukin-6, and interleukin-8 in critically ill patients admitted with suspected sepsis. Am J Respir Crit Care Med 2001;164(3):396–402.

[33] Cho SY, Choi JH. Biomarkers of sepsis. Infect Chemotherapy 2014;46:1–12.

[34] Kojic D, Siegler B, Uhle F, Lichtenstern C, Nowroth P. Are there new approaches for diagnosis, therapy guidance and outcome prediction of sepsis? WJEM 2015;20:50–63.

[35] Meisner M. Update on procalcitonin measurements. Ann Lab Med 2014;34:263–73.

[36] Meynar M. In critically il patients, serum procalcitonin is more useful in differentiating between sepsis and SRIS than CRP, Il-6, and LBP. CCRP 2011;34.

[37] Vincent JL, Bakker J. Blood lactate levels in sepsis: in 8 questions. Curr Opin Crit Care 2021;27(3):298–302.

[38] Dombrovskiy VY, Martin AA, Sunderram J, et al. Rapid increase in hospitalization and mortality rates for severe sepsis in the United States: a trend analysis from 1993 to 2003. Crit Care Med 2007;35(5):1244–50.

[39] Castellanos-Ortega A, Suberviola B, García-Astudillo LA, et al. Impact of the Surviving Sepsis Campaign protocols on hospital length of stay and mortality in septic shock patients: results of a three-year follow-up quasi-experimental study. Crit Care Med 2010;38(4):1036–43.

[40] Abella Álvarez A, Torrejón Pérez I, Enciso Calderón V, et al. ICU without walls project. Effect of the early detection of patients at risk. Med Intensiva 2013;37(1):12–8.

[41] Micek ST, Roubinian N, Heuring T, et al. Before-after study of a standardized hospital order set for the management of septic shock. Crit Care Med 2006;34(11):2707–13.

[42] Makam AN, Nguyen OK, Auerbach AD. Diagnostic accuracy and effectiveness of automated electronic sepsis alert systems: a systematic review. J Hosp Med June 2015;10(6):396–402. https://doi.org/10.1002/jhm.2347. Epub 2015 Mar 11.

[43] Despins LA. Automated detection of sepsis using electronic medical record data: a systematic review. J Healthc Qual 2017 Nov/Dec;39(6):322–33. https://doi.org/10.1097/JHQ.0000000000000066.

[44] Warttig S, Alderson P, Evans DJ, Lewis SR, et al. Automated monitoring compared to standard care for the early detection of sepsis in critically ill patients. Cochrane Database Syst Rev June 25, 2018;6(6):CD012404. https://doi.org/10.1002/14651858.CD012404.pub2.

[45] Hwang MI, Bond WF, Powell ES. West J. Sepsis alerts in emergency departments: a systematic review of accuracy and quality measure impact. Emerg Med August 24, 2020;21(5):1201–10. https://doi.org/10.5811/westjem.2020.5.46010.

[46] Seetharaman S, Wilson C, Landrum M, Qasba S, Katz M, Ladikos N, Harris JE, Galiatsatos P, Yousem DM, Knight AM, Pearse DB, Blanding R, Bennett R, Galai N, Perl TM, Sood G. Does use of electronic alerts for systemic inflammatory response syndrome (SIRS) to identify patients with sepsis improve mortality? Am J Med July 2019;132(7):862–8. https://doi.org/10.1016/j.amjmed.2019.01.032. Epub 2019 Mar 2. PMID: 30831065.

[47] Guirgis FW, Jones L, Esma R, Weiss A, et al. Managing sepsis: electronic recognition, rapid response teams, and standardized care save lives. J Crit Care August 2017;40:296–302. https://doi.org/10.1016/j.jcrc.2017.04.005. Epub 2017 Apr 8. PMID: 28412015; PMCID: PMC5563264.

[48] Arabi YM, Al-Dorzi HM, Alamry A, Hijazi R, et al. The impact of a multifaceted intervention including sepsis electronic alert system and sepsis response team on the outcomes of patients with sepsis and septic shock. Ann Intensive Care December 2017;7(1):57. https://doi.org/

10.1186/s13613-017-0280-7. Epub 2017 May 30. PMID: 28560683; PMCID: PMC5449351.

[49] Arabi YM, Alsaawi A, Al Zahrani M, Al Khathaami AM, et al. SCREEN Trial Group. Electronic early notification of sepsis in hospitalized ward patients: a study protocol for a stepped-wedge cluster randomized controlled trial. Trials October 11, 2021;22(1):695. https://doi.org/10.1186/s13063-021-05562-5. PMID: 34635151; PMCID: PMC8503718.

[50] Ackermann K, Baker J, Green M, Fullick M, et al. Computerized clinical decision support systems for the early detection of sepsis among adult inpatients: scoping review. J Med Internet Res February 23, 2022;24(2): e31083. https://doi.org/10.2196/31083.

[51] Gatewood MO, Wemple M, Greco S, Kritek PA, Durvasula R. A quality improvement project to improve early sepsis care in the emergency department. BMJ Qual Saf December 2015;24(12):787–95. https://doi.org/10.1136/bmjqs-2014-003552. Epub 2015 Aug 6.

[52] Panch T, Szolovits P, Atun R. Artificial intelligence, machine learning and health systems. J Glob Health 2018; 8. https://doi.org/10.7189/jogh.08.020303.

[53] Schinkel M, Paranjape K, Nannan Panday RS, Skyttberg N, Nanayakkara PWB. Clinical applications of artificial intelligence in sepsis: a narrative review. Comput Biol Med 2019;115. https://doi.org/10.1016/j.compbiomed.2019.103488.

[54] Fleuren LM, Klausch TLT, Zwager CL, Schoonmade LJ, Guo T, Roggeveen LF, et al. Machine learning for the prediction of sepsis: a systematic review and meta-analysis of diagnostic test accuracy. Intensive Care Med 2020;46: 383–400. https://doi.org/10.1007/s00134-019-05872-y.

[55] Mao Q, Jay M, Hoffman JL, Calvert J, Barton C, Shimabukuro D, et al. Multicentre validation of a sepsis prediction algorithm using only vital sign data in the emergency department, general ward and ICU. BMJ Open 2018;8:e017833.

[56] Nemati S, Holder A, Razmi F, Stanley MD, Clifford GD, Buchman TG. An interpretable machine learning model for accurate prediction of sepsis in the ICU. Crit Care Med 2018;46:547–53.

[57] Desautels T, Calvert J, Hoffman J, Jay M, Kerem Y, Shieh L, et al. Prediction of sepsis in the intensive care unit with minimal electronic health record data: a machine learning approach. JMIR Med Informatics 2016;4:e28.

[58] Delahanty RJ, Alvarez J, Flynn LM, Sherwin RL, Jones SS. Development and evaluation of a machine learning model for the early identification of patients at risk for sepsis. Ann Emerg Med 2019;73(4):334–44.

[59] Giannini HM, Ginestra JC, Chivers C, Draugelis M, et al. A machine learning algorithm to predict severe sepsis and septic shock: development, implementation, and impact on clinical practice. Crit Care Med November 2019; 47(11):1485–92. https://doi.org/10.1097/CCM.0000000000003891. PMID: 31389839; PMCID: PMC8635476.

[60] Seymour CW, Kennedy JN, Wang S, Chang C-CH, et al. Derivation, validation, and potential treatment implications of novel clinical phenotypes for sepsis. JAMA 2019;321:2003. https://doi.org/10.1001/jama.2019.5791.

CHAPTER 8

Diagnosis and Monitoring of Sepsis

PIETRO ARINA • MERVYN SINGER

INTRODUCTION

Sepsis is a complex syndrome characterized by profound physiological, pathological, and biochemical alterations. The lack of a specific diagnostic test has led to considerable challenges, both for clinical diagnosis and in epidemiological descriptor studies. In the clinical setting, the diagnosis of sepsis remains problematic as confirmation of an underlying infection is frequently lacking and the clinical and biochemical signs of sepsis are often nonspecific. Given the complexity of sepsis pathophysiology and its evolution, no single biomarker or test has yet provided sufficient sensitivity and specificity for a firm diagnosis. Furthermore, sepsis is a syndrome representing an umbrella term for a wide range of clinical conditions. It originates from a wide range of pathogens, from different sites, and across many patient populations ranging from neonate to elderly, healthy to comorbid, frail and immunosuppressed, medical to surgical, and varying ethnic, cultural, and social backgrounds. Sepsis also presents several types of clinical and biological subphenotypes/endotypes. These are only being explored in recent years, and there is no current consensus as to which specific systems should be formally adopted by clinicians [1]. An important future prospective is to tailor treatments to specific subphenotypes/endotypes in the hope this will reduce morbidity and mortality and avoid unnecessary or even harmful treatments.

Prompt and accurate diagnosis of sepsis often represents a considerable challenge, especially for the gray cases where the patient is a poor historian, infection may or may not be present, and the type of infecting organism is uncertain. Infection source control is a key component of sepsis treatment as is appropriate antibiotic therapy. However, the evidence base on the speed of delivery of antibiotics remains weak in terms of patient benefit [2]. This must also be balanced against the risks of overprescribing with needless prescription for nonbacterial cases and the risks of side effects, and the contribution toward increasing antimicrobial resistance. Indeed, up to 40% of cases of sepsis originate from nonbacterial infections [3], where antibacterial agents offer no advantage. As microbiological results are rarely available in the first hours after patient presentation, there is, at present, significant clinical uncertainty as to best treatment [4].

SEPSIS DEFINITIONS AND CONTROVERSIES

The sepsis definition has changed over three millennia (Fig. 8.1). The current "Sepsis-3" iteration defines sepsis as a *"life-threatening organ dysfunction caused by a dysregulated host response to infection"* [5]. The clinical criteria used to identify this condition is a ≥ 2 point rise in the Sequential Organ Failure Assessment (SOFA) score from the patient's normal baseline. Septic shock is defined as a *"subset of sepsis in which underlying circulatory, cellular, and metabolic abnormalities are associated with a greater risk of mortality than sepsis alone."* This is described clinically as persisting hypotension requiring vasopressors to maintain a mean arterial pressure (MAP) ≥ 65 mmHg and having a concurrent serum lactate level >2 mmol/L (18 mg/dL) despite adequate volume resuscitation [5].

The Sepsis-3 definitions [5] have moved the focus away from the presence of infection and more toward the underlying host response which, if severe enough, can lead to multiorgan dysfunction (MOD). Indeed, it is now generally accepted that organ dysfunction is not merely a consequence of the infection itself and subsequent hyperinflammation, but it has a complex, multifactorial host-driven etiology [6].

The earlier iterations of the sepsis definitions [7,8] defined sepsis as infection and at least two of the four systemic inflammatory response syndrome (SIRS) criteria. Severe sepsis was when sepsis was accompanied

The Sepsis Codex. https://doi.org/10.1016/B978-0-323-88271-2.00037-7

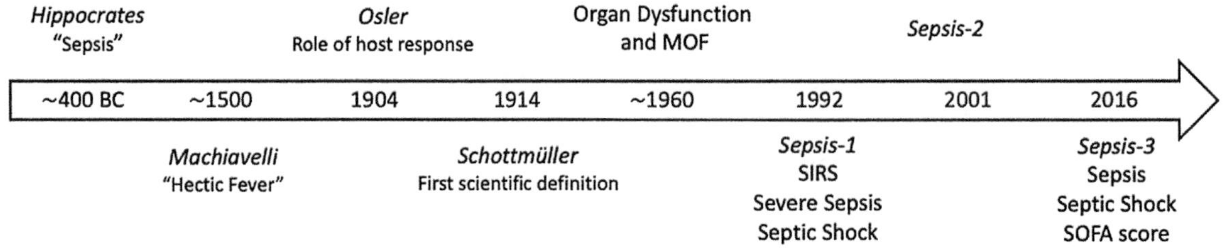

Hippocrates "Sepsis"		Osler Role of host response		Organ Dysfunction and MOF		Sepsis-2	
~400 BC	~1500	1904	1914	~1960	1992	2001	2016
	Machiavelli "Hectic Fever"		Schottmüller First scientific definition		Sepsis-1 SIRS Severe Sepsis Septic Shock		Sepsis-3 Sepsis Septic Shock SOFA score

FIG. 8.1 Timeline of sepsis descriptions and definitions.

by ill-defined *"organ dysfunction, hypoperfusion, or hypotension,"* and septic shock by the presence of hypotension despite adequate fluid resuscitation plus the ill-defined presence of perfusion abnormalities that could include *"lactic acidosis, oliguria, or an acute alteration in mental status."* The lack of precise descriptors of what constituted organ dysfunction, hypoperfusion, or even hypotension contributed to different researchers adopting highly variable criteria to describe *"severe sepsis"* and *"septic shock."* Accordingly, the control group mortality in 65 septic shock trials ranged from 15% to 80% [9]. As explained below, SIRS has been dropped from the Sepsis-3 definition as it does not usefully discriminate between infection and sepsis. *"Severe sepsis"* has now been replaced by *"sepsis"* to simplify the nomenclature into infection, infection with organ dysfunction (*sepsis*), and infection with organ dysfunction plus fluid-resistant hypotension and hyperlactatemia (*septic shock*).

Sepsis-3 cannot be the definitive answer, but it does provide an important updating of the concept of sepsis that takes into account current understanding and which provides a more consistent approach with clearly defined criteria for what constitutes organ dysfunction and shock. These criteria have changed the epidemiology of sepsis [10,11], but they should offer a stronger base to enable better comparisons to be drawn between hospitals, countries, and longitudinally. It maintains the umbrella syndrome concept and does not segment types and sites of infection nor categories of patients. The same term will thus include a previously well 20-year-old patient with urosepsis, a frail 80-year-old with multiple comorbidities presenting with fecal peritonitis, and a 50-year-old chemotherapy patient developing sepsis from a hospital-acquired pneumonia. Mortality risk will obviously differ in these individual patients, so Sepsis-3 offers more of a population-based tool to improve coding and epidemiology.

Sepsis-3 can however be used for categorization in trials. Post hoc analyses of the Vasopressin and Septic

Shock Trial (VASST) trial [12] and the Hyperoxia and hypertonic saline in patients with septic shock (HYPERS2S) trial [13] showed markedly different outcomes to vasopressin and hyperoxia depending on whether the patient was hypotensive with a normal blood lactate or fulfilled the Sepsis-3 shock criteria.

Another criticism of the Sepsis-3 definition is that it does not offer facilitate precision medicine therapies based on specific genomic and cellular alterations that accompany an individual patient's disease process [14]. However, the current lack of suitable biomarkers, especially those that are readily available at or near the bedside, the still-developing field of subphenotype identification, and the need to offer a definition that can be applied more globally rather than restricted to a few highly resourced hospitals makes this aspirational rather than a current-day reality. Evolution will embrace new technology and understanding, but any such technology must be affordable, quickly accessed, and widely available.

SIRS AND SURROUNDING CONTROVERSIES

The concept of SIRS was first introduced by Roger Bone and colleagues in the first Sepsis (Sepsis-1) definitions published in 1992 to assist the identification of suitable patients for early immunomodulatory trials in sepsis [7]. They recognized that a similar physiological response could arise following infection or multiple other inflammatory conditions such as trauma, pancreatitis, ischemia, autoimmune diseases, burns, and complications of therapy. They thus coined the term SIRS to describe this systemic inflammatory process which was agnostic of cause. SIRS required at least two of [1]: a body temperature >38°C or <36°C [2]; a heart rate >90 beats/min [3]; tachypnoea, with a respiratory rate >20 breaths/min, or hyperventilation indicated by a $PaCO_2$ value <32 mm Hg; and [4] a white cell count >12,000 or <4000 mm^3 or the presence of >10% immature neutrophils ("bands").

While an increasing number of SIRS criteria are associated with increasing disease severity and mortality risk [7], the use of SIRS suffers for a number of important reasons. First, inflammation is usually an appropriate and protective host response to any external insult; its presence does not necessarily indicate pathology. Inflammation activates the body's immune response both locally and systemically and modifies multiple other physiological and behavioral systems to react appropriately to the insult. Second, SIRS criteria are often fulfilled by mild infections that do not result in organ dysfunction, let alone death. A common cold is one such example where a high temperature and a low-grade tachycardia are commonly seen. Third, SIRS criteria are present in many hospitalized patients who suffer from varied noninfectious inflammatory conditions and who do not incur adverse outcomes (i.e., poor *discriminant validity*) [15]. On the other hand, one in eight patients requiring admission to Australasian critical care units with infection and organ failure lacked the requisite minimum of two SIRS criteria to fulfill prior definitions of sepsis (i.e., poor *concurrent validity*), yet these patients still often suffered significant morbidity and mortality [16]. *Discriminant validity* and *convergent validity* are the two domains of *construct validity*; the SIRS criteria perform poorly on both. As a consequence, SIRS has been dropped from the latest Sepsis-3 definitions.

ORGAN DYSFUNCTION/FAILURE CRITERIA

Dysfunction and failure are often used interchangeably to describe altered functionality of a specific organ system and its consequences on homeostasis. Dysfunction is a more accurate descriptor as failure implies a binary yes-no cutoff point which does not exist, whereas dysfunction describes a continuum from mild to severe. The presence of two or more organ dysfunctions is defined as MOD.

Organ systems involved in sepsis vary in terms of severity, number, and type of organs affected. Such organ systems include cardiovascular, respiratory, neurological, renal, hepatic, muscular, bioenergetic-metabolic, hematological, hormonal, and immune. Standardized criteria have been developed to help clinicians diagnose organ dysfunction and its severity, and to monitor disease progression and the response to interventions. The ideal criteria for organ dysfunction would have high sensitivity and specificity and able to be assessed temporally and readily at low cost.

Cardiovascular Criteria

Cardiovascular failure criteria represent a keystone of Sepsis-3 definitions that utilize the need for vasopressors to reverse hypotension plus concurrent hyperlactatemia. This is reflected by the frequent use of blood pressure (systolic or mean) ± vasopressor use in scoring systems. While decreased stroke volume, cardiac output, and oxygen delivery are evident in sepsis-induced cardiomyopathy, no specific values are used to define it. An arbitrary value of cardiac index <2.2 L/min/m^2 with support, or <1.8 L/min/m^2 without support, is often cited to raise suspicion of cardiogenic shock. Plasma lactate rises with any causes of hypoperfusion; however, this is a nonspecific marker as it also increases with multiple other causes including liver dysfunction, cellular poisoning, catecholamine use, and thiamine deficiency. A capillary refill time of >2 s is used as a clinical guide indicative of poor peripheral perfusion.

Bedside echocardiography is often used to identify sepsis-induced cardiomyopathy which may involve systolic and/or diastolic dysfunction [17]. Studies have often used cutoff thresholds of left ventricular ejection of 40%–50%. Although easy to assess noninvasively, this measure does depend substantially on loading conditions. Global longitudinal strain is a more sensitive measure of left ventricular performance, but optimal cutoffs remain uncertain. Troponin, B-type natriuretic peptide, and heart-type fatty acid-binding protein (h-FABP) have been proposed as clinical criteria of septic cardiomyopathy, but despite high sensitivity, they all have low specificity [17,18].

Respiratory Criteria

Respiratory failure—coined the acute respiratory distress syndrome (ARDS)—is frequently seen in sepsis [19]. The Berlin ARDS criteria are generally used to characterize respiratory dysfunction [20]. These use specified cutoffs for the ratio of partial pressure of O_2 to fractional inspired O_2 (P:F ratio) to identify mild (201–300 mmHg), moderate (101–200 mm Hg), and severe (≤ 100 mm Hg) lung injury, with a positive end-expiratory pressure or continuous positive airway pressure ≥ 5 cm water. In addition, an ARDS diagnosis requires the presence of bilateral radiographic opacities, noncardiogenic pulmonary edema, and occurrence within a week of a known clinical insult. Other parameters such as arterial–alveolar gradient and calculations of dead space, shunt and ventilation-perfusion mismatch are not routinely calculated and used clinically. Scoring systems often incorporate the need or otherwise for mechanical respiratory support.

Neurological Criteria

The Glasgow Coma Scale (GCS), first developed in 1974 [21], is the common standard used to characterize neurological dysfunction. Markers of brain injury such as serum S100B [22] and nonspecific enolase [23] are used to suggest the presence of sepsis-related encephalopathy. A rise in insulin-like growth factor-1 is associated with the development of delirium in intensive care patients [24]. The CAM-ICU score is often used as a bedside score for identifying delirium.

Renal Criteria

Acute kidney injury is very common in sepsis [25]. A variety of scores (AKIN, RIFLE) have been generally supplanted by the simplified KDIGO criteria [26], namely an increase in serum creatinine ≥ 0.3 mg/dL within 48 h, or an increase in serum creatinine to $\geq 1.5\times$ baseline within seven days, or urine output <0.5 mL/kg/h for 6 h. Multiple novel biomarkers are proposed to identify acute kidney injury, such as neutrophil gelatinase-associated lipocalin (NGAL), kidney injury molecule-1 (KIM-1), cystatin-C, interleukin (IL)-18, and liver-type fatty acid binding protein (L-FABP); however, a recent consensus statement concluded that more research was needed [27].

Hepatic Criteria

Acute liver dysfunction criteria in sepsis are numerous and not specific for sepsis. These include an increase in international normalized ratio, a rise $1.5\times$ above baseline in liver enzymes or bilirubin, and hypoalbuminemia. Elevations in hyaluronic acid (HA) and bilirubin are associated with an increased risk of death in sepsis [28]. CAAP48, the C-terminal fragment of alpha-1-antitrypsin, has also been recently proposed as a new biomarker [29].

Hematological Criteria

Acute hematological disfunction is present in many septic patients and may include some or all of anemia, leukocytosis or leukopenia, thrombocytopenia, and markers (coagulopathic, fibrinolytic) of increased activation of the hemostatic system [30]. These include increases in prothrombin and activated partial thromboplastin time and D-dimers, and falls in protein C and ADAMTS-13. All, however, are nonspecific for sepsis.

Immune Criteria

The immune dysfunction is a complex and bimodal process, characterized by early hyperinflammatory process and concomitant immunosuppression [31]. Lymphopenia is an easily accessed biomarker of immune dysfunction; however, the need for more sophisticated, nonautomated flow cytometric tests have generally precluded the routine use of a range of biomarkers such as HLA-DR, neutrophil CD64, VLA-3, CCR2, and CX3CR1 [32].

Endocrine Criteria

Sepsis induces a pan-endocrine dysfunction, with altered production and/or release and/or metabolism of multiple hormones, or up-/downregulation of their receptors or binding proteins [33]. In the acute phase of sepsis, there is usually an increase in plasma levels of "catabolic" hormones such as cortisol, glucagon, and catecholamines and a decrease in circulating sex hormones. Later on, these trends often invert, with decreased levels of active thyroid hormones such as triiodothyronine, a fall in growth hormone, and a blunted rise in cortisol following exogenous stimulation.

SEVERITY SCORES: A CRITICAL ASSESSMENT

Severity scores represent a useful tool of describing the degree of critical illness. The perfect severity scoring system should be based on routinely measured variables, calibrated to assess different types of patients, and should be usable in different settings. It should have the capacity for daily monitoring and provide prognostication capability. No single score can necessarily achieve all these requirements, but different scores can be gainfully combined to assist both clinicians and researchers. Severity scores can be classified according to the type of data used (Table 8.1). Some are used at a precise point or time interval in the patient's ICU stay, e.g., admission or first 24-hour Acute Physiology and Chronic Health Evaluation (APACHE) II or Simplified Acute Physiology Score (SAPS) score, whereas others can be used to serially monitor disease progression (e.g., SOFA, Multiorgan Dysfunction Score [MODS] scores).

While SOFA clearly predominates, and will thus be described in more detail below, multiple other scores have also been developed to predict mortality risk [34]. It is beyond the scope of this article to detail them, and we would refer the interested reader to an excellent recent analysis by Keuning et al. [35].

The SOFA Score (Table 8.2)

The SOFA score is a composite score based on the degree of dysfunction in six organ systems—respiratory, coagulation, hepatic, cardiovascular, central nervous system, and renal [36]. Each organ dysfunction scores from 0 to 4, with increasing scores reflecting more

TABLE 8.1
Scoring Systems Based on Type of Data Used [35]

Score	Data used to calculate the score
Anatomical	Score based on anatomical part of the body involved. These are used mainly for surgical and trauma purposes, e.g., the Trauma and Injury Severity Score (TRISS) and are not routinely used in ICU patients.
Therapeutic weighted	Score based on the amount of intervention needed for the patient, e.g., Therapeutic Intervention Scoring System (TISS). This assuming the sicker or more demanding patients will need more intervention.
Organ-specific	Score that assesses the degree ± number of organ dysfunction/failures, e.g., Glasgow Coma Score, Sequential Organ Failure Assessment (SOFA), and Multiorgan Dysfunction Score (MODS)
Physiological	Score based on the degree of alteration of physiological and laboratory variables, e.g., Acute Physiology and Chronic Health Evaluation (APACHE), Simplified Acute Physiology Score (SAPS)
Disease-specific	Score based on specific disease or condition, e.g., Glasgow-Imrie for pancreatitis severity, Child-Pugh score for cirrhosis mortality risk

abnormal physiology and biochemistry or an increasing degree of intervention. SOFA utilizes (i) physiological variables such as urine output and blood pressure, (ii) biochemical values such as $PaO_2:FiO_2$ ratio, creatinine, bilirubin, and platelets, and (iii) therapeutic interventions such as dosage of vasopressors. While physiology and intervention data are immediately available to the clinician, there is a necessary albeit short delay until laboratory-based results are forthcoming. This delay should not however detract from any immediate necessary therapeutic intervention as a sick patient needs prompt treatment irrespective of any score.

The SOFA score was developed in a consensus meeting held in 1994 *"to describe quantitively and as objectively as possible the degree of organ dysfunction/failure over time in groups of patients or even individual patients"* [36]. The cutoffs for each point score were determined arbitrarily, and no weighting was ascribed to specific organ systems in terms of prognostic risk. Nonetheless, despite this, it has been validated as a good prognosticator in multiple settings including upper, middle- and low-income countries [37]. The SOFA score on admission has been shown to closely reflect mortality risk [36,38]; however, the absolute level of risk will generally vary between richer and poorer countries [39,40]. Because of its repeatability and use of standardized terminology, the SOFA score also represents a useful longitudinal illness severity stratification tool [41].

There is clearly room for further improvement with the SOFA score, for example, determining optimal cutoffs for each point rise and weighting individual organ scores for mortality. There are also the obvious ongoing challenges such as scoring Glasgow Coma Score on the basis of the last presedation value, even though this may have been weeks prior. Several studies have indicated that SOFA score proved to be a better predictor of 30-day sepsis mortality compared with SIRS or Sepsis-2 criteria [42,43].

Other Illness Severity Scores
Many are in existence, but we briefly describe the main ones still in use today.

APACHE I, II, III (Physiological score, first 24 hours from ICU admission, prognostication)
The first widely used score in critical care was the APACHE score. This was first introduced in 1981 [44] with updated iterations in 1985, 1991, and 2006. It was initially based on abnormalities in 34 physiological and laboratory variables with extra points given for increasing age and severe chronic comorbidities [44–47]. However, this proved overly complex, so the APACHE II score reduced the physiological/biochemical variables to a more manageable 12. The APACHE score uses the worst values obtained from the first 24 h from ICU admission. The composite score correlates with ICU mortality [45]. APACHE III further refined the calibration of the score, including HIV and oncological malignancy in the chronic assessment of the patient [46]. Its widespread adoption enabled a standardized, reliable classification system for patients admitted to the ICU and comparison of outcomes between different ICUs and over time. However, it is not

TABLE 8.2
Sequential Organ Failure Assessment (SOFA) Score

	SOFA POINTS				
	0	1	2	3	4
Respiratory: PaO_2/FiO_2 kPa (mmHg)	≥ 53.3 (400)	<53.3 (400)	<39.9 (300)	<26.7 (200) with respiratory support	<13.3 (100) with respiratory support
Coagulation: Platelets $\times 10^3/\mu$L	≥ 150	<150	<100	<50	<20
Hepatic: Bilirubin μmol/L (mg/dL)	<20 (1.2)	20–32 (1.2–1.9)	33–101 (2.0–5.9)	102–204 (6.0–11.9)	>204 (>12)
Cardiovascular[a]	MAP>70 mmHg	MAP<70 mmHg	Dopamine <5 μg/kg/min, or Dobutamine (any dose)	Dopamine 5–15 μg/kg/min Epinephrine ≤ 0.1 μg/kg/min Norepinephrine ≤ 0.1 μg/kg/min	Dopamine >15 μg/kg/min Epinephrine >0.1 μg/kg/min Norepinephrine >0.1 μg/kg/min
Central nervous system: GCS	15	13–14	10–12	6–9	<6
Renal system: • Creatinine μmol/L (mg/dL) • Urine output mL/day	<110 (<1.2)	111–170 (1.2–1.9)	171–299 (2.0–3.4)	300–440 (3.5–4.9) <500	>440 (>5) <200

Abbreviations: *FiO₂*, fraction of inspired Oxygen; *MAP*, mean arterial pressure; *PaO₂*, partial pressure of oxygen.
[a] Catecholamines are given for at least one hour.

designed for immediate scoring of a critically ill patient, nor longitudinal scoring of individuals.

SAPS (Physiological score, first 24 hours from ICU admission, prognostication)
The SAPS is similar to the APACHE score. Introduced in 1984 with the assessment of 14 variables, it was subsequently upgraded to SAPS II and then SAPS III version which introduced more details of the patient's past medical history [48–50]. As with APACHE, it is based on variables collected over the first 24 h from ICU admission and can be used to prognosticate for ICU mortality.

MODS (Multiorgan Dysfunction Score)
Similar to SOFA, MODS is an organ dysfunction score which offers mortality prediction [51]. It was developed in the early 1990s and assesses dysfunctions in six different organ systems (respiratory, hematological, hepatic, cardiovascular, neurological, and renal) with each system scoring from 0 to 4 depending on the degree of dysfunction. The higher the value, the greater the degree of dysfunction, with a total of 24 maximal points. It is fairly similar to SOFA except for cardiovascular dysfunction. Whereas SOFA uses MAP and vasoactive agents, MODS uses the pressure-adjusted heart rate using the formula (HR x CVP)/MAP. A single-center prospective observational study enrolling more than 900 patients showed both MODS and SOFA were reliable outcome predictors though cardiovascular dysfunction was better correlated to outcome with SOFA [52].

LODS (Logistic Organ Dysfunction Score)
The Logistic Organ Dysfunction System score (LODS score) was developed in 1996. It is similar to SOFA and MODS, but here it identifies three levels of organ

dysfunction for six organ systems: neurological, cardio-vascular, renal, pulmonary, hematological, and hepatic. One to five points are assigned to each level of severity, and the resulting total score can range from 0 to 22 points [53].

MPM (prediction of mortality in ICU)
Mortality prediction model (MPM), iterations I and II, are based on multiple chronic health variables, acute variables, and the current diagnosis to predict ICU mortality. It could be calculated sequentially with patient data at 0, 24, 48, and 72h from ICU admission to recalibrate the risk. It does not provide an illness stratification [54].

Bedside Illness Severity Scores
The above scores are reliant on preillness information and laboratory values. For rapid assessment, a number of bedside scores have been developed which rely purely on readily measurable physiological variables.

MEWS, NEWS, and NEWS-2 (2012 and 2017) (Early assessment score)
The Modified Early Warning Score (MEWS) was developed in the United Kingdom to assess the deterioration of patients in surgical wards and to assess their need for ICU admission, mostly due to sepsis. It is based on the degree of alteration of vital signs from their normal values [55,56]. It has been superseded by the National Early Warning Score (NEWS); the first version was published in 2012 and NEWS-2 was released in 2017 [57]. It utilizes seven variables—respiratory rate, pulse oximetry-measured oxygen saturation, need for oxygen, systolic blood pressure, heart rate, conscious level (ACVPU score), and core temperature, with scores ranging from 0 to 3 depending on the degree of abnormality. It is now recommended for use in the United Kingdom across all healthcare settings—from care homes and general practice to emergency departments and hospital wards. Its use is rapidly being adopted in other countries. The frequency of monitoring is dictated by the score as is the need and urgency to triage to outreach teams, medical (and senior medical) review. While not validated in advance, multiple studies have now confirmed its utility in identifying patient deterioration and mortality risk [58,59].

quickSOFA score
The quickSOFA score was developed as part of the Sepsis-3 definitions work to aid clinicians rapidly identify patients with presumed infection who at risk of having sepsis (organ dysfunction) before laboratory confirmation that dysfunction is present. It was developed after interrogation of large patient databases from which approximately 850,000 patients with suspected infection were extracted [10]. Three clinical criteria—low systolic blood pressure (<100 mmHg), high respiratory rate (>22 breaths/min), or altered mentation (GCS <15)—were the best indicators for identifying subsequent deterioration. Each criterion was ascribed a single point. The presence of 2 or 3 points was present in approximately 24% of non-ICOU encounters and was associated with a greater risk of death or prolonged intensive care unit stay. Seventy percent of all poor outcomes were contained within this group. It is important to stress that this study only focused on patients with presumed infection, so specificity is not claimed for infectious versus noninfectious conditions. Many comparator studies have been performed subsequently [60]; the overall conclusion was that qSOFA significantly outperforms SIRS in predicting sepsis outcomes. However, though it was much more specific, it was less sensitive compared with SIRS. The authors concluded that neither SIRS nor qSOFA are ideal screening tools for sepsis. The three qSOFA variables are contained within the seven variables of the NEWS-2 score, so whether a more comprehensive score such as NEWS is superior for identifying subsequent deterioration merits further study. In a single-center study of over 30,000 patients, NEWS-2 was superior at risk stratification to MEWS, qSOFA, and SIRS [61].

Machine learning and artificial intelligence
With the increasing utilization of electronic healthcare record (EHR) systems, and availability of large population databases, there has been a proliferation of studies using machine learning and AI that claim to identify sepsis in advance of clinical identification (e.g. Refs. [62,63]). Some have already been incorporated into commercial EHR system as a "sepsis alert" to aid the clinician in early identification. While these clearly show significant promise and an indication of the way forward, it is important to stress that these have been developed on retrospective analyses of patient databases. Few, if any, have been prospectively validated and shown to actually work. An excellent example of an external multicenter validation cohort study was recently published assessing the EPIC Sepsis Model (ESM) [64]. It found that the ESM has poor discrimination and calibration in predicting the onset of sepsis. Sensitivity of the model was poor, only identifying 7% who did not receive timely administration of antibiotics. The model also failed to identify 67% of patients

with sepsis and generated a large number of false-positive alerts, creating a large burden of alert fatigue.

REFERENCES

[1] Reddy K, Sinha P, O'Kane CM, Gordon AC, Calfee CS, McAuley DF. Subphenotypes in critical care: translation into clinical practice. Lancet Respir Med 2020;8:631–43.

[2] Evans L, Rhodes A, Alhazzani W, et al. Surviving sepsis campaign: international guidelines for management of sepsis and septic shock 2021. Intensive Care Med 2021. https://doi.org/10.1007/s00134-021-06506-y.

[3] Lin G-L, McGinley JP, Drysdale SB, Pollard AJ. Epidemiology and immune pathogenesis of viral sepsis. Front Immunol 2018;9:2147.

[4] Fitzpatrick F, Tarrant C, Hamilton V, Kiernan FM, Jenkins D, Krockow EM. Sepsis and antimicrobial stewardship: two sides of the same coin. BMJ Qual Saf 2019;28:758–61.

[5] Singer M, Deutschman CS, Seymour CW, Shankar-Hari M, Annane D, Bauer M, et al. The third international consensus definitions for sepsis and septic shock (Sepsis-3). JAMA 2016;315:801–10.

[6] Arina P, Singer M. Pathophysiology of sepsis. Curr Opin Anaesthesiol 2021;34:77–84.

[7] Bone RC, Balk RA, Cerra FB, Dellinger RP, Fein AM, Knaus WA, et al. Definitions for sepsis and organ failure and guidelines for the use of innovative therapies in sepsis. The ACCP/SCCM consensus conference committee. American college of Chest Physicians/Society of Critical Care medicine. Chest 1992;101:1644–55.

[8] Levy MM, Fink MP, Marshall JC, Abraham E, Angus D, Cook D, et al. 2001 SCCM/ESICM/ACCP/ATS/SIS international sepsis definitions conference. Crit Care Med 2003;31:1250–6.

[9] de Grooth H-J, Postema J, Loer SA, Parienti J-J, Oudemans-van Straaten HM, Girbes AR. Unexplained mortality differences between septic shock trials: a systematic analysis of population characteristics and control-group mortality rates. Intensive Care Med 2018; 44:311–22.

[10] Seymour CW, Liu VX, Iwashyna TJ, Brunkhorst FM, Rea TD, Scherag A, et al. Assessment of clinical criteria for sepsis. JAMA 2016;315:762–74.

[11] Fujishima S. Organ dysfunction as a new standard for defining sepsis. Inflamm Regen 2016;36:24.

[12] Russell JA, Lee T, Singer J, Boyd JH. Walley KR for the vasopressin and septic shock trial (VASST) group. The septic shock 3.0 definition and trials: a vasopressin and septic shock trial experience. Crit Care Med 2017;45: 940–8.

[13] Demiselle J, Wepler M, Hartmann C, Radermacher P, Schortgen F, Meziani F, et al. Hyperoxia toxicity in septic shock patients according to the Sepsis-3 criteria: a post hoc analysis of the HYPER2S trial. Ann Intensive Care 2018;8:90.

[14] Abraham E. New definitions for sepsis and septic shock: continuing evolution but with much still to be done. JAMA 2016;315:757–9.

[15] Churpek MM, Zadravecz FJ, Winslow C, Howell MD, Edelson DP. Incidence and prognostic value of the systemic inflammatory response syndrome and organ dysfunctions in ward patients. Am J Respir Crit Care Med 2015;192:958–64.

[16] Kaukonen K-M, Bailey M, Pilcher D, Cooper DJ, Bellomo R. Systemic inflammatory response syndrome criteria in defining severe sepsis. N Engl J Med 2015; 372:1629–38.

[17] Hollenberg SM, Singer M. Pathophysiology of sepsis-induced cardiomyopathy. Nat Rev Cardiol 2021;315: 801–11.

[18] Kim J-S, Kim M, Kim Y-J, Ryoo SM, Sohn CH, Ahn S, et al. Troponin testing for assessing sepsis-induced myocardial dysfunction in patients with septic shock. J Clin Med 2019;8:239.

[19] Mikkelsen ME, Shah CV, Meyer NJ, Gaieski DF, Lyon S, Miltiades AN, et al. The epidemiology of acute respiratory distress syndrome in patients presenting to the emergency department with severe sepsis. Shock 2013;40:375–81.

[20] ARDS Definition Task Force, Ranieri VM, Rubenfeld GD, Thompson BT, Ferguson ND, Caldwell E, et al. Acute respiratory distress syndrome: the Berlin Definition. JAMA 2012;307:2526–33.

[21] Teasdale G, Jennett B. Assessment of coma and impaired consciousness. A practical scale. Lancet 1974;ii:81–4.

[22] Wu L, Feng Q, Ai M-L, Deng S, Liu Z-Y, Huang L, et al. The dynamic change of serum S100B levels from day 1 to day 3 is more associated with sepsis-associated encephalopathy. Sci Rep 2020;10:7718.

[23] Anderson BJ, Reilly JP, Shashaty MGS, Palakshappa JA, Wysoczanski A, Dunn TG, et al. Admission plasma levels of the neuronal injury marker neuron-specific enolase are associated with mortality and delirium in sepsis. J Crit Care 2016;36:18–23.

[24] Khan BA, Zawahiri M, Campbell NL, Boustani MA. Biomarkers for delirium - a review. J Am Geriatr Soc 2011; 59:S256–61.

[25] Kellum JA, Romagnani P, Ashuntantang G, Ronco C, Zarbock A, Anders H-J. Acute kidney injury. Nat Rev Dis Prim 2021;7:1–17.

[26] Kidney Disease: Improving Global Outcomes (KDIGO) Acute Kidney Injury Work Group. KDIGO clinical practice guideline for acute kidney injury. Kidney Int 2012; 2(Suppl. l):1–138.

[27] Ostermann M, Zarbock A, Goldstein S, Kashani K, Macedo E, Murugan R, et al. Recommendations on acute kidney injury biomarkers from the acute disease quality initiative consensus conference: a consensus statement. JAMA Netw Open 2020;3:e2019209.

[28] Jensen J-US, Peters L, Itenov TS, Bestle M, Thormar KM, Mohr TT, et al. Biomarker-assisted identification of sepsis-related acute liver impairment: a frequent and deadly condition in critically ill patients. Clin Chem Lab Med 2019;57:1422–31.

[29] Blaurock-Möller N, Gröger M, Siwczak F, Dinger J, Schmerler D, Mosig AS, et al. CAAP48, a new sepsis biomarker, induces hepatic dysfunction in an in vitro liver-on-chip model. Front Immunol 2019;10:273.

[30] Iba T, Levy JH, Warkentin TE, Thachil J, van der Poll T, Levi M. Scientific and standardization committee on DIC, and the scientific and standardization committee on perioperative and critical care of the international society on thrombosis and haemostasis. Diagnosis and management of sepsis-induced coagulopathy and disseminated intravascular coagulation. J Thromb Haemostasis 2019;17:1989−94.

[31] Hotchkiss RS, Monneret G, Payen D. Sepsis-induced immunosuppression: from cellular dysfunctions to immunotherapy. Nat Rev Immunol 2013;13:862−74.

[32] Trzeciak A, Pietropaoli AP, Kim M. Biomarkers and associated immune mechanisms for early detection and therapeutic management of sepsis. Immune Netw 2020;20:e23.

[33] Wasyluk W, Wasyluk M, Zwolak A. Sepsis as a pan-endocrine illness - endocrine disorders in septic patients. J Clin Med 2021;10:2075.

[34] Bouch DC, Thompson JP. Severity scoring systems in the critically ill. Cont Educ Anaesth Crit Care Pain 2008;8:181−5.

[35] Keuning BE, Kaufmann T, Wiersema R, Granholm A, Pettilä V, Møller MH, et al. Mortality prediction models in the adult critically ill: a scoping review. Acta Anaesthesiol Scand 2020;64:424−42.

[36] Vincent JL, de Mendonça A, Cantraine F, Moreno R, Takala J, Suter PM, et al. Use of the SOFA score to assess the incidence of organ dysfunction/failure in intensive care units: results of a multicenter, prospective study. Working group on "sepsis-related problems" of the European Society of Intensive Care Medicine. Crit Care Med 1998;26:1793−800.

[37] Moreno R, Vincent JL, Matos R, Mendonça A, Cantraine F, Thijs L, et al. The use of maximum SOFA score to quantify organ dysfunction/failure in intensive care. Results of a prospective, multicentre study. Working Group on Sepsis related Problems of the ESICM. Intensive Care Med 1999;25:686−96.

[38] Ferreira FL, Bota DP, Bross A, Mélot C, Vincent JL. Serial evaluation of the SOFA score to predict outcome in critically ill patients. JAMA 2001;286:1754−8.

[39] Raith EP, Udy AA, Bailey M, McGloughlin S, MacIsaac C, Bellomo R, et al. Prognostic accuracy of the SOFA score, SIRS criteria, and qSOFA score for in-hospital mortality among adults with suspected infection admitted to the intensive care unit. JAMA 2017;317:290−300.

[40] Lie KC, Lau C-Y, Van Vinh Chau N, West TE, Limmathurotsakul D, for Southeast Asia Infectious Disease Clinical Research Network. Utility of SOFA score, management and outcomes of sepsis in Southeast Asia: a multinational multicenter prospective observational study. J Intensive Care 2018;6:9.

[41] Lambden S, Laterre PF, Levy MM, Francois B. The SOFA score - development, utility and challenges of accurate assessment in clinical trials. Crit Care 2019;23:374.

[42] Freund Y, Lemachatti N, Krastinova E, Van Laer M, Claessens Y-E, Avondo A, et al. Prognostic accuracy of Sepsis-3 criteria for in-hospital mortality among patients with suspected infection presenting to the emergency department. JAMA 2017;317:301−8.

[43] Poutsiaka DD, Porto MC, Perry WA, Hudcova J, Tybor DJ, Hadley S, et al. Prospective observational study comparing Sepsis-2 and Sepsis-3 definitions in predicting mortality in critically ill patients. Open Forum Infect Dis 2019;6:ofz271.

[44] Knaus WA, Zimmerman JE, Wagner DP, Draper EA, Lawrence DE. APACHE-acute physiology and chronic health evaluation: a physiologically based classification system. Crit Care Med 1981;9:591−7.

[45] Knaus WA, Draper EA, Wagner DP, Zimmerman JE. APACHE II: a severity of disease classification system. Crit Care Med 1985;13:818−29.

[46] Knaus WA, Wagner DP, Draper EA, Zimmerman JE, Bergner M, Bastos PG, et al. The APACHE III prognostic system: risk prediction of hospital mortality for critically III hospitalized adults. Chest 1991;100:1619−36.

[47] Zimmerman JE, Kramer AA, McNair DS, Malila FM. Acute Physiology and Chronic Health Evaluation (APACHE) IV: hospital mortality assessment for today's critically ill patients. Crit Care Med 2006;34:1297−310.

[48] Abizanda R, Marse P, Abadal JM. Simplified acute physiology score. Crit Care Med 1985;13:517.

[49] Le Gall JR, Lemeshow S, Saulnier F. A new Simplified Acute Physiology Score (SAPS II) based on a European/North American multicenter study. JAMA 1993;270:2957−63.

[50] Vazquez G, Benito S, Rivera R. Spanish Project for the Epidemiological Analysis of Critical Care Patients. Simplified Acute Physiology Score III: a project for a new multidimensional tool for evaluating intensive care unit performance. Crit Care 2003;7:345−6.

[51] Marshall JC, Cook DJ, Christou NV, Bernard GR, Sprung CL, Sibbald WJ. Multiple organ dysfunction score: a reliable descriptor of a complex clinical outcome. Crit Care Med 1995;23:1638−52.

[52] Peres Bota D, Melot C, Lopes Ferreira F, Nguyen BV, Vincent J-L. The multiple organ dysfunction score (MODS) versus the sequential organ failure assessment (SOFA) score in outcome prediction. Intensive Care Med 2002;28:1619−24.

[53] Le Gall JR, Klar J, Lemeshow S, Saulnier F, Alberti C, Artigas A, et al. The Logistic Organ Dysfunction system. A new way to assess organ dysfunction in the intensive care unit. ICU Scoring Group. JAMA 1996;276:802−10.

[54] Timsit J-F, Fosse J-P, Troché G, De Lassence A, Alberti C, Garrouste-Orgeas M, et al. Calibration and discrimination by daily Logistic Organ Dysfunction scoring comparatively with daily Sequential Organ Failure Assessment scoring for predicting hospital mortality in critically ill patients. Crit Care Med 2002;30:2003−13.

[55] Gardner-Thorpe J, Love N, Wrightson J, Walsh S, Keeling N. The value of Modified Early Warning Score (MEWS) in surgical in-patients: a prospective observational study. Ann R Coll Surg Engl 2006;88:571–5.

[56] Subbe CP, Kruger M, Rutherford P, Gemmel L. Validation of a modified early warning score in medical admissions. QJM 2001;94:521–6.

[57] National early warning score (NEWS) 2 [Internet]. RCP London; 2017 [cited 2021 Sep 10]. Available from: https://www.rcplondon.ac.uk/projects/outputs/national-early-warning-score-news-2.

[58] Smith GB, Prytherch DR, Jarvis S, Kovacs C, Meredith P, Schmidt PE, et al. A comparison of the ability of the physiologic components of medical emergency team criteria and the U.K. National Early Warning Score to discriminate patients at risk of a range of adverse clinical outcomes. Crit Care Med 2016;44:2171–81.

[59] Masson H, Stephenson J. Investigation into the predictive capability for mortality and the trigger points of the National Early Warning Score 2 (NEWS2) in emergency department patients. Emerg Med J June 9, 2021. emermed-2020-210190 (ePub).

[60] Herwanto V, Shetty A, Nalos M, Chakraborty M, McLean A, Eslick GD, et al. Accuracy of quick sequential organ failure assessment score to predict sepsis mortality in 121 studies including 1,716,017 individuals: a systematic review and meta-analysis. Crit Care Explor 2019;1:e0043.

[61] Churpek MM, Snyder A, Han X, Sokol S, Pettit N, Howell MD, et al. Quick sepsis-related organ failure assessment, systemic inflammatory response syndrome, and early warning scores for detecting clinical deterioration in infected patients outside the intensive care unit. Am J Respir Crit Care Med 2017;195:906–11.

[62] Horng S, Sontag DA, Halpern Y, Jernite Y, Shapiro NI, Nathanson LA. Creating an automated trigger for sepsis clinical decision support at emergency department triage using machine learning. PLoS One 2017;12:e0174708.

[63] Henry KE, Hager DN, Pronovost PJ, Saria S. A targeted real-time early warning score (TREWScore) for septic shock. Sci Transl Med 2015;7:299ra122.

[64] Wong A, Otles E, Donnelly JP, Krumm A, McCullough J, DeTroyer-Cooley O, et al. External validation of a widely implemented proprietary sepsis prediction model in hospitalized patients. JAMA Intern Med 2021;181:1065–70.

CHAPTER 9

Sepsis: Molecular Diagnostics and Biomarkers

JOHN LYONS • CRAIG COOPERSMITH

INTRODUCTION

Sepsis is defined as a life-threatening organ dysfunction caused by a dysregulated host response to infection [1]. While there is inherent intellectual appeal to the definition in explaining the essence of sepsis, it has no practical utility at the bedside. Unfortunately, there is no easy way to diagnose what is an inherently heterogeneous syndrome. This contrasts significantly with other common diseases. For instance, a myocardial infarction can be diagnosed by an abnormal electrocardiogram and troponin, and cancer can be diagnosed by identifying neoplasia on a biopsy. For sepsis, each element in the definition is either impossible to measure or fairly nonspecific. Infection can be suspected by fever and leukocytosis, but these can both be markers of inflammation rather than infection. Further, many septic patients do not have a fever (and many are hypothermic) or elevated white blood cell count. There is no common method to measure dysregulated host response in use at the bedside currently. While organ dysfunction can be measured by the Sequential Organ Failure Assessment (SOFA) score, this is not specific for sepsis and presupposes that the treating clinician is familiar with the SOFA score (which many are not) and also knows the baseline score. As such, the timely diagnosis of sepsis continues to challenge clinicians. Since the dysregulated host response to infection is inherently variable, patients can exhibit a variety of clinical presentations that may not readily be labeled as "septic." Ambiguity in diagnosis may lead to delay in life-saving therapy, thereby increasing septic mortality. In contrast, overdiagnosis of sepsis triggers unnecessary antibiotic use, exacerbating the worldwide problem of drug-resistant organisms [2]. Rapid, accurate diagnosis of sepsis is thus key to combating sepsis morbidity and mortality. To that end, considerable research effort has been dedicated to the discovery of novel sepsis diagnostics and biomarkers, with the ultimate goal of quickly identifying those patients who are truly battling infection and those with a noninfectious pathology whose clinical presentation only mirrors sepsis [3].

Sepsis is initiated by a microorganism whose elements constitute pathogen-associated molecular patterns (PAMPs). PAMPs are recognized by both pattern-recognition receptors and nonpattern recognition receptors that, in turn, trigger multiple signaling pathways that produce pro- and antiinflammatory mediators aimed at controlling the initiating pathogen. The resultant inflammatory milieu results in the release of endogenous danger-associated molecular patterns, which further modulates the host response. While an overview of the complex inflammatory response is outside the scope of this chapter, it is relevant that ultimately the differences between infected and noninfected patients may hold diagnostic significance which can be measured as biomarkers. Importantly, a biomarker might potentially also function as a mediator of outcomes in sepsis—in which case it may also be a therapeutic target for treatment—or a biomarker may have utility solely as a marker to distinguish disease states.

Unfortunately, despite the identification of countless promising biomarkers, few new diagnostic tools have made their way into clinical practice. In short, no single biomarker reliably differentiates sepsis from noninfectious inflammation. However, advancing technologies offer hope of coming breakthroughs. This chapter will provide an overview of existing septic biomarkers and discuss evolving diagnostic strategies with potential to substantially impact the clinical diagnosis and management of sepsis.

BIOMARKERS AS CLINICAL TOOLS

A biomarker is something that may be objectively measured and evaluated as an indicator of normal

The Sepsis Codex. https://doi.org/10.1016/B978-0-323-88271-2.00001-8

physiology, the presence of pathology, a response to treatment, or as a predictor of clinical outcomes [4,5]. This definition is inherently broad and not only emphasizes that many different biologic quantities, patterns, or characteristics may serve as biomarkers but also highlights that biomarkers have clinical utility beyond solely aiding in the diagnosis of conditions like sepsis. Normalization of pathologic biomarkers may argue for cessation of therapy just as persistent elevation of the same measurements may suggest a lack of therapeutic response and a need for alternative approaches. Further, the degree of deviation from normal for a given biomarker may be correlated with the severity of disease, allowing its measurement to predict clinical trajectory and potentially guide strategies of care. With each of these possibilities, it is important to bear in mind that biomarkers are often functioning as surrogate measurements for something else, and there are many ways in which a given measurement may fail to accurately reflect an underlying process or predict a clinical endpoint [5]. The potentially misleading nature of biomarkers is particularly relevant in the context of sepsis, as the wide-ranging dysregulation of both pro- and anti-inflammatory host responses to infection [6] creates the clear possibility that an isolated change in a single protein, chemical, or other marker in the bloodstream may not have much use in guiding clinical decision-making. In the treatment of atherosclerotic disease, serum cholesterol levels have proven to be effective biomarkers; increased cholesterol levels portend increased risk of coronary artery disease, and correction of cholesterol levels both confirms treatment response to lipid-lowering agents and reduces the risk of myocardial infarction [4]. With regard to sepsis, such effective and precise biomarkers are not yet described, and targeted therapies aimed at correcting the fundamental immune dysregulation in the host response do not exist. As knowledge of septic pathobiology grows, emphasis must be placed on diagnostic signals that accurately reflect and mediate the underlying disease state while offering reliable guideposts for branches in clinical management.

ESTABLISHED BIOMARKERS
Lactate

Lactate is a ubiquitous hydrocarbon that is produced from pyruvate during glycolysis [7,8]. In a broad clinical context, lactate has historically been considered a byproduct of anaerobic respiration and thereby an indicator of potential tissue hypoxia [8]. While indeed lack of available oxygen at a cellular level will increase lactate production via anaerobic glycolysis, lactate concentration is ultimately dependent on the equilibrium between production and clearance, and impaired hepatic or renal function may complicate the interpretation of elevated lactate levels [9]. Further, research suggests the idea that lactate levels rise during shock states as a result of deranged oxygen utilization is flawed. Lactate is transported freely around the body and in and out of cells, and its ability to interconvert with glucose provides metabolic flexibility to body tissues [7]. Circulating lactate directly supports function of the Krebs cycle and the production of adenosine triphosphate (ATP) [10], may be used by cells as a preferred fuel despite abundant oxygen and glucose [11], and may even facilitate homeostasis of the body's overall redox state [7,12,13]. The increased lactate levels associated with sepsis are therefore more likely to indicate an altered metabolic strategy in an organism battling infection [14,15] as opposed to impaired oxygen handling at a cellular level [16].

Despite some uncertainty surrounding the etiology of increased serum lactate during sepsis, its use as a biomarker features prominently in modern management of the disease. The Surviving Sepsis Guidelines recommend measuring serum lactate within the first hour of diagnosis, as part of the "hour-one" care bundle, as significant elevation predicts increased mortality [17,18]. Furthermore, randomized controlled trials and metaanalyses suggest resuscitation strategies aimed at lactate normalization do improve survival [19–23], leading to a suggestion in Surviving Sepsis that resuscitation be tailored to decrease lactate in patients with elevated levels [18].

Measurement and trending of serum lactate thus provides some utility as a biomarker in evaluating the clinical course of septic patients. Obviously, given that multiple processes or conditions other than sepsis may elevate lactate levels or alter its clearance, its isolated use as a diagnostic tool is limited [24]. Lactate levels, like most other diagnostic studies and biomarkers, are best considered as additional pieces of information to be evaluated and considered in the management of sepsis.

Procalcitonin

Calcitonin is a calcium-regulating protein whose serum elevation was initially described in the context of medullary thyroid cancer, as was its precursor protein, procalcitonin (PCT) [25,26]. Unlike mature calcitonin, however, PCT is produced widely in mammalian tissues beyond the thyroid, and increases in serum PCT values have been described in numerous settings including bacterial infection, trauma, pancreatitis, tissue ischemia, and other inflammatory conditions [27–29]. PCT therefore functions as an acute phase protein, a nonspecific indicator of inflammation. Given the numerous conditions that may increase serum PCT, it is ill-suited for use as a confirmatory or "rule-in" test for sepsis. Though PCT concentrations above 0.25 or 0.5 ng/mL are consistent with bacterial infection, such results are by no means exclusive to a diagnosis of sepsis [30]. Rather, measurement of PCT appears to have utility in determining when bacterial sepsis is not a likely diagnosis or when it has been sufficiently treated with antibiotics.

Bacterial infection increases serum PCT, and the degree of increase correlates with disease severity [31,32]. Further, a rise in PCT is less commonly associated with viral or fungal infections [27,33]. In theory, a low or normal PCT level may provide an argument against initiation of empiric antibiotic therapy in the appropriate clinical setting [30]. Serum PCT has indeed been shown to be generally accurate at ruling out bacteremia in this fashion [34]. However, since PCT may rise during viral or fungal infections and PCT elevations are nonspecific in nature, PCT is not recommended to delineate bacterial from nonbacterial infection or to determine if antibiotics should be initiated [18,35]. What appears consistent in recent studies is that persistently elevated levels predict worsened clinical outcomes and that lack of normalization is consistently correlated with increased sepsis mortality [36–40]. Therefore, while an isolated PCT value may have limited use as an up-front diagnostic tool, it nonetheless has proven to be a relevant biomarker for evaluating therapeutic response in sepsis.

Along this line, PCT has been widely studied in the de-escalation or cessation of antibiotic treatment. Patients being treated with empiric, broad-spectrum antibiotics on intensive care unit (ICU) admission frequently do not have their treatments narrowed in a timely fashion [41], contributing to the growing issue of drug-resistant organisms. Normalization of PCT would suggest resolution of bacterial infection, potentially offering a marker that antibiotics could be stopped. Prior metaanalyses have indeed found PCT-guided antibiotic de-escalation to be safe [42–44] and in some instances associated with reduced mortality [44,45]. As might be expected, PCT guidance also specifically reduces infection and death attributable *Clostridium difficile* or multidrug-resistant organisms [46]. While adherence to PCT-guided algorithms is inconsistent among physicians [47], expert panel recommendations do endorse utilization of PCT for antibiotic

de-escalation and cessation [18,30]. As with other biomarkers in sepsis, PCT functions best not as a stand-alone test to diagnose sepsis or definitively state the need for antibiotics, but rather provides value as an additional point of information considered in balance with other clinical data. Finally, it should be noted that PCT is partially cleared by continuous renal replacement therapy (CRRT), and thus interpretation of this and other sepsis biomarkers much be approached with caution in patients undergoing CRRT, as apparent reduction in serum concentrations may be misleading [48].

C-Reactive Protein

C-reactive protein (CRP) was initially identified as an acute phase reactant binding to the capsular (C) polysaccharide found on *Streptococcus pneumoniae*, and elevation in serum CRP has long been known as a nonspecific indicator of inflammation [49–51]. Synthesized primarily in hepatocytes and known to exist in both multimeric and monomeric isoforms, CRP concentrations may increase over 1000-fold under conditions of infection or inflammation, with such elevations serving as both a marker of inflammation and likely providing functional contributions to inflammatory and immune signaling [52]. Clinically, elevated CRP concentrations may denote a generally more proinflammatory state, one associated with diverse consequences such as increased risk of cardiovascular events or progression of rheumatoid arthritis [53,54].

As a sepsis biomarker, CRP generally mirrors the pattern exhibited by PCT. Increased CRP thus may have some degree of utility in arguing for the presence bacterial versus nonbacterial infection [35], and similar to PCT, a persistently elevated CRP during sepsis predicts increased septic mortality [55–57]. Though less well studied than PCT-based guidelines, antibiotic therapy guided by CRP levels similarly appears to reduce overall antibiotic exposure [58,59]. Importantly, CRP kinetics are delayed compared to PCT, taking longer to rise and fall over the course of infection, perhaps limiting its utility as a sepsis biomarker [60,61]. In general, CRP may be regarded as a nonspecific inflammatory biomarker whose ultimate clinical utility in managing sepsis at present is limited.

EMERGING MOLECULAR APPROACHES
Transcriptomics

As gene sequencing technology has advanced, so too has the hope that analysis of the transcriptome, the complete set of RNA transcripts present in a given moment, might identify unique gene expression signatures and provide a more accurate understanding of underlying disease processes [62,63]. To this end, there are some data to suggest that analysis of RNA transcripts may eventually provide an effective tool for modern sepsis diagnosis. Patterns of gene expression do indeed vary significantly between infected and noninfected patients, and novel RNA assays have been developed to recognize specific gene activity and identify septic patients [64−67]. In some preliminary studies, transcriptome analysis has been as good or better than PCT at distinguishing between bacterial and nonbacterial infection, suggesting the potential for future incorporation into antibiotic prescribing guidelines [68−70]. Furthermore, RNA signatures may also predict sepsis survival or death, providing an additional means of stratifying high-risk patient groups [71,72].

Notably, not all RNA sequences are translated into proteins, and substantial growth in our knowledge of noncoding RNA (ncRNA) has revealed an enormous potential contribution of these molecules to the pathophysiology of sepsis. Despite not coding for proteins, 90% of noncoding gene sequences are nonetheless transcribed in ncRNA. Previously considered largely nonfunctional, these ncRNA molecules are now understood to bind DNA, protein, and other RNA molecules, thereby regulating gene expression and protein synthesis and exerting effects on a wide range of biologic processes [73,74]. ncRNA modulates Toll-like receptor signaling, alters cytokine elaboration, and impacts immune cell proliferation and death, thus regulating the host response to pathogens [74−77]. Patterns of ncRNA expression may correlate with sepsis severity and may eventually serve a diagnostic function [78−82]. Future investigations of septic gene expression may not only identify advanced molecular biomarkers for the diagnosis and monitoring of sepsis but may also shed light on fundamental drivers of septic immune dysregulation to guide development of novel therapeutics.

Epigenetics

Epigenetics refers to the regulation of gene expression that does not involve alterations to the underlying DNA code. Rather, epigenetic processes include DNA methylation, histone modifications, and nucleosome positioning, phenomena that regulate how and if a given region of DNA is transcribed into RNA [83]. These factors are now understood to contribute substantially to cell differentiation, organism development, and human disease, as they help govern the ultimate makeup of cells and tissues by dictating which genes are active and which remain silent [84]. Thus, while genetic

makeup correlates poorly with septic outcomes, constellations of epigenetic findings, acquired via the interaction of genome and environment, may directly impact septic pathophysiology [83,85]. Though research into the epigenetics of sepsis is still preliminary, recent studies have demonstrated that epigenetic information can readily be obtained from septic patients and that such data have potential diagnostic and prognostic utility, as methylation patterns and other epigenetic modifications differ between infected and noninfected patients and between patients infected with different pathogens [86−88]. With the advance of epigenetic science, these assays have the potential to feature not only in acute sepsis management but also in the care of long-term sepsis survivors and even their offspring, as stress-induced genetic modifications have been shown to be heritable and may confer disease risk to future generations [84].

Proteomics and Metabolomics

Proteomic and metabolomic studies seek to understand disease states by creating a detailed picture of proteins and metabolites present in a tissue at a given time. This approach has the potential to more accurately reflect active biologic processes, as rates of mRNA translation, posttranslational protein modification, and protein degradation are not reflected in gene expression assays, and proteins are generally more participatory in performing biologic processes than DNA or RNA [89]. The initial promise of proteomics research was limited by technical difficulty in consistently identifying low-abundance proteins of interest in samples containing large volumes of other proteins [89−91]. As the technology of mass spectrometry and high-throughput protein analysis has improved, evidence has accumulated that proteomic analysis may eventually find clinical applications. Proteomic and combined proteomic/metabolomic signatures can identify relevant protein biomarkers and may predict mortality in animal models of infection, and modified proteomic approaches have also identified novel protein biomarkers in human patients that show promise in separating sepsis from noninfectious inflammation [92,93]. Understanding of patient trajectory may also be aided by assaying the proteome, as protein modification patterns are distinct in sepsis survivors and nonsurvivors [94].

Similar to proteomics, metabolomic techniques can analyze thousands of small molecules at once in a small sample volume, providing a direct view of active biochemical pathways and potentially identifying novel disease signals or therapeutic targets [95,96]. Additionally, because metabolites are the direct byproducts of active cell biochemistry and are not subject to forces regulating gene expression or protein function, they may potentially be more easily correlated with phenotypes [95]. Numerous metabolic alterations have been associated with sepsis [96,97]. In small studies, several metabolic signatures have reliably identified sepsis and nonseptic inflammation [98,99], and surveillance of the metabolome may provide early warning signs that patients are becoming septic or deteriorating [100−102]. Combined metabolomic and proteomic markers may be combined to improve future diagnostic or prognostic accuracy, particularly as improved microfluidic chip technology permits rapid turnaround for multiplex assays [103].

NONDIAGNOSTIC UTILITY OF BIOMARKERS

While biomarkers are often thought of for their role in diagnosis, they can also be used to identify patients with sepsis who are at risk for poor outcome, to identify subgroups of patients based on biological commonalities or for clinical trial enrichment [104,105]. While the reasons the vast majority of clinical trials for sepsis have been negative are assuredly multifactorial, one key reason is likely that enrollment is quite broad enrolling patients with sepsis or septic shock, despite the fact that there are certainly differences at a cellular level in the host response in patients who look grossly similar to a clinician at the bedside.

Numerous strategies to distinguish septic patients for the purposes of moving the field toward precision medicine have recently been published. These specifics of these range from very simple to remarkably complex, but each shares the goal of distinguishing patient populations that may respond differently to the same therapeutic intervention despite an inability to determine this from examining the patient and elements of their electronic medical record. A pioneering example of this was using 100 genes in a subclass corresponding to adaptive immunity and glucocorticoid receptors signaling to distinguish pediatric patients into two septic shock classes [106]. A total of 300 patients in both a training set and a validation set demonstrated that using methods meeting the time constraints of a critical care environment, patients could be distinguished into subsets that predict increased mortality to being prescribed corticosteroids. A further study on over 300 adult patients with sepsis due to community acquired pneumonia examined the potential of performing a transcriptomic analysis of peripheral blood leukocytes [71]. Two sepsis response signatures were identified including an immunosuppressed phenotype that included features of endotoxin tolerance, T-cell

exhaustion, and downregulation of HLA-class II. Notably, patients in this subgroup had a higher 14-day mortality. Further, a study enrolled septic patients in a discovery set in two ICUs in the Netherlands for genome-wide blood gene expression profiling which it then validated in a set of patients specifically with sepsis from community acquired pneumonia in 29 ICUs in the United Kingdom [107]. A 140-gene expression signature reliably separated patients into four different endotypes, and to facilitate possible clinical use, a biomarker was derived for each endotype.

More recent studies have tried to identify phenotypes of sepsis using simpler techniques. A retrospective analysis using machine learning of over 20,000 patients who met Sepsis-3 criteria within 6 h of admission to 12 different US hospitals identified four clinical phenotypes using 29 clinical and laboratory variables available in the electronic medical record [108]. These phenotypes correlated with host response patterns and clinical outcomes and were validated in a database of over 40,000 patients, with different mortality in the different phenotypes. Notably, when simulation was performed changing the proportion of each phenotype in randomized controlled trials, the results of the trials changed from potential benefit to likely harm. Remarkably, even vital signs have been shown to have predictive significance. Four different subgroups were identified in a 30,000-patient study examining body temperature trajectories over the first 72 h of admission, associated with different mortalities [109]. Notably, these temperature subphenotypes correlate with immune responses in septic patients [110].

SUMMARY

For all of the research effort that has been put forth to improve the care of septic patients, biomarkers play only a limited role currently in the diagnosis of sepsis. Transcriptomics, epigenetics, proteomics, and metabolomics each offer enticing new approaches to improve our understanding of sepsis. Modern biomarker and molecular diagnostic investigations have the potential to highlight pathways, processes, and effector molecules that are central to disease pathophysiology, producing the potential of improved diagnostic biomarkers and identification of novel targets for future therapies. While incremental improvements have been made by combining inherently nonspecific markers into multiplex assays [111−113], emerging science promises to better define the specific molecular fingerprints of sepsis, ideally leading to more accurate diagnoses and more precise clinical care.

REFERENCES

[1] Singer M, et al. The third international consensus definitions for sepsis and septic shock (Sepsis-3). JAMA 2016; 315(8):801−10.

[2] Jee Y, et al. Antimicrobial resistance: a threat to global health. Lancet Infect Dis 2018;18(9):939−40.

[3] Coopersmith CM, et al. Surviving sepsis campaign: research priorities for sepsis and septic shock. Crit Care Med 2018;46(8):1334−56.

[4] Lesko LJ, Atkinson Jr AJ. Use of biomarkers and surrogate endpoints in drug development and regulatory decision making: criteria, validation, strategies. Annu Rev Pharmacol Toxicol 2001;41:347−66.

[5] Frank R, Hargreaves R. Clinical biomarkers in drug discovery and development. Nat Rev Drug Discov 2003; 2(7):566−80.

[6] Hotchkiss RS, Monneret G, Payen D. Sepsis-induced immunosuppression: from cellular dysfunctions to immunotherapy. Nat Rev Immunol 2013;13(12): 862−74.

[7] Rabinowitz JD, Enerback S. Lactate: the ugly duckling of energy metabolism. Nat Metab 2020;2(7):566−71.

[8] Gladden LB. Lactate metabolism: a new paradigm for the third millennium. J Physiol 2004;558(Pt 1):5−30.

[9] Levy B. Lactate and shock state: the metabolic view. Curr Opin Crit Care 2006;12(4):315−21.

[10] Hui S, et al. Glucose feeds the TCA cycle via circulating lactate. Nature 2017;551(7678):115−8.

[11] Lottes RG, et al. Lactate as substrate for mitochondrial respiration in alveolar epithelial type II cells. Am J Physiol Lung Cell Mol Physiol 2015;308(9):L953−61.

[12] Patgiri A, et al. An engineered enzyme that targets circulating lactate to alleviate intracellular NADH:NAD(+) imbalance. Nat Biotechnol 2020;38(3):309−13.

[13] Nocito L, et al. The extracellular redox state modulates mitochondrial function, gluconeogenesis, and glycogen synthesis in murine hepatocytes. PLoS One 2015;10(3): e0122818.

[14] Levy B, et al. Relation between muscle Na+K+ ATPase activity and raised lactate concentrations in septic shock: a prospective study. Lancet 2005;365(9462): 871−5.

[15] Luchette FA, et al. Hypoxia is not the sole cause of lactate production during shock. J Trauma 2002;52(3):415−9.

[16] Boekstegers P, et al. Skeletal muscle partial pressure of oxygen in patients with sepsis. Crit Care Med 1994; 22(4):640−50.

[17] Casserly B, et al. Lactate measurements in sepsis-induced tissue hypoperfusion: results from the Surviving Sepsis Campaign database. Crit Care Med 2015;43(3):567−73.

[18] Evans L, et al. Surviving sepsis campaign: international guidelines for management of sepsis and septic shock 2021. Crit Care Med 2021;49(11):e1063−143.

[19] Jansen TC, et al. Early lactate-guided therapy in intensive care unit patients: a multicenter, open-label, randomized controlled trial. Am J Respir Crit Care Med 2010; 182(6):752−61.

[20] Jones AE, et al. Lactate clearance vs central venous oxygen saturation as goals of early sepsis therapy: a randomized clinical trial. JAMA 2010;303(8):739−46.

[21] Rhodes A, et al. Surviving sepsis campaign: international guidelines for management of sepsis and septic shock: 2016. Crit Care Med 2017;45(3):486−552.

[22] Gu WJ, Zhang Z, Bakker J. Early lactate clearance-guided therapy in patients with sepsis: a meta-analysis with trial sequential analysis of randomized controlled trials. Intensive Care Med 2015;41(10):1862−3.

[23] Simpson SQ, et al. Early goal-directed therapy for severe sepsis and septic shock: a living systematic review. J Crit Care 2016;36:43−8.

[24] Vincent JL, Bakker J. Blood lactate levels in sepsis: in 8 questions. Curr Opin Crit Care 2021;27(3):298−302.

[25] Bihan H, et al. Calcitonin precursor levels in human medullary thyroid carcinoma. Thyroid 2003;13(8):819−22.

[26] Tashijan Jr AH, et al. Immunoassay of human calcitonin. N Engl J Med 1970;283(17):890−5.

[27] Becker KL, Snider R, Nylen ES. Procalcitonin assay in systemic inflammation, infection, and sepsis: clinical utility and limitations. Crit Care Med 2008;36(3):941−52.

[28] Snider Jr RH, Nylen ES, Becker KL. Procalcitonin and its component peptides in systemic inflammation: immunochemical characterization. J Invest Med 1997;45(9): 552−60.

[29] Muller B, et al. Ubiquitous expression of the calcitonin-i gene in multiple tissues in response to sepsis. J Clin Endocrinol Metab 2001;86(1):396−404.

[30] Schuetz P, et al. Procalcitonin (PCT)-guided antibiotic stewardship: an international experts consensus on optimized clinical use. Clin Chem Lab Med 2019;57(9): 1308−18.

[31] Huang DT, et al. Risk prediction with procalcitonin and clinical rules in community-acquired pneumonia. Ann Emerg Med 2008;52(1):48−58 e2.

[32] Muller B, et al. Diagnostic and prognostic accuracy of clinical and laboratory parameters in community-acquired pneumonia. BMC Infect Dis 2007;7:10.

[33] Assicot M, et al. High serum procalcitonin concentrations in patients with sepsis and infection. Lancet 1993;341(8844):515−8.

[34] Hoeboer SH, et al. The diagnostic accuracy of procalcitonin for bacteraemia: a systematic review and meta-analysis. Clin Microbiol Infect 2015;21(5):474−81.

[35] Kapasi AJ, et al. Host biomarkers for distinguishing bacterial from non-bacterial causes of acute febrile illness: a comprehensive review. PLoS One 2016;11(8): e0160278.

[36] Schuetz P, et al. Serial procalcitonin predicts mortality in severe sepsis patients: results from the multicenter procalcitonin MOnitoring SEpsis (MOSES) study. Crit Care Med 2017;45(5):781−9.

[37] Pieralli F, et al. Procalcitonin kinetics in the first 72 hours predicts 30-day mortality in severely ill septic patients admitted to an intermediate care unit. J Clin Med Res 2015;7(9):706−13.

[38] Ruiz-Rodriguez JC, et al. Usefulness of procalcitonin clearance as a prognostic biomarker in septic shock. A prospective pilot study. Med Intensiva 2012;36(7): 475–80.

[39] Karlsson S, et al. Predictive value of procalcitonin decrease in patients with severe sepsis: a prospective observational study. Crit Care 2010;14(6):R205.

[40] Kutz A, et al. Prognostic value of procalcitonin in respiratory tract infections across clinical settings. Crit Care 2015;19:74.

[41] De Bus L, et al. Antimicrobial de-escalation in the critically ill patient and assessment of clinical cure: the DIANA study. Intensive Care Med 2020;46(7): 1404–17.

[42] de Jong E, et al. Efficacy and safety of procalcitonin guidance in reducing the duration of antibiotic treatment in critically ill patients: a randomised, controlled, open-label trial. Lancet Infect Dis 2016;16(7):819–27.

[43] Iankova I, et al. Efficacy and safety of procalcitonin guidance in patients with suspected or confirmed sepsis: a systematic review and meta-analysis. Crit Care Med 2018;46(5):691–8.

[44] Lam SW, et al. Systematic review and meta-analysis of procalcitonin-guidance versus usual care for antimicrobial management in critically ill patients: focus on subgroups based on antibiotic initiation, cessation, or mixed strategies. Crit Care Med 2018;46(5):684–90.

[45] Wirz Y, et al. Effect of procalcitonin-guided antibiotic treatment on clinical outcomes in intensive care unit patients with infection and sepsis patients: a patient-level meta-analysis of randomized trials. Crit Care 2018; 22(1):191.

[46] Kyriazopoulou E, et al. Procalcitonin to reduce long-term infection-associated adverse events in sepsis. A randomized trial. Am J Respir Crit Care Med 2021;203(2): 202–10.

[47] Huang DT, et al. Procalcitonin-guided use of antibiotics for lower respiratory tract infection. N Engl J Med 2018; 379(3):236–49.

[48] Honore PM, et al. Procalcitonin is useful for antibiotic deescalation in sepsis and septic shock: beware of some confounders! Crit Care Med 2021;49(6):e659.

[49] Abernethy TJ, Avery OT. The occurrence during acute infections of a protein not normally present in the blood: I. Distribution of the reactive protein in patients' sera and the effect of calcium on the flocculation reaction with C polysaccharide of pneumococcus. J Exp Med 1941;73(2):173–82.

[50] Volanakis JE, Kaplan MH. Specificity of C-reactive protein for choline phosphate residues of pneumococcal C-polysaccharide. Proc Soc Exp Biol Med 1971;136(2): 612–4.

[51] Tillett WS, Francis T. Serological reactions in pneumonia with a non-protein somatic fraction of pneumococcus. J Exp Med 1930;52(4):561–71.

[52] Sproston NR, Ashworth JJ. Role of C-reactive protein at sites of inflammation and infection. Front Immunol 2018;9:754.

[53] Pai JK, et al. Inflammatory markers and the risk of coronary heart disease in men and women. N Engl J Med 2004;351(25):2599–610.

[54] Lindqvist E, et al. Prognostic laboratory markers of joint damage in rheumatoid arthritis. Ann Rheum Dis 2005; 64(2):196–201.

[55] Ryu JA, et al. Clinical usefulness of procalcitonin and C-reactive protein as outcome predictors in critically ill patients with severe sepsis and septic shock. PLoS One 2015;10(9):e0138150.

[56] Hoeboer SH, Groeneveld AB. Changes in circulating procalcitonin versus C-reactive protein in predicting evolution of infectious disease in febrile, critically ill patients. PLoS One 2013;8(6):e65564.

[57] Lisboa T, et al. C-reactive protein correlates with bacterial load and appropriate antibiotic therapy in suspected ventilator-associated pneumonia. Crit Care Med 2008; 36(1):166–71.

[58] Petel D, et al. Use of C-reactive protein to tailor antibiotic use: a systematic review and meta-analysis. BMJ Open 2018;8(12):e022133.

[59] Oliveira CF, et al. Procalcitonin versus C-reactive protein for guiding antibiotic therapy in sepsis: a randomized trial. Crit Care Med 2013;41(10):2336–43.

[60] Kataria Y, Remick D. Sepsis biomarkers. Methods Mol Biol 2021;2321:177–89.

[61] Simon L, et al. Serum procalcitonin and C-reactive protein levels as markers of bacterial infection: a systematic review and meta-analysis. Clin Infect Dis 2004;39(2): 206–17.

[62] Chaussabel D, Pascual V, Banchereau J. Assessing the human immune system through blood transcriptomics. BMC Biol 2010;8:84.

[63] Wang Z, Gerstein M, Snyder M. RNA-Seq: a revolutionary tool for transcriptomics. Nat Rev Genet 2009; 10(1):57–63.

[64] Holcomb ZE, et al. Host-based peripheral blood gene expression analysis for diagnosis of infectious diseases. J Clin Microbiol 2017;55(2):360–8.

[65] McHugh L, et al. A molecular host response assay to discriminate between sepsis and infection-negative systemic inflammation in critically ill patients: discovery and validation in independent cohorts. PLoS Med 2015;12(12):e1001916.

[66] Sweeney TE, et al. A comprehensive time-course-based multicohort analysis of sepsis and sterile inflammation reveals a robust diagnostic gene set. Sci Transl Med 2015;7(287):287ra71.

[67] Sweeney TE, Khatri P. Comprehensive validation of the FAIM3:PLAC8 ratio in time-matched public gene expression data. Am J Respir Crit Care Med 2015;192(10): 1260–1.

[68] Tsalik EL, et al. Host gene expression classifiers diagnose acute respiratory illness etiology. Sci Transl Med 2016; 8(322):322ra11.

[69] Suarez NM, et al. Superiority of transcriptional profiling over procalcitonin for distinguishing bacterial from viral

lower respiratory tract infections in hospitalized adults. J Infect Dis 2015;212(2):213−22.

[70] Sweeney TE, Wong HR, Khatri P. Robust classification of bacterial and viral infections via integrated host gene expression diagnostics. Sci Transl Med 2016;8(346): 346ra91.

[71] Davenport EE, et al. Genomic landscape of the individual host response and outcomes in sepsis: a prospective cohort study. Lancet Respir Med 2016;4(4):259−71.

[72] Wong HR, et al. Improved risk stratification in pediatric septic shock using both protein and mRNA biomarkers. PERSEVERE-XP. Am J Respir Crit Care Med 2017; 196(4):494−501.

[73] Cech TR, Steitz JA. The noncoding RNA revolution-trashing old rules to forge new ones. Cell 2014;157(1): 77−94.

[74] Wang W, et al. Long noncoding RNA: regulatory mechanisms and therapeutic potential in sepsis. Front Cell Infect Microbiol 2021;11:563126.

[75] O'Neill LA, Sheedy FJ, McCoy CE. MicroRNAs: the fine-tuners of Toll-like receptor signalling. Nat Rev Immunol 2011;11(3):163−75.

[76] Iro MA, Soundara Pandi SP. Clinical application of non-coding RNAs in sepsis. Curr Opin Infect Dis 2020;33(6): 530−9.

[77] Beltran-Garcia J, et al. Circular RNAs in sepsis: biogenesis, function, and clinical significance. Cells 2020;9(6).

[78] Huang S, et al. Diagnostic value of the lncRNA NEAT1 in peripheral blood mononuclear cells of patients with sepsis. Dis Markers 2017;2017:7962836.

[79] He F, Zhang C, Huang Q. Long noncoding RNA nuclear enriched abundant transcript 1/miRNA-124 axis correlates with increased disease risk, elevated inflammation, deteriorative disease condition, and predicts decreased survival of sepsis. Medicine (Baltim) 2019;98(32): e16470.

[80] Geng F, Liu W, Yu L. Potential role of circulating long noncoding RNA MALAT1 in predicting disease risk, severity, and patients' survival in sepsis. J Clin Lab Anal 2019;33(8):e22968.

[81] Reyes M, et al. An immune-cell signature of bacterial sepsis. Nat Med 2020;26(3):333−40.

[82] Correia CN, et al. Circulating microRNAs as potential biomarkers of infectious disease. Front Immunol 2017; 8:118.

[83] Binnie A, et al. Epigenetics of sepsis. Crit Care Med 2020; 48(5):745−56.

[84] Portela A, Esteller M. Epigenetic modifications and human disease. Nat Biotechnol 2010;28(10):1057−68.

[85] Clark MF, Baudouin SV. A systematic review of the quality of genetic association studies in human sepsis. Intensive Care Med 2006;32(11):1706−12.

[86] Binnie A, et al. Epigenetic profiling in severe sepsis: a pilot study of DNA methylation profiles in critical illness. Crit Care Med 2020;48(2):142−50.

[87] Tendl KA, et al. DNA methylation pattern of CALCA in preterm neonates with bacterial sepsis as a putative epigenetic biomarker. Epigenetics 2013;8(12):1261−7.

[88] Dhas DB, et al. Comparison of genomic DNA methylation pattern among septic and non-septic newborns - an epigenome wide association study. Genom Data 2015;3:36−40.

[89] Mann M, et al. The coming age of complete, accurate, and ubiquitous proteomes. Mol Cell 2013;49(4): 583−90.

[90] Pernemalm M, Lehtio J. Mass spectrometry-based plasma proteomics: state of the art and future outlook. Expert Rev Proteomics 2014;11(4):431−48.

[91] Tirumalai RS, et al. Characterization of the low molecular weight human serum proteome. Mol Cell Proteomics 2003;2(10):1096−103.

[92] Claxton AJ, et al. Efficacy and safety of procalcitonin guidance in patients with suspected or confirmed sepsis: a systematic review and meta-analysis: author correction. Crit Care Med 2018;46(9):1560.

[93] Hayashi N, et al. Multiple biomarkers of sepsis identified by novel time-lapse proteomics of patient serum. PLoS One 2019;14(9):e0222403.

[94] DeCoux A, et al. Plasma glycoproteomics reveals sepsis outcomes linked to distinct proteins in common pathways. Crit Care Med 2015;43(10):2049−58.

[95] Patti GJ, Yanes O, Siuzdak G. Innovation: metabolomics: the apogee of the omics trilogy. Nat Rev Mol Cell Biol 2012;13(4):263−9.

[96] Eckerle M, et al. Metabolomics as a driver in advancing precision medicine in sepsis. Pharmacotherapy 2017; 37(9):1023−32.

[97] Beloborodova NV, Olenin AY, Pautova AK. Metabolomic findings in sepsis as a damage of host-microbial metabolism integration. J Crit Care 2018;43:246−55.

[98] Langley RJ, et al. Integrative "omic" analysis of experimental bacteremia identifies a metabolic signature that distinguishes human sepsis from systemic inflammatory response syndromes. Am J Respir Crit Care Med 2014; 190(4):445−55.

[99] Lin ZY, et al. A metabonomic approach to early prognostic evaluation of experimental sepsis by (1)H NMR and pattern recognition. NMR Biomed 2009;22(6): 601−8.

[100] Fanos V, et al. Urinary (1)H-NMR and GC-MS metabolomics predicts early and late onset neonatal sepsis. Early Hum Dev 2014;90(Suppl. 1):S78−83.

[101] Blaise BJ, et al. Metabolic phenotyping of traumatized patients reveals a susceptibility to sepsis. Anal Chem 2013;85(22):10850−5.

[102] Langley RJ, et al. An integrated clinico-metabolomic model improves prediction of death in sepsis. Sci Transl Med 2013;5(195):195ra95.

[103] Zhang Y, et al. Microfluidics for sepsis early diagnosis and prognosis: a review of recent methods. Analyst 2021;146(7):2110−25.

[104] Wong HR. Sepsis biomarkers. J Pediatr Intensive Care 2019;8(1):11−6.

[105] DeMerle KM, et al. Sepsis subclasses: a framework for development and interpretation. Crit Care Med 2021; 49(5):748−59.

[106] Wong HR, et al. Developing a clinically feasible personalized medicine approach to pediatric septic shock. Am J Respir Crit Care Med 2015;191(3):309—15.

[107] Scicluna BP, et al. Classification of patients with sepsis according to blood genomic endotype: a prospective cohort study. Lancet Respir Med 2017;5(10):816—26.

[108] Seymour CW, et al. Derivation, validation, and potential treatment implications of novel clinical phenotypes for sepsis. JAMA 2019;321(20):2003—17.

[109] Bhavani SV, et al. Identifying novel sepsis subphenotypes using temperature trajectories. Am J Respir Crit Care Med 2019;200(3):327—35.

[110] Bhavani SV, et al. Temperature trajectory subphenotypes correlate with immune responses in patients with sepsis. Crit Care Med 2020;48(11):1645—53.

[111] Abasiyanik MF, et al. Ultrasensitive digital quantification of cytokines and bacteria predicts septic shock outcomes. Nat Commun 2020;11(1):2607.

[112] Berger J, et al. Simultaneous electrical detection of IL-6 and PCT using a microfluidic biochip platform. Biomed Microdevices 2020;22(2):36.

[113] Liu J, et al. Mortality prediction using a novel combination of biomarkers in the first day of sepsis in intensive care units. Sci Rep 2021;11(1):1275.

CHAPTER 10

Hemodynamic Monitoring: Current Practice and New Perspectives

CHRISTOPHER LAI • JEAN-LOUIS TEBOUL

INTRODUCTION

Septic shock is defined as a sepsis associated with an acute circulatory failure [1]. Clinically, this situation is characterized by an increase in lactatemia >2 mmol/L and hypotension requiring vasopressor therapy to maintain a mean arterial pressure (MAP) $\geq$ 65 mmHg despite fluid administration. Three pathophysiological mechanisms can be involved in septic shock: hypovolemia, vasoplegia, and cardiac dysfunction. In-hospital mortality associated with septic shock still ranges from 30% to 50% [2,3]. Septic shock represents thus a medical emergency. The Surviving Sepsis Campaign (SSC) 2021 suggests beginning resuscitation immediately with at least 30 mL/kg of intravenous crystalloids within the first 3 h and starting vasopressors if necessary, in order to aim a target of MAP of at least 65 mmHg [4]. However, after the early phase of resuscitation and once the patient is admitted in intensive care unit (ICU), fluid administration should be closely monitored [5]. Indeed, if fluid therapy can be used to improve cardiac output (CO) and enhance microvascular blood flow, excessive fluid administration can be harmful and impair patient's outcome [6−9]. It is therefore logical to use a hemodynamic monitoring in order to identify the type of shock, to guide therapy, and to assess its effectiveness. In this chapter, we will review the current practice based on experts' recommendations for hemodynamic monitoring in shock but also the perspectives that we can expect in the coming years to improve the management of these patients.

CURRENT PRACTICE BASED ON INTERNATIONAL EXPERTS' RECOMMENDATIONS

Careful clinical examination is essential to identify the presence of circulatory failure. Mottling [10−13] and increased capillary refill time (CRT) [14] represent markers of low CO and tissue hypoperfusion, and they are related with poor outcome [11,12,14]. In a multicenter randomized controlled trial called ANDROMEDA-SHOCK, performed in the first eight hours of resuscitation of patients with septic shock, a therapy guided on normalization of CRT—evaluated every 30 min—was compared to a strategy guided by a decrease in lactate level assessed every 2 h [15]. The 28-day mortality rates were 43.4% in the lactate level-guided group and 34.9% in the CRT-guided group ($P = .06$). There was less organ dysfunction at 72 h in the CRT-guided group, as evidenced by a mean Sequential Organ Failure Assessment (SOFA) score of 5.6 versus 6.6, although the lactate-guided group received more fluids [15]. In an ancillary study, the two resuscitation strategies had comparable effects on regional and microcirculatory flow parameters and tissue hypoxia surrogates [16]. Although guiding resuscitation on CRT is promising, many questions remain unsolved such as which mechanisms determine an abnormal CRT or how vasoactive agents influence this bedside marker. Moreover, the methodology to assess CRT is not well defined and must be standardized (e.g., level and duration of pressure, location, use of specific device).

Current guidelines recommend using arterial and central venous catheters [4,17] to manage patients with circulatory shock (Fig. 10.1). The arterial catheter allows continuous measurement of arterial blood pressure and of its different components. A low diastolic arterial pressure (e.g., <40 mmHg) as a marker of a low vascular tone suggests introducing vasopressor early. A low arterial pulse pressure reflects a low stroke volume, secondary to hypovolemia or to reduced cardiac contractility. In patients under mechanical ventilation, pulse pressure ventilation (PPV) can also be calculated to predict fluid responsiveness [18−20], although several limitations apply such as

The Sepsis Codex. https://doi.org/10.1016/B978-0-323-88271-2.00010-9

necessity of no spontaneous breathing [21], tidal volume ≥ 8 mL/kg, or sinus rhythm [22]. In patients ventilated with a low tidal volume (e.g., 6 mL/kg), the tidal volume challenge, consisting in a transient increase in tidal volume from 6 to 8 mL/kg, can be reliably used to predict fluid responsiveness [23].

The central venous catheter also provides important hemodynamic variables such as the central venous pressure (CVP) and central venous oxygen saturation ($ScvO_2$). Although the CVP is not reliable to detect preload responsiveness [24] or preload unresponsiveness [25], it can detect right ventricular dysfunction, which can be confirmed by echocardiography. Additionally, CVP, as a reflection of the downstream pressure of most vital organs, can be used to calculate the organ perfusion pressure (difference between the MAP and the CVP). This is helpful to define the appropriate MAP value to target, in the way that in case of high CVP, a higher MAP should be targeted than in case of low CVP, to ensure adequate organ perfusion. The central venous catheter also provides the $ScvO_2$, which reflects the adequacy between oxygen consumption and oxygen delivery, and the central venous carbon dioxide tension ($PcvCO_2$). The $ScvO_2$ has been used in a protocol developed by Rivers et al. known as the "early goal-directed therapy" and aimed at achieving a $ScvO_2$ $\geq 70\%$ [26]. In this monocentric study, the authors showed that fluid administration guided by $ScvO_2$ resulted in a decrease in mortality rate from 49% to 33%. However, these data have not been confirmed in multicenter studies [27–29], and $ScvO_2$ is no longer part of the 2021 SSC guidelines [4]. Moreover, $ScvO_2$ can be normal or abnormally high in cases of alteration of oxygen extraction such as in septic shock. In this situation, the venoarterial difference in CO_2 pressure (PCO_2 gap) obtained using $PcvCO_2$ and arterial $PaCO_2$ can be helpful, since it reliably indicates the adequacy of CO with the metabolic condition. A PCO_2 gap higher than 6 mmHg suggests than CO is inadequate (not high enough) and would incite to increase it in case of shock [17,30]. The ratio of the PCO_2 gap over the arteriovenous difference of oxygen content (PCO_2 gap/$C_{a\text{-}v}O_2$) is considered a marker of anaerobiosis [31].

Echocardiography is a noninvasive and easy-to-perform technique that enables to assess the left ventricular function, the right ventricular function, and CO through measurement of velocity-time integral of the flow through the aortic valve [32]. Preload responsiveness can be assessed by measuring the response of velocity-time integral to passive leg raising (PLR) or to a combination of end-expiratory and end-inspiratory occlusions in patients under mechanical ventilation [33]. However, echocardiographic CO evaluation is intermittent and requires a specific training (Table 10.1).

In most situations, manipulating all the above-mentioned variables is sufficient for improving the patient's hemodynamic condition. Nevertheless, if the

TABLE 10.1
Advantage and Inconvenience of Different Hemodynamic Monitoring Techniques. CO: Cardiac Output, ICU: Intensive Care Unit

Technique	Invasiveness	Reliability in ICU	Easy to use	Calibration	Real-time CO measurement	Other Variables than CO
Pulmonary artery catheter	+++	+++	−	+++	−	+++
Transpulmonary thermodilution	+++	+++	++	+++	+++	+++
Echocardiography	0	++	++	−	++	++
Uncalibrated pulse wave analysis	++	+	+++	−	++	+
Bioreactance	0	+/−	+++	−	+	−
Volume-clamp	0	+/−	+++	−	++	−
Radial-artery applanation tonometry	0	+/−	+++	−	++	−
Pulse index	0	++	+++	−	−	−

Adapted from Jozwiak M, Monnet X, Teboul J-L. Less or more hemodynamic monitoring in critically ill patients. Curr Opin Crit Care 2018;24(2018): 309–315. https://doi.org/10.1097/MCC.0000000000000516, with permission.

hemodynamic response is not sufficient or when a severe acute respiratory distress syndrome (ARDS) is associated, using an advanced hemodynamic monitoring is recommended [17,35,36] (Fig. 10.1).

The pulmonary artery catheter (PAC) allows measuring right atrial pressure, pulmonary arterial pressure, pulmonary artery occlusion pressure, and mixed venous blood oxygen saturation (SvO_2). The PAC also provides intermittent CO measurements through pulmonary artery thermodilution, which represents the "gold standard" of CO measurement. Some catheters also provide automatic calculation of CO in a semicontinuous way, but this does not represent a real-time CO monitoring per se, and thus cannot serve to assess preload responsiveness. Its high invasiveness, the frequent errors in pressure measurement, and the lack of demonstrated outcome benefits [37] have made its use decreasing in the recent years [38] (Table 10.1). Nevertheless, the variables provided by the PAC could be informative in cases of right ventricular dysfunction

accompanying cardiogenic shock [17] or ARDS [17,35,36].

The transpulmonary thermodilution (TPTD) systems provide intermittent measurements of CO after bolus injection of cold saline in a vein of the superior vena cava territory. The changes in blood temperature induced by this injection are detected by a thermistor located at the tip of a femoral arterial catheter. The thermodilution curve allows calculation of CO using the Stewart−Hamilton principle [39,40]. The TPTD also calibrates the arterial pulse contour analysis. This technique allows a real-time monitoring of CO [41], which is precise as the least significant change with this technique is only 1% [42]. Thus, it allows the use of several preload responsiveness tests [43] such as the PLR test [44−47], the end-expiratory occlusion test [48−50], or the mini-fluid challenge [50−52]. In addition to intermittent and continuous CO measurements, the TPTD devices provide the values of: (1) global end-diastolic volume, a marker of global cardiac preload,

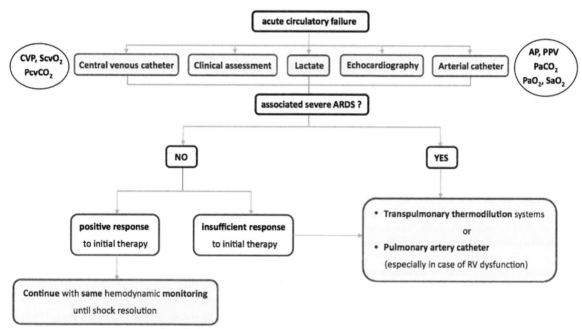

FIG. 10.1 **Choice of hemodynamic monitoring in patients with acute circulatory failure.** AP: arterial pressure, ARDS: acute respiratory distress syndrome, CVP: central venous pressure, $PaCO_2$: carbon dioxide pressure in the arterial blood, PaO_2: oxygen pressure in the arterial blood, $PcvCO_2$: carbon dioxide pressure in the central venous blood, PPV: pulse pressure variation, RV: right ventricular, SaO_2: arterial blood oxygen saturation, $ScvO_2$: central venous blood oxygen saturation. (Cited from Teboul J-L, Saugel B, Cecconi M, De Backer D, Hofer CK, Monnet X, Perel A, Pinsky MR, Reuter DA, Rhodes A, Squara P, Vincent J-L, Scheeren TW. Less invasive hemodynamic monitoring in critically ill patients. Intensive Care Med 2016; 42(2016):1350−1359. https://doi.org/10.1007/s00134-016-4375-7, with permission.)

(2) extravascular lung water (EVLW), a marker of the amount of lung edema, (3) cardiac function index and global ejection fraction, which are markers of the global cardiac systolic function, and (4) pulmonary vascular permeability index (PVPI), a marker of lung capillary leak. The EVLW and PVPI are independent prognostic factors in patients with ARDS [53]. The pulse contour analysis technique also allows monitoring of PPV and stroke volume variation (SVV), which are reliable predictors of preload responsiveness in patients ventilated with a tidal volume of at least 8 mL/kg, without cardiac arrhythmias and spontaneous breathing activity. A European pre- and postquestionnaire study showed that intensivists had limited ability to correctly assess the hemodynamic status of patients and adapted their decision in 33% concerning fluid administration and 22% concerning vasopressors when information from TPTP systems was provided [54]. The TPTD systems are more often used in patients with both acute circulatory failure and ARDS, as suggested by experts from the European Society of Intensive Care Medicine [17,35] (Fig. 10.1, Table 10.1). In a recent international survey carried out in 1000 intensivists involved in the care of COVID-19 patients, physicians declared to use TPTD in 43% of patients and PAC in 13% [38], whereas advanced hemodynamic monitoring was used in less than 15% of critically ill patients in the early 2010s [55]. In the context of ARDS, the use of TPTD systems is relevant because they provide EVLW and PVPI, which can be viewed as markers of lung tolerance to fluid administration. Moreover, use of TPTD allows assessment of preload responsiveness (PPV and its response to a tidal volume challenge, continuous CO response to PLR, or to end-expiratory occlusion). These systems can thus provide assessment of the benefit/risk balance of fluid infusion: preload responsiveness markers to assess the benefits and EVLW and PVPI to assess the risks. The same markers can be used to guide fluid removal after the initial resuscitation efforts have started. Consequently, the TPTD systems allow personalization of fluid management.

IMPROVEMENT OF AVAILABLE MINIMALLY OR NONINVASIVE TECHNOLOGIES
Uncalibrated Pulse Wave Analysis Devices
Whereas recommended in most severe patients, advanced hemodynamic monitoring is not always used in such patients [38] mainly because of its cost and/or its invasiveness. Alternatively, different devices that use the pulse wave analysis have been developed [41,56] (Fig. 10.2). Although attractive, these CO monitoring systems should be interpreted with caution as they are not calibrated and could not be reliable in critically ill patients, especially in those suffering from sepsis or those receiving vasoactive agents. In addition, the values of CO are averaged and refreshed over several seconds, which are moreover, not necessarily set at the same rate. Shortening of refreshment rate and averaging time should increase reliability of these CO monitoring systems, particularly to perform preload responsiveness tests or assess the efficacy of fluid administration [57−60] (Table 10.1).

Bioreactance
Technologies using bioreactance also improved over the last years. These systems work after placing four dual sensors on the patient's chest, which send a low-amplitude, high-frequency electrical current, only affected by pulsatile flow. Extrapolation of stroke volume, and thus CO, is made using variations in the transthoracic electrical impedance (Table 10.1). Reduction in the period over which the CO is averaged has enhanced reliability of bioreactance device making it more suitable for performing preload responsiveness tests such as PLR or end-expiratory occlusion test [61−63]. However, bioreactance CO measurements can be disturbed by a variety of factors, such as edema, pleural effusions, pulmonary edema, arrhythmias, electrical interference, internal or external pacemakers, or patient's movement.

Pulse Oximetry and Perfusion Index
The peripheral perfusion index (PI), derived from the plethysmography signal of pulse oximetry, has been proposed to track changes of CO during dynamic tests aimed at detecting preload responsiveness [64−66]. The plethysmography signal has a pulsatile component and a nonpulsatile component. The pulsatile component is a variable amount of light absorbed by the pulsatile arterial blood flow. It reflects changes in the finger blood volume during one cardiac cycle, which may also reflect changes in stroke volume. The nonpulsatile component is supposed to be a constant amount of light absorbed by skin, bone, and tissues. The PI is calculated as the ratio of the amplitude of the pulsatile signal over that of the nonpulsatile signal [67]. Precision and least significant change values for PI measurement are 1.6% and 1.2%, respectively [65]. A study performed in ICU patients showed that an increase in PI more than 9% during PLR could detect an increase in pulse contour CO during PLR more than 10% with a sensitivity of 91% (76%−98%), a specificity of 79% (63%−90%), and an area under receiver operating characteristic curve (AUROC) of 0.89 (0.80−0.95) [65].

These first results were confirmed in another study, in which changes in PI also demonstrated to be a reliable surrogate of changes in CO for performing the end-expiratory occlusion test that can predict preload responsiveness [64]. An increase in PI ≥ 2.5% during end-expiratory occlusion detected a positive PLR test with an AUROC of 0.95 ± 0.03 [64]. In the operating room setting, changes in PI during lung recruitment maneuvers can also accurately predict preload responsiveness [66]. Although very promising, these results should be confirmed by further studies (Table 10.1).

Noninvasive Methods

Nowadays, noninvasive devices are available to obtain a continuous arterial pressure waveform signal and thus to provide a real-time CO monitoring (Fig. 10.2).

The volume clamp method derives the finger arterial pressure waveform from the cuff pressure that is needed to keep the blood volume (assessed by photoplethysmography) in the finger arteries constant throughout the cardiac cycle [68] (Fig. 10.2, Table 10.1). In the perioperative context, the volume clamp method showed acceptable agreement and trending ability when compared to references techniques. However, several limitations of the volume clamp technique exist as peripheral edema or vasoconstriction, limiting its application in critically ill patients [69].

The continuous radial artery applanation tonometry technique records the arterial pressure waveform using a sensor that is electromechanically driven over the radial artery [70] (Fig. 10.2). Position of the sensor is crucial, and patient's movements can impair the quality of the signal. Thus, application of this technique might be more applicable in patients under general anesthesia rather than in ICU patients [69] (Table 10.1). Improvement in the quality of signal acquisition is mandatory in order to use these devices in critically ill patients.

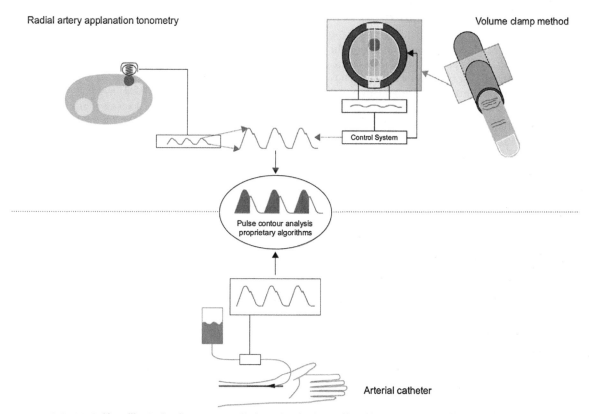

FIG. 10.2 **Uncalibrated pulse wave analysis technologies.**   (Cited from Teboul J-L, Saugel B, Cecconi M, De Backer D, Hofer CK, Monnet X, Perel A, Pinsky MR, Reuter DA, Rhodes A, Squara P, Vincent J-L, Scheeren TW. Less invasive hemodynamic monitoring in critically ill patients. Intensive Care Med 2016;42(2016): 1350–1359. https://doi.org/10.1007/s00134-016-4375-7, with permission.)

NEW NONINVASIVE HEMODYNAMIC MONITORING TECHNOLOGIES

The future of hemodynamic monitoring should probably at least use the derivation of noninvasive monitoring of arterial blood pressure and hence of CO when coupled with uncalibrated pulse wave analysis. It is easier to perform than echocardiography and allows a rapid response before more invasive monitoring (e.g., arterial catheter or advanced hemodynamic monitoring) can be set-up. Wireless, noninvasive, wearable devices for continuous monitoring of hemodynamic parameters are in development [71]. Using chest, radial, or carotid sensors, these new devices could monitor heart rate, arterial blood pressure, and CO through pulse wave analysis. Nevertheless, most of these devices are still in their feasibility and clinical validation stage, with limited evidence on their clinical effectiveness [72].

CLINICAL APPLICATION OF TECHNOLOGIES ASSESSING MICROCIRCULATION CURRENTLY USED FOR RESEARCH PURPOSE

Restoring adequate tissue oxygenation is the goal of hemodynamic resuscitation of patients with acute circulatory failure. Estimation of global oxygen delivery (DO_2) is important to be made through measurements of CO, hemoglobin concentration, and arterial blood oxygen saturation (SaO_2). Adequacy of DO_2 to oxygen demand is even more important to assess than the value of DO_2 per se. Knowledge of SvO_2 or $ScvO_2$ is a way to assess the adequacy of DO_2 to oxygen consumption (VO_2) but not to oxygen demand, particularly in the situations where oxygen extraction is altered such as sepsis. In such situations, the distribution of CO and DO_2 within the organs can be severely impaired [73] so that monitoring only markers of macrocirculation is insufficient. In this regard, a value of $ScvO_2$ within the normal range can be misleading as it can be associated with profound tissue hypoxia due to alteration of microcirculation or impairment of cellular oxygen utilization. Over the last 10 years, much research has been undertaken to better explore microvascular hemodynamics and tissue oxygenation.

Sublingual Microcirculation Assessment

Several methods exist to explore the microcirculation [74], including the laser Doppler that measures red blood cell velocity in small vessels, intravital microvideo-surface microscopy applied directly on organs, microvideo-surface microscopy by orthogonal polarization spectral or sidestream darkfield imaging, and nail capillaro-videoscopy. Hand-held vital microscopes assessing the sublingual microcirculation have been the most widely studied method and has enabled the description of microcirculatory alterations in patients with septic shock [73]. Persistent microvascular impairment has been frequently observed even after normalization of macrovascular variables [75,76]. This approach was used to assess the effects of various interventions on the microcirculation, including the titration of norepinephrine [77]. However, the clinical utility of these measurements to guide resuscitation remains to be proven. Although the potential use of this technique has been mentioned in the European consensus on circulatory shock [17], this method is rarely used because it is not easy to perform and to interpret the results [78]. Hopefully, this technique should be improved in the future, and its bedside use simplified and facilitated by automation of the interpretation.

Muscle Tissue Oxygenation

Peripheral oxygenation can be assessed through near-infrared spectroscopy (NIRS) allowing the measurement of the muscle tissue oxygenation (StO_2). When the NIRS sensor is placed at the thenar eminence, it is also possible to obtain the StO_2 recovery slope, which reflects the capacity of microvessels to dilate or to be recruited in response to a local hypoxic stimulus induced by a vascular occlusion using a brachial cuff [79]. In patients with septic shock, the StO_2 recovery slope, unlike the StO_2, was shown to be an independent prognostic factor [80,81]. A multicentric randomized controlled trial evaluated whether targeting an StO_2 value $\geq 80\%$ at a minimum of two different sites in patients with septic shock, as well as maintaining CVP >8 mmHg, MAP >65 mmHg, and $ScvO_2$ > 70%, would improve seven-day mortality or organ dysfunction [82]. Unfortunately, the study ended prematurely due to lack of funding after enrollment of 103/190 patients with no difference in the primary criteria. More recently, assessment of StO_2 and its recovery slope to personalize the target of MAP has been investigated [83]. In this study, decreasing MAP from 81 [78,84] to 68 [68,70] mmHg, whereas cardiac index did not change, led to a decrease in StO_2 recovery slope but with a large interindividual variability [83], suggesting that a unique MAP target may not be suitable for all patients with septic shock as its impact on peripheral oxygenation may widely differ among patients. It could make sense to personalize the MAP target through a multimodal assessment including peripheral oxygenation. Although this fully noninvasive approach is seducing, strong outcome data are still lacking to implement the use of StO_2 to guide resuscitation in patients with septic shock. It should be noted that the NIRS device dedicated to the thenar eminence is no longer commercialized. This is regrettable as the vascular occlusion test provides important information about the microvascular reactivity, an important characteristic that cannot be easily explored at the bedside by other methods. We can hope that in the very next future, industrial companies will invest in this interesting technology.

AUTOMATION/ARTIFICIAL INTELLIGENCE/ MACHINE LEARNING

In an increasingly digital world, the future in hemodynamic monitoring will likely also come from the artificial intelligence, automatic calculation and assessment, big data, and machine learning [84].

Automation and Integrative Assessment

The automatic calculation of PPV and SVV enables real-time monitoring of preload responsiveness when conditions of validity of these variables are ensured. Presence of extrasystoles precludes any valid interpretation of PPV or SVV. Improvement of the algorithm, recognizing and excluding extrasystoles, has shown to better predict fluid responsiveness [85]. This software is now used in the latest version of some devices such as the FloTrac 4.0 (Edwards LifeScience) for instance. Dynamic tests to assess preload responsiveness such as the tidal volume challenge or the end-expiratory occlusion test could also be automated in the future. Coupling the ventilator with the hemodynamic monitor is necessary for that, but this should not represent a real technical difficulty.

Closed Loop

A closed-loop control system is a system in which relevant biological parameters are continuously monitored in real time to continuously adjust a therapy with the aim to achieve a predefined physiological state without human interaction. In the ICU setting, closed-loop systems could be used to administer and titrate fluids or norepinephrine.

However, studies evaluating closed-loop systems were mainly performed in the operating room setting. Implementation of closed-loop goal-directed fluid therapy was associated with a decrease in fluid administration during major abdominal surgery and a decrease in hospital length of stay [86]. In a randomized controlled trial, intraoperative management (fluids and anesthetic drugs) using multiple closed-loop systems was associated with a significant decrease in postoperative neurocognitive impairment [87]. In animal model of hemorrhagic shock, closed-loop resuscitation with combination of fluid and norepinephrine was similar to physician-guided therapy with the aim of targeting MAP [88,89]. However, these systems, which aim at achieving a predefined hemodynamic goal cannot "understand" yet the underlying pathophysiology of a hemodynamic situation, and thus cannot intelligently select the most appropriate treatment (e.g., fluids or norepinephrine). It is likely that in the next years, these systems can improve and be applicable to critically ill patients, for whom hemodynamic assessment is much more complex than in surgical patients.

Machine Learning

Machine learning can be defined as various statistical methods used to predict and make decisions based on similarities in what is being analyzed to what has previously been observed. While machine learning and artificial intelligence have already deeply transformed many industries, healthcare and especially intensive care are still lagging behind. Indeed, setting up large databases, inter- and intraoperability variations, and incomplete, spurious, and artifact data are very difficult to deal with to build these complex models. Nevertheless, major advances have been made in the last years. Several models based on retrospective data of thousands of patients have shown good performance to predict the onset of septic shock [90,91]. The LiSep model was able to predict septic shock with an AUROC 0.83 (95%CI: 0.82–0.84). In another model, a machine learning algorithm could predict septic shock with low sensitivity (26%) but very high specificity (98%). However, prepost impact evaluation of this algorithm did not show any difference in mortality, discharge proportion, or transfer in the ICU, although there was a significant decrease in time-to-ICU transfer with the machine learning [92].

Algorithms have also been newly developed, with the aim to predict hypotensive events. The first study conducted by Hatib et al. developed an algorithm based on the arterial pressure waveform analysis in surgical patients [93]. The mathematical analysis provided a variable, the "hypotension predictive index," which was able to predict hypotension 15 min before its occurrence in 84% of hypotensive events [93]. This index was also tested in mechanically ventilated patients with COVID-19 [94] with an AUROC of 0.95 (0.93–0.97), although it could predict the hypotensive episode only 4 min before its occurrence [94]. Recently, another group also demonstrated that a model, including the analysis of 112 variables (demographic, clinical, biological variables and those obtained from multiple monitoring systems) was able to predict more than 2 h in advance the occurrence of hypotension in ICU patients with an AUROC of 0.94 ± 0.004 [95].

Komorowski et al. built and validated a novel computational learning model to optimize hemodynamic therapy and decrease mortality in adult patients with sepsis [96]. This model was based on the retrospective analysis of data sets from nearly 100,000 ICU patients, with time series analysis of 40 demographic and clinical variables, to model patient trajectories and outcome in response to therapeutic strategies. The algorithm recommended lower doses of intravenous fluids and higher doses of vasopressors than the clinician did. Interestingly, the mortality rate was lower when the doses of either therapy were closer to the doses recommended by the model [96]. These results are encouraging for the future but need to be validated in further prospective studies.

Machine learning has the potential both to support the workflow inherent in interpreting vital signs as well as providing insights into data patterns and complexities that are beyond the perceptive capabilities of the normal human observer. Nevertheless, irrespective of the quality of the algorithm, human clinical knowledge would always remain necessary for caring at best the ICU patients. It must be used not to replace but to help the physician in the clinical decision-making processes.

CONCLUSION

Today, arterial catheter, central venous catheter, and echocardiography are the first-line monitoring in patients with shock. Such a basic hemodynamic monitoring provides intensivists with a lot of valuable information to manage patients with circulatory failure. In cases of complex shock states, advanced hemodynamic monitoring is recommended as it is more reliable and it provides more information of interest than uncalibrated CO monitoring methods. In the next years, improvement in remote mini- or noninvasive continuous monitoring could also be helpful and easier to use for the clinician. Future hemodynamic monitoring should also help the clinician to choose the most appropriate treatment and to predict its effectiveness through machine learning, automation, or closed-loop systems in order to adapt and personalize the hemodynamic management of critically ill patients.

REFERENCES

[1] Singer M, Deutschman CS, Seymour CW, Shankar-Hari M, Annane D, Bauer M, Bellomo R, Bernard GR, Chiche J-D, Coopersmith CM, Hotchkiss RS, Levy MM, Marshall JC, Martin GS, Opal SM, Rubenfeld GD, van der Poll T, Vincent J-L, Angus DC. The third international consensus definitions for sepsis and septic shock (Sepsis-3). JAMA 2016;315:801. https://doi.org/10.1001/jama.2016.0287.

[2] Bauer M, Gerlach H, Vogelmann T, Preissing F, Stiefel J, Adam D. Mortality in sepsis and septic shock in Europe, North America and Australia between 2009 and 2019—results from a systematic review and meta-analysis. Crit Care 2020;24:239. https://doi.org/10.1186/s13054-020-02950-2.

[3] Shankar-Hari M, Phillips GS, Levy ML, Seymour CW, Liu VX, Deutschman CS, Angus DC, Rubenfeld GD, Singer M. For the sepsis definitions task force, developing a new definition and assessing new clinical criteria for septic shock: for the third international consensus definitions for sepsis and septic shock (Sepsis-3). JAMA 2016; 315:775. https://doi.org/10.1001/jama.2016.0289.

[4] Evans L, Rhodes A, Alhazzani W, Antonelli M, Coopersmith CM, French C, Machado FR, Mcintyre L, Ostermann M, Prescott HC, Schorr C, Simpson S, Wiersinga WJ, Alshamsi F, Angus DC, Arabi Y, Azevedo L, Beale R, Beilman G, Belley-Cote E, Burry L, Cecconi M, Centofanti J, Coz Yataco A, De Waele J, Dellinger RP, Doi K, Du B, Estenssoro E, Ferrer R, Gomersall C, Hodgson C, Møller MH, Iwashyna T, Jacob S, Kleinpell R, Klompas M, Koh Y, Kumar A, Kwizera A, Lobo S, Masur H, McGloughlin S, Mehta S, Mehta Y, Mer M, Nunnally M, Oczkowski S, Osborn T, Papathanassoglou E, Perner A, Puskarich M, Roberts J, Schweickert W, Seckel M, Sevransky J, Sprung CL, Welte T, Zimmerman J, Levy M. Surviving sepsis campaign: international guidelines for management of sepsis and septic shock 2021. Intensive Care Med 2021; 47:1181—247. https://doi.org/10.1007/s00134-021-06506-y.

[5] Vincent J-L, De Backer D. Circulatory shock. N Engl J Med 2013;369:1726—34. https://doi.org/10.1056/NEJMra1208943.

[6] Vincent J-L, Sakr Y, Sprung CL, Ranieri VM, Reinhart K, Gerlach H, Moreno R, Carlet J, Le Gall J-R, Payen D. Sepsis occurrence in acutely ill patients investigators, sepsis in European intensive care units: results of the SOAP study. Crit Care Med 2006;34:344—53. https://doi.org/10.1097/01.ccm.0000194725.48928.3a.

[7] Boyd JH, Forbes J, Nakada T, Walley KR, Russell JA. Fluid resuscitation in septic shock: a positive fluid balance and elevated central venous pressure are associated with increased mortality. Crit Care Med 2011;39:259—65. https://doi.org/10.1097/CCM.0b013e3181feeb15.

[8] Malbrain MLNG, Van Regenmortel N, Saugel B, De Tavernier B, Van Gaal P-J, Joannes-Boyau O, Teboul J-L, Rice TW, Mythen M, Monnet X. Principles of fluid management and stewardship in septic shock: it is time to

consider the four D's and the four phases of fluid therapy. Ann Intensive Care 2018;8:66. https://doi.org/10.1186/s13613-018-0402-x.

[9] Legrand M, Dupuis C, Simon C, Gayat E, Mateo J, Lukaszewicz A-C, Payen D. Association between systemic hemodynamics and septic acute kidney injury in critically ill patients: a retrospective observational study. Crit Care 2013;17:R278. https://doi.org/10.1186/cc13133.

[10] Dumas G, Lavillegrand J-R, Joffre J, Bigé N, de-Moura EB, Baudel J-L, Chevret S, Guidet B, Maury E, Amorim F, Ait-Oufella H. Mottling score is a strong predictor of 14-day mortality in septic patients whatever vasopressor doses and other tissue perfusion parameters. Crit Care 2019; 23:211. https://doi.org/10.1186/s13054-019-2496-4.

[11] Ait-Oufella H, Lemoinne S, Boelle PY, Galbois A, Baudel JL, Lemant J, Joffre J, Margetis D, Guidet B, Maury E, Offenstadt G. Mottling score predicts survival in septic shock. Intensive Care Med 2011;37:801−7. https://doi.org/10.1007/s00134-011-2163-y.

[12] de Moura EB, Amorim FF, da Cruz Santana AN, Kanhouche G, de Souza Godoy LG, de Jesus Almeida L, Rodrigues TA, da Silveira CDG, de Oliveira Maia M. Skin mottling score as a predictor of 28-day mortality in patients with septic shock. Intensive Care Med 2016;42: 479−80. https://doi.org/10.1007/s00134-015-4184-4.

[13] Hariri G, Joffre J, Leblanc G, Bonsey M, Lavillegrand J-R, Urbina T, Guidet B, Maury E, Bakker J, Ait-Oufella H. Narrative review: clinical assessment of peripheral tissue perfusion in septic shock. Ann Intensive Care 2019;9: 37. https://doi.org/10.1186/s13613-019-0511-1.

[14] Ait-Oufella H, Bige N, Boelle PY, Pichereau C, Alves M, Bertinchamp R, Baudel JL, Galbois A, Maury E, Guidet B. Capillary refill time exploration during septic shock. Intensive Care Med 2014;40:958−64. https://doi.org/10.1007/s00134-014-3326-4.

[15] Hernández G, Ospina-Tascón GA, Damiani LP, Estenssoro E, Dubin A, Hurtado J, Friedman G, Castro R, Alegría L, Teboul J-L, Cecconi M, Ferri G, Jibaja M, Pairumani R, Fernández P, Barahona D, Granda-Luna V, Cavalcanti AB, Bakker J. For the ANDROMEDA-SHOCK investigators and the Latin America intensive care network (LIVEN), effect of a resuscitation strategy targeting peripheral perfusion status vs serum lactate levels on 28-day mortality among patients with septic shock: the ANDROMEDA-SHOCK randomized clinical trial. JAMA 2019;321:654. https://doi.org/10.1001/jama.2019.0071.

[16] Castro R, Kattan E, Ferri G, Pairumani R, Valenzuela ED, Alegría L, Oviedo V, Pavez N, Soto D, Vera M, Santis C, Astudillo B, Cid MA, Bravo S, Ospina-Tascón G, Bakker J, Hernández G. Effects of capillary refill time-vs.-lactate-targeted fluid resuscitation on regional, microcirculatory and hypoxia-related perfusion parameters in septic shock: a randomized controlled trial. Ann Intensive Care 2020;10:150. https://doi.org/10.1186/s13613-020-00767-4.

[17] Cecconi M, De Backer D, Antonelli M, Beale R, Bakker J, Hofer C, Jaeschke R, Mebazaa A, Pinsky MR, Teboul JL, Vincent JL, Rhodes A. Consensus on circulatory shock and hemodynamic monitoring. Task force of the European Society of Intensive Care Medicine. Intensive Care Med 2014;40:1795−815. https://doi.org/10.1007/s00134-014-3525-z.

[18] Yang X, Du B. Does pulse pressure variation predict fluid responsiveness in critically ill patients? A systematic review and meta-analysis. Crit Care Lond Engl 2014;18: 650. https://doi.org/10.1186/s13054-014-0650-6.

[19] Teboul J-L, Monnet X, Chemla D, Michard F. Arterial pulse pressure variation with mechanical ventilation. Am J Respir Crit Care Med 2019;199:22−31. https://doi.org/10.1164/rccm.201801-0088CI.

[20] Michard F, Chemla D, Richard C, Wysocki M, Pinsky MR, Lecarpentier Y, Teboul J-L. Clinical use of respiratory changes in arterial pulse pressure to monitor the hemodynamic effects of PEEP. Am J Respir Crit Care Med 1999;159:935−9. https://doi.org/10.1164/ajrccm.159.3.9805077.

[21] Hamzaoui O, Shi R, Carelli S, Sztrymf B, Prat D, Jacobs F, Monnet X, Gouëzel C, Teboul J-L. Changes in pulse pressure variation to assess preload responsiveness in mechanically ventilated patients with spontaneous breathing activity: an observational study. Br J Anaesth 2021;127: 532−8. https://doi.org/10.1016/j.bja.2021.05.034.

[22] Michard F, Chemla D, Teboul J-L. Applicability of pulse pressure variation: how many shades of grey? Crit Care 2015;19:144. https://doi.org/10.1186/s13054-015-0869-x.

[23] Myatra SN, Prabu NR, Divatia JV, Monnet X, Kulkarni AP, Teboul J-L. The changes in pulse pressure variation or stroke volume variation after a "tidal volume challenge" reliably predict fluid responsiveness during low tidal volume ventilation. Crit Care Med 2017;45:415−21. https://doi.org/10.1097/CCM.0000000000002183.

[24] Osman D, Ridel C, Ray P, Monnet X, Anguel N, Richard C, Teboul J-L. Cardiac filling pressures are not appropriate to predict hemodynamic response to volume challenge. Crit Care Med 2007;35:64−8. https://doi.org/10.1097/01.CCM.0000249851.94101.4F.

[25] Hamzaoui O, Gouëzel C, Jozwiak M, Millereux M, Sztrymf B, Prat D, Jacobs F, Monnet X, Trouiller P, Teboul J-L. Increase in central venous pressure during passive leg raising cannot detect preload unresponsiveness. Crit Care Med 2020;48:e684−9. https://doi.org/10.1097/CCM.0000000000004414.

[26] Rivers E, Nguyen B, Havstad S, Resslers J, Muzzin A, Knoblich B, Peterson E, Tomlanovich M. Early goal-directed therapy in the treatment of severe sepsis and septic shock. N Engl J Med 2001:10.

[27] Mouncey PR, Osborn TM, Power GS, Harrison DA, Sadique MZ, Grieve RD, Jahan R, Harvey SE, Bell D, Bion JF, Coats TJ, Singer M, Young JD, Rowan KM. Trial of early, goal-directed resuscitation for septic shock. N Engl J Med 2015;372:1301−11. https://doi.org/10.1056/NEJMoa1500896.

[28] The ARISE Investigators and the ANZICS Clinical Trials Group. Goal-directed resuscitation for patients with early septic shock. N Engl J Med 2014;371:1496–506. https://doi.org/10.1056/NEJMoa1404380.

[29] The P.CESS Investigators. A randomized trial of protocol-based care for early septic shock. N Engl J Med 2014;370:1683–93. https://doi.org/10.1056/NEJMoa1401602.

[30] Gavelli F, Teboul J-L, Monnet X. How can CO2-derived indices guide resuscitation in critically ill patients? J Thorac Dis 2019;11:S1528–37. https://doi.org/10.21037/jtd.2019.07.10.

[31] Monnet X, Julien F, Ait-Hamou N, Lequoy M, Gosset C, Jozwiak M, Persichini R, Anguel N, Richard C, Teboul J-L. Lactate and venoarterial carbon dioxide difference/arterial-venous oxygen difference ratio, but not central venous oxygen saturation, predict increase in oxygen consumption in fluid responders. Crit Care Med 2013;41:1412–20. https://doi.org/10.1097/CCM.0b013e318275cece.

[32] Vignon P. Critical care echocardiography: diagnostic or prognostic? Ann Transl Med 2020;8:909. https://doi.org/10.21037/atm-20-3208.

[33] Jozwiak M, Depret F, Teboul J-L, Alphonsine J-E, Lai C, Richard C, Monnet X. Predicting fluid responsiveness in critically ill patients by using combined end-expiratory and end-inspiratory occlusions with echocardiography. Crit Care Med 2017;45:e1131–8. https://doi.org/10.1097/CCM.0000000000002704.

[34] Jozwiak M, Monnet X, Teboul J-L. Less or more hemodynamic monitoring in critically ill patients. Curr Opin Crit Care 2018;24:309–15. https://doi.org/10.1097/MCC.0000000000000516.

[35] Teboul J-L, Saugel B, Cecconi M, De Backer D, Hofer CK, Monnet X, Perel A, Pinsky MR, Reuter DA, Rhodes A, Squara P, Vincent J-L, Scheeren TW. Less invasive hemodynamic monitoring in critically ill patients. Intensive Care Med 2016;42:1350–9. https://doi.org/10.1007/s00134-016-4375-7.

[36] Vignon P, Evrard B, Asfar P, Busana M, Calfee CS, Coppola S, Demiselle J, Geri G, Jozwiak M, Martin GS, Gattinoni L, Chiumello D. Fluid administration and monitoring in ARDS: which management? Intensive Care Med 2020;46:2252–64. https://doi.org/10.1007/s00134-020-06310-0.

[37] Richard C, Warszawski J, Anguel N, Deye N, Combes A, Barnoud D, Boulain T, Lefort Y, Fartoukh M, Baud F, Boyer A, Brochard L, Teboul J-L. Early use of the pulmonary artery catheter and outcomes in patients with shock and acute respiratory distress syndrome. JAMA 2003;290:2713–20.

[38] Michard F, Malbrain ML, Martin GS, Fumeaux T, Lobo S, Gonzalez F, Pinho-Oliveira V, Constantin J-M. Haemodynamic monitoring and management in COVID-19 intensive care patients: an International survey. Anaesth. Crit. Care Pain Med. 2020;39:563–9. https://doi.org/10.1016/j.accpm.2020.08.001.

[39] Monnet X, Teboul J-L. Transpulmonary thermodilution: advantages and limits. Crit Care 2017;21:147. https://doi.org/10.1186/s13054-017-1739-5.

[40] Beurton A, Teboul J-L, Monnet X. Transpulmonary thermodilution techniques in the haemodynamically unstable patient. Curr Opin Crit Care 2019;25(3):273–9. https://doi.org/10.1097/MCC.0000000000000608.

[41] Jozwiak M, Monnet X, Teboul J-L. Pressure waveform analysis. Anesth Analg 2018;126:1930–3. https://doi.org/10.1213/ANE.0000000000002527.

[42] de Courson H, Ferrer L, Cane G, Verchère E, Sesay M, Nouette-Gaulain K, Biais M. Evaluation of least significant changes of pulse contour analysis-derived parameters. Ann Intensive Care 2019;9:116. https://doi.org/10.1186/s13613-019-0590-z.

[43] Shi R, Monnet X, Teboul J-L. Parameters of fluid responsiveness. Curr Opin Crit Care 2020;26:319–26. https://doi.org/10.1097/MCC.0000000000000723.

[44] Monnet X, Rienzo M, Osman D, Anguel N, Richard C, Pinsky MR, Teboul J-L. Passive leg raising predicts fluid responsiveness in the critically ill. Crit Care Med 2006;34:1402–7. https://doi.org/10.1097/01.CCM.0000215453.11735.06.

[45] Monnet X, Teboul J-L. Passive leg raising: five rules, not a drop of fluid. Crit Care Lond Engl 2015;19:18. https://doi.org/10.1186/s13054-014-0708-5.

[46] Monnet X, Marik P, Teboul J-L. Passive leg raising for predicting fluid responsiveness: a systematic review and meta-analysis. Intensive Care Med 2016;42:1935–47. https://doi.org/10.1007/s00134-015-4134-1.

[47] Cherpanath TGV, Hirsch A, Geerts BF, Lagrand WK, Leeflang MM, Schultz MJ, Groeneveld ABJ. Predicting fluid responsiveness by passive leg raising: a systematic review and meta-analysis of 23 clinical trials. Crit Care Med 2016;44:981–91. https://doi.org/10.1097/CCM.0000000000001556.

[48] Monnet X, Osman D, Ridel C, Lamia B, Richard C, Teboul J-L. Predicting volume responsiveness by using the end-expiratory occlusion in mechanically ventilated intensive care unit patients. Crit Care Med 2009;37:951–6. https://doi.org/10.1097/CCM.0b013e3181968fe1.

[49] Gavelli F, Teboul J-L, Monnet X. The end-expiratory occlusion test: please, let me hold your breath. Crit Care 2019;23:274. https://doi.org/10.1186/s13054-019-2554-y.

[50] Messina A, Dell'Anna A, Baggiani M, Torrini F, Maresca GM, Bennett V, Saderi L, Sotgiu G, Antonelli M, Cecconi M. Functional hemodynamic tests: a systematic review and a metanalysis on the reliability of the end-expiratory occlusion test and of the mini-fluid challenge in predicting fluid responsiveness. Crit Care Lond Engl 2019;23:264. https://doi.org/10.1186/s13054-019-2545-z.

[51] Muller L, Toumi M, Bousquet P-J, Riu-Poulenc B, Louart G, Candela D, Zoric L, Suehs C, de La Coussaye J-E, Molinari N, Lefrant J-Y. An increase in aortic blood flow after an infusion of 100 ml colloid over 1 minute can predict fluid responsiveness: the mini-fluid challenge study. Anesthesiology 2011;115:541–7. https://doi.org/10.1097/ALN.0b013e318229a500.

[52] Biais M, de Courson H, Lanchon R, Pereira B, Bardonneau G, Griton M, Sesay M, Nouette-Gaulain K.

Mini-fluid challenge of 100 ml of crystalloid predicts fluid responsiveness in the operating room. Anesthesiology 2017;127:450−6. https://doi.org/10.1097/ALN.0000000000001753.

[53] Jozwiak M, Silva S, Persichini R, Anguel N, Osman D, Richard C, Teboul J-L, Monnet X. Extravascular lung water is an independent prognostic factor in patients with acute respiratory distress syndrome. Crit Care Med 2013;41:472−80. https://doi.org/10.1097/CCM.0b013e31826ab377.

[54] Perel A, Saugel B, Teboul J-L, Malbrain MLNG, Belda FJ, Fernández-Mondéjar E, Kirov M, Wendon J, Lussmann R, Maggiorini M. The effects of advanced monitoring on hemodynamic management in critically ill patients: a pre and post questionnaire study. J Clin Monit Comput 2016;30:511−8. https://doi.org/10.1007/s10877-015-9811-7.

[55] Funcke S, Sander M, Goepfert MS, Groesdonk H, Heringlake M, Hirsch J, Kluge S, Krenn C, Maggiorini M, Meybohm P, Salzwedel C, Saugel B, Wagenpfeil G, Wagenpfeil S, Reuter DA. For the ICU-CardioMan Investigators, Practice of hemodynamic monitoring and management in German, Austrian, and Swiss intensive care units: the multicenter cross-sectional ICU-CardioMan Study. Ann Intensive Care 2016;6:49. https://doi.org/10.1186/s13613-016-0148-2.

[56] Kouz K, Scheeren TWL, de Backer D, Saugel B. Pulse wave analysis to estimate cardiac output. Anesthesiology 2021;134:119−26. https://doi.org/10.1097/ALN.0000000000003553.

[57] Monnet X, Anguel N, Naudin B, Jabot J, Richard C, Teboul J-L. Arterial pressure-based cardiac output in septic patients: different accuracy of pulse contour and uncalibrated pressure waveform devices. Crit Care 2010;14.

[58] Monnet X, Anguel N, Jozwiak M, Richard C, Teboul J-L. Third-generation FloTrac/Vigileo does not reliably track changes in cardiac output induced by norepinephrine in critically ill patients. Br J Anaesth 2012;108:615−22. https://doi.org/10.1093/bja/aer491.

[59] Slagt C, Malagon I, Groeneveld ABJ. Systematic review of uncalibrated arterial pressure waveform analysis to determine cardiac output and stroke volume variation. Br J Anaesth 2014;112:626−37. https://doi.org/10.1093/bja/aet429.

[60] Monnet X, Vaquer S, Anguel N, Jozwiak M, Cipriani F, Richard C, Teboul J-L. Comparison of pulse contour analysis by Pulsioflex and Vigileo to measure and track changes of cardiac output in critically ill patients. Br J Anaesth 2015;114:235−43. https://doi.org/10.1093/bja/aeu375.

[61] Kupersztych-Hagege E, Teboul J-L, Artigas A, Talbot A, Sabatier C, Richard C, Monnet X. Bioreactance is not reliable for estimating cardiac output and the effects of passive leg raising in critically ill patients. Br J Anaesth 2013;111:961−6. https://doi.org/10.1093/bja/aet282.

[62] Galarza L, Mercado P, Teboul J-L, Girotto V, Beurton A, Richard C, Monnet X. Estimating the rapid haemodynamic effects of passive leg raising in critically ill patients using bioreactance. Br J Anaesth 2018;121:567−73. https://doi.org/10.1016/j.bja.2018.03.013.

[63] Gavelli F, Beurton A, Teboul J-L, De Vita N, Azzolina D, Shi R, Pavot A, Monnet X. Bioreactance reliably detects preload responsiveness by the end-expiratory occlusion test when averaging and refresh times are shortened. Ann Intensive Care 2021;11:133. https://doi.org/10.1186/s13613-021-00920-7.

[64] Beurton A, Gavelli F, Teboul J-L, De Vita N, Monnet X. Changes in the plethysmographic perfusion index during an end-expiratory occlusion detect a positive passive leg raising test. Crit Care Med 2021;49:e151−60. https://doi.org/10.1097/CCM.0000000000004768.

[65] Beurton A, Teboul J-L, Gavelli F, Gonzalez FA, Girotto V, Galarza L, Anguel N, Richard C, Monnet X. The effects of passive leg raising may be detected by the plethysmographic oxygen saturation signal in critically ill patients. Crit Care 2019;23:19. https://doi.org/10.1186/s13054-019-2306-z.

[66] de Courson H, Michard F, Chavignier C, Verchère E, Nouette-Gaulain K, Biais M. Do changes in perfusion index reflect changes in stroke volume during preload-modifying manoeuvres? J Clin Monit Comput 2019;34(6):1193−8. https://doi.org/10.1007/s10877-019-00445-2.

[67] Coutrot M, Joachim J, Dépret F, Millasseau S, Nougué H, Matéo J, Mebazaa A, Gayat E, Vallée F. Noninvasive continuous detection of arterial hypotension during induction of anaesthesia using a photoplethysmographic signal: proof of concept. Br J Anaesth 2019;122:605−12. https://doi.org/10.1016/j.bja.2019.01.037.

[68] Truijen J, van Lieshout JJ, Wesselink WA, Westerhof BE. Noninvasive continuous hemodynamic monitoring. J Clin Monit Comput 2012;26:267−78. https://doi.org/10.1007/s10877-012-9375-8.

[69] Kim S-H, Lilot M, Sidhu KS, Rinehart J, Yu Z, Canales C, Cannesson M. Accuracy and precision of continuous noninvasive arterial pressure monitoring compared with invasive arterial pressure. Anesthesiology 2014;120:1080−97. https://doi.org/10.1097/ALN.0000000000000226.

[70] Meidert AS, Huber W, Müller JN, Schöfthaler M, Hapfelmeier A, Langwieser N, Wagner JY, Eyer F, Schmid RM, Saugel B. Radial artery applanation tonometry for continuous non-invasive arterial pressure monitoring in intensive care unit patients: comparison with invasively assessed radial arterial pressure. Br J Anaesth 2014;112:521−8. https://doi.org/10.1093/bja/aet400.

[71] Nachman D, Constantini K, Poris G, Wagnert-Avraham L, Gertz SD, Littman R, Kabakov E, Eisenkraft A, Gepner Y. Wireless, non-invasive, wearable device for continuous remote monitoring of hemodynamic parameters in a swine model of controlled hemorrhagic shock. Sci Rep 2020;10:17684. https://doi.org/10.1038/s41598-020-74686-6.

[72] Michard F. A sneak peek into digital innovations and wearable sensors for cardiac monitoring. J Clin Monit Comput 2017;31:253−9. https://doi.org/10.1007/s10877-016-9925-6.

[73] De Backer D, Creteur J, Preiser J-C, Dubois M-J, Vincent J-L. Microvascular blood flow is altered in patients with sepsis. Am J Respir Crit Care Med 2002;166:98−104. https://doi.org/10.1164/rccm.200109-016OC.

[74] De Backer D, Durand A. Monitoring the microcirculation in critically ill patients. Best Pract Res Clin Anaesthesiol 2014;28:441−51. https://doi.org/10.1016/j.bpa.2014.09.005.

[75] Sakr Y, Dubois M-J, De Backer D, Creteur J, Vincent J-L. Persistent microcirculatory alterations are associated with organ failure and death in patients with septic shock. Crit Care Med 2004;32:1825−31. https://doi.org/10.1097/01.CCM.0000138558.16257.3F.

[76] De Backer D, Donadello K, Sakr Y, Ospina-Tascon G, Salgado D, Scolletta S, Vincent J-L. Microcirculatory alterations in patients with severe sepsis: impact of time of assessment and relationship with outcome. Crit Care Med 2013;41:791−9. https://doi.org/10.1097/CCM.0b013e3182742e8b.

[77] Fiorese Coimbra KT, de Freitas FGR, Bafi AT, Pinheiro TT, Nunes NF, de Azevedo LCP, Machado FR. Effect of increasing blood pressure with noradrenaline on the microcirculation of patients with septic shock and previous arterial hypertension. Crit Care Med 2019;47:1033−40. https://doi.org/10.1097/CCM.0000000000003795.

[78] Ince C, Boerma EC, Cecconi M, De Backer D, Shapiro NI, Duranteau J, Pinsky MR, Artigas A, Teboul J-L, Reiss IKM, Aldecoa C, Hutchings SD, Donati A, Maggiorini M, Taccone FS, Hernandez G, Payen D, Tibboel D, Martin DS, Zarbock A, Monnet X, Dubin A, Bakker J, Vincent J-L, Scheeren TWL. On behalf of the Cardiovascular Dynamics Section of the ESICM, Second consensus on the assessment of sublingual microcirculation in critically ill patients: results from a task force of the European Society of Intensive Care Medicine. Intensive Care Med 2018;44:281−99. https://doi.org/10.1007/s00134-018-5070-7.

[79] Mayeur C, Campard S, Richard C, Teboul J-L. Comparison of four different vascular occlusion tests for assessing reactive hyperemia using near-infrared spectroscopy. Crit Care Med 2011;39:695−701. https://doi.org/10.1097/CCM.0b013e318206d256.

[80] Creteur J, Carollo T, Soldati G, Buchele G, De Backer D, Vincent J-L. The prognostic value of muscle StO$_2$ in septic patients. Intensive Care Med 2007;33:1549−56. https://doi.org/10.1007/s00134-007-0739-3.

[81] Shapiro NI, Arnold R, Sherwin R, O'Connor J, Najarro G, Singh S, Lundy D, Nelson T, Trzeciak SW, Jones AE. The Emergency Medicine Shock Research Network (EMShockNet), the association of near-infrared spectroscopy-derived tissue oxygenation measurements with sepsis syndromes, organ dysfunction and mortality in emergency department patients with sepsis. Crit Care 2011;15:R223. https://doi.org/10.1186/cc10463.

[82] Nardi O, Zavala E, Martin C, Nanas S, Scheeren T, Polito A, Borrat X, Annane D. Targeting skeletal muscle tissue oxygenation (StO$_2$) in adults with severe sepsis and septic shock: a randomised controlled trial (OTO-StS Study).

BMJ Open 2018;8:e017581. https://doi.org/10.1136/bmjopen-2017-017581.

[83] Jozwiak M, Chambaz M, Sentenac P, Monnet X, Teboul J-L. Assessment of tissue oxygenation to personalize mean arterial pressure target in patients with septic shock. Microvasc Res 2020;132:104068. https://doi.org/10.1016/j.mvr.2020.104068.

[84] Scheeren TWL, Ramsay MAE. New developments in hemodynamic monitoring. J Cardiothorac Vasc Anesth 2019;33: S67−72. https://doi.org/10.1053/j.jvca.2019.03.043.

[85] Cannesson M, Tran NP, Cho M, Hatib F, Michard F. Predicting fluid responsiveness with stroke volume variation despite multiple extrasystoles. Crit Care Med 2012;40:193−8. https://doi.org/10.1097/CCM.0b013e31822ea119.

[86] Joosten A, Coeckelenbergh S, Delaporte A, Ickx B, Closset J, Roumeguere T, Barvais L, Van Obbergh L, Cannesson M, Rinehart J, Van der Linden P. Implementation of closed-loop-assisted intra-operative goal-directed fluid therapy during major abdominal surgery: a case−control study with propensity matching. Eur J Anaesthesiol 2018;35:650−8. https://doi.org/10.1097/EJA.0000000000000827.

[87] Joosten A, Rinehart J, Bardaji A, Van der Linden P, Jame V, Van Obbergh L, Alexander B, Cannesson M, Vacas S, Liu N, Slama H, Barvais L. Anesthetic management using multiple closed-loop systems and delayed neurocognitive recovery. Anesthesiology 2020;132:253−66. https://doi.org/10.1097/ALN.0000000000003014.

[88] Libert N, Chenegros G, Harrois A, Baudry N, Cordurie G, Benosman R, Vicaut E, Duranteau J. Performance of closed-loop resuscitation of haemorrhagic shock with fluid alone or in combination with norepinephrine: an experimental study. Ann Intensive Care 2018;8:89. https://doi.org/10.1186/s13613-018-0436-0.

[89] Libert N, Chenegros G, Harrois A, Baudry N, Decante B, Cordurie G, Benosman R, Mercier O, Vicaut E, Duranteau J. Performance of closed-loop resuscitation in a pig model of haemorrhagic shock with fluid alone or in combination with norepinephrine, a pilot study. J Clin Monit Comput 2021;35:835−47. https://doi.org/10.1007/s10877-020-00542-7.

[90] Nemati S, Holder A, Razmi F, Stanley MD, Clifford GD, Buchman TG. An interpretable machine learning model for accurate prediction of sepsis in the ICU. Crit Care Med 2018;46:547−53. https://doi.org/10.1097/CCM.0000000000002936.

[91] Fagerström J, Bång M, Wilhelms D, Chew MS, LiSep LSTM. A machine learning algorithm for early detection of septic shock. Sci Rep 2019;9:15132. https://doi.org/10.1038/s41598-019-51219-4.

[92] Giannini HM, Ginestra JC, Chivers C, Draugelis M, Hanish A, Schweickert WD, Fuchs BD, Meadows L, Lynch M, Donnelly PJ, Pavan K, Fishman NO, Hanson CW, Umscheid CA. A machine learning algorithm to predict severe sepsis and septic shock: development, implementation, and impact on clinical practice. Crit Care Med 2019;47:1485−92. https://doi.org/10.1097/CCM.0000000000003891.

[93] Hatib F, Jian Z, Buddi S, Lee C, Settels J, Sibert K, Rinehart J, Cannesson M. Machine-learning algorithm to predict hypotension based on high-fidelity arterial pressure waveform analysis. Anesthesiology 2018;129:663—74. https://doi.org/10.1097/ALN.0000000000002300.

[94] van der Ven WH, Terwindt LE, Risvanoglu N, Ie ELK, Wijnberge M, Veelo DP, et al. Performance of a machine-learning algorithm to predict hypotension in mechanically ventilated patients with COVID-19 admitted to the intensive care unit: a cohort study. J Clin Monit Comput 2021 Nov 13:1—9. https://doi.org/10.1007/s10877-021-00778-x.

[95] Hyland SL, Faltys M, Hüser M, Lyu X, Gumbsch T, Esteban C, Bock C, Horn M, Moor M, Rieck B, Zimmermann M, Bodenham D, Borgwardt K, Rätsch G, Merz TM. Early prediction of circulatory failure in the intensive care unit using machine learning. Nat Med 2020;26:364—73. https://doi.org/10.1038/s41591-020-0789-4.

[96] Komorowski M, Celi LA, Badawi O, Gordon AC, Faisal AA. The Artificial Intelligence Clinician learns optimal treatment strategies for sepsis in intensive care. Nat Med 2018;24:1716—20. https://doi.org/10.1038/s41591-018-0213-5.

CHAPTER 11

Point of Care Ultrasound in the Management of Sepsis

THARWAT AISA • SAAD MAHDY • AHMED F. HEGAZY

OBJECTIVES

- To highlight the role of point of care ultrasound (POCUS) in the diagnosis of sepsis.
- To review the role of POCUS in fluid resuscitation in sepsis.
- Discuss the role of POCUS in the diagnosis of left ventricular and right ventricular dysfunction in septic patients.
- Elaborate on POCUS-guided management in septic shock.

INTRODUCTION

Septic shock is a very common admission diagnosis in the intensive care unit (ICU). It can present with a multitude of pathophysiological derangements including hypovolemia, hemodynamic failure, left and right ventricular (RV) dysfunction, and cardiomyopathy. Sepsis-induced cardiomyopathy (SICM) (also known as sepsis-induced cardiac dysfunction) can be univentricular, biventricular, or regional in patients without underlying cardiac disease. As an entity, SICM carries mortality implications, and its incidence has been described to range between 10% and 70% [1]. SICM usually occurs in the second or third day of sepsis diagnosis and resolves, if sepsis is adequately treated, after 7—10 days [1].

There is consensus among all critical care societies that critical care echocardiography (CCE) is indicated in all hemodynamically unstable patients admitted to the ICU [2,3]. Point of care ultrasound (POCUS) is a noninvasive tool which can help the clinician at the bedside discern sepsis etiology, cardiac function, volume responsiveness, and periodically revisit fluid management in these often complicated patients. POCUS has therefore evolved to be an important tool in the armamentarium of intensivists managing patients with sepsis and septic shock. This chapter reviews the use of POCUS in the diagnosis of sepsis, source identification, in addition to management of fluid resuscitation, and cardiovascular dysfunction associated with septic shock.

CASE PRESENTATION

A 64-year-old female patient with a history of diabetes mellitus and hypertension presents to the emergency department (ED) with right upper quadrant abdominal pain and feeling generally unwell. Her vital signs on presentation included a blood pressure of 80/47, heart rate 116 beat per minute, temperature 39.4 C, respiratory rate 28/minute, and an oxygen saturation of 94% on room air. She is confused, jaundiced, and has had no urine output since bladder catheter insertion. Her bloodwork reveals leukocytosis, elevated C-reactive protein, acute kidney injury, and deranged liver function tests. With a working diagnosis of sepsis, the ED team start their sepsis management protocol.

IS POCUS HELPFUL IN MANAGING THIS PATIENT?

As per the institutional care pathway, this patient undergoes a full septic screen, cultures are withdrawn, early empiric antibiotics are administered, aggressive fluid resuscitation is initiated, and a noradrenaline infusion is commenced. Despite these initial attempts at stabilization, she remained hypotensive. The intensivist performed a comprehensive POCUS exam in the ED which revealed decreased left ventricular (LV) contractility (ejection fraction [EF] estimated at 30%—40%), global hypokinesia, a markedly collapsible inferior vena cava (IVC), dry lungs with no evidence of lung consolidation, a dilated gall bladder with multiple

The Sepsis Codex. https://doi.org/10.1016/B978-0-323-88271-2.00022-5

stones, and no evidence of obstructive uropathy/hydronephrosis. Further fluid boluses were therefore deemed appropriate, and a dobutamine infusion was added. Given the findings, gastroenterology and general surgery were both consulted, and a decision was made to arrange for an endoscopic retrograde cholangiopancreatography on an urgent basis. After undergoing source control and a further three days of intensive care, markers of organ dysfunction showed signs of improvement. She was eventually transferred out of the ICU in stable condition. A follow-up echocardiogram after 10 days of admission showed normalization of LV systolic function. This case highlights the pivotal role of POCUS in confirming the diagnosis of septic shock, guiding hemodynamic management (fluid resuscitation and vasoactive support), and in the early identification of a septic source.

ROLE OF POCUS IN THE DIAGNOSIS OF SEPSIS

All patients presenting with undifferentiated shock to the ICU warrant CCE. The value of CCE in shock patients lies not only in confirming the provisional diagnosis of septic shock but also in ruling out other potential causes of hemodynamic instability. This is especially important if competing diagnoses are deemed possible. For instance, an elderly nonambulatory patient presenting in shock thought to be secondary to urosepsis is likely to benefit from a POCUS examination to rule out a massive/submassive pulmonary embolism (PE) as a possible alternative or codiagnosis. Timely CCE can help discern with greater certainty shock etiology and expedite management; hence, its importance in this population cannot be overemphasized.

Another equally important role for POCUS in sepsis patients lies in identifying the source. Early source control is of paramount importance in the management of sepsis and should be undertaken in a timely fashion. This is endorsed by the recent Surviving Sepsis Campaign guidelines, which recommend pursuing an anatomic diagnosis for the infection and emergently identifying whether any source control interventions are needed. Once identified, source control interventions should be implemented as soon as medically and logistically practical [4].

POCUS can help diagnose sepsis of intraabdominal origin (e.g., acute cholecystitis, liver abscess, pyelonephritis), pulmonary origin (e.g., pneumonia or empyema), and cardiac origin (infective endocarditis). Cortellaro F et al. found that POCUS-implemented

diagnosis is an effective and reliable tool for the identification of a septic source and found it to be superior to initial clinical evaluation alone with a sensitivity of 73% and a specificity of 95% [5].

Lung ultrasound was also demonstrated to be a powerful tool in diagnosing a myriad of common pulmonary pathologies (e.g., pneumonias, pleural effusions, empyema). Its sensitivity and specificity were shown to be superior to chest radiography and comparable to chest computerized tomography (CT) scans. Furthermore, it can be easily repeated at the bedside allowing serial follow-up of lung pathologies and evaluating the response to treatment. Lastly, POCUS can guide and contribute to the safety of certain interventions like drainage of a pleural effusions [6].

The seminal work of Daniel Lichtenstein laid the foundation of modern point-of-care lung ultrasound [7]. Two types of lung consolidation can be identified; nontranslobar and translobar. Each type has its own specific and distinct features. Nontranslobar consolidation represents most cases and can be distinguished by the "shred sign." The border between consolidated and aerated lung is irregular, forming a fractal line, fully opposed to the lung line. Translobar consolidation can be identified by the "tissue-like" sign. When alveoli of an entire lobe become fluid-filled, a tissue-like sonographic pattern is created also known as lung hepatization (liver-like appearance). When examined adequately, these signs have 90% sensitivity and 98% specificity for diagnosing pneumonia [8]. Ultrasound can also help distinguish a primary lung consolidative process (i.e., pneumonia) with a concomitant effusion versus compressive lung atelectasis secondary to a large pleural effusion. Findings such as dynamic or static air bronchograms, a complex effusion with a plankton sign, and pleural effusion size being less than or equal to the size of the consolidation all favor a primary pneumonic consolidation process [8].

Assessment of pleural effusions is another important application of pulmonary ultrasound. Dickman E and colleagues [9] reported 93% sensitivity and specificity of the extended spine sign to diagnose pleural effusions. Lichtenstein [7] used the posterolateral alveolar or pleural syndrome (PLAPS) point for locating small dependent pleural effusions. His approach generated standardized signs namely the quad sign and the sinusoid sign. The quad sign seen on two-dimensional (2D) imaging consists of a quadrangle of fluid bordered by rib shadows on either side with the parietal pleura in the near-field and the visceral pleura overlying the lung in the far-field. The sinusoid sign is the dynamic equivalent of the quad sign generated on examining pleural effusions using M-mode. Movement of the visceral pleura overlying the lung toward the parietal pleura with each inspiration can generate a sinusoidal appearance. Ultrasound is superior to chest X-rays in diagnosing pleural effusions; ultrasound sensitivity 96%, specificity 100% compared with chest X-ray, sensitivity of 39%, and a specificity of 85% [10]. In general, sonographically complex pleural effusions favor an exudative process and warrant urgent drainage for both diagnostic and therapeutic purposes (source control). Sonographic features of effusion complexity include fluid layering with different fluid densities, floating debris in the effusion known as the plankton sign, and septations and fibrin stranding. Septations within an effusion can progress to forming loculations, we therefore recommend involving thoracic surgery early in the management of these patients [11].

Skin and soft tissue infections, including abscesses and cellulitis, are not uncommon causes of sepsis. POCUS is a valuable tool in the diagnosis and management of soft tissue infections. It can evaluate the extent and depth of infection in addition to the presence of a collection requiring incision and drainage. In a systematic review, it was found that the sensitivity of ultrasound for diagnosing soft tissue infections ranged from 89% to 98% and the specificity ranged from 64% to 88% [12,13].

CCE may detect cardiac valve vegetations, especially if large, making a case for infective endocarditis as the source of sepsis. A thorough 2D examination of valve structure should aim at assessing for vegetations which classically appear as oscillating masses arising from the low pressure side of the leaflets [14]. Vegetations can cause valve destruction or impede valve closure causing acute valvular regurgitation. This can be demonstrated with color flow Doppler interrogation. Caution should be exercised, however, as normal findings of the aortic valve, such as Lambl's excrescences or Arantius nodules, should not be confused for vegetations [15]. In addition, focused transthoracic cardiac ultrasound should not be used to rule out endocarditis as false-negative exams can occur in up to 15% of patients [16]. If clinical suspicion for endocarditis is high, comprehensive transesophageal echocardiography should be performed [17].

Focused abdominal ultrasound may support the diagnosis of acute calculous or acalculous cholecystitis. Most cases of cholecystitis are calculous (90%–95%). Detection of gall bladder stones has therefore been demonstrated to be the most important sonographic feature of cholecystitis [18]. A sonographic Murphy's sign has also been demonstrated to be sensitive for cholecystitis [19]. Other findings suggestive of cholecystitis include gall bladder wall thickening (>3 mm) and the presence of pericholecystic fluid [20].

Ultrasound examination of the kidneys and bladder may provide useful information when obstructive uropathy associated with urosepsis is suspected. Hydronephrosis can be mild, moderate, or severe and is characterized by dilation of the pelvicalyceal system. This usually appears as an anechoic fluid collection within a hyperechoic renal sinus [21]. Unilateral hydronephrosis can be secondary to external ureteral compression or an obstructing ureteric stone. Bilateral hydronephrosis can be caused by bladder outlet obstruction. Ultrasound, however, has a low sensitivity for visualizing ureteric stones [22]. Utilizing ultrasound for the imaging abdominal structures, in general, requires training and expertise. Clinical suspicion for an abdominal source of sepsis, therefore, warrants expert consultation and may necessitate additional imaging.

PRELOAD SENSITIVITY AND VOLUME RESPONSIVENESS

Sepsis is associated with hypotension and hypovolemia due to arterial and venous vasodilation, increased endothelial permeability, and a subsequent capillary leak into the interstitial space. Septic shock patients, therefore, usually require aggressive fluid resuscitation. Responsiveness to volume administration and tolerance to fluid loading could often be predicted with POCUS at the bedside. Fluid responsiveness and fluid tolerance, however, are two distinct concepts. Clinicians involved in the resuscitation of patients with sepsis should have a clear understanding of the difference.

In broad terms, fluid responsiveness refers to the ability of a fluid bolus to produce a favorable hemodynamic response in a patient in shock. The precise definition of fluid responsiveness that we adopt is an increase in stroke volume (SV) by at least 10% after receiving a fluid bolus of 6 mL/kg over a 10-minute period [23]. Volume tolerance, however, refers to the safety margin beyond which adverse events from fluid administration can be encountered. Patients who have limited volume tolerance are likely to develop pulmonary edema, organ congestion, and possibly a prolonged ICU length of stay with excessive volume loading [24]. Certain CCE findings should raise suspicion for a reduced volume tolerance. These include CCE findings of severe RV dilation, severe LV systolic dysfunction, or bilateral diffuse B-lines of the lungs. Such findings warrant either withholding further intravenous fluid boluses, or at a minimum, a very judicious and cautious approach to volume loading [25].

INFERIOR VENA CAVA ASSESSMENT

Evaluating the IVC comprises assessing its absolute diameter and its variability with respiration. In general, diameter of the IVC is affected by right atrial pressure, vessel wall compliance, and intraabdominal pressure. A small IVC diameter (<10 mm [mm] in a spontaneously breathing patients and <15 mm in a mechanically ventilated patient) suggests volume responsiveness. This is especially true if found to be in keeping with the clinical context and other features supportive of volume responsiveness. However, as with most static parameters, absolute IVC diameter has less of a predictive value for fluid responsiveness compared to dynamic parameters [26].

Understanding normal respirophasic variability in IVC size is an essential first step for the clinician performing an ultrasound-informed volume status assessment. In spontaneously breathing patients, chest expansion results in negative intrathoracic pressure drawing blood into the thorax leading to IVC collapse. Conversely, in patients who are mechanically ventilated, inspiratory positive pressure leads to a decrease in venous return causing the IVC to distend. These normally occurring changes in IVC diameter become exaggerated in hypovolemic patients. In a nonintubated spontaneously breathing patient, IVC variability of >50% predicts volume responsiveness. In a mechanically ventilated patient who is completely passive on the ventilator, IVC collapsibility >12% to 18% predicts volume responsiveness. Alternatively, distensibility of the superior vena cava by > 31% on transesophageal echocardiography also predicts volume responsiveness in patients on controlled mechanical ventilation.

Measuring IVC collapsibility can be accomplished using a curvilinear (abdominal) probe or a phased-array (cardiac) probe. The probe is positioned just below the xiphoid process in the subcostal window in a longitudinal orientation, index mark pointed cephalad. If the aorta is visualized, a slight tilt of the probe or moving the probe very subtly to the patient's right will usually result in IVC visualization. It is common for learners and beginners to mistakenly label the descending thoracic aorta as the IVC. Cardinal sonographic features used to identify the IVC include demonstrating the hepatic vein as it joins the IVC, visualizing IVC entry into the right atrium, and clearly visualizing the IVC's intrahepatic course (aorta is retro hepatic). An alternative window to visualize the IVC is the transhepatic (right upper quadrant) window. Normal IVC diameters using this window, however, remain to be established [27]. A very small, flat IVC in septic shock patients can sometimes be difficult to visualize and requires ultrasound expertise and finesse.

Once an adequate longitudinal image of the IVC from the subcostal window is obtained, measuring IVC diameter and variability is best accomplished using M-mode. The M-mode interrogation beam should fall perpendicular on the IVC just next to the hepatic vein approximately 1–2 cm from the cava right atrial junction. After visually inspecting the M-mode screen for IVC variability with respiration, the maximum and minimum IVC diameter should be measured. A collapsibility index of 18% or more is indicative of fluid responsiveness [26]. The collapsibility index can then be calculated for a mechanically ventilated patient using the following equation:

$$\Delta \text{IVC diameter} = \frac{\text{Dmax insp} - \text{Dmin exp}}{\text{Dmin exp}} \times 100$$

Other investigators reported an IVC variability index. These investigators found a change of 12% or more to be indicative of fluid responsiveness [28].

$$\Delta \text{IVC diameter} = \frac{\text{Dmax insp} - \text{Dmin exp}}{\text{Dmean}} \times 100$$

There are multiple limitations that need to be considered when assessing the IVC in the clinical setting. First, for intubated patients, these variability cutoff values that predict volume responsiveness have only been validated in patients who are completely passive on mechanical ventilation. There are no evidence-based variability cutoff values for patients who are triggering on the ventilator (e.g., on pressure support ventilation). Second, while variability values above these cutoffs are often very predictive, obtaining values below these cutoffs does not necessarily rule out volume responsiveness. It is therefore very common for an isolated IVC assessment of volume status to yield an indeterminate result. A multifaceted volume status assessment approach incorporating clinical assessment with multiple sonographic features is therefore preferred. Lastly, examining the IVC with accuracy and reproducibility requires training. The IVC is a cylindrical structure and measuring its true diameter requires the incident ultrasound beam to fall on its center. It is common for learners and beginners to image the IVC off-axis with an oblique incident beam producing a falsely small diameter. We therefore recommend certain tips and tricks to help attain better confidence in sonographic findings.

TIPS AND TRICKS

- Visualizing the descending thoracic aorta on applying the probe means you need to tilt or move your probe slightly to the right.

- It is important not to confuse the descending thoracic aorta with the IVC. The IVC is distinguished from the aorta by demonstrating the hepatic vein as it joins, the IVC's intrahepatic course, and the IVC as it enters the right atrium.
- Volume responsiveness is predicted by assessing the IVC diameter and excessive IVC variability with respiration. Different IVC variability cutoffs have been validated in patients who are extubated and in patients who are completely passive on controlled mechanical ventilation. No validated cutoff values exist for patients who are triggering on the ventilator.
- Off-axis visualization of the IVC can lead to foreshortening (the cylinder effect); hence, very subtle tilting of the probe back and forth until the maximal diameter of the IVC is captured is recommended.
- Vigorous movements of the diaphragm may make assessing IVC diameter at a fixed point along its course extremely challenging. Beware of this translational artifact contributing to what may be misinterpreted as respirophasic variability.

Other applications for IVC assessment include evaluation for tamponade physiology and RV failure. In the right clinical context, a distended noncollapsible IVC is an essential feature of tamponade physiology and can be supportive of the diagnosis of RV failure. Conversely, a small collapsible IVC in a patient with a pericardial effusion effectively rules out tamponade physiology.

VARIATIONS IN THE LEFT VENTRICULAR OUTFLOW TRACT VELOCITY TIME INTERVAL

Patients on mechanical ventilation normally experience an increase in left-sided venous return, LV preload, and SV during positive pressure inspiration. During expiration, however, intrathoracic pressure drops and capacitance of the pulmonary vascular bed increases leading to a drop in LV preload and SV. These respirophasic effects on left-sided cardiac output (COP) tend to be exaggerated in patients who are hypovolemic and volume responsive.

Measurement of LV SV can be easily performed using transthoracic or transesophageal echocardiography. Forward flow though the left ventricular outflow tract (LVOT) with each cardiac cycle approximates the LV SV. This approximation is valid provided there is no significant mitral regurgitation (backward flow) or shunting. Given these prerequisites, SV can be calculated by multiplying the LV cross-sectional area by the LVOT velocity time integral (VTI). The LVOT VTI is obtained using pulse wave Doppler with the interrogation point

placed in the LVOT, 1–2 cm proximal to the aortic valve. In practice, the LVOT VTI can be used as a surrogate for SV alone (normal LVOT VTI: 18–22 cm), given that LVOT cross-sectional area remains largely unchanged throughout the cardiac cycle. Using transthoracic echocardiography, adequate alignment of the pulse wave Doppler beam in the LVOT is necessary and is best achieved in a five-chamber view or three-chamber view. From a transesophageal echocardiography standpoint, adequate LVOT alignment is achieved in either a deep transgastric view or a transgastric long axis view.

Exaggerated respiratory variation in aortic (LVOT) peak velocity could predict volume responsiveness in patients with septic shock [28].

$$\Delta \text{Aortic peak velocity} = \frac{\text{Vpeak max} - \text{Vpeak min}}{\text{Vpeak average}} \times 100$$

LVOT peak velocity variability $\geq 10\%$ was found to be predictive of fluid responsiveness in patients with septic shock with reasonable sensitivity (79%) andand specificity (64%) [29]. This cutoff value, however, is only valid if the patient is on controlled mechanical ventilation and passive on the ventilator (not triggering), with tidal volumes of at least 8 mL/kg, in normal sinus rhythm, and with normal intrabdominal pressure.

When examining different variability cutoffs for volume responsiveness, high variability cutoff values tend to yield better specificity but low sensitivity. Conversely, lower cutoff values tend to yield higher sensitivity but much lower specificity. We therefore do not advocate for a single measurement or cutoff value per se, rather a multifaceted assessment approach incorporating several dynamic parameters and the clinical context.

PASSIVE LEG RAISE TEST

The passive leg raise (PLR) test has been the historic gold standard for assessing volume responsiveness. Passive leg raising causes transient autotransfusion of blood from the peripheral circulation to the central circulation increasing the venous return to the heart. Therefore, it can predict the response to a bolus of 300 mL of blood in a quick and reversible fashion, thus avoiding the risk of circulatory overload. The response to a PLR can be assessed by measuring LVOT VTI at baseline and 1–2 min post-PLR. This approach has been validated in patients who are spontaneously breathing, triggering on the ventilator, and in patients with atrial fibrillation provided multiple LVOT VTI measurements are obtained and averaged out (POCUS book).

An increase in the SV and COP in response to PLR is predictive of fluid responsiveness. Different cutoffs for a predictive SV increase in response to PLR have been reported in the literature. In general, choosing higher cutoff values yield greater specificity but lower sensitivity. Preau et al. evaluated the changes in SV, pulse pressure, and femoral artery velocities in response to the PLR in septic patients and found an increase of ≥10% in SV to be predictive of fluid responsiveness [30]. Conversely, Maisel et al. found PLR to be predictive of fluid responsiveness in mechanically ventilated patients with spontaneous breathing efforts when an increase of >12.5% in SV was observed [31].

TIPS AND TRICKS FOR PERFORMING AN ACCURATE PLR TEST

- Start from the semirecumbent position (head of the bed elevated at 30°), then measure the SV using transthoracic echo assessment of LVOT VTI. Consider averaging out five measurements if patient is in atrial fibrillation.
- Adjust the bed position to supine then elevate the leg of the bed to 45° without touching the patient or inducing any discomfort, pain, or awakening.
- Repeat LVOT VTI measurement after one minute in this legs up position in the same manner and calculate the percentage increase.
- Return patient to semirecumbent position.

LEFT VENTRICLE SYSTOLIC DYSFUNCTION

It is demonstrated in the evidence that myocardial contractility is depressed in septic shock. The process is explained by many mechanisms, such as the effects of circulating cytokines particularly the IL-1, IL-6, and TNF-α, nitric oxide, myocardial edema, and cardiomyocyte apoptosis are also involved. The LV dysfunction can compromise further the hemodynamics instability associated with septic shock. The sepsis-induced systolic dysfunction may include global hypokinesia or regional wall motion abnormalities [32–35]. Since the septic shock is associated with vasodilatation and relative hypovolemia, the LV systolic function might be normal in the initial assessment. Thus, it is suggested to repeat the echocardiographic evaluation after fluid resuscitation and vasopressor initiation. Reduced EF below 40%–45% was reported; however, unlike cardiogenic shock, without elevated filling pressures [36]. In patients with no underling structural heart disease at baseline, LV dimensions are usually normal in patients with sepsis-induced cardiac dysfunction. Normal LV dimensions are typical of acute systolic dysfunction unlike chronic dysfunction where the left ventricle tends to dilate over time.

Evaluation of LV systolic function can be achieved from the apical four-chamber, subcostal, and parasternal long and short axis views. The assessment could be quantitatively by estimating the EF or fractional shortening using M-mode or qualitatively by eyeballing. It is found in the studies that the qualitative evaluation is equivalent to the quantitative one if the echocardiography is performed by experienced operator. The basic echocardiographer, however, can appreciate the LV function as severely impaired, moderately impaired, normal, or hyperdynamic. Fractional shortening of LV cavity can be estimated using the M-mode through the cavity during end systole and end diastole. EF can be estimated using M-mode in the parasternal views or by Simpson method in the apical four-chamber and two-chamber views. These changes are usually reversible; however, it should guide the clinician at the bedside to adjust the fluid management in addition to the vasopressor or inotropic usage.

LEFT VENTRICLE DIASTOLIC DYSFUNCTION

It has been reported in several studies that septic shock is associated with LV diastolic dysfunction, and it has been associated with high mortality [37–39]. It can occur as an isolated abnormality or in conjunction with systolic dysfunction. Although the role and significance of diastolic dysfunction in sepsis is still unclear, but its assessment might help estimate the LV and left atrial pressures and subsequently the pulmonary capillary pressure. This could help the clinician to guide the fluid resuscitation in septic patients.

HOW TO ASSESS?

The latest guidelines of the American Society of Echocardiography and European Association of Cardiovascular Imaging recommended to measure four variables and their cutoff values to diagnose diastolic dysfunction.

Those variables are annular e′ velocity: septal e′ < 7 cm/s, lateral e′ < 10 cm/s, average E/e′ ratio >14, left atrium volume index >34 mL/m^2, and peak tricuspid regurgitation velocity >2.8 m/s. LV diastolic function is normal if more than half of the available variables do not meet the cutoff values for identifying abnormal function. LV diastolic dysfunction is present if more than half of the available parameters meet these cutoff values. The study is inconclusive if half of the parameters do not meet the cutoff values [40].

The measurements can be obtained from the apical four-chamber view. By using the pulsed wave Doppler and applying it at the tip of mitral valve leaflets, you can get the E/A ratio.

TIPS AND TRICKS

To get accurate measurement, we need to avoid being too apical.

Keep the Doppler angle below 20°.

Average measurements of three cycles are required.

To obtain the e', we need to get the apical four-chamber view, by applying the tissue Doppler image at the septal or lateral mitral annulus. The septal mitral annulus is usually easier to use for measurement, and the velocity is slower than the lateral one.

RIGHT VENTRICLE DYSFUNCTION IN SEPSIS

Sepsis can affect the RV function directly or indirectly. The patient with sepsis can present with pneumonia and/or acute respiratory distress syndrome, which is subsequently associated with increased pulmonary vascular resistance leading to RV dysfunction. Additionally, mechanical ventilation with high positive end-expiratory pressure can worsen the RV function by increasing the RV afterload. Direct depression of the RV contractility may be related to the circulating inflammatory mediators as occurs in LV dysfunction. The incidence of RV dilation in sepsis ranges between 11% and 32% [36].

Qualitative assessment of the RV function can be obtained by in the apical four-chamber view and parasternal views. We can appreciate the global movement and contractility of RV free wall, interventricular septal movement throughout the cardiac cycle, alongside with its size. The bulging of the interventricular septum toward the LV is indicative of pressure or volume overload. This creates the classic D-shaped LV cavity in the short-axis view.

Quantitative assessment of the RV systolic function can be obtained by measuring the tricuspid annular plane systolic excursion (TAPSE) in the longitudinal direction [41]. By using the M-mode, the TAPSE can be measured in the apical four-chamber view, which is normally more than 16 mm. Values less than 16 mm indicate poor function. Another way of evaluating the RV displacement motion is by measuring the systolic excursion of the tricuspid peak velocity using the pulsed wave Doppler. RV dimensions can be obtained in all apical, subcostal, and parasternal views.

POCUS-GUIDED MANAGEMENT IN SEPTIC SHOCK

Implementing POCUS early in the management of sepsis is of paramount importance for many reasons. It is crucial to have a tool which is portable, repeatable, and handy to get a lot of information at the bedside especially for unstable, unmovable critically ill patient. The POCUS can help identify the source of sepsis and guide its control, like ultrasound-guided drainage of a collection or drain insertion. It can guide the fluid resuscitation using the echocardiographic parameters, IVC collapsibility index, VTI variability, using the PLR test to determine the need for further volume resuscitation or not. Furthermore, the echocardiography can help evaluate the LV function and so guide the use of inotropic or vasopressor support. Additionally, the intensivist can rule out other causes of shock like the obstructive shock (e.g., cardiac tamponade, tension pneumothorax, or in case of massive PE), cardiogenic shock, significant valvular pathology, or wall motion abnormalities, which raise the concern of ischemic heart disease or hemorrhagic shock (extended focused assessment with sonography in trauma). Many comprehensive and focused protocols have been published and validated for using POCUS in the critically ill patients with different underlying pathologies including BLUE (beside lung ultrasound in emergency) protocol for lung diseases [42], RUSH (rapid ultrasound in shock) protocol for the shocked patients [43], and FATE (focus-assessed transthoracic echocardiography) protocol for hemodynamic assessment and optimization [44,45]. Therefore, POCUS can answer many questions at the bedside for the critically ill patients especially in septic shock.

KEY POINTS

- POCUS is found to be helpful in the diagnosis and source control of sepsis.
- CCE as a part of POCUS is a validated tool to manage the fluid responsiveness in sepsis.
- LV and RV dysfunction is not uncommon in sepsis, and it is easily identifiable abnormalities by CCE.
- Applying the integrated approaches using POCUS can answer many questions at the bedside for the management of critically ill patients.

REFERENCES

[1] L'Heureux M, Sternberg M, Brath L, Turlington J, Kashiouris MG. Sepsis-induced cardiomyopathy: a comprehensive review. Curr Cardiol Rep May 6, 2020; 22(5):35. https://doi.org/10.1007/s11886-020-01277-2.

[2] Vieillard-Baron A, Millington SJ, Sanfilippo F, Chew M, DiazGomez J, McLean A, et al. A decade of progress in critical care echocardiography: a narrative review. Intensive Care Med 2019;45:770—88 [Extensive review of critical care echocardiography].

[3] Alhamid S, Balik M, Beaulieu Y, Breitkreutz R. Expert round table on echocardiography in ICU. International consensus statement on training standards for advanced critical care echocardiography. Intensive Care Med 2014;40:654—66.

[4] Rhodes A, Evans LE, Alhazzani W, Levy MM, Antonelli M, Ferrer R, et al. Surviving sepsis campaign: international guidelines for management of sepsis and septic shock: 2016. Intensive Care Med March 2017;43(3):304—77. https://doi.org/10.1007/s00134-017-4683-6. Epub 2017 Jan 18.

[5] Cortellaro F, Ferrari L, Molteni F, et al. Accuracy of point of care ultrasound to identify the source of infection in septic patients: a prospective study. Intern Emerg Med 2017;12:371—8. https://doi.org/10.1007/s11739-016-1470-2.

[6] Shrestha GS, Weeratunga D, Baker K. Point-of-care lung ultrasound in critically ill patients. Rev Recent Clin Trials January 31, 2018;13(1):15—26. https://doi.org/10.2174/1574887112666170911125750. PMID: 28901850.

[7] Lichtenstein DA. Lung ultrasound in the critically ill. Ann Intensive Care January 9, 2014;4(1):1. https://doi.org/10.1186/2110-5820-4-1. PMID: 24401163; PMCID: PMC3895677.

[8] Lichtenstein D, Lascols N, Mezière G, Gepner A. Ultrasound diagnosis of alveolar consolidation in the critically ill. Intensive Care Med 2004;30:276—81.

[9] Dickman E, Terentiev V, Likourezos A, Derman A, Haines L. Extension of the thoracic spine sign: a new sonographic marker of pleural effusion. J Ultrasound Med September 2015;34(9):1555—61. https://doi.org/10.7863/ultra.15.14.06013. Epub 2015 Aug 12. PMID: 26269297.

[10] Soni NJ, Franco R, Velez MI, Schnobrich D, Dancel R, Restrepo MI, Mayo PH. Ultrasound in the diagnosis and management of pleural effusions. J Hosp Med December 2015;10(12):811—6. https://doi.org/10.1002/jhm.2434. Epub 2015 Jul 28. PMID: 26218493; PMCID: PMC4715558.

[11] Ludwig N, Hegazy A. Pulmonary ultrasound. In: Slinger P, editor. Principles and practice of anesthesia for thoracic surgery. Springer International Publishing; 2019. p. 457—69. https://doi.org/10.1007/978-1-4419-0184-2.

[12] Alsaawi A, Alrajhi K, Alshehri A, Ababtain A, Alsolamy S. Ultrasonography for the diagnosis of patients with clinically suspected skin and soft tissue infections: a systematic review of the literature. Eur J Emerg Med June 2017;24(3):162—9. https://doi.org/10.1097/MEJ.0000000000000340.

[13] Barbic D, Chenkin J, Cho DD, Jelic T, Scheuermeyer FX. In patients presenting to the emergency department with skin and soft tissue infections what is the diagnostic accuracy of point-of-care ultrasonography for the diagnosis of abscess compared to the current standard of care? A systematic review and meta-analysis. BMJ Open January 10, 2017;7(1):e013688. https://doi.org/10.1136/bmjopen-2016-013688.

[14] Hegazy AF. In: Soni NJ, Arntfield R, Kory P, editors. "Valves" in point-of-care ultrasound. 2nd ed. Elsevier; 2020. p. 167—75. 13: 978-0323544702.

[15] Ho SY. Structure and anatomy of the aortic root. Eur J Echocardiogr 2009;10(1):i3—10. https://doi.org/10.1093/ejechocard/jen243.

[16] Habib G, Badano L, Tribouilloy C, et al. Recommendations for the practice of echocardiography in infective endocarditis. Eur J Echocardiogr 2010;11(2):202—19. https://doi.org/10.1093/ejechocard/jeq004.

[17] Baddour LM, Wilson WR, Bayer AS, et al. American heart association committee on rheumatic fever, endocarditis, and kawasaki disease of the council on cardiovascular disease in the young, council on clinical cardiology, council on cardiovascular surgery and anesthesia, and stroke council. Infective endocarditis in adults: diagnosis, antimicrobial therapy, and management of complications: a scientific statement for healthcare professionals from the American heart association. Circulation October 13, 2015;132(15):1435—86. https://doi.org/10.1161/CIR.0000000000000296.

[18] Villar J, Summers SM, Menchine MD, Fox JC, Wang R. The absence of gallstones on point-of-care ultrasound rules out acute cholecystitis. J Emerg Med October 2015; 49(4):475—80. https://doi.org/10.1016/j.jemermed.2015.04.037. Epub 2015 Jul 7. PMID: 26162764.

[19] Summers SM, Scruggs W, Menchine MD, Lahham S, Anderson C, Amr O, Lotfipour S, Cusick SS, Fox JC. A prospective evaluation of emergency department bedside ultrasonography for the detection of acute cholecystitis. Ann Emerg Med August 2010;56(2): 114—22. https://doi.org/10.1016/j.annemergmed.2010.01.014. PMID: 20138397.

[20] Ralls PW, Colletti PM, Lapin SA, Chandrasoma P, Boswell Jr WD, Ngo C, Radin DR, Halls JM. Real-time sonography in suspected acute cholecystitis. Prospective evaluation of primary and secondary signs. Radiology June 1985;155(3):767—71. https://doi.org/10.1148/radiology.155.3.3890007. PMID: 3890007.

[21] Noble VE, Brown DF. Renal ultrasound. Emerg Med Clin August 2004;22(3):641—59. https://doi.org/10.1016/j.emc.2004.04.014. PMID: 15301843.

[22] Fowler KA, Locken JA, Duchesne JH, Williamson MR. US for detecting renal calculi with nonenhanced CT as a reference standard. Radiology January 2002;222(1): 109—13. https://doi.org/10.1148/radiol.2221010453. PMID: 11756713.

[23] Cherpanath TG, Aarts LP, Groeneveld JA, Geerts BF. Defining fluid responsiveness: a guide to patient-tailored volume titration. J Cardiothorac Vasc Anesth June 2014;28(3):745—54. https://doi.org/10.1053/j.jvca.2013.12.025. PMID: 24917061.

[24] Vincent JL, Gerlach H. Fluid resuscitation in severe sepsis and septic shock: an evidence-based review. Crit Care

Med November 2004;32(11 Suppl. l):S451–4. https://doi.org/10.1097/01.ccm.0000142984.44321.a4. PMID: 15542955.

[25] [Chapter 21]: Hemodynamics in PoCUS textbook by Soni, Arntfield, Perry. ISBN-13: 978-0323544702.

[26] Barbier C, Loubieres Y, Schmit C, et al. Respiratory changes in inferior vena cava diameter are helpful in predicting fluid responsiveness in ventilated septic patients. Intensive Care Med 2004;30:1740–6.

[27] Qasem F, Hegazy AF, Fuller JG, Lavi R, Singh SI. Inferior vena cava assessment in term pregnant women using ultrasound: a comparison of the subcostal and right upper quadrant views. Anaesth Intensive Care September 2021; 49(5):389–94. https://doi.org/10.1177/0310057X2110 34181.

[28] Feissel M, Michard F, Faller JP, Teboul JL. The respiratory variation in inferior vena cava diameter as a guide to fluid therapy. Intensive Care Med September 2004;30(9): 1834–7. https://doi.org/10.1007/s00134-004-2233-5. Epub 2004 Mar 25. PMID: 15045170.

[29] Vignon P, Repessé X, Bégot E, Léger J, Jacob C, Bouferrache K, Slama M, Prat G, Vieillard-Baron A. Comparison of echocardiographic indices used to predict fluid responsiveness in ventilated patients. Am J Respir Crit Care Med April 15, 2017;195(8):1022–32. https://doi.org/10.1164/rccm.201604-0844OC. PMID: 27653798.

[30] Préau S, Saulnier F, Dewavrin F, Durocher A, Chagnon JL. Passive leg raising is predictive of fluid responsiveness in spontaneously breathing patients with severe sepsis or acute pancreatitis. Crit Care Med March 2010;38(3):819–25. https://doi.org/10.1097/CCM.0b013e3181c8fe7a.

[31] Maizel J, Airapetian N, Lorne E, Tribouilloy C, Massy Z, Slama M. Diagnosis of central hypovolemia by using passive leg raising. Intensive Care Med July 2007;33(7): 1133–8. https://doi.org/10.1007/s00134-007-0642-y.

[32] Yu P, Boughner DR, Sibbald WJ, keys J, Dunmore J, Martin CM. Myocardial collagen changes and edema in rats with hyperdynamic sepsis. Crit Care Med 1997;25:657–62.

[33] Neviere R, Fauvel H, Chopin C, Formstecher P, Marchetti P. Caspase inhibition prevents cardiac dysfunction and heart apoptosis in a rat model of sepsis. Am J Respir Crit Care Med 2001;163:218–25.

[34] Krishnagopalan S, Kumar A, Parrillo JE. Myocardial dysfunction in the patient with sepsis. Curr Opin Crit Care 2002;8:376–88.

[35] Kumar A, Krieger A, Symeoneides S, Parrillo JE. Myocardial dysfunction in septic shock: Part II. Role of cytokines and nitric oxide. J Cardiothorac Vasc Anesth 2001;15:485–511.

[36] Kanji HD, McCallum J, Sirounis D, MacRedmond R, Moss R, Boyd JH. Limited echocardiography-guided therapy in subacute shock is associated with change in management and improved outcomes. J Crit Care October 2014; 29(5):700–5. https://doi.org/10.1016/j.jcrc.2014.04.008.

[37] Etchecopar-Chevreuil C, Francois B, Clavel M, Pichon N, Gastinne H, Vignon P. Cardiac morphological and functional changes during early septic shock: a transesophageal echocardiographic study. Intensive Care Med 2008;34:250–6.

[38] Jafri SM, Lavine S, Field BE, Bahorozian MT, Carlson RW. Left ventricular diastolic function in sepsis. Crit Care Med 1990;18:709–14.

[39] Munt B, Jue J, Gin K, Fenwick J, Tweeddale M. Diastolic filling in human severe sepsis: an echocardiographic study. Crit Care Med 1998;26:1829–33.

[40] Nagueh SF, Smiseth OA, Appleton CP, Byrd 3rd BF, Dokainish H, Edvardsen T, Flachskampf FA, Gillebert TC, Klein AL, Lancellotti P, Marino P, Oh JK, Popescu BA, Waggoner AD. Recommendations for the evaluation of left ventricular diastolic function by echocardiography: an update from the American society of echocardiography and the European association of cardiovascular imaging. J Am Soc Echocardiogr April 2016;29(4):277–314. https://doi.org/10.1016/j.echo.2016.01.011.

[41] Ueti OM, Camargo EE, Ueti A de A, Lima-Filho E C de, Nogueira EA. Assessment of right ventricular function with Doppler echocardiographic indices derived from tricuspid annular motion: comparison with radionuclide angiography. Heart 2002;88:244–8.

[42] Lichtenstein DA. BLUE-protocol and FALLS-protocol: two applications of lung ultrasound in the critically ill. Chest June 2015;147(6):1659–70. https://doi.org/10.1378/chest.14-1313.

[43] (28) Perera P, Mailhot T, Riley D, Mandavia D. The RUSH exam: rapid Ultrasound in SHock in the evaluation of the critically Ill. Emerg Med Clin February 2010;28(1): 29–56. https://doi.org/10.1016/j.emc.2009.09.010. vii.

[44] Breitkreutz R, Walcher F, Seeger FH. Focused echocardiographic evaluation in resuscitation management: concept of an advanced life support-conformed algorithm. Crit Care Med May 2007;35(5 Suppl. l):S150–61. https://doi.org/10.1097/01.CCM.0000260626.23848.FC.

[45] Jensen MB, Sloth E, Larsen KM, Schmidt MB. Transthoracic echocardiography for cardiopulmonary monitoring in intensive care. Eur J Anaesthesiol September 2004;21(9): 700–7. https://doi.org/10.1017/s0265021504009068.

CHAPTER 12

New Approaches and Understanding of Sepsis

VANESSA FONSECA-FERRER • SULIMAR MORALES-COLÓN •
LUIS GERENA-MONTANO • WILLIAM RODRÍGUEZ-CINTRÓN •
GLORIA M. RODRÍGUEZ-VEGA

INTRODUCTION

The definition of sepsis has evolved since the early 1990s [1]. It is defined as a dysregulated host response to an otherwise ordinary infection, characterized by various biological, physiological, and biochemical abnormalities. It is one of the oldest described illnesses and is the leading cause of death secondary to an infection among hospitalized patients in the intensive care unit (ICU). Diagnosis is sometimes difficult, given the multiple comorbidities and underlying disease that are present in most patients [2].

The word sepsis is derived from the ancient Greek term "make rotten," and it was described by Hippocrates around the year 400 BC to describe the natural process of meat decay and swaps where gas is released, but also through which infected wounds become purulent. It was about 2000 years later where the first hypothesis was set up, in which it is not the pathogen itself but rather the host response which is responsible for the symptoms that characterized sepsis [3].

In August of 1991, the American College of Chest Physicians/Society of Critical Care Medicine (ACCP/SCCM) held the first consensus conference with the objective to define sepsis, its sequelae, and guidelines for the use of innovative therapies in sepsis. At that time, a broad framework was done to define systemic inflammatory response syndrome (SIRS), sepsis, and severe sepsis. These conditions were thought to be a continuum of worsening inflammation starting with SIRS and evolving to the point of septic shock. By 2001, a sepsis definition conference was held to decide if new updates in sepsis definition would be made based on new data [4]. In 2002, the SCCM and the European Society of Intensive Care Medicine announced the Barcelona Declaration with the launch the Surviving Sepsis Campaign (SSC) with the goal of reducing mortality from sepsis by 25%.

The Global Sepsis Alliance estimates that sepsis affects between 47 and 50 million individuals every year of which at least 11 million die. This makes sepsis a global health crisis, impacting millions of people around the world each year, and depending on the country, mortality rates vary from 15% to over 50%. Early recognition and diagnosis of sepsis is required to avoid transition into septic shock, which has a high mortality rate of 40% or higher. Improvements in standards of care have decreased mortality rates since the first publication of the SSC Guidelines in 2004 [5]. Throughout the years, literature has been making changes, and the focus has shifted to early identification, proper management, and treatment in the initial hours after the development of sepsis. Based on this, we have seen that many patients are surviving sepsis, some patients do well, and they are being discharged from hospital quickly, while others may suffer from the long-term consequences of sepsis and become chronically ill, experiencing many challenges in recovery. Based on this, newer guidelines have addressed this issue and emphasized improving the care of sepsis patients' post-ICU and hospital discharge.

MONITORING CLINICAL SIGNS

Sepsis may affect everyone, but it has a particular risk in patients who suffer from preexisting medical comorbidities such as pulmonary diseases, diabetes, obesity, kidney disease, and cancer. Other risks include patients older than 65 years old, pregnant, weakened immune system such as those patients with AIDS, asplenia, and hepatic and renal failure, burn patient, patients with bacteremia, hospitalized patients, those with intravenous catheters, indwelling foley, and mechanical ventilation.

The Sepsis Codex. https://doi.org/10.1016/B978-0-323-88271-2.00013-4

The clinical signs and symptoms that characterize sepsis mostly depend on the involved or affected organ, for example, cough when the underlying disease is a pneumonia or acute abdominal pain noted when a patient develops sepsis secondary to an acute appendicitis or pancreatitis. Still common symptoms include fever or hypothermia, shaking chills, confusion or disorientation, tachycardia, tachypnea, and chills. Clinical signs are nonspecific and may include low platelet count, acidosis, leukopenia (<4000 mL^{-1}) or leukocytosis ($>12,000$mL^{-1}), hyperglycemia, arterial hypoxemia, elevated plasma C-reactive protein (CRP) and lactate levels (>2 mmol/L), abnormal coagulation panel, adrenal insufficiency, hyperbilirubinemia, acute kidney injury, liver dysfunction, and, in some cases, a positive blood culture.

In those cases, where the disease progresses to septic shock, sphygmomanometer may be unreliable requiring the insertion of an arterial catheter to monitor blood pressure more precisely. Patient with septic shock will show signs of end-organ perfusion such as cool extremities, decreased capillary refill, cyanosis, and, in some cases, mottling. Obtundation and oliguria, as well as absent bowel sounds are seen at the end stage of hypoperfusion. It is important to highlight that a patient with an underlying use of beta blockers secondary to a diabetic or heart condition may not exhibit the common signs of tachycardia. Physical examination and knowledge of patient's medical history are vital to achieve diagnosis as soon as possible.

Early detection is key to impact mortality. It has been documented that every hour of delayed care worsens outcomes by 6%, and about 30% of those who lapse into septic shock end up dying. Technology has focused in reducing the time of detection and initiation of treatment. For example, electronic health record–based sepsis phenotyping showed better performance when compared with other automated definitions of sepsis [6].

Mobile health (mHealth) focuses on obtaining information immediately to diagnose illness, track diseases, and provide timely information. The emergence of mHealth has proven important in remote areas where healthcare providers may not be present to provide treatment. To assist clinicians at the bedside, mHealth companies and health systems are targeting sepsis with mobile monitoring platforms designed to identify the condition at its earliest stages, while others are developing mobile-accessible clinical decision support platforms and even games designed to help clinicians identify sepsis as soon as possible.

Clinical decision support interventions continue to have a role in the complex critical care environment.

Evolving artificial intelligence and machine learning models hold promise to improve patient outcomes by being applied in the multiple stages of sepsis [7].

DIAGNOSIS

Diagnosis of sepsis is highly based on clinical suspicion and the presence of organ dysfunction. Diagnosis does not require any radiographic or microbiological evidence, but it aids in identifying the possible source of infection. In those cases, where notable hypotension is not noted, elevated levels of lactate are a sign of tissue hypoperfusion, requiring aggressive medical therapy.

Sepsis-3 challenged the original conceptualization of sepsis as defined by the SIRS criteria since it focused solely on the inflammatory response [8] and not necessarily reflected the dysregulated or exaggerated host response to an infection [9]. The Sepsis-3 Task Force recommended the use of the Sepsis-related Organ Failure Assessment (SOFA) score as a simple screening tool to identify dysfunction resulting from sepsis [10]. Currently the quick SOFA (qSOFA) was developed and implemented as a bedside tool to predict death and prolong intensive care admission in patients with known or suspected sepsis. The qSOFA consists of three easy to identify criteria, which consist of altered level of consciousness (Glasgow score equal to or less than 13), systolic blood pressure equal to or less than 100 mmHg, and a respiratory rate equal to or more than 22 breaths per minute. A score of 2 or higher as a similar predictive value as the original SOFA in the identification of patient with sepsis and poor outcome. Data suggest that regardless of the initial SOFA score, those who have an increase in the first 48 h of admission, have a higher mortality rate of at least 50% [11]. Other scores such as the National Early Warning Score (NEWS) and the Modified Early Warning Score (MEWS) have been developed, but the SSC of 2021 recommends against using qSOFA compared to SIRS, NEWS, or MEWS as a single screening tool for sepsis or septic shock [12,13]. The qSOFA is more specific but less sensitive to the SIRS criteria in the identification of organ dysfunction, for which clinicians need to understand the limitation of all four [4] screening tools. In those with suspected sepsis, measuring of lactate levels is recommended as an adjunctive test to modify the pretest probability of sepsis in patients with suspected but not confirmed diagnosis of sepsis [12,13].

The diagnosis of sepsis also requires biochemical, hematological, and microbiological studies to monitor for acid-base disturbances, blood oxygenation, and organ dysfunction. Imaging studies such as X-rays, ultrasound, and computerized tomography scans are commonly used for better evaluation of organ involvement and monitoring of complications. As the microbiological studies are not always conclusive and are slow to grow, several efforts are being made in the use of biomarkers as a tool for early diagnosis of sepsis. Most studied markers are related to the inflammatory phase of sepsis and include CRP and procalcitonin (PCT). Still all these tools need to be correlated with other laboratory studies and clinician medical evaluation and assessment [14].

MONITORING WITH BIOMARKERS AND PRACTICAL APPLICATION OF MONITORING SYSTEMS IN THE DIFFERENT PHASES OF SEPSIS

What exactly is a biomarker? According to the National Institute of Health, a biomarker is an objectively measured indicator of a biologic, pathogenic, or pharmacological reaction [15]. In clinical practice, it is used as a diagnostic or prognostication tool and in some cases to determine which patients may benefit from a particular therapeutic option. The use of biomarkers for the diagnosis of sepsis and septic shock has risen over the years and varies depending on the disease phase.

Over the years, it was noticed that although the 1991 consensus conference laid the framework to define sepsis, it had important limitations. The definition of SIRS required at least 2 of 4 criteria; however, this criterion did not include biochemical markers, such as CRP, PCT, or interleukin 6 (IL-6), all of which are elevated in sepsis. Based on this, the Sepsis-2 definition was introduced in 2001 expanding the list of signs and symptoms of sepsis. Sepsis arises through the activation of an innate immune response, with changes in the expression and activation of thousands of endogenous mediators of inflammation, coagulation, and intermediary metabolism. Components of this response are attractive targets of therapy. More than 100 distinct molecules have been proposed as useful biological markers of sepsis; however, it is not known which of these provides truly useful information or utility. The utility of a biomarker lies in its capacity to provide timely information beyond that which is readily available from routine physiologic data and clinical examination. A biomarker may serve one or more of five overlapping roles, which are screening, diagnosis, risk stratification, monitoring, and surrogate end point. In 2005, the International Sepsis Forum Colloquium on Biomarkers of Sepsis developed a systematic framework for the identification

and validation of biomarkers in sepsis [16]. They proposed that the use of biomarkers could potentially change our view of sepsis, from one broad physiologic syndrome to a group of diverse biochemical disorders. Based on this view, this would help in the therapeutic decision-making and improve the prognosis of septic patients.

Sepsis may be divided into two phases, one that is characterized by a proinflammatory phase that sometimes resolves with no progression to shock and a second phase which is an immunosuppressive phase characterized by organ dysfunction and that is commonly known as a compensatory antiinflammatory syndrome. Both phases are marked by different biomarkers. Among the proinflammatory phase is the CRP, which is commonly synthesized by alveolar macrophages or the liver after an inflammation, trauma, or tissue damage. It is usually released by stimulus of tumor necrosis factor (TNF-alpha), IL-6 and interleukin 1. Its short half-life of 19 h aids in its use as a monitoring tool for infection, response to antibiotic therapy, and assessment of sepsis severity [17]. In cases of neonatal sepsis, it is commonly used as a diagnostic tool for early onset sepsis (within 24 h). PCT is another useful marker. It is usually at low levels in the plasma and increased as a result of cytokines and bacterial endotoxins secondary to infection. It has the potential to discriminate between noninfectious and infectious inflammation in patient with low acuity, as well as to distinct between the presence of a viral or bacterial infection [18]. When comparing both markers, PCT's kinetics and half-life make it a better biomarker for early diagnosis of sepsis and disease progression.

At the immunosuppressive phase, studies have shown a decreased expression of human leukocyte antigen (HLA)-DR and functional inactivation of monocytes. The HLA classes are responsible for antigen presentation to CD4-T lymphocyte to initiate an immune response. In sepsis, the decreased expression of HLA-DR may serve as a sign of severe immunosuppression, as myocytes will not secrete cytokines and present antigen essential for antibacterial response and prevention of complications associated with such infections [19].

INFECTIOUS MONITORING

Sepsis has been commonly associated with bacteria as the predominant pathogen in those cases where an organism is identified. Among the most common organisms identified are Gram-positive bacteria, followed by Gram-negative bacteria. Over the years, the incidence of multidrug resistance organisms and resistant strains of methicillin-resistant *Staphylococcus aureus*, extended spectrum B lactamase, and vancomycin-resistant enterococci are commonly found in critically ill patients. Causes of sepsis by viruses are usually underdiagnosed. Fungal sepsis is becoming more common over time, and in half of the cases, an organism is never identified, known as culture-negative sepsis.

The viruses commonly identified are influenza A and B, respiratory syncytial virus, parainfluenza type 1 and 3, coronavirus, enterovirus, adenovirus, and rhinovirus. There is also an emerging organism as the novel corona virus (SARS-CoV-2) that forms part of the recent pandemic that started in the year 2019 [20].

Organism may affect any organ, but most cases arise from infection to the respiratory tract leading to pneumonia. Other infections include abdominal skin, central nervous system, endocarditis, and the genitourinary tract infections.

MONITORING ACCORDING WITH ORGAN DYSFUNCTION

Throughout the years, the understanding of the pathophysiology of sepsis has evolved from a simple activation of anti- and proinflammatory response to a more complex activation of nonimmunological pathways involving autonomic, cardiovascular, metabolic, hormonal, and clotting system. This knowledge led to the new definition in 2016 as a life-threatening organ dysfunction secondary to a host response to an infection and that of septic shock, defined as a complication of sepsis, which involved metabolic/circulatory abnormalities which increase overall patient's mortality [8].

Organ dysfunction results from damage to the epithelial lining of the lungs, kidneys, intestines, and liver. Epithelial and endothelial dysfunction result from the increased permeability and loss of the epithelial barriers that may result in acute lung injury or acute respiratory distress syndrome, for example. Impairment of the endothelial system leads to activation of the coagulation cascade and increase of the nitric oxide, which results in vascular dilation, tissue hypoperfusion, hypotension and increase permeability, which characterizes septic processes.

When monitoring for organ dysfunction, lactate levels are always a key component. Hyperlactatemia is considered a marker of poor tissue perfusion and aids in the stratification of sepsis, and also provides guidance for the use of vasoactive drugs. It has been established that those patients with significant hypoperfusion classified as a lactate level >4 mmol/L are

considered for a diagnosis of shock even in those cases where hypotension is not noted. Lactate levels are also used to monitor disease prognosis, and its elevated levels correlate with organ dysfunction as its clearance depends on the kidney and liver function [21].

Another useful marker for organ dysfunction is the venous to arterial carbon dioxide pressure difference (ΔpCO_2), which serve to monitor those patients in septic shock. CO_2 levels are usually produced during both the aerobic and anaerobic metabolism where bicarbonate buffers the produced acidic metabolites. Its high solubility into the venous system makes it a sensitive marker for hypoperfusion, providing an index of tissue oxygenation. CO_2 levels above 6 mmHg within 24 h of a critically ill patient correlate with poor outcomes. Still several studies are exploring its usefulness [22]. Another marker is the cell-free DNA which is commonly released after tissue necrosis or apoptosis. Cell death is commonly seen in septic process but is still nonspecific as it is seen in other inflammatory processes, for such reason, it is mainly studied as a prognostic rather than a diagnostic biomarker. Given the complex pathophysiology of septic process, there is no single biomarker to be considered as the ideal, rather diagnosis should be prompt in a combination of multiple biomarkers to increase result specificity and reliability [23].

TREATMENT

Once a sepsis or septic shock process is identified, management is mainly focused on hemodynamic resuscitation, antimicrobial management, and control of infectious process. Selection of antimicrobial therapy must be done as quickly as possible, but de-escalation of therapy should also be done on a promptly manner to avoid the development of multidrug-resistant organisms. Those patients that present with hypotension in sepsis should be initiated in an antimicrobial therapy within the first hour of identification to increased survival and overall mortality [24,25]. It is important to note that infectious control includes not only the initiation of a drug therapy but also the removal of an infected catheter, drainage of an abscess or fluid collection, or tissue resection/debridement of an infected wound.

The SSC states that all therapeutic steps including obtaining blood culture and lactate levels, as well as administration of broad-spectrum antibiotics and fluid administration of balanced crystalloid, rather than normal saline at a rate of 30mL/kg in hypotensive patient and those with lactate> 4 mmol/L should be done within the first hour of recognition of a septic process. Fluid resuscitation should be evaluated through dynamic monitoring, capillary refill timing, and serum lactate measurement. Other time-sensitive recommendations include the use of vasopressors such as norepinephrine as the first line therapy, maintaining a goal mean arterial pressure (MAP) equal to or greater than 65 mmHg. If unable to achieve MAP goal, vasopressin could be added and thirdly epinephrine. In cases of cardiac dysfunction, dobutamine may be added to norepinephrine. The use of vasopressors may be initiated via peripheral line distal to the antecubital fossa for at least 6 h, until a central line access is safely secured. In those cases, where patient is on ongoing requirement of vasopressors, intravenous administration of corticosteroids is recommended as it accelerates resolution of shock and decrease days on vasopressor therapy. In those cases, where infection is not identified, differential diagnosis should be evaluated to discontinue antibiotic therapy as soon as possible. Venous thromboembolism and stress prophylaxis are recommended in patients with sepsis and septic shock [13].

Oxygen administration via noninvasive ventilation or high-flow nasal canula should be done to optimize oxygen consumption and in those with impaired conscious for airway protection. Once blood culture results are obtained, antimicrobial therapy from broad-spectrum antibiotic to organism-specific therapy should be addressed to avoid resistance, minimize drug side effects, reduce risk of reinfection, toxicity, and treatment cost [26].

LONG-TERM OUTCOME AND MORTALITY

The mortality associated with sepsis is markedly high and ranges from 10% to 52%. These rates correlate with disease severity from sepsis to more severe septic shock, which poses a mortality of more than 40%. Mortality tends to be lower in those patients who are less than 50 years old and with no comorbidities, been around 10%. During hospitalization, patient with diagnosed sepsis is more vulnerable to nosocomial infections such as pneumonia, abdominal infections, or catheter-associated infections. Prognosis in the long term is also affected as studies suggest that following discharge, patients are at an increased risk of death within the first six months to two years (20%), further sepsis and readmission (10%), and in many cases, patients required discharge to long-term care facilities due to decrease quality of life secondary to sepsis infection. Cognitive, physical, and emotional surveillance are also recommended upon hospital discharge.

REFERENCES

[1] Martin GS, Mannino DM, Eaton S, Moss M. The epidemiology of sepsis in the United States from 1979 through 2000. N Engl J Med 2003;348:1546.

[2] Vincent J-L, Rello J, Marshall J, et al. International study of the prevalence and outcomes of infection in intensive care units. JAMA 2009;302(21):1303–10. https://doi.org/10.1001/jama.2009.1754.

[3] American College of Chest Physicians/Society of Critical Care Medicine Consensus Conference: definitions for sepsis and organ failure and guidelines for the use of innovative therapies in sepsis. Crit Care Med 1992;20:864.

[4] Levy M, et al. SCCM/ESICM/ACCP/ATS/SIS international sepsis definitions conference. Crit Care Med 2003;31:1250.

[5] Dellinger RP, Carlet JM, Masur H, Gerlach H, Calandra T, Cohen J, Gea-Banacloche J, Keh D, Marshall JC, Parker MM, Ramsay G, Zimmerman JL, Vincent JL, Levy MM, Surviving Sepsis Campaign Management Guidelines Committee. Surviving sepsis campaign guidelines for management of severe sepsis and septic shock. Crit Care Med March 2004;32(3):858–73. https://doi.org/10.1097/01.ccm.0000117317.18092.e4. Erratum in: Crit Care Med. June 2004;32(6):1448. Dosage error in article text. Erratum in: Crit Care Med. October 2004;32(10):2169–2873. PMID: 15090974.

[6] Henry KE, Hager DN, Osborn TM, Wu AW, Saria S. Comparison of automated sepsis identification methods and electronic health record-based sepsis phenotyping: improving case identification accuracy by accounting for confounding comorbid conditions. Crit Care Explor 2019;1(10):e0053. https://doi.org/10.1097/CCE.0000000000000053. Published 2019 Oct 30.

[7] Wu M, Du X, Gu R, Wei J. Artificial intelligence for clinical decision support in sepsis. Front Med May 13, 2021;8:665464. https://doi.org/10.3389/fmed.2021.665464. PMID: 34055839; PMCID: PMC8155362.

[8] Singer M, Deutschman CS, Seymour CW, Shankar-Hari M, Annane D, Bauer M, Bellomo R, Bernard GR, Chiche JD, Coopersmith CM, Hotchkiss RS, Levy MM, Marshall JC, Martin GS, Opal SM, Rubenfeld GD, van der Poll T, Vincent JL, Angus DC. The third international consensus definitions for sepsis and septic shock (Sepsis-3). JAMA February 23, 2016;315(8):801–10. https://doi.org/10.1001/jama.2016.0287. PMID: 26903338; PMCID: PMC4968574.

[9] Novosad SA, Sapiano MRP, Grigg C, et al. Vital signs: epidemiology of sepsis: prevalence of health care factors and opportunities for prevention. Morb Mortal Wkly Rep 2016;65(33):864–9. https://doi.org/10.15585/mmwr.mm6533e1.

[10] Seymour CW, Liu VX, Iwashyna TJ, Brunkhorst FM, Rea TD, Scherag A, Rubenfeld G, Kahn JM, Shankar-Hari M, Singer M, Deutschman CS, Escobar GJ, Angus DC. Assessment of clinical criteria for sepsis: for the third international consensus definitions for sepsis

and septic shock (Sepsis-3). JAMA February 23, 2016; 315(8):762−74. https://doi.org/10.1001/jama.2016. 0288. Erratum in: JAMA. 2016 May 24-31;315(20): 2237. PMID: 26903335; PMCID: PMC5433435.

[11] Doerr F, Badreldin AM, Heldwein MB, et al. A comparative study of four intensive care outcome prediction models in cardiac surgery patients. J Cardiothorac Surg 2011;6:21. https://doi.org/10.1186/1749-8090-6-21.

[12] Wagenlehner F, Dittmar F. Re: surviving sepsis campaign: international guidelines for management of sepsis and septic shock 2021. Eur Urol 2022;81(2):213. https:// doi.org/10.1016/j.eururo.2021.11.014.

[13] Evans L, et al. Surviving sepsis campaign: international guidelines for management of sepsis and septic shock. Crit Care Med November 2021;49(Issue 11):1064.

[14] Faix JD. Biomarkers of sepsis. Crit Rev Clin Lab Sci 2013; 50(1):23−36. https://doi.org/10.3109/10408363.2013. 764490.

[15] Atkinson AJ, Colburn WA, DeGruttola VG, et al. Biomarkers and surrogate endpoints: preferred definitions and conceptual framework. Clin Pharmacol Ther 2001;69(3):89−95. https://doi.org/10.1067/mcp.2001. 113989.

[16] Biron BM, et al. Biomarkers for sepsis: what is and what might be? Biomark Insights September 15, 2015; 10(Suppl. 4):7−17. https://doi.org/10.4137/BMI.S29519.

[17] Miglietta F, Faneschi ML, Lobreglio G, Palumbo CRA. Procalcitonin, C-reactive protein and serum lactate dehydrogenase in the diagnosis of bacterial sepsis, SIRS and systemic candidiasis. Le Infez Med 2015;3:230−7.

[18] Watt DG, Horgan PG, McMillan DC. Routine clinical markers of the magnitude of the systemic inflammatory response after elective operation: a systematic review. Surgery 2015;157:362−80.

[19] Juskewitch JE, Abraham RS, League SC, et al. Monocyte HLA-DR expression and neutrophil CD64 expression as biomarkers of infection in critically ill neonates and infants. Pediatr Res 2015;78(6):683−90. https://doi.org/ 10.1038/pr.2015.164.

[20] Gu X, Zhou F, Wang Y, et al. Respiratory viral sepsis: epidemiology, pathophysiology, diagnosis and treatment. Eur Respir Rev 2020;29:200038.

[21] Bolvardi E, Malmir J, Reihani H, et al. The role of lactate clearance as a predictor of organ dysfunction and mortality in patients with severe sepsis. Mater Sociomed 2016;28(1): 57−60. https://doi.org/10.5455/msm.2016.28.57-60.

[22] Naumann DN, Midwinter MJ, Hutchings S. Venous-to-arterial CO_2 differences and the quest for bedside point-of-care monitoring to assess the microcirculation during shock. Ann Transl Med 2016;4(2):37.

[23] Saukkonen K, Lakkisto P, Pettilä V, et al. Cell-free plasma DNA as a predictor of outcome in severe sepsis and septic shock. Clin Chem 2008;54(6):1000−7. https://doi.org/ 10.1373/clinchem.2007.101030.

[24] Levy MM, Evans LE, Rhodes A. The surviving sepsis campaign bundle: 2018 update, critical care medicine. Crit Care Med June 2018;46(6):997−1000.

[25] Sterling SA, Miller WR, Pryor J, Puskarich MA, Jones AE. The impact of timing of antibiotics on outcomes in severe sepsis and septic shock: a systematic review and meta-analysis. Crit Care Med 2015;43:1907−15. https:// doi.org/10.1097/CCM.0000000000001142.

[26] Garnacho-Montero J, Garcia-Garmendia JL, Barrero-Almodovar A, Jimenez-Jimenez FJ, Perez-Paredes C, Ortiz-Leyba C. Impact of adequate empirical antibiotic therapy on the outcome of patients admitted to the intensive care unit with sepsis. Crit Care Med 2003;31(12):2742−51. https://doi.org/10.1097/01.CCM.0000098031.24329.10.

CHAPTER 13

Sepsis Quality Indicators in the Emergency Department

LUIS ANTONIO GORORDO-DELSOL • GRACIELA MERINOS-SÁNCHEZ

INTRODUCTION

Quality indicators (QIs) are measurement tools that record the presence of a phenomenon or event and its magnitude; these must be objective, measurable, widely accepted, relevant, and evidence-based [1]. In the field of health, the QIs are used to analyze processes, that is, sets of planned or unplanned actions that are part of health care, these are also used to evaluate the implementation of procedures, obtain certifications, carry out research with the objective of executing improvement programs, and even to compare homologous areas inside and outside a health system, always with the main objective of improving the quality of care and the outcomes of users; these are patients, families, and healthcare professionals (HCP) and institutions [2].

In health care, these QIs can be very diverse, but there are some basic ones that every health system and its subsystems—service, unit, department, etc—must have, to which are added others planned for an area, process, and/or specific pathology [1,3]. The Emergency Department (ED) receives a huge number of consultations in proportion (beds-patient, nurse-patient, doctor-patient, resources-patient ratios) to what other services receive individually, patients who will or will not be hospitalized through this same door, so measuring the quality of care and redesigning processes that improve outcomes while reducing errors and ED saturation is a priority that impacts the entire hospital system [4−7].

Although QIs are normally divided into those of structure, process, or result [1,3], for the purposes of this chapter, they have been grouped differently according to the stages of care, so that leaders can focus on different points with its "champions" in each area, even adding other specialties and hospital departments that can focus on a particular goal. We are also going to ignore the QIs and other general indicators such as the type and number of staff, standard patient safety measures, length of stay in the ED, intensive care unit, and/or hospitalization, morbidity and mortality because these are already measured routinely, since these are not exclusive to the care of patients with sepsis, but global indicators to all health institutions, so they must be measured and their ideal goals must be established according to each area and organization [8].

INFECTION PREVENTION INDICATORS

Due to the fast-paced and, sometimes, belligerent number of procedures performed in the ED [6,7], there is a high probability that barriers and security processes for the infection prevention and control (IPC) could be omitted, for this reason, the QIs of IPC like the implementation of bundles should be measured [8]; the fundamental axes are the protection of HCP and the reduction of healthcare-associated infections (HAIs) during the stay in the ED [9,10].

In this area, the most important QIs are:

- Hands hygiene compliance in the five moments: it is expected that the percentage of adherence exceeds 80% of the hands' hygiene/handwashing opportunities and that the consumption of solutions such as soap, alcohol gel, or other products overcome 20 L for every 1000 days of stay [11].
- Isolation-type indications: consists of the prescription and compliance with the type of isolation that each patient requires to prevent them from infecting or being infected during their stay in the ED. These are: standard precautions, by contact, by drops, by aerosols, and inverse isolation [11−13],
- Bloodstream infection event (Central line-associated bloodstream infection [CLABSIs] and noncentral line-associated bloodstream infection): consists of compliance with packages of measures for the installation and maintenance of any intravascular devices—understood as central or peripheral venous

catheters, dialysis catheters, arterial lines, etc—as well as the incidence of CLABSIs which is reported internationally among 4.0 and 16.1 per 1000 device days [11,12,14].

- Ventilator-associated pneumonia (VAP): consists of compliance with packages of measures for the installation and maintenance of advanced airway management devices—orotracheal, nasotracheal, tracheostomy cannula, and even noninvasive ventilation—as well as the incidence of VAP that in previous works is reported from 2.9 to 24.1 per 1000 days of ventilation [11,12,15],
- Catheter-associated urinary tract infection (CAUTIs): consists of compliance with packages for the installation and maintenance of bladder catheters, as well as the incidence of CAUTIs that range from 3.1 to 8.9 per 1000 days of use of the catheter [11,12,16].
- Surgical site infection (SSI): consists of compliance with SSI prevention packages for surgical procedures performed in the ED, such as cricotomies, tracheostomies, thoracostomies for endopleural tubes, etc., as well as the incidence of SSI that should be less than 2% of all postoperative patients [12,17].

These six QIs encompass at least 12 points, some related to the availability of resources to comply with the bundles, others to devices placement process, and others to the result (the low incidence of HAIs), all of these related to quality and the safety of care.

TIMING INDICATORS

These are the most "popular" indicators, since the saturation of the ED [5,7,8] has led many to believe that the success of this service is in the speed, however, for the "attention times" to be reliable, they must be measured and contrasted with other outcomes, since often exaggeratedly short times do not necessarily translate into better results and can reveal oversights in healthcare protocols, while times that are too long can be considered delays in care with some impact on outcomes [3]. Therefore, there are no "standard" times for sepsis care, but the evidence suggests windows of opportunity that are widely accepted as goals. The three most relevant moments are:

- Antibiotic door time: this is measured from the time the infectious clinical syndrome is diagnosed, that is, the trigger for sepsis, until the first dose of the prescribed antimicrobial regimen is administered; this must be measured from the triage, and it is suggested that it be within the first 60 min [18–20], although some studies suggest that they can be administered in

the first 3 h without negatively affecting mortality [20–22]. To this item must be added the proper selection of the antimicrobial based on local epidemiology, type of infection, and the particularities of pharmacodynamics and pharmacokinetics of each of these drugs [19,22,23],

- Hypotension to vasopressor time: this is measured from the detection of arterial hypotension, clinical and/or biochemical data of hypoperfusion, even when there may be a need to continue resuscitation with fluids, until the start of vasopressor infusion. Although there is no established standard time, some studies suggest that each hour of delay increases mortality significantly [22,24–27]; it can be said that the same indicator is applicable to the use of inotropes, steroids, and other adjuvant therapies.
- Door to operating room time: this period is measured from the detection of the infectious clinical syndrome that requires surgical management until the patient is admitted to the operating room; this should be prioritized in the first 6 h of care [28–30].

DIAGNOSTIC INDICATORS

These QIs are relevant to establish new diagnostic approach protocols and must be contrasted with the "attention times" to determine if the sample collection and reporting of complementary studies is adequate, in which some of these may be more specific by type of study or by diagnostic intention according to the infectious clinical syndrome of each patient with sepsis. The most relevant are:

- Completion of general studies: these QIs are more related to resources access such as basic laboratory studies, but it can also help determine if they were performed properly, if the necessary ones for the diagnostic approach were taken, and the time it took to process them and obtain a result for the HCP to make decisions [3,30,31].
- Sampling for microbiological approach: these QIs analyze several aspects, among which the access to a microbiology laboratory and other microbiological approach tests, the sampling of directed cultures, the timing of samples (preferably prior to the first dose of antimicrobial), the collection of results and their adequate reporting (including the antibiogram), and finally the local epidemiology reports and antibiotic resistance profiles that can serve to create local guides for the rational use of antimicrobials [23, 30–32].
- Measurement of biomarkers: another QI that records from access to the resource, the correct use, the

appropriate decision-making derived from each biomarker that is considered appropriate for the care of infection, organ failure, and sepsis [22,29,30].

PERSPECTIVES

This chapter described 12 QIs that can provide information on at least 30 structural, process, or outcome determinants related to the care of patients with sepsis and septic shock in the ED, many of which are suitable to other departments or as part of the global evaluation of the patient with sepsis, to which must be added other widely known general indicators such as length of stay, morbidity, sequelae, and mortality, all aimed at improving ED performance for the benefit of patients and healthcare systems.

REFERENCES

[1] Martín MC, Cabré L, Ruiz J, Blanch L, Blanco J, Castillo F, et al. Indicadores de calidad en el enfermo crítico. Med Intensiva 2008;32(1):23−32. https://doi.org/10.1016/S0210-5691(08)70899-4.

[2] Drynda S, Shindler W, Slagman A, Pollmanns J, Horenkamp-Sonntag D, Schirrmeister W, et al. Evaluation of outcome relevance of quality indicators in the emergency department (ENQuIRE): study protocol for a prospective multicentre cohort study. DOI: 10.1136/bmjopen-2020-038776.

[3] Aaronson EL, Marsh RH, Guha M, Schuur JD, Rouhani SA. Emergency department quality and safety indicators in resource-limited settings: an environmental survey. Int J Emerg Med 2015;8:39. https://doi.org/10.1186/s12245-015-0088-x.

[4] McDonald CM, West S, Dushenski D, Lapinsky SE, Soong C, van der Broek K, et al. Sepsis now a priority: a quality improvements initiative for early sepsis recognition and care. Int J Qual Health Care 2018;30(1):802−9. https://doi.org/10.1093/intqhc/mzy121.

[5] Castañón-González JA, Polanco-González C, Camacho-Juárez S. La sobresaturación de los servicios de urgencais médicas. Cir Cir 2014;82(2):127−8.

[6] Polanco-González C, Castañón-González JA, Buhse T, Samaniego-Mendoza JL, Arreguín-Nava R, Villanueva-Martínez S. Índice de saturación modificado en el servicio de urgencais médicas. Gac Med Mex 2013;149(4):417−24.

[7] Marley C, Unwin M, Peterson GM, Stankovich J, Kinsman L. Emergency Department crowding: a systematic review of causes, consequences and solutions. PLoS

One 2018;13(8):e0203316. https://doi.org/10.1371/journal.pone.0203316.

[8] The Royal College of Emergency Medicine. Improving quality indicators and system metrics for Emergency Departments in England. EEC 2019. https://rcem.ac.uk/clinical-guidelines/.

[9] Liang SY, Theodoro DL, Schuur JD, Marschall J. Infection prevention in the emergency department. Ann Emerg Med 2014;64(3):299−313. https://doi.org/10.1016/j.annemergmed.2014.02.024.

[10] Stewart S, Robertson C, Pan J, Kennedy S, Dancer S, Haahr L, et al. Epidemiology of healthcare-associated infection reported from a hospital-wide incidence study: considerations for infection prevention and control planning.

[11] WHO guidelines on hand hygiene in health care: first flobal patient safety challenge clean care is safer care. Geneva: World Health Organizacion; 2009. Available from: https://www.who.int/publications/i/item/9789241597906.

[12] Haque M, Sartelli M, McKimm J, Abu Bakar M. Healthcare-associated infections − an overview. Infect Drug Resist 2018;11:2321−33. https://doi.org/10.2147/IDR.S177247.

[13] Siegel JD, Rhinehart E, Jackson M, Chiarello L and the Healthcare Infection Control Practices Advisory Committee. 2007 guidelines for isolation precautions: preventing transmission of infectious agents in healthcare settings. http://www.cdc.gov/infectioncontrol/guidelines/isolation/index.html.

[14] Rosenthal VD, Maki DG, Jamulitrat S, Medeiros EA, Todi SK, Gómez DY, et al. International nosocomial infection control consortium (INICC) report, data summary for 2003-2008. Am J Infect Control 2010;38(2):95−104. https://doi.org/10.1016/j.ajic.2009.12.004.

[15] National Nosocomial Infections Surveillance (NNIS) system report, data summary from January 1992 through June 2004. Am J Infect Control 2004;32:470−85.

[16] Gould CV, Umscheid CA, Agarwal RK, Kuntz G, Pegues DA, and the healthcare infection control practices advisory committee (HICPAC). Guideline for prevention of catheter-associated urinary tract infections 2009. Centers for Disease Control and Prevention. 2009. Available from: https://www.cdc.gov/infectioncontrol/guidelines/cauti/index.html.

[17] Gillespie BM, Harbeck E, Rattray M, Liang R, Walker R, Latimer S, et al. Worldwide incidence of surgical site infections in general surgical patients: a systematic review and meta-analysis of 488,594 patients. Int J Surg 2021;95:106136. https://doi.org/10.1016/j.ijsu.2021.106136.

[18] Mixon M, Dietrich S, Floren M, Rogosxewsi R, Kane L, Nudell N, et al. Time to antibiotic administration: sepsis

alerts called in emergency department versus in the field via emergency medical services. Am J Emerg Med 2021; 44:291—5. https://doi.org/10.1016/j.ajem.2020.04.008.

[19] Denny KJ, Gartside JG, Alcorn K, Cross JW, Maloney S, Keijzers G. Appropriateness of antibiotic prescribing in the emergency department. J Antimicrob Chemother 2019;74(2):515—20. https://doi.org/10.1093/jac/dky447.

[20] Seymour CW, Gesten F, Prescott HC, Friedrich ME, Iwashyma TJ, et al. Time to treatment and mortality during mandate emergency care for sepsis. N Engl J Med 2017; 376:2235—44. https://doi.org/10.1056/NEJMoa1703058.

[21] Fee C, Webee EJ, Maak CA, Bacchetti P. Effect of emergency department crowding on time to antibiotics in patients admitted with community-acquired pneumonia. Ann Emerg Med 2007;50(5):501—9. https://doi.org/10.1016/j.annemergmed.2007.08.003.

[22] Evans L, Rhodes A, Alhazzani W, Antonelli M, Coopersmith CM, French C, et al. Surviving sepsis campaign: international guidelines for management of sepsis and septic shock 2021. Intensive Care Med 2021; 47(11):1181—247. https://doi.org/10.1007/s00134-021-06506-y.

[23] Dixit D, Ranka R, Kumar Panda P. Compliance with the 4Ds of antimicrobial stewardship practice in a tertiary care centre. JAC Antimicrob Resist 2021;3(3):dlab135. https://doi.org/10.1093/jacamr/dlab135.

[24] Bai X, Yu W, Ji W, Lin Z, Tan S, Duan K, et al. Early versus delayed administration of norepinephrine in patients with septic shock. Crit Care 2014;18(5):532. https://doi.org/10.1186/s13054-014-0532-y.

[25] Shi R, Hamzaoui O, de Vita N, Monnet X, Teboul JL. Vasopressors in septic shock: which, when, and how much? Ann Transl Med 2020;8(12):764. https://doi.org/10.21037/atm.2020.04.24.

[26] Black LP, Puskarich MA, Smotherman C, Miller T, Fernandez R, Guirgis FW. Time to vasopressor initiation and organ failure progression in early septic shock. J Am Coll Emerg Physicians Open 2020;1(3):222—30. https://doi.org/10.1002/emp2.12060.

[27] Beck V, Chateau D, Bryson GL, Pisipati A, Zanotti S, Parrillo JE, et al. Timing of vasopressor initiation and mortality in septic shock: a cohort study. Crit Care 2014;18:R97. https://doi.org/10.1186/cc13868.

[28] Azuhata T, Kinoshita K, Kawano D, Komatsu T, Sakurai A, Chiba Y, et al. Time from admission to initiation of surgery for source control is a critical determinant of survival in patients with gastrointestinal perforation with associated septic shock. Crit Care 2014;18:R87. https://doi.org/10.1186/cc13854.

[29] Gorordo-Delsol LA, Merinos-Sánchez G, Estrada-Escobar RA, Medveczky-Ordoñez NI, Amezcua-Gutiérrez MA, Morales-Segura MA, et al. Sepsis and septic shock in emergency departments of México: a multicenter point prevalence study. Gac Med Mex 2020;156(6): 486—92. https://doi.org/10.24875/GMM.M21000492.

[30] Julián-Jiménez A, Supino M, López-Tapia JA, Ulloa-González C, Vargas-Téllez LE, González-del Castillo J, et al. Sepsis in the emergency department: key points, controversies, and proposals for improvements in Latin America. Emergencias 2019;31(2):123—35.

[31] Broccoli MC, Moresky R, Dixon J, Muya I, Taubman C, Wallis LA, et al. Defining quality indicators for emergency care delivery: findings of an expert consensus process by emergency care practitioners in Africa. BMJ Glob Health 2018;3(1):e000479. https://doi.org/10.1136/bmhgh-2017-000479.

[32] Gatewood MO, Wemple M, Greco S, Kritek PA, Durvasula R. A quality improvement project to improve early sepsis care in the emergency department. BMJ Qual Saf 2015;24(12):787—95. https://doi.org/10.1136/bmjqs-2014-003552.

FURTHER READING

[1] Sangorrin-Iranzo A. Precaucioens de aislamiento en la atención sanitaria. An Pediatr Contin 2014;12(6):340—3.

CHAPTER 14

Sepsis Treatment: Fluids

MICHAËL MEKEIRELE • DOMIEN VANHONACKER • MANU L.N.G. MALBRAIN

INTRODUCTION

Due to vasodilatation and capillary leak, sepsis induces a functional hypovolemic state. This combined with an increased energy expense leads to an insufficient supply of oxygen and nutrients. To restore these imbalanced scales of supply and demand, fluids remain the backbone of resuscitation during sepsis [1,2]. However, in recent years, awareness grew on the harmful effects of inappropriate fluid administration [3–5].

This led to the idea that fluids, like antibiotics, should be considered as drugs. One has to choose the right drug, apply an adequate dose, administer it for the correct duration, and de-escalate timely. This concept is known as the four D's of fluid therapy. Furthermore, fluid therapy should also be tailored to the phase of the disease. Specifically in sepsis, four distinct phases forming the acronym ROSE can typically be distinguished: Resuscitation, Optimization, Stabilization, and Evacuation (Fig. 14.1). Each of these phases requires a specific approach [6]. A thorough understanding of the four D's concept and ROSE framework should lead to better fluid stewardship.

In this chapter, we will first dig deeper into the background of fluid therapy while explaining the four D's concept. Next, we will elaborate the basics of fluid therapy during sepsis by focusing on its four phases forming the ROSE acronym. In the final part of this chapter, we will provide an in-depth description of the available types of fluids and their place in sepsis.

BACKGROUND: THE FOUR D'S OF FLUID THERAPY

In 2001, Rivers et al. showed a revolutionary decrease in sepsis mortality by using protocolized early goal-directed therapy. One of the cornerstones in this protocol was an early aggressive fluid administration of 20–30 mL/kg fluid over 30 min followed by 500 mL per 30 min until the central venous pressure (CVP) was between 8 and 12 mmHg [7]. Subsequent studies, PROCESS, PROMISE, ARISE, and SEPSISPAM by other researchers could not confirm a significant reduction in mortality when using this protocol as compared to the standard of care [8–11]. On one hand by the time these repeat studies had been performed, the standard of care was much influenced by the Rivers' study. The Rivers' protocol was already integrated into the surviving sepsis campaign guidelines [12]. On the other hand, these studies support that one does not need to blindly adhere to a protocol with fixed numbers to deliver optimal care and that there might still be room for optimization in sepsis care [8–11].

Since the Rivers' trial, the CVP that had a prominent place in the initial protocol has been refuted as a predictor of fluid responsiveness [13]. At the end of the last millennium, the SOAP study retrospectively showed an important association between positive fluid balances and mortality [3]. As stated earlier, the Rivers' trial and subsequent surviving sepsis campaign advocate the administration of large amounts of fixed dose boluses [1,7]. However, more recent studies showed that unthoughtful aggressive administration of fluids in sepsis can also increase mortality, even when compared to administering no bolus therapy at all [14].

It was increasingly recognized that one should not just give fluids or withhold fluids but rather see fluids as an often-prescribed drug—like antibiotics—where the choice of *drug, dose, duration,* and *de-escalation* are all equally important. Given the extensive literature on the fluid of choice in sepsis, the "D" for drug is discussed separately in the last section. We will now zoom in on the remaining three D's.

Dose

Paracelsus stated that "all things are poison, and nothing is without poison; only the dose permits

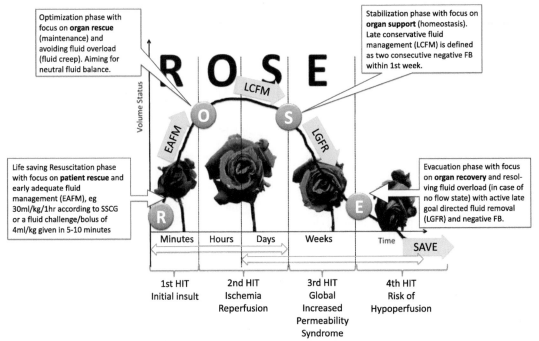

Optimization phase with focus on **organ rescue** (maintenance) and avoiding fluid overload (fluid creep). Aiming for neutral fluid balance.

Stabilization phase with focus on **organ support** (homeostasis). Late conservative fluid management (LCFM) is defined as two consecutive negative FB within 1st week.

Life saving Resuscitation phase with focus on **patient rescue** and early adequate fluid management (EAFM), eg 30ml/kg/1hr according to SSCG or a fluid challenge/bolus of 4ml/kg given in 5-10 minutes

Evacuation phase with focus on **organ recovery** and resolving fluid overload (in case of no flow state) with active late goal directed fluid removal (LGFR) and negative FB.

Volume Status

ROSE
LCFM
EAFM
O
S
LGFR
R
E
SAVE

Minutes	Hours	Days	Weeks	Time

| 1st HIT | 2nd HIT | 3rd HIT | 4th HIT |
| Initial insult | Ischemia Reperfusion | Global Increased Permeability Syndrome | Risk of Hypoperfusion |

FIG.14.1 **Visualization of the ROSE conceptual model.** Graph showing the four-hit model of shock with evolution of patients' cumulative fluid volume status over time during the five distinct phases of resuscitation: Resuscitation (R), Optimization (O), Stabilization (S), and Evacuation (E) (ROSE), followed by a possible risk of Hypoperfusion in case of too aggressive deresuscitation. On admission, patients are hypovolemic, followed by normovolemia after fluid resuscitation (EAFM, early adequate fluid management), and possible fluid overload, again followed by a phase going to normovolemia with late conservative fluid management (LCFM) and late goal-directed fluid removal (LGFR) or deresuscitation. In case of hypovolemia, O_2 cannot get into the tissue because of convective problems; in case of hypervolemia, O_2 cannot get into the tissue because of diffusion problems related to interstitial and pulmonary edema, gut edema (ileus and abdominal hypertension). (Adapted according to the Open Access CC BY Licence 4.0 with permission from Malbrain MLNG, Van Regenmortel N, Saugel B, De Tavernier B, Van Gaal PJ, Joannes-Boyau O, et al. Principles of fluid management and stewardship in septic shock: it is time to consider the four D's and the four phases of fluid therapy. Ann Intensive Care. 2018;8(1):66.)

something not to be poisonous." In the case of fluids, both the necessity of fluids in sepsis, as shown by Rivers, and the detrimental effects of too much fluids, as shown by SOAP and FEAST are well established [3,7,14]. In order to apply a correct dose, one has to take into account both pharmacodynamics and pharmacokinetics.

Pharmacodynamics involves the interaction of a drug to its specific effect. The dose-effect curve for fluids, as seen for other drugs, is described by the Frank–Starling relationship between preload and cardiac output. Given the nonlinear shape of this curve, the effect of fluids on cardiac output is not constant. Optimal fluid therapy from a pharmacodynamic point of view requires determining an individual patient's position on the Frank–Starling curve to predict the effect of fluid administration [15].

Pharmacokinetics describes the interaction of the body with a drug. Each type of fluids remains intravascular for a specific amount and time period, theoretically favoring fluids with higher tonicity. In vasoplegic shock, it has been well established that these characteristics can be altered [16,17].

Pharmacodynamics and pharmacokinetics are not static and depend on both individual factors as well as the timing of fluid administration This implies that there is no one-size-fits-all dose of fluids to be administered. As described in a different chapter, dynamic tests for assessing fluid responsiveness can be a helpful tool in administering an adequate dose of fluids [6].

When administering fluids during resuscitation, a bolus approach is preferred. It implies the quick infusion (5–10 min) of a small amount of fluid. The administered volume is highly clinician-dependent varying between 500 mL (over 10 min) and 1000 mL (over 15–20 min) [18]. The minimal volume required to increase the venous return is around 4 mL/kg/5 min [19]. We would advocate using small boluses during close clinical observation and repeating these smaller boluses depending on the observed changes.

Duration

Starting resuscitation in sepsis as early as possible remains quintessential. Murphy et al. showed that delaying fluid administration in septic shock patients leads to increased levels of microcirculatory hypoperfusion and subsequent organ damage related to ischemia-reperfusion [20]. In a retrospective analysis of patients with septic shock, they studied the effect of either early adequate or early conservative fluid therapy combined with either late conservative or late liberal fluid administration. They reported that the best outcomes were observed in patients treated with the combination of early adequate and late conservative fluid management [20]. Other studies suggest that a late conservative strategy might have the biggest impact on outcome [21–24].

Concerning the duration of fluid therapy, we would like to point out that it is a misconception that fluids should be administered as long as dynamic tests indicate fluid responsiveness. Resuscitation fluids should be given to treat shock and restore the DO_2/VO_2 imbalance, but not continued to treat the numbers (e.g., low CVP, cardiac output, blood pressure, or urine output). It is safe to stop fluid resuscitation once the initial signs and symptoms of hypovolemia and shock have resolved.

De-escalation

De-escalation of fluid therapy implies not only limiting fluid administration but also active fluid removal. In the case of sepsis, de-escalation should be applied at the latest during the evacuation phase of the ROSE conceptual model. It is essential to prevent fluid overload, defined as a 10% increase in body weight from baseline through the accumulation of fluids and the adverse events associated herewith.

The FACTT trial supports the approach of restrictive fluid therapy after initial resuscitation in patients with ARDS. In this trial, 1000 patients were treated with conservative or liberal fluid management for seven consecutive days. While there was no difference in mortality, the conservative strategy resulted in improved lung function, a shorter duration of mechanical ventilation, and a shorter length of stay in the ICU without increasing nonpulmonary organ failures [25].

The retrospective RADAR trial revealed an association between a negative fluid balance on day three and a positive outcome. Limiting fluid intake by reducing maintenance fluids, minimizing fluid creep through administered drug diluents, and active fluid evacuation are all essential to achieving this goal [26].

In contrast to the RADAR trial, the RELIEF trial, a pragmatic prospective trial in 3000 patients undergoing major abdominal surgery, showed that a restrictive fluid strategy was associated with increased acute kidney injury (AKI). There was no mortality difference nor significant difference in disability between the two groups [27]. In our opinion, this study should be read as a warning against blind fluid removal, while it should not necessarily lead to abandoning controlled active fluid removal.

The CLASSIC pilot study evaluated the impact of very early de-escalation using a restrictive fluid resuscitation strategy in the initial phase. This study was designed as a feasibility trial. As such, the administered volume of fluid was significantly different, but no significant difference in outcome was observed. We eagerly await the final results of the larger CLASSIC-2 trial [23].

BASICS OF THE FLUID TREATMENT IN SEPSIS: THE ROSE PRINCIPLE AND FOUR PHASES OF FLUID RESUSCITATION

When applying fluids in sepsis, one must be aware of not only the type of fluid but also the fluid–patient interaction as well as the phase of illness. In 2014, Malbrain proposed the mnemonic ROSE after an initial paper by Vincent describing four distinct phases in sepsis patients [6,28] (Table 14.1).

During the initial phase, aggressive fluid administration is needed to rescue the patient. Following the *resuscitation* phase, a more thoughtful administration of fluid is in order. Supplementary fluid administration to *optimize* organ perfusion and counteract organ damage while avoiding fluid overload is usually necessary. After a few days, during the *stabilization* phase, neutral fluid balances should be aimed for. Accumulated fluids should be actively eliminated during the fourth and final phase, the evacuation phase.

Resuscitation Phase

Following the paper by Rivers, the sepsis guidelines still favor liberal use of resuscitation fluids by proposing 30 mL/kg in the first hour of septic shock [2,7]. However, as clearly shown by PROCESS, PROMISE, ARISE, and SEPSISPAM, the blind adherence to these protocols

TABLE 14.1
The ROSE Conceptual Model Avoiding Fluid Overload.

	Resuscitation	Optimization	Stabilization	Evacuation
Hit sequence	First hit	Second hit	Second hit	Third hit
Time frame	Minutes	Hours	Days	Days to weeks
Underlying mechanism	Inflammatory insult	Ischemia and reperfusion	Ischemia and reperfusion	Global increased permeability syndrome
Clinical presentation	Severe shock	Unstable shock	Absence of shock or threat of shock	Recovery from shock, possible global increased permeability syndrome
Goal	Early adequate goal-directed fluid management	Focus on organ support and maintaining tissue perfusion	Late conservative fluid management	Late goal-directed fluid removal (de-resuscitation)
Fluid therapy	Early administration with fluid boluses, guided by indices of fluid responsiveness	Fluid boluses guided by fluid responsiveness indices and indices of the risk of fluid administration	Only for normal maintenance and replacement	Reversal of the positive fluid balance, either spontaneous or active
Fluid balance	Positive	Neutral	Neutral to negative	Negative
Primary result of treatment	Salvage or patient rescue	Organ rescue	Organ support (homeostasis)	Organ recovery
Main risk	Insufficient resuscitation	Insufficient resuscitation and fluid overload (e.g., pulmonary edema, intraabdominal hypertension)	Fluid overload (e.g., pulmonary edema, intraabdominal hypertension)	Excessive fluid removal, possibly inducing hypotension, hypoperfusion, and a "fourth hit"

Adapted with permission from Malbrain ML, Marik PE, Witters I, Cordemans C, Kirkpatrick AW, Roberts DJ, et al. Fluid overload, de-resuscitation, and outcomes in critically ill or injured patients: a systematic review with suggestions for clinical practice. Anaesthesiol Intensive Ther. 2014;46(5): 361–80.

does not improve outcomes [8–11]. This topic will be further discussed in another chapter.

Cohort studies and smaller trials support a more restrictive resuscitation strategy in septic shock [23,27,29]. In low-income countries, early aggressive fluid therapy was even associated with increased mortality [14,30]. Critics might argue that these results depend on the lack of access to mechanical ventilation or patient- and disease-specific parameters. However, the SOAP and VASST trials in high-income countries also identified a link between positive fluid balances and increased mortality rates [3,31].

It has been long suggested that early application of vasopressors might reduce the amount of fluids required to restore adequate perfusion, especially given the mainly vasoplegic nature of septic shock. We are eagerly awaiting the results from the CLOVER trial,

hopefully answering the question of whether this physiological plausible strategy will stand the test.

In summary, it remains important to quickly obtain the desired hemodynamic goals during the resuscitation phase. However, one size does not fit all. A patient-tailored approach, keeping their premorbid condition in mind, seems desirable [32–34]. The dynamic tests described in earlier chapters as well as repeated postinterventional clinical evaluations play a key role in individualizing therapy.

Optimization Phase

Several hours after initial resuscitation, reperfusion of previously ischemic cells occurs, leading to a second hit. Fluid management at this stage is aimed at optimizing organ perfusion. In this phase, it is often less evident whether a patient will benefit from additional fluid administration. Dynamic tests for fluid responsiveness could help to make the right decision. In this phase, the risks of fluid overload must not be overlooked when deciding if administering extra fluids is appropriate. The evolution of lung impairment should certainly warn against overaggressive fluid administration. In daunting cases, advanced hemodynamic monitoring can help to take the plunge [35,36].

Stabilization

Within a few days, patients usually enter the stabilization phase characterized by the absence of shock or organ function deterioration. There should be no more need for fluid boluses at this stage. The retrospective SOAP trial showed an important association between positive fluid balances and mortality [3]. The prospective randomized controlled trial FACTT showed that a restrictive fluid strategy resulted in fewer ventilation days and a shorter ICU length of stay [5]. These studies suggest that one should aim for neutral fluid balances in this phase of sepsis [3].

To obtain this goal, and avoid the detrimental effects of fluid overload, it is important to take all administered fluids into account [3,26]. The RADAR study showed that maintenance fluids, replacement fluids for ongoing losses, feeding fluids as well as fluid creep by fluids administered along with medication account for more fluid input than resuscitation fluids [26]. This implies that adequate fluid therapy during the stabilization phase often requires the cessation of redundant maintenance fluids.

Evacuation

At a further stage, fluids that accumulated in the second and third space earlier need to be evacuated. While some patients progress spontaneously to this phase, others remain in a state of "no flow," retaining all administered fluids. In the latter case, also known as globally increased permeability syndrome, a third hit that can occur due to impaired oxygen diffusion and nutrient absorption [37]. The main risk of removing fluids too aggressively is inducing a fourth hit by causing hypovolemia and hypoperfusion [27].

Murphy et al. defined late conservative fluid administration as two consecutive days with a negative fluid balance during the first week of ICU stay [20]. Late goal-directed fluid removal is the aggressive use of diuretics or renal replacement therapy (RRT) resulting in a net ultrafiltration to actively remove the accumulated fluids. Both late conservative fluid administration and

late goal-directed fluid removal are often required to obtain negative fluid balances [22].

Retrospective literature suggested an independent survival benefit when obtaining either a negative fluid balance by day three or two consecutive days with a negative fluid balance within the first week of admission [20,26]. However, given the retrospective nature of these papers, we can only conclude there is an association but not derive causality. It could well be that positive fluid balances are merely a biomarker of disease severity [4]. We hope that the prospective RCT's RADAR-2 and CLASSIC-2 will shed a better light on this matter.

FLUIDS AND THEIR DIFFERENCE: CHOOSING THE RIGHT DRUG

Following the earlier described four D's concept, this section will provide an in-depth review of the available fluids (*drug*) in sepsis. We will first describe the colloids, differentiating synthetic colloids and human albumin. Next, we will discuss the different crystalloids dividing them according to tonicity and reviewing the literature on balanced and unbalanced crystalloids.

Colloids
Introduction

Until recently, synthetic colloids have been used in abundance in septic shock. It was assumed that by using colloids only half the volume was required to expand the intravascular blood compartment sufficiently to obtain hemodynamic stabilization. However, recent studies have shown that the true ratio of volume sparing effect is 1.3:1 or even 1:1 in case of acute shock, after induction of anesthesia, and during surgery where fluid distribution, elimination, and excretion are altered [16,17]. Aside from this refuted advantage, concerns arose about the safety of some colloids [38–41].

Hydroxyethyl Starches

While hydroxyethyl starch (HES) has long been the favorite resuscitation fluid, strong evidence grew regarding its negative effects.

In the VISEP study, a two-by-two factorial randomized controlled clinical trial (RCCT) including 537 patients, HES ($n = 262$) was compared to crystalloids, mainly Ringer's lactate ($n = 275$), to obtain a CVP of 8 mm Hg [40]. This complex study also compared intensive insulin therapy ($n = 247$) to conventional insulin therapy ($n = 290$). The group treated with HES showed higher rates of acute renal failure and/or need for RRT: 24.9% versus 22.8% ($P=0.002$). HES 10% was administered with an intended maximum limit of 20 mL/kg/day; however, more than 10% of the patients exceeded this limit. In the HES group, more patients developed heart failure or received emergency surgery. The study was prematurely stopped due to a higher incidence of hypoglycemia in the intensive insulin group.

A second noteworthy study often cited to support the increased need for RRT in HES is the CHEST trial. This pragmatic trial included 7000 patients and compared administration of HES with saline [41]. There was no difference in 90-day mortality nor in the incidence of AKI (according to RIFLE scoring). On one hand, the patients treated with 6% HES had a reduction of RIFLE-R and RIFLE-I, and similarly RIFLE-F. On the other hand, the (subjective) need for RRT was significantly different: 7.0% in the HES group versus 5.8% in the saline group (RR 1.21; 95% CI 1−1.45; $P = 0.04$). Patient randomization occurred after an average of 11 ± 156 h suggesting large differences between patients and non-Gaussian distribution. The CHEST study has been criticized a lot, moreover since the authors refused to share the raw data [42,43].

Stronger evidence was provided by the 6S study in 2012. This study, including 798 patients showed that administration of HES did not only increase the need for RRT when compared to Ringer's acetate (relative risk 1.35; 95% CI 1.01 to 1.8; $P = .04$) but also significantly increased mortality in the patients treated with HES (relative risk 1.17; 95% CI 1.01 to 1.36; $P = .03$) [39].

At first sight, the CRYSTMAS study seemed to support a good safety profile of HES. 196 patients were randomly resuscitated with either 6% HES 130/0.4 or NaCl 0.9%. The authors claimed there was no difference in adverse events between the two groups while a lower volume of fluids was required when using HES [44]. However, when the full data set was reassessed after publication, it was pointed out that there was no volume-saving effect when using HES. Power calculation also proved the study was underpowered to identify differences in the need for RRT. The trend of both mortality and time to RRT was one against treatment with HES, showing a doubling in the need for RRT in the patients treated with HES [45].

In patients with hypovolemia, the CRISTAL study also seemed to support similar outcomes when administering crystalloids, mainly NaCl 0.9%, or colloids. It was an open-label trial including 2847 patients over nine years where mainly HES was used as a colloid besides gelatins, dextran, and human albumin. It should be pointed out that all colloids were analyzed as one group. Subgroup analyses were reported, although they are underpowered to prove significant differences in renal failure or mortality [46]. Furthermore, mainly NaCl 0.9% was administered to the control group. As explained later, we now know the latter fluid also has detrimental effects on renal function [47,48].

Following this evidence, the Pharmacovigilance Risk Assessment Committee (PRAC) of the European Medicines Agency (EMA) stated starches must not be used anymore in burn injuries, renal failure, sepsis, and septic shock [38].

Dextran

Few data exist on the effectiveness and complications of dextran in sepsis. Old data showed tissue deposition of dextran in hemodialysis patients after receiving this type of fluid [49]. A retrospective study of 332 patients also suggested dextran 70 caused increased usage of blood products due to an increased bleeding risk [50]. These findings were not confirmed by a more recent study including 778 propensity score-matched patients [51]. Although one could argue that dextran is not unequivocally proven worse than other resuscitation fluids, we would not recommend using dextran given the cheaper and proven safe alternatives.

Gelatins

Gelatins have always been a less popular colloid. Recently, a systematic review concluded that gelatins increase the risk of anaphylaxis, may increase renal failure, mortality, and bleeding due to extravascular uptake and coagulation impairment [52]. The GENIUS study, a large prospective phase 4 trial, comparing administration of gelatin or crystalloids in sepsis was launched in 2016. To this day, only the protocol was published, but according to the researchers, the final data analysis is due December 2021 [53]. At this time, we would advise against using gelatins given the cheaper and safer alternatives.

Human albumin

As evidence against synthetic colloids grew, concerns arose over the safety profile of albumin. The SAFE study is a double-blinded RCCT comparing administration of fluid boluses of either albumin 4% to boluses of saline 0.9% as a resuscitation fluid in ICU. It was a robust trial showing no difference in mortality or length of stay when albumin 4% was applied. Only the subgroup of patients with head injuries treated with albumin had a significantly worse outcome, while there was a trend toward mortality benefit in the subgroup of sepsis patients.

The researchers acknowledged that the study was underpowered for thorough subgroup analysis. Furthermore, it is noteworthy that inclusion for this trial was performed in ICU, often after initial resuscitation (during the optimization phase) explaining the relatively low administered fluid volumes in both groups [54].

The ALBIOS trial included 1818 patients with sepsis or septic shock. In this trial, resuscitation with crystalloids was performed in both arms, at the investigator's discretion. The intervention was the administration of 300 mL albumin 20% daily to obtain a target above 30 g/L. There was no difference in 28- or 90-day mortality nor in the amount of administered fluids. A post hoc analysis showed a trend toward lower mortality in patients with septic shock. The authors concluded that albumin administration was safe but did not provide a survival advantage. However, as the mortality in this study was much lower than anticipated, this could be due to a type 2 error, not identifying a real difference in mortality when there is one [55].

The EARSS study, by Charpentier and Mira, is a third trial on the use of albumin in septic shock. All patients were resuscitated with NaCl 0.9%. As an intervention, either 100 mL of albumin 20% or 100 mL of NaCl 0.9% was administered every eight hours for three days. Unfortunately, this study was only published as an abstract. According to the provided data, there was no significant difference in mortality between the group treated with albumin (24.1%) and the saline group (26.3%) [56].

While all these trials can at best prove that albumin is not harmful in septic shock, Wiedermann analyzed the combined data of all three trials on albumin use in sepsis. He calculated a pooled relative risk of 0.92 (CI $0.84-1.00; P = .046$) suggesting a mortality benefit [56].

A final trial worth mentioning on the use of albumin is the FEAST trial. It is an RCCT that was performed in children with febrile illness and impaired perfusion. This study had three arms: administration of albumin 5% boluses, administration of NaCl 0.9% boluses, and administration of no fluid boluses. In the bolus group, 20 mL/kg was administered to the patients without hypotension and 40 mL/kg was administered to patients with hypotension over the first hour. This initial treatment was followed by another 20 mL/kg in case of signs of impaired perfusion or by another 40 mL/kg in case of hypotension. After a protocol amendment, the initial boluses were further increased

by 50%. The study was prematurely stopped due to increased mortality in the treatment arms using fluid boluses [14]. While technically this study could be identified as a study on albumin resuscitation, in our opinion, it should mainly be seen as a study warning against uncontrolled fixed administration of large fluid boluses.

Taking these data into account, albumin 4% or 20% could be viable options in a subset of patients with severe sepsis or septic shock in case of low serum albumin levels (<30 g/L). However, given the broad use of NaCl 0.9% as a crystalloid in all these trials, it is also possible that the effects seen in the abovementioned trials are based on harm caused by the control strategy rather than benefit of albumin as an intervention. As with all fluids or drugs in general, appropriate dosing is always important.

Crystalloids

Crystalloids are less expensive and often a better choice in sepsis compared to the much-debated colloids. However, the term crystalloids encompass a large variety of fluids with different properties. We will cover the crystalloids according to tonicity, since this will influence their initial distribution volume.

Since *hypotonic* crystalloids have a large distribution volume, these fluids are not suitable as resuscitation fluids. In the absence of contraindications such as craniocerebral trauma or ischemic stroke, these fluids are preferred as maintenance fluids. Maintenance fluids are due when daily fluid needs are not met by enteral or parenteral nutritional intake [57–59].

Administration of *hypertonic* fluids should theoretically increase the intravascular volume more than isotonic infusions due to a fluid flux toward the intravascular space caused by the higher tonicity. The HYPERS2S trial was performed to investigate this hypothesis. In this trial, sepsis patients were randomized and either treated with boluses of 280 mL hypertonic saline 3.0% or treated with boluses of 280 mL NaCl 0.9%. There was no positive effect on cumulative fluid balances nor specific outcome parameters. While there was an initial fluid sparing effect during resuscitation, this effect was completely nullified by supplementary fluid administration due to hypernatremia [60]. The HERACLES trial described similar findings in patients treated with hypertonic saline admitted to the ICU after cardiac surgery [61].

Regarding the *isotonic* fluids, a distinction must be made between unbalanced (hyperchloremic) fluids and balanced fluids. The detrimental effects of hyperchloremic solutions have been well established in preclinical studies. Administration of (ab)normal NaCl 0.9% was consistently associated with decreased renal perfusion, AKI, and metabolic acidosis [62–69].

In the clinical setting, the SPLIT trial compared the occurrence of AKI when applying either NaCl 0.9% or balanced crystalloids whenever fluids were indicated. While no difference in outcome could be shown due to power issues, it proved the feasibility of comparing balanced and unbalanced fluids [70].

Two large RCTs followed soon after: the SMART and SALT-ED trials [47,48]. The SMART trial was an unblinded pragmatic RCT during which 15,802 patients admitted to ICU either received balanced crystalloids (Plasmalyte or Ringer's lactate) or NaCl 0.9% when fluids were indicated [48]. The SALT-ED trial included 13,347 noncritically ill patients to be treated with either balanced crystalloids (95.3% Ringer's lactate and 4.7% Plasmalyte) or NaCl 0.9% when clinically indicated [47]. Both studies showed administration of crystalloids rather than NaCl 0.9% resulted in a reduction in MAKE 30 (**M**ajor **A**dverse **K**idney **E**vents within **30** days), a composite endpoint for death, need for RRT, and persisting renal disfunction. The effect was largest in patients with sepsis or septic shock in the SMART trial with a number needed to treat of 20 [48]. For the population of the SALT-ED trial, the number needed to treat was 111 [47].

In August 2021, the BaSICS trial was published. In this trial, 11,056 patients were included. It was a two-by-two factorial trial comparing infusion rates of 333 and 999 mL/h at one hand and administration of either Plasmalyte or NaCl 0.9% in bolus whenever administration of a bolus was clinically deemed appropriate on the other hand. There was no significant difference in mortality in this trial. However, important weaknesses were present: the mortality was lower than anticipated compromising the power of this study. Furthermore, 50% of the patients were elective postoperative admissions resulting in a low medium SOFA score of 4 and APACHE II score of 12. The administered fluid volume was less than 1 L a day, and 68% received fluids prior to randomization and following randomization, while 30% of the administered fluid was nonrandomized crystalloid. Although this study might indicate administration of NaCl 0.9% is not detrimental from the first drop in less ill patients, in our opinion, it does not prove these fluids can be safely used in large amounts in sepsis [71].

At the time of writing, the results of the PLUS trial are awaited later in 2021. This study intends to answer the question of whether administration of Plasmalyte or NaCl 0.9% as a sole resuscitation fluid, maintenance fluid, and drug dilution fluid influences 90-day mortality [72].

In conclusion, balanced crystalloids are generally the fluid of choice in sepsis resuscitation, while there might be a place for human albumin in patients with septic shock and an albumin level below 30 g/L. Hypotonic crystalloids are the maintenance fluids of choice when enteral or parenteral feeding is insufficient. There is strong evidence against using HES or NaCl 0.9% in sepsis. There is no convincing evidence to support the use of gelatins or dextran.

REFERENCES

[1] Rhodes A, Evans LE, Alhazzani W, Levy MM, Antonelli M, Ferrer R, et al. Surviving sepsis campaign: international guidelines for management of sepsis and septic shock: 2016. Intensive Care Med 2017;43(3):304–77.

[2] Levy MM, Evans LE, Rhodes A. The surviving sepsis campaign bundle: 2018 update. Intensive Care Med 2018;44(6):925–8.

[3] Vincent JL, Sakr Y, Sprung CL, Ranieri VM, Reinhart K, Gerlach H, et al. Sepsis in European intensive care units: results of the SOAP study. Crit Care Med 2006;34(2):344–53.

[4] Bagshaw SM, Brophy PD, Cruz D, Ronco C. Fluid balance as a biomarker: impact of fluid overload on outcome in critically ill patients with acute kidney injury. Crit Care 2008;12(4):169.

[5] Wiedemann HP, Wheeler AP, Bernard GR, Thompson BT, Hayden D, deBoisblanc B, et al. Comparison of two fluid-management strategies in acute lung injury. N Engl J Med 2006;354(24):2564–75.

[6] Malbrain MLNG, Van Regenmortel N, Saugel B, De Tavernier B, Van Gaal PJ, Joannes-Boyau O, et al. Principles of fluid management and stewardship in septic shock: it is time to consider the four D's and the four phases of fluid therapy. Ann Intensive Care 2018;8(1):66.

[7] Rivers E, Nguyen B, Havstad S, Ressler J, Muzzin A, Knoblich B, et al. Early goal-directed therapy in the treatment of severe sepsis and septic shock. N Engl J Med 2001;345(19):1368–77.

[8] Yealy DM, Kellum JA, Huang DT, Barnato AE, Weissfeld LA, Pike F, et al. A randomized trial of protocol-based care for early septic shock. N Engl J Med 2014;370(18):1683–93.

[9] Peake SL, Delaney A, Bailey M, Bellomo R, Cameron PA, Cooper DJ, et al. Goal-directed resuscitation for patients with early septic shock. N Engl J Med 2014;371(16):1496–506.

[10] Rowan KM, Angus DC, Bailey M, Barnato AE, Bellomo R, Canter RR, et al. Early, goal-directed therapy for septic shock - a patient-level meta-analysis. N Engl J Med 2017;376(23):2223–34.

[11] Asfar P, Meziani F, Hamel JF, Grelon F, Megarbane B, Anguel N, et al. High versus low blood-pressure target in patients with septic shock. N Engl J Med 2014; 370(17):1583–93.

[12] Dellinger RP, Carlet JM, Masur H, Gerlach H, Calandra T, Cohen J, et al. Surviving Sepsis Campaign guidelines for management of severe sepsis and septic shock. Crit Care Med 2004;32(3):858–73.

[13] Marik PE, Cavallazzi R. Does the central venous pressure predict fluid responsiveness? An updated meta-analysis and a plea for some common sense. Crit Care Med 2013;41(7):1774–81.

[14] Maitland K, Kiguli S, Opoka RO, Engoru C, Olupot-Olupot P, Akech SO, et al. Mortality after fluid bolus in African children with severe infection. N Engl J Med 2011;364(26):2483–95.

[15] Monnet X, Marik PE, Teboul JL. Prediction of fluid responsiveness: an update. Ann Intensive Care 2016; 6(1):111.

[16] Hahn RG. Volume kinetics for infusion fluids. Anesthesiology 2010;113(2):470–81.

[17] Hahn RG, Lyons G. The half-life of infusion fluids: an educational review. Eur J Anaesthesiol 2016;33(7): 475–82.

[18] Cecconi M, Hofer C, Teboul JL, Pettila V, Wilkman E, Molnar Z, et al. Fluid challenges in intensive care: the FENICE study: a global inception cohort study. Intensive Care Med 2015;41(9):1529–37.

[19] Aya HD, Rhodes A, Chis Ster I, Fletcher N, Grounds RM, Cecconi M. Hemodynamic effect of different doses of fluids for a fluid challenge: a quasi-randomized controlled study. Crit Care Med 2017;45(2):e161–8.

[20] Murphy CV, Schramm GE, Doherty JA, Reichley RM, Gajic O, Afessa B, et al. The importance of fluid management in acute lung injury secondary to septic shock. Chest 2009;136(1):102–9.

[21] Cordemans C, De Laet I, Van Regenmortel N, Schoonheydt K, Dits H, Martin G, et al. Aiming for a negative fluid balance in patients with acute lung injury and increased intra-abdominal pressure: a pilot study looking at the effects of PAL-treatment. Ann Intensive Care 2012; 2(Suppl. 1):S15.

[22] Cordemans C, De Laet I, Van Regenmortel N, Schoonheydt K, Dits H, Huber W, et al. Fluid management in critically ill patients: the role of extravascular lung water, abdominal hypertension, capillary leak, and fluid balance. Ann Intensive Care 2012;2(Suppl. 1):S1.

[23] Hjortrup PB, Haase N, Bundgaard H, Thomsen SL, Winding R, Pettilä V, et al. Restricting volumes of resuscitation fluid in adults with septic shock after initial management: the CLASSIC randomised, parallel-group, multicentre feasibility trial. Intensive Care Med 2016; 42(11):1695–705.

[24] Silversides JA, Perner A, Malbrain MLNG. Liberal versus restrictive fluid therapy in critically ill patients. Intensive Care Med 2019;45(10):1440–2.

[25] Semler MW, Wheeler AP, Thompson BT, Bernard GR, Wiedemann HP, Rice TW, et al. Impact of initial central venous pressure on outcomes of conservative versus liberal fluid management in acute respiratory distress syndrome. Crit Care Med 2016;44(4):782–9.

[26] Silversides JA, Fitzgerald E, Manickavasagam US, Lapinsky SE, Nisenbaum R, Hemmings N, et al. Deresuscitation of patients with iatrogenic fluid overload is associated with reduced mortality in critical illness. Crit Care Med 2018;46(10):1600–7.

[27] Myles PS, Bellomo R, Corcoran T, Forbes A, Peyton P, Story D, et al. Restrictive versus liberal fluid therapy for major abdominal surgery. N Engl J Med 2018;378(24): 2263–74.

[28] Vincent JL, De Backer D. Circulatory shock. N Engl J Med 2013;369(18):1726–34.

[29] Perner A, Singer M. Fixed minimum fluid volume for resuscitation: Con. Intensive Care Med 2017;43(11): 1681–2.

[30] Andrews B, Muchemwa L, Kelly P, Lakhi S, Heimburger DC, Bernard GR. Simplified severe sepsis protocol: a randomized controlled trial of modified early goal-directed therapy in Zambia. Crit Care Med 2014; 42(11):2315–24.

[31] Boyd JH, Forbes J, Nakada TA, Walley KR, Russell JA. Fluid resuscitation in septic shock: a positive fluid balance and elevated central venous pressure are associated with increased mortality. Crit Care Med 2011;39(2):259–65.

[32] Saugel B, Trepte CJ, Heckel K, Wagner JY, Reuter DA. Hemodynamic management of septic shock: is it time for "individualized goal-directed hemodynamic therapy" and for specifically targeting the microcirculation? Shock 2015;43(6):522–9.

[33] Marik PE, Malbrain MLNG. The SEP-1 quality mandate may be harmful: how to drown a patient with 30 mL per kg fluid. Anaesthesiol Intensive Ther 2017;49(5): 323–8.

[34] Vandervelden S, Malbrain ML. Initial resuscitation from severe sepsis: one size does not fit all. Anaesthesiol Intensive Ther 2015;47:44–55.

[35] Bernards J, Mekeirele M, Hoffmann B, Peeters Y, De Raes M, Malbrain ML. Hemodynamic monitoring: to calibrate or not to calibrate? Part 2–Non-calibrated techniques. Anaesthesiol Intensive Ther 2015;47(5):501–16.

[36] Peeters Y, Bernards J, Mekeirele M, Hoffmann B, De Raes M, Malbrain ML. Hemodynamic monitoring: to calibrate or not to calibrate? Part 1–Calibrated techniques. Anaesthesiol Intensive Ther 2015;47(5):487–500.

[37] Malbrain ML, De Laet I. AIDS is coming to your ICU: be prepared for acute bowel injury and acute intestinal distress syndrome. Intensive Care Med 2008;34(9): 1565–9.

[38] Malbrain MLNG, Langer T, Annane D, Gattinoni L, Elbers P, Hahn RG, et al. Intravenous fluid therapy in the perioperative and critical care setting: executive

summary of the International Fluid Academy (IFA). Ann Intensive Care 2020;10(1):64.

[39] Perner A, Haase N, Guttormsen AB, Tenhunen J, Klemenzson G, Åneman A, et al. Hydroxyethyl starch 130/0.42 versus Ringer's acetate in severe sepsis. N Engl J Med 2012;367(2):124−34.

[40] Brunkhorst FM, Engel C, Bloos F, Meier-Hellmann A, Ragaller M, Weiler N, et al. Intensive insulin therapy and pentastarch resuscitation in severe sepsis. N Engl J Med 2008;358(2):125−39.

[41] Myburgh JA, Finfer S, Bellomo R, Billot L, Cass A, Gattas D, et al. Hydroxyethyl starch or saline for fluid resuscitation in intensive care. N Engl J Med 2012; 367(20):1901−11.

[42] Priebe HJ, Malbrain ML, Elbers P. The great fluid debate: methodology, physiology and appendicitis. Anaesthesiol Intensive Ther 2015;47(5):437−40.

[43] Doshi P. Data too important to share: do those who control the data control the message? BMJ 2016;352:i1027.

[44] Guidet B, Martinet O, Boulain T, Philippart F, Poussel JF, Maizel J, et al. Assessment of hemodynamic efficacy and safety of 6% hydroxyethylstarch 130/0.4 vs. 0.9% NaCl fluid replacement in patients with severe sepsis: the CRYSTMAS study. Crit Care 2012;16(3):R94.

[45] Hartog CS, Reinhart K. CRYSTMAS study adds to concerns about renal safety and increased mortality in sepsis patients. Crit Care 2012;16(6):454.

[46] Annane D, Siami S, Jaber S, Martin C, Elatrous S, Declère AD, et al. Effects of fluid resuscitation with colloids vs crystalloids on mortality in critically ill patients presenting with hypovolemic shock: the CRISTAL randomized trial. JAMA 2013;310(17):1809−17.

[47] Self WH, Semler MW, Wanderer JP, Wang L, Byrne DW, Collins SP, et al. Balanced crystalloids versus saline in noncritically ill adults. N Engl J Med 2018;378(9): 819−28.

[48] Semler MW, Self WH, Rice TW. Balanced crystalloids versus saline in critically ill adults. N Engl J Med 2018; 378(20):1951.

[49] Bergonzi G, Paties C, Vassallo G, Zangrandi A, Poisetti PG, Ballocchi S, et al. Dextran deposits in tissues of patients undergoing haemodialysis. Nephrol Dial Transplant 1990;5(1):54−8.

[50] Hvidt LN, Perner A. High dosage of dextran 70 is associated with severe bleeding in patients admitted to the intensive care unit for septic shock. Dan Med J 2012; 59(11):A4531.

[51] Bentzer P, Broman M, Kander T. Effect of dextran-70 on outcome in severe sepsis; a propensity-score matching study. Scand J Trauma Resuscitation Emerg Med 2017; 25(1):65.

[52] Moeller C, Fleischmann C, Thomas-Rueddel D, Vlasakov V, Rochwerg B, Theurer P, et al. How safe is gelatin? A systematic review and meta-analysis of gelatin-containing plasma expanders vs crystalloids and albumin. J Crit Care 2016;35:75−83.

[53] Marx G, Zacharowski K, Ichai C, Asehnoune K, Černý V, Dembinski R, et al. Efficacy and safety of early target-controlled plasma volume replacement with a balanced gelatine solution versus a balanced electrolyte solution in patients with severe sepsis/septic shock: study protocol, design, and rationale of a prospective, randomized, controlled, double-blind, multicentric, international clinical trial : GENIUS-Gelatine use in ICU and sepsis. Trials 2021;22(1):376.

[54] Finfer S, Bellomo R, Boyce N, French J, Myburgh J, Norton R, et al. A comparison of albumin and saline for fluid resuscitation in the intensive care unit. N Engl J Med 2004;350(22):2247−56.

[55] Caironi P, Tognoni G, Masson S, Fumagalli R, Pesenti A, Romero M, et al. Albumin replacement in patients with severe sepsis or septic shock. N Engl J Med 2014; 370(15):1412−21.

[56] Wiedermann CJ, Joannidis M. Albumin replacement in severe sepsis or septic shock. N Engl J Med 2014; 371(1):83.

[57] Van Regenmortel N, De Weerdt T, Van Craenenbroeck AH, Roelant E, Verbrugghe W, Dams K, et al. Effect of isotonic versus hypotonic maintenance fluid therapy on urine output, fluid balance, and electrolyte homeostasis: a crossover study in fasting adult volunteers. Br J Anaesth 2017;118(6):892−900.

[58] Van Regenmortel N, Hendrickx S, Roelant E, Baar I, Dams K, Van Vlimmeren K, et al. 154 compared to 54 mmol per liter of sodium in intravenous maintenance fluid therapy for adult patients undergoing major thoracic surgery (TOPMAST): a single-center randomized controlled double-blind trial. Intensive Care Med 2019; 45(10):1422−32.

[59] Lobo DN, Stanga Z, Simpson JA, Anderson JA, Rowlands BJ, Allison SP. Dilution and redistribution effects of rapid 2-litre infusions of 0.9% (w/v) saline and 5% (w/v) dextrose on haematological parameters and serum biochemistry in normal subjects: a double-blind crossover study. Clin Sci (Lond). 2001;101(2):173−9.

[60] Asfar P, Schortgen F, Boisramé-Helms J, Charpentier J, Guérot E, Megarbane B, et al. Hyperoxia and hypertonic saline in patients with septic shock (HYPERS2S): a two-by-two factorial, multicentre, randomised, clinical trial. Lancet Respir Med 2017;5(3):180−90.

[61] Pfortmueller CA, Kindler M, Schenk N, Messmer AS, Hess B, Jakob L, et al. Hypertonic saline for fluid resuscitation in ICU patients post-cardiac surgery (HERACLES): a double-blind randomized controlled clinical trial. Intensive Care Med 2020;46(9):1683−95.

[62] Chowdhury AH, Cox EF, Francis ST, Lobo DN. A randomized, controlled, double-blind crossover study on the effects of 2-L infusions of 0.9% saline and plasma-lyte® 148 on renal blood flow velocity and renal cortical tissue perfusion in healthy volunteers. Ann Surg 2012;256(1):18−24.

[63] Hasman H, Cinar O, Uzun A, Cevik E, Jay L, Comert B. A randomized clinical trial comparing the effect of rapidly infused crystalloids on acid-base status in dehydrated patients in the emergency department. Int J Med Sci 2012; 9(1):59−64.

[64] Kellum JA. Fluid resuscitation and hyperchloremic acidosis in experimental sepsis: improved short-term survival and acid-base balance with Hextend compared with saline. Crit Care Med 2002;30(2):300—5.

[65] Orbegozo D, Su F, Santacruz C, He X, Hosokawa K, Creteur J, et al. Effects of different crystalloid solutions on hemodynamics, peripheral perfusion, and the microcirculation in experimental abdominal sepsis. Anesthesiology 2016;125(4):744—54.

[66] Potura E, Lindner G, Biesenbach P, Funk GC, Reiterer C, Kabon B, et al. An acetate-buffered balanced crystalloid versus 0.9% saline in patients with end-stage renal disease undergoing cadaveric renal transplantation: a prospective randomized controlled trial. Anesth Analg 2015;120(1): 123—9.

[67] Waters JH, Gottlieb A, Schoenwald P, Popovich MJ, Sprung J, Nelson DR. Normal saline versus lactated Ringer's solution for intraoperative fluid management in patients undergoing abdominal aortic aneurysm repair: an outcome study. Anesth Analg 2001;93(4): 817—22.

[68] Jaynes MP, Murphy CV, Ali N, Krautwater A, Lehman A, Doepker BA. Association between chloride content of intravenous fluids and acute kidney injury in critically ill medical patients with sepsis. J Crit Care 2018;44: 363—7.

[69] Langer T, Santini A, Scotti E, Van Regenmortel N, Malbrain ML, Caironi P. Intravenous balanced solutions: from physiology to clinical evidence. Anaesthesiol Intensive Ther 2015;47:s78—88.

[70] Young P, Bailey M, Beasley R, Henderson S, Mackle D, McArthur C, et al. Effect of a buffered crystalloid solution vs saline on acute kidney injury among patients in the intensive care unit: the SPLIT randomized clinical trial. JAMA 2015;314(16):1701—10.

[71] Zampieri FG, Machado FR, Biondi RS, Freitas FGR, Veiga VC, Figueiredo RC, et al. Effect of intravenous fluid treatment with a balanced solution vs 0.9% saline solution on mortality in critically ill patients: the BaSICS randomized clinical trial. JAMA 2021;326(9):1—12. https:// doi.org/10.1001/jama.2021.11684.

[72] Hammond NE, Bellomo R, Gallagher M, Gattas D, Glass P, Mackle D, et al. The Plasma-Lyte 148 v Saline (PLUS) study protocol: a multicentre, randomised controlled trial of the effect of intensive care fluid therapy on mortality. Crit Care Resusc 2017;19(3):239—46.

[73] Malbrain ML, Marik PE, Witters I, Cordemans C, Kirkpatrick AW, Roberts DJ, et al. Fluid overload, de-resuscitation, and outcomes in critically ill or injured patients: a systematic review with suggestions for clinical practice. Anaesthesiol Intensive Ther 2014;46(5): 361—80.

CHAPTER 15

Vasopressor Therapy in Septic Shock

AHSINA JAHAN LOPA • SULAGNA BHATTACHARJEE •
RAJESH CHANDRA MISHRA • AHSAN AHMED • SHARMILI SINHA

INTRODUCTION

Septic shock is characterized by a profound abnormality in circulatory and cellular metabolism which substantially increases mortality. It is diagnosed as persistent hypotension requiring vasopressors to maintain mean arterial pressure (MAP) >65 mmHg and hyperlactatemia (serum lactate > 2 mmol/L) despite adequate fluid resuscitation in patients presenting with the clinical construct of sepsis. In-hospital mortality in such patients exceeds 40%. Therefore, septic shock is a medical emergency and warrants immediate treatment and resuscitation [1].

Vasopressors are hormones that constrict blood vessels, by acting through a myriad of receptors on vascular smooth muscles, cardiac myocytes, or other neurohumoral targets. Use of vasopressors is central to the management of septic shock. Over the last two decades, the role of vasopressors in sepsis has evolved from being used in early goal-directed therapy, to hourly bundles, and more recently to individualized hemodynamic targets.

This chapter will review on the relevant pathophysiology of septic shock, specific vasopressor pharmacology, dose, indications, adverse effects, pivotal trials, clinical monitoring and weaning of vasopressor therapy, vasopressor-sparing strategies, and directions of future research.

UNDERSTANDING THE RELEVANT PATHOPHYSIOLOGY OF SEPTIC SHOCK

Dysregulated host immune system in sepsis releases cytokines in response to pathogen-associated molecular patterns and the damage-associated molecular patterns, causing vasodilation by direct action, synthesis of nitric oxide (NO), direct myocardial depression, and loss of intravascular volume by endothelial disruption, all of which contribute to hypotension in sepsis [2]. Other mediators of vasodilation include prostaglandins and adrenomedullin [3]. A disbalance oxygen supply and delivery at the global (systemic hypoperfusion) and/or regional level (organ-specific, microcirculatory dysfunction) coupled with sepsis-induced mitochondrial dysfunction leads to shock and organ dysfunction in sepsis [4].

Although the initial response to vasodilation triggers the release of endogenous vasoconstrictors and hormones such as endogenous norepinephrine, epinephrine, vasopressin, angiotensin II (AT II), aldosterone, and cortisol, causing increased inotropy and contractility, failure to achieve homeostasis results from factors such as adrenergic receptor downregulation, genotype differences in sensitivity, and variable hormone metabolism [3]. Profound vasopressin deficiency is also found in later stages of septic shock [5].

The hallmark of circulatory failure in sepsis is peripheral vasodilation and shunting at the arterial and capillary level. The early phase of septic shock is hyperdynamic or warm shock, which is marked by high cardiac output, low systemic vascular resistance (SVR), and warm peripheries, with normal capillary refill time (<1 s). The late phase or the cold phase is characterized by hypodynamic shock with persistent hypotension, low cardiac output, cold peripheries, and delayed capillary refill time (>3 s) [6]. Sepsis-induced myocardial dysfunction is present in about 25%−50% of adults with septic shock. It is characterized by both decreased systolic contractility and impaired diastolic function and is associated with adverse clinical outcomes [7].

Vasopressors: Mechanism of action, clinical evidence, doses, and adverse effects (Table 15.1).

Catecholamines: The endogenous catecholamines namely norepinephrine, epinephrine, and dopamine are secreted from the adrenal medulla and act on adrenergic and dopaminergic receptors [8].

Alpha adrenergic receptors: Located on the vascular smooth muscles, their activation causes intense

The Sepsis Codex. https://doi.org/10.1016/B978-0-323-88271-2.00011-0

TABLE 15.1
Receptor Binding, Dose, Major Adverse Events, and Additional Effects of Vasopressors [8,18,35]

Vasopressor	Receptor affinity	Dose	Immunologic/other effects	Major adverse effects
Catecholamines				
Noradrenaline	$\alpha1$, $\alpha2$, $\beta1>$ $\beta2$	0.01–3 µg/kg/min (5–100 µg/min)	↑IL-10, ↑IL-1β in vivo in rats	Organ and digital ischemia, tachycardia, tachyarrhythmia, inadvertent immunomodulation
Adrenaline	$\alpha1$, $\alpha2$, $\beta1$, $\beta2$	0.01–0.1 µg/kg/min 1 mg IV every 3–5 min for cardiac arrest, unresponsive bradycardia (5–60 µg/min)	In humans ↓ TNF-α, ↑IL-10	Tachycardia, tachyarrhythmia, ischemia, increased myocardial oxygen demand, hyperglycemia, lactic acidosis
Dopamine	D1, D2 Low dose D1 Moderate dose $\beta1$ Higher doses $\alpha1$ [9]	1–5 µg/kg/min low dose 5–10 µg/kg/min moderate 10–20 µg/kg/min higher doses (max 50 µg/kg/min) [36]	Affects cell-mediated immunity	Tachycardia, tachyarrhythmia
Phenylephrine	$\alpha1$	0.1–1.5 µg/kg/min Bolus 50–100 µg	↑Circulating TNF-α in canine model	Decreased cardiac output, reflex bradycardia
Non catecholamines				
Vasopressin	V1, V2	0.01–0.04 U/min	↓ IL-6, TNF-α, IL-10 in pig model	Organ and digital ischemia, thromboembolism, antidiuresis
Selepressin	V1a	1.25–2.5 ng/kg/min in phase 2 1.25–5 ng/kg/min in phase 3	↓ IL-6 in sheep model, ↓ angiopoietin 2, vascular permeability	Organ and digital ischemia, decreased cardiac output
Terlipressin	V1a > V2	1.3 µg/kg/hr or 20–160 µg/hr Bolus dose 1 mg	Immune activity?	Organ and digital ischemia, decreased cardiac output
Angiotensin II	AT1, AT2	5–200 ng/kg/min for 3 h; 1.25–40 ng/kg/min upto 7 days [33]	↑Vasopressin, ↑ Erythropoietin	Organ digital ischemia
Methylene blue	NO-cGMP pathway	1–2 mg/kg infusion for 15 min ± infusion		Bluish discoloration of skin and urine, methemoglobinemia, falsely low pulse oximetry readings

vasoconstriction leading to increased SVR [8]. Alpha 1 receptor is the major site for action of sympathetic vasopressor. Alpha 2 receptors located on the vascular smooth muscles also mediate vasopressor effects [9].

Beta adrenergic receptors: Located on the vascular cardiac myocytes, β1 stimulation leads to increased inotropy and chronotropy, whereas in vascular smooth muscles cells, β2 stimulation leads to vasodilation [8].

Dopaminergic receptors: D1 and D2 receptors located in the renal and splanchnic vasculature lead to vasodilation [8].

NORADRENALINE

It is the major endogenous catecholamine secreted by postganglionic adrenergic nerves. It is a potent $\alpha 1$ as well as $\alpha 2$ receptor agonist with modest β agonism, which renders it a powerful vasoconstrictor increasing systolic, diastolic and pulse pressures, with some inotropic activity, with minimal effect on net cardiac output and heart rate. It enhances coronary blood flow by increasing diastolic pressure and release of local mediators by cardiac myocytes. Prolonged use of noradrenaline infusion can cause direct myocardial toxicity by inducing apoptosis via protein kinase A pathway [8].

The Surviving Sepsis Campaign 2016 (SSC 16) guidelines recommend noradrenaline is the first line vasopressor for the management of septic shock (strong recommendation, moderate quality of evidence [10]). The multicentric SOAP II study (2010) by De backer et al. was one of the pivotal randomized control trials (RCTs) that compared dopamine ($n = 858$) and noradrenaline ($n = 821$) as the first-line agents for shock. Although the groups showed no statistically significant difference in terms of 28-day mortality, dopamine group reported more arrhythmic events. A subgroup analysis showed that dopamine was associated with increased risk of death in patients with cardiogenic shock but not with septic or hypovolemic shock [11].

The Surviving Sepsis Campaign bundle 2018 recommends applying vasopressors with persistent hypotension during the first hour of initial fluid resuscitation [12]. A recent RCT comparing administration of early noradrenaline infusion versus standard treatment ($n = 310$) within the first hour of septic shock found earlier control of shock and lower incidence of cardiogenic pulmonary edema and new onset arrhythmias in the intervention group [13]. A metaanalysis by Liu et al. including 929 patients demonstrated that the early use of noradrenaline was associated with reduced short-term mortality, shorter time to achieve MAP, and reduced fluid requirement during the initial 6 h of resuscitation of septic shock [14]. In the systematic review and metanalysis by Avni et al. noradrenaline use was associated with reduced all-cause mortality (absolute risk reduction of 11%), and lower risk of major adverse events and tachycardia, as compared to dopamine. Also, it was associated with a better hemodynamic profile [15].

ADRENALINE

Adrenaline is an endogenous catecholamine which is a potent agonist of $\alpha 1$, $\alpha 2$, $\beta 1$, and $\beta 2$ receptors, with β action prominent at low doses and α action at higher doses [8,9]. Coronary blood flow is enhanced by increasing the relative diastolic time and release of local vasodilatory mediators. Pulmonary arterial and venous pressures are increased by pulmonary vasoconstriction and increased pulmonary blood flow. Sustained use can lead to direct myocardial toxicity and apoptosis [8].

The SSC 16 guideline uses adrenaline as a second line agent for raising MAP to target range (weak recommendation, low quality of evidence [10]). Although, evidence from human and animal studies reveal deleterious effects of adrenaline like reduced splanchnic perfusion and hyperlactatemia, clinically significant adverse outcomes are unknown [10]. The CAT randomized controlled trial comparing epinephrine to norepinephrine in critically ill patients revealed no difference in mortality but an increase in transient metabolic events and tachycardia in adrenaline group [16].

The CATS trial that compared adrenaline infusion to noradrenaline plus dobutamine infusion in 330 patients with septic shock demonstrated no difference in the primary end point of 28-day mortality or in other secondary end points like 90-day mortality, time to hemodynamic success, time to vasopressor withdrawal, and in SOFA scores [17].

Also, a metaanalysis involving four clinical trials found no mortality benefit of norepinephrine compared to epinephrine [15].

PHENYLEPHRINE

It is a potent $\alpha 1$ agonist commonly used for immediate correction of profound hypotension. It can cause baroreceptor reflex-mediated severe bradycardia and splanchnic vasoconstriction, which precludes its use as a first-line agent in resuscitation of septic shock [18]. A retrospective cohort study revealed that during the noradrenaline shortage phase in United States in 2011, patients with septic shock treated with phenylephrine had a higher mortality as compared to noradrenaline [19].

DOPAMINE

Dopamine is an endogenous neurotransmitter and the immediate precursor to noradrenaline.

It acts on dopaminergic and adrenergic receptors to exert a multitude of effects (Table 15.1). At low doses, it acts on postsynaptic presynaptic D1 receptors located in the renal, coronary, mesenteric, and cerebral beds, and D2 receptors in the vasculature and renal beds, causing vasodilation and increased perfusion. At intermediate doses, dopamine acts on β1 receptor, promoting norepinephrine release, thereby increasing cardiac contractility and SVR. At higher doses, it acts on α1 receptor, causing predominant vasoconstriction [8].

Although previously it was a first line vasopressor in septic shock, it is currently used as an alternative agent to noradrenaline in highly selected patients who are at a lower risk of tachyarrhythmia or with absolute or relative bradycardia [10]. A large randomized controlled clinical trial by Bellomo R et al. and a metaanalysis by Marik P found no difference of low-dose dopamine versus placebo for peak serum creatinine concentration, need for renal replacement therapy (RRT), urine output, renal recovery, cardiac arrhythmias, mortality, length of intensive care unit (ICU) stay, and hospital stay [20,21].

NONCATECHOLAMINES
Vasopressin: V1a receptors on the vascular smooth muscles mediates vasoconstriction. V2 receptors, located in the renal collecting tubules, cause water reabsorption by increasing the density of apical aquaporin channels. V2 receptor stimulation also mediates vasodilation through NO release and procoagulant action by release of Von Willebrand factor and clotting factors from the liver [22].

By stimulation of V3 (V1b) receptors located in the anterior pituitary and hippocampus, vasopressin increases adrenocorticotrophic hormone release [5]. Vasopressin has less direct effects on cerebral or coronary vessels, compared to catecholamines, and has a neutral or inhibitory effect on cardiac output, depending on the increase in SVR. It may act on direct pathways of vasodilation such as inhibition of potassium sensitive ATP channels, upregulation of adrenergic receptors, and attenuation of NO production. The pressor effects of vasopressin are augmented by the modulation of vascular sensitivity to norepinephrine. Also, vasopressin effects are relatively retained during hypoxia and acidosis [8].

Vasopressin levels in septic shock are reported to be lower than expected for the degree of shock, a phenomenon called relative vasopressin deficiency, which is thought to be secondary to the depletion of stored vasopressin in early septic shock, as well as a sustained impaired synthesis and release of vasopressin after the onset of septic shock. Earlier clinical studies had indicated vasopressin infusion led to improvement in blood pressure, urine output, and noradrenaline requirement [5].

The VASST trial comparing noradrenaline plus vasopressin (0.03 U/min) to noradrenaline alone found no significant difference in short term or 90-day mortality in between the groups. However, in the predefined subgroup of less severe septic shock (<15 μg/min of noradrenaline requirement), mortality was lower in the vasopressin group [23].

The VANISH trial randomized patients in a factorial 2 × 2 design, comparing vasopressin with hydrocortisone or placebo and noradrenaline with hydrocortisone or placebo. Although the vasopressin group required less RRT, there was no significant difference in death or kidney failure–free days [24].

An updated metaanalysis, compiling data from nine trials comparing norepinephrine versus vasopressin or terlipressin, revealed no significant difference in mortality (relative risk [RR] 0.89, confidence interval [CI] 0.77–1.02) [10].

In a systematic review and metaanalysis of 23 trials that included 3088 patients, addition of vasopressin to a catecholamine seemed to prevent atrial fibrillation (RR 0.77) [25].

VASOPRESSIN ANALOGS
Terlipressin is a long-acting synthetic analog of vasopressin with action on V1a, V1b, and V2 receptors [22].

In the TERLIVAP randomized control pilot trial ($N = 45$), terlipressin infusion (1.3 μg/kg/min) was compared with vasopressin (0.03 U/min) and noradrenaline as the initial vasopressor in septic shock patients. Open label noradrenaline was given to all the three groups as necessary. Although there was no difference in the groups in terms of systemic and regional hemodynamics, terlipressin resulted in lower noradrenaline requirement across all groups and less incidence of rebound hypotension [26].

In 2018, Liu et al. published the largest multicentric RCT from China, evaluating the safety and efficacy of continuous terlipressin infusion in patients with septic shock. It included 526 patients randomized to the terlipressin ($n = 260$) group or the noradrenaline group ($n = 266$) to receive terlipressin (2–160 μg/h, maximum up to 4 mg/day) or noradrenaline 4–30 μg/min as the initial vasopressor. There was no significant difference in the primary end point of 28-day mortality (40% in the terlipressin and 38% in the NE group), [OR 0.93, 95% CI 0.55–1.56]; $P = .80$). Change in SOFA score at day 7 was similar in the two groups. However, serious adverse events like digital ischemia were higher in the terlipressin group [27]. This was followed by a metaanalysis by Zhu et al. that demonstrated that compared to catecholamines, terlipressin did not reduce the risk of mortality, had similar ICU and hospital stay, similar rate of adverse events, but resulted in shorter duration of mechanical ventilation and reduced noradrenaline requirement [28].

SELEPRESSIN

It is a novel short-acting selective V1a receptor agonist. In a phase IIa randomized placebo-controlled clinical trial, selepressin infusion at 2.5 ng/kg/min was an effective substitute for noradrenaline and appeared to improve fluid balance and shorten duration of mechanical ventilation [29]. Early administration of selepressin has been associated with reduced vascular leak and extravascular lung water [22].

The SEPSIS-ACT was an adaptive design phase 2 b/3 RCT that compared selepressin infusion regimens to placebo in 828 septic shock patients requiring >5 µg/min of noradrenaline. There was no difference in primary end point between selepressin and placebo groups (median ventilator and vasopressor-free days 15 vs. 14.5 days; difference 0.6, 95% CI 1.3−2.4) or key secondary end points (90-day mortality, kidney replacement−free days or ICU-free days. The trial was stopped after part 1 for futility [30].

ANGIOTENSIN II

AT II is the most important product of renin-angiotensin-aldosterone axis, which is synthesized from angiotensinogen by the action of renin. It acts on G protein-coupled receptors AT1 and AT2. AT1 receptors are located in the kidney, heart, adrenal glands, skeletal muscles, brain, and peripheral blood mononuclear cells. The major hemodynamic effects include vasoconstriction, release of aldosterone and vasopressin, and remodeling of the heart. AT1 receptor stimulation can also lead to proinflammatory and procoagulant mediators, and increased vascular permeability. Significance of AT2 receptor stimulation is still uncertain and is believed to inhibit vascular smooth muscle [31].

The pilot randomized ATHOS trial evaluated infusion of AT II versus placebo with standard care for patients ($N = 20$) with distributive shock. AT II infusion (2−10 ng/kg/min) caused marked reduction in noradrenaline requirement, without any difference in 30-day mortality [32].

This was followed by the ATHOS-3 trial by Khanna et al. which randomized 344 patients with vasodilatory shock (noradrenaline dose> 0.2 µg/kg/min) to either required receive infusion of either AT II or placebo. The primary end point, which was increase in MAP >10 mmHg or MAP> 75 mmHg at 3 h of start of infusion, was achieved in significantly higher number of patients than placebo (69.9% vs. 23.4%, odds ratio 7.95; 95% CI 4.76−13.3). Secondary end points like 48- cardiovascular SOFA score and 28-day mortality were significantly higher in the AT II group. The incidence of serious adverse effects was also fewer in the AT II group. Therefore, the ATHOS-3 trial demonstrated that AT II was effective in controlling blood pressure in vasodilatory shock that did not respond to high doses of conventional vasopressors [33].

METHYLENE BLUE

It blocks the NO-cyclic guanosine monophosphate pathway (cGMP), by inhibiting NO synthase and soluble guanyl cyclase, thereby counteracting the NO-mediated vasodilation in sepsis. It increases mean arterial and pulmonary arterial pressures. Use of methylene blue has been reported in refractory distributive shock states such as septic shock, anaphylactic shock, and postcardiopulmonary bypass vasoplegic states. However, effect of methylene blue on clinical outcome and mortality remains uncertain [34].

SIDE EFFECTS OF VASOPRESSOR THERAPY

The most common side effects of vasopressor therapy are digital and organ ischemia, tachyarrhythmias, and atrial fibrillation. Higher cumulative dose of vasopressor is associated with higher mortality. Ischemia is mediated by the α1 and V1a receptors and is seen with noradrenaline, adrenaline, vasopressin, and dopamine. Tachyarrhythmias are primarily β1-mediated, seen with adrenaline, noradrenaline, dopamine, and dobutamine, less frequently with vasopressin. Hyperglycemia and hyperlactatemia are also mediated via β1and is more common with adrenaline than noradrenaline. Although mentioned in some earlier reports, acute kidney injury due to noradrenaline infusion seems to be unfounded at clinically used doses [37]. V2 receptor stimulation by vasopressin or terlipressin can lead to vasodilation, thromboembolism, and antidiuresis [22]. Current data from in vitro and animal studies suggest that noradrenaline use can lead to immunosuppression and increased bacterial growth. Future human studies are warranted [35].

Some pivotal trials on vasopressors are discussed in Table 15.2.

TABLE 15.2
Pivotal Randomized Controlled Trials in Vasopressor Therapy

Trial name (year)	Design	Patient population	Total no of patients (N)	Intervention (n)	Control (n)	Intervention mortality	Control mortality	Absolute difference [95% CI]	Other outcomes
SOAP II (2010) [11]	Multicentric RCT	Undifferentiated shock	1679	Noradrenaline (821)	Dopamine (858)	48.5%	52.5%	OR for dopamine 1.17 [0.97 to 1.42], P = .12	More arrhythmogenic events in dopamine group (24.1%) versus noradrenaline (12.4%)
CAT (2008) [16]	Multicentric RCT	ICU patients requiring vasopressors	277	Adrenaline (139)	Noradrenaline (138)	28 day-22.5%	28 day-26.1%	HR 0.86 [0.57–1.31] P = .48	No difference in primary outcome of achievement of MAP goal, increased transient metabolic side effects in the epinephrine group
CATS (2007) [17]	Multicentric RCT	Septic shock	330	Adrenaline (161)	Dobutamine plus noradrenaline (169)	28 day-40%	28 day-34%	RR0.86 [0.65–1.14], P = .31	No difference in 90-day mortality, time to hemodynamic success, time to vasopressor withdrawal
VAAST (2008) [23]	Multicentric RCT	Septic shock with ≥5 μ/min noradrenaline	778	Vasopressin (396)	Noradrenaline (382)	28 day-35.4%	28 day-39.3%	ARR 3.9 [-2.9 to 10.7] P = .26	Lower mortality in less severe septic shock
VANISH (2016) [24]	Multicentric RCT factorial 2 × 2	Septic shock	409	Vasopressin (hydrocortisone vs. placebo) (205)	Noradrenaline (hydrocortisone vs. placebo) (204)	28 day-30.9%	28 day-27.5%	-3.4% [-5.4% to 12.3%]	No difference in primary outcome kidney failure–free days

Study	Design	Population	N	Intervention	Comparator				Outcome
ATHOS3 (2017) [33]	Multicentric RCT	Vasodilatory shock	321	Angiotensin II (163)	Placebo (154)	28 day-46%	28 day-54%	HR-0.78 [0.57 to 1.07] $P = .12$	Primary outcome response of MAP at 3 h was significantly higher for intervention group ($P < .001$)
SEPSIS ACT (2019) [30]	Multicentric adaptive phase 2 b/3 RCT	Septic shock requiring ≥5 µ/min noradrenaline	828	Selepressin 3 regimens (562)	Placebo (266)	90 day-40.6%	90 day-39.4%	Difference 1.1 [−6.5 to 8.8] $P = .77$	No difference in primary outcome ventilator and vasopressor-free days $P = .30$
Liu et al. (2018) [27]	Multicentric RCT	Septic shock	526	Terlipressin	Noradrenaline	28 day-40%	28 day-38%	OR-0.93 [0.55–1.56] $P = .80$	Higher incidence of serious adverse effects in terlipressin group

ARR, absolute risk reduction; *CI*, confidence interval; *HR*, hazard ratio; *OR*, odds ratio; *RR*, relative risk.

PRINCIPLES OF VASOPRESSOR THERAPY

Initial evaluation and management should focus on optimizing the airway, breathing, and circulation, based on brief history, clinical assessment of volume status, fluid responsiveness (dynamic indices), as well as laboratory (hematology, liver, renal function tests, arterial blood gases), microbiology, and imaging studies. According to the Surviving Sepsis Campaign Bundle 2018, vasopressor therapy should be initiated within the first hour if adequate fluid resuscitation (30 mL/kg or more) fails to achieve MAP $\geq$ 65 mmHg [12]. Vasopressor-sparing strategies should be applied in case of refractory septic shock, which is characterized by high vasopressor requirements (noradrenaline >0.5μ/kg/min) and is associated with mortality of 60%–90% [38] (Fig. 15.1).

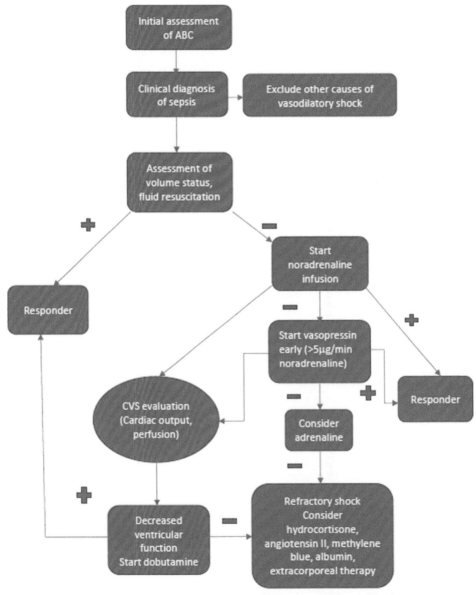

FIG. 15.1 Algorithm for Vasopressor Management in Septic Shock.

CLINICAL MONITORING OF VASOPRESSOR THERAPY

Bedside clinical and hemodynamic monitoring is of utmost importance in the management of septic shock. Arterial cannulation with beat-to-beat monitoring of invasive blood pressure is recommended for patients on vasopressors (weak recommendation). Bedside echocardiography, minimally invasive cardiac output monitoring or pulmonary arterial catheter should be used appropriately [39].

The SSC 16 recommends initial target MAP of 65 mmHg in patients requiring vasopressors. Resuscitation should be guided to normalize lactate or capillary refill time (<2 s). However, the optimal MAP for patients with septic shock should be individualized [40]. A recent retrospective cohort study involving 4689 patients from a single health care system suggests that target MAP should be personalized based on premorbid blood pressure (80−85 mmHg in patients with premorbid hypertension, 65 mmHg in normotension, and lower target [approx. 55 mm Hg in hypotension]) [41,42].

WEANING OF VASOPRESSOR THERAPY

Discontinuation of vasopressor therapy is equally important as they are associated with adverse events. Results of prospective as well as retrospective studies [43−46] indicate that discontinuation of vasopressin prior to noradrenaline may be associated with a higher incidence of hypotension. Use of a hemodynamic algorithm based on ventriculo-arterial coupling, using echocardiography or continuous hemodynamic monitoring system can guide optimal timing of discontinuation. Artificial intelligence−based algorithms can assist the clinicians in the weaning of vasopressors in the coming days [47].

VASOPRESSOR SPARING STRATEGIES

As vasopressor therapy is associated with serious adverse effects and increased cost of ICU stay, numerous vasopressor-sparing strategies have been investigated so far. In a recent scoping review by Guinot et al. the strategies that were found to be associated with decreased vasopressor therapy were implementation of a weaning strategy, systemic corticosteroids, vasopressin use, beta blockers, and normothermia. Strategies such as early goal-directed fluid therapy, vitamin C use, oral vasopressors, and RRT were not associated with increased vasopressor-free days [47]

1. Corticosteroids:
   Sepsis and septic shock are associated with absolute or relative adrenal insufficiency, termed as critical illness-related corticosteroid insufficiency, which is contributed by hypothalamo-pituitary axis activation, adrenal hypo responsiveness, and glucocorticoid resistance.
   SSC 2016 guidelines recommend using intravenous hydrocortisone 200 mg/day if adequate fluid resuscitation and vasopressors fail to achieve hemodynamic stability (weak recommendation, low quality of evidence) based on earlier studies [10].
   With advent of the recent ADRENAL and APROCCHSS trial, updated metanalyses have revealed that systemic corticosteroids offer no or minimal mortality benefit in septic shock. However, steroids can shorten the duration of shock.

2. Inotropes
   Septic shock is commonly associated with myocardial dysfunction and may require inotrope therapy along with vasopressors and fluid resuscitation to maintain adequate tissue perfusion.
   SSC 16 guidelines advocate the use of dobutamine in such scenarios (weak recommendation, low quality of evidence). Dobutamine is a synthetic catecholamine with predominant $\beta1>\beta2$ action [8]. Milrinone is a phosphodiesterase inhibitor with inodilator properties, with limited data clinical efficacy in septic shock [10].
   Levosimendan acts as calcium sensitizer in cardiac myocytes and a potassium channel opener, causing positive inotropy and vasodilation. Pooled estimates from small RCTs did not show any survival benefit of levosimendan over dobutamine [10]. Although limited by trial design, the LeoPARDS trial did not show any advantage of levosimendan for improving organ dysfunction or mortality in patients with sepsis [48].

3. Addition of nonadrenergic vasopressor like vasopressin to norepinephrine is recommended in refractory shock.

4. Albumin administration is recommended in addition to crystalloids in patients with septic shock, who require substantial amounts of fluids. Albumin expands the plasma volume, has protective effects on vessel wall integrity, has antioxidant effects and renal protective effects [49].
   The subgroup analysis of the ALBIOS trial of 1121 patients with septic shock demonstrated a reduced mortality with albumin resuscitation [50].

5. Cardio-selective beta blockers have been shown to reduce vasopressor doses in patients with sepsis and tachycardia, a phenomenon explained by the ventriculo-arterial coupling [51]. In a small proof of concept RCT, esmolol infusion after initial

hemodynamic optimization in septic shock patients maintained heart rates, increased stroke volume, reduced noradrenaline requirement, and was associated with improved 28-day survival [52].

6. Implementing hemodynamic objectives and strategies to achieve targets, as well as strategies to wean vasopressors.

7. Maintaining normothermia: Targeting normothermia may decrease the duration of vasopressor therapy. In a small randomized controlled trial of 200 septic shock patients, external cooling to treat fever resulted in 50% reduction in vasopressor dose and significantly lower day 14 mortality as compared to no cooling [53].

DIRECTIONS OF FUTURE RESEARCH

Although septic shock is the commonest cause of shock requiring ICU admission, the mechanisms of vascular responsiveness to various vasopressors at different stages of septic shock and shock resolution remain largely elusive to the clinician at the bedside. We demarcate a few evolving areas of future research (Fig. 15.2).

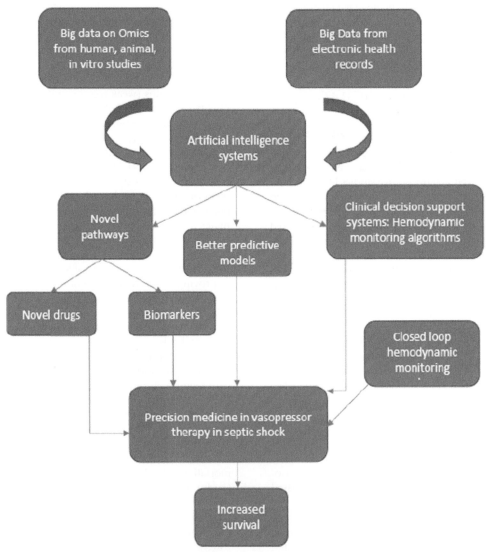

FIG. 15.2 Future Directions of Research in Vasopressor Therapy in Septic Shock.

1. Biomarkers in septic shock: Catecholamine receptor single nucleotide polymorphism (SNP) can detect norepinephrine responsiveness. Angiopoietin 2, SNP of V1a receptor can be potentially used as biomarkers for vasopressin and analogs. Future studies are needed [18].
2. Racial variability in response to vasopressors.
3. Biological mechanisms of vascular responsiveness and genomic mechanisms of neurohumoral responses to septic shock.
4. Immunomodulatory effects of vasopressors.
5. Developing clinical prediction models for septic shock.
6. Defining the thresholds for starting second vasopressor, determining the order of adding vasopressors, optimal combinations as well as for weaning vasopressor therapy.
7. Defining optimal resuscitation targets in septic shock.

CONCLUSION

To summarize, vasopressor therapy forms the cornerstone in the management of septic shock. Vasopressors should be used early in the resuscitation phase of septic shock. Noncatecholamine vasopressors like vasopressin should be added as the second vasopressor early in the course of hemodynamic resuscitation at lower thresholds for noradrenaline to prevent receptor desensitization and adverse effects associated with catecholamine use. Individualized blood pressure targets should be established in resuscitated septic shock patients to ensure adequate end organ perfusion. Vasopressor-sparing strategies used should be instituted, including pharmacological therapy and hemodynamic algorithms. Finally, future research involving omics and artificial intelligence to discover novel pathways, drugs, and biomarkers, along with advanced closed-loop monitoring systems, should pave the way for precision medicine in vasopressor therapy, which will ultimately translate into improved survival.

KEY POINTS

- Vasopressors should be used early in the resuscitation phase of septic shock.
- Noncatecholamine vasopressors like vasopressin should be added as the second vasopressor early in the course of hemodynamic resuscitation at lower thresholds for noradrenaline.
- Individualized blood pressure targets should be established in resuscitated septic shock patients to ensure adequate end-organ perfusion.

- Vasopressor-sparing strategies used should be instituted, including pharmacological therapy and hemodynamic algorithms.

REFERENCES

[1] Singer M, Deutschman CS, Seymour CW, et al. The third international consensus definitions for sepsis and septic shock (Sepsis-3). JAMA 2016;315(8):801−10.
[2] Hotchkiss R, Moldawer L, Opal S, et al. Sepsis and septic shock. Nat Rev Dis Prim 2016;2:16045.
[3] Russel JA, Gordon AC, Williams MD, et al. Vasopressor therapy in the intensive care unit. Semin Respir Crit Care Med 2021;42(01):059−77.
[4] Cecconi M, Evans L, Levy M, Rhodes A. Sepsis and septic shock. Lancet July 7, 2018;392(10141):75−87. https://doi.org/10.1016/S0140-6736(18)30696-2.
[5] Russell JA. Bench-to-bedside review: vasopressin in the management of septic shock. Crit Care 2011;15(4):226. https://doi.org/10.1186/cc8224. Published 2011 Aug 11.
[6] Kakihana Y, Ito T, Nakahara M, et al. Sepsis-induced myocardial dysfunction: pathophysiology and management. J Intensive Care 2016;4:22.
[7] Walley KR. Sepsis-induced myocardial dysfunction. Curr Opin Crit Care August 2018;24(4):292−9.
[8] Overgaard CB, Dzavík V. Inotropes and vasopressors: review of physiology and clinical use in cardiovascular disease. Circulation September 2, 2008;118(10):1047−56.
[9] Giovannitti Jr JA, Thoms SM, Crawford JJ. Alpha-2 adrenergic receptor agonists: a review of current clinical applications. Anesth Prog 2015;62(1):31−9. https://doi.org/10.2344/0003-3006-62.1.31.
[10] Rhodes A, Evans LE, Alhazzani W, et al. Surviving sepsis Campaign: international guidelines for management of sepsis and septic shock: 2016. Intensive Care Med 2017;43:304−77.
[11] De Backer D, Biston P, Devriendt J, Madl C, Chochrad D, Aldecoa C, Brasseur A, Defrance P, Gottignies P, Vincent JL, SOAP II Investigators. Comparison of dopamine and norepinephrine in the treatment of shock. N Engl J Med March 4, 2010;362(9):779−89.
[12] Levy MM, Evans LE, Rhodes A. The surviving sepsis Campaign bundle: 2018 update. Intensive Care Med June 2018;44(6):925−8.
[13] Permpikul C, Tongyoo S, Viarasilpa T, Trainarongsakul T, Chakorn T, Udompanturak S. Early use of norepinephrine in septic shock resuscitation (censer). A randomized trial. Am J Respir Crit Care Med May 1, 2019;199(9):1097−105.
[14] Li Y, Li H, Zhang D. Timing of norepinephrine initiation in patients with septic shock: a systematic review and meta-analysis. Crit Care 2020;24:488.
[15] Avni T, Lador A, Lev S, Leibovici L, Paul M, Grossman A. Vasopressors for the treatment of septic shock: systematic review and meta-analysis. PLoS One August 3, 2015;10(8):e0129305.

[16] Myburgh JA, Higgins A, Jovanovska A, et al. A comparison of epinephrine and norepinephrine in critically ill patients. Intensive Care Med 2008;34:2226.

[17] Annane D, Vignon P, Renault A, Bollaert PE, Charpentier C, Martin C, Troché G, Ricard JD, Nitenberg G, Papazian L, Azoulay E, Bellissant E, CATS Study Group. Norepinephrine plus dobutamine versus epinephrine alone for management of septic shock: a randomised trial. Lancet August 25, 2007;370(9588):676–84. https://doi.org/10.1016/S0140-6736(07)61344-0.

[18] Russell JA. Vasopressor therapy in critically ill patients with shock. Intensive Care Med November 2019; 45(11):1503–17.

[19] Vail E, Gershengorn HB, Hua M, Walkey AJ, Rubenfeld G, Wunsch H. Association between US norepinephrine shortage and mortality among patients with septic shock. JAMA April 11, 2017;317(14):1433–42.

[20] Bellomo R, Chapman M, Finfer S, Hickling K, Myburgh J. Low-dose dopamine in patients with early renal dysfunction: a placebo-controlled randomised trial: Australian and New Zealand Intensive Care Society (ANZICS) Clinical Trials Group. Lancet 2000;356:2139–43.

[21] Marik P. Low-dose dopamine: a systematic review. Intensive Care Med 2002;28:877–83.

[22] Saad AF, Maybauer MO. The role of vasopressin and the vasopressin type V1a receptor agonist selepressin in septic shock. J Crit Care August 2017;40:41–5.

[23] Russell JA, Walley KR, Singer J, Gordon AC, Hébert PC, Cooper DJ, Holmes CL, Mehta S, Granton JT, Storms MM, Cook DJ, Presneill JJ, Ayers D, VASST Investigators. Vasopressin versus norepinephrine infusion in patients with septic shock. N Engl J Med February 28, 2008;358(9):877–87.

[24] Gordon AC, Mason AJ, Thirunavukkarasu N, Perkins GD, Cecconi M, Cepkova M, Pogson DG, Aya HD, Anjum A, Frazier GJ, Santhakumaran S, Ashby D, Brett SJ, VANISH Investigators. Effect of early vasopressin vs norepinephrine on kidney failure in patients with septic shock: the VANISH randomized clinical trial. JAMA August 2, 2016;316(5):509–18.

[25] McIntyre WF, Um KJ, Alhazzani W, et al. Association of vasopressin plus catecholamine vasopressors vs catecholamines alone with atrial fibrillation in patients with distributive shock: a systematic review and meta-analysis. JAMA 2018;319(18):1889–900.

[26] Morelli A, Ertmer C, Rehberg S, Lange M, Orecchioni A, Cecchini V, Bachetoni A, D'Alessandro M, Van Aken H, Pietropaoli P, Westphal M. Continuous terlipressin versus vasopressin infusion in septic shock (TERLIVAP): a randomized, controlled pilot study. Crit Care 2009;13(4): R130.

[27] Liu ZM, Chen J, Kou Q, et al. Terlipressin versus norepinephrine as infusion in patients with septic shock: a multicentre, randomised, double-blinded trial. Intensive Care Med 2018;44:1816–25.

[28] Zhu Y, Huang H, Xi X, et al. Terlipressin for septic shock patients: a meta-analysis of randomized controlled study. J Intensive Care 2019;7:16.

[29] Russell JA, Vincent JL, Kjølbye AL, Olsson H, Blemings A, Spapen H, Carl P, Laterre PF, Grundemar L. Selepressin, a novel selective vasopressin V$_{1A}$ agonist, is an effective substitute for norepinephrine in a phase IIa randomized, placebo-controlled trial in septic shock patients. Crit Care August 15, 2017;21(1):213.

[30] Laterre PF, Berry SM, Blemings A, Carlsen JE, François B, Graves T, Jacobsen K, Lewis RJ, Opal SM, Perner A, Pickkers P, Russell JA, Windeløv NA, Yealy DM, Asfar P, Bestle MH, Muller G, Bruel C, Brulé N, Decruyenaere J, Dive AM, Dugernier T, Krell K, Lefrant JY, Megarbane B, Mercier E, Mira JP, Quenot JP, Rasmussen BS, Thorsen-Meyer HC, Vander Laenen M, Vang ML, Vignon P, Vinatier I, Wichmann S, Wittebole X, Kjølbye AL, Angus DC. SEPSIS-ACT investigators. Effect of selepressin vs placebo on ventilator- and vasopressor-free days in patients with septic shock: the SEPSIS-ACT randomized clinical trial. JAMA October 15, 2019;322(15):1476–85.

[31] Antonucci E, Gleeson PJ, Annoni F, Agosta S, Orlando S, Taccone FS, Velissaris D, Scolletta S. Angiotensin II in refractory septic shock. Shock May 2017;47(5):560–6.

[32] Chawla LS, Busse L, Brasha-Mitchell E, et al. Intravenous angiotensin II for the treatment of high-output shock (ATHOS trial): a pilot study. Crit Care 2014;18:534.

[33] Khanna A, English SW, Wang XS, Ham K, Tumlin J, Szerlip H, Busse LW, Altaweel L, Albertson TE, Mackey C, McCurdy MT, Boldt DW, Chock S, Young PJ, Krell K, Wunderink RG, Ostermann M, Murugan R, Gong MN, Panwar R, Hästbacka J, Favory R, Venkatesh B, Thompson BT, Bellomo R, Jensen J, Kroll S, Chawla LS, Tidmarsh GF, Deane AM. ATHOS-3 investigators. Angiotensin II for the treatment of vasodilatory shock. N Engl J Med August 3, 2017;377(5):419–30.

[34] Jang DH, Nelson LS, Hoffman RS. Methylene blue for distributive shock: a potential new use of an old antidote. J Med Toxicol 2013;9(3):242–9.

[35] Stolk RF, van der Poll T, Angus DC, van der Hoeven JG, Pickkers P, Kox M. Potentially inadvertent immunomodulation: norepinephrine use in sepsis. Am J Respir Crit Care Med September 1, 2016;194(5):550–8.

[36] Marinosci GZ, De Robertis E, De Benedictis G, Piazza O. Dopamine use in intensive care: are we ready to turn it down? Transl Med UniSa 2012;4:90–4.

[37] Bellomo R, Giantomasso DD. Noradrenaline and the kidney: friends or foes? Crit Care 2001;5(6):294–8.

[38] Nandhabalan P, Ioannou N, Meadows C, et al. Refractory septic shock: our pragmatic approach. Crit Care 2018;22: 215.

[39] Cecconi M, De Backer D, Antonelli M, et al. Consensus on circulatory shock and hemodynamic monitoring. Task force of the European Society of Intensive Care Medicine. Intensive Care Med 2014;40(12):1795–815.

[40] Leone M, Asfar P, Radermacher P, Vincent JL, Martin C. Optimizing mean arterial pressure in septic shock: a critical reappraisal of the literature. Crit Care March 10, 2015;19(1):101.

[41] Gershengorn HB, Stelfox HT, Niven DJ, Wunsch H. Association of premorbid blood pressure with vasopressor

infusion duration in patients with shock. Am J Respir Crit Care Med 2020;202:91–9.

[42] Russell JA. Personalized blood pressure targets in shock: what if your normal blood pressure is "low"? Am J Respir Crit Care Med 2020;202(1):10–2.

[43] Song X, Liu X, Evans KD, et al. The order of vasopressor discontinuation and incidence of hypotension: a retrospective cohort analysis. Sci Rep 2021;11:16680.

[44] Hammond DA, McCain K, Painter JT, Clem OA, Cullen J, Brotherton AL, Chopra D, Meena N. Discontinuation of vasopressin before norepinephrine in the recovery phase of septic shock. J Intensive Care Med October 2019; 34(10):805–10.

[45] Jeon K, Song JU, Chung CR, et al. Incidence of hypotension according to the discontinuation order of vasopressors in the management of septic shock: a prospective randomized trial (DOVSS). Crit Care 2018;22:131.

[46] Musallam N, Altshuler D, Merchan C, Zakhary B, Aberle C, Papadopoulos J. Evaluating vasopressor discontinuation strategies in patients with septic shock on concomitant norepinephrine and vasopressin infusions. Ann Pharmacother August 2018;52(8):733–9.

[47] Guinot P-G, Martin A, Berthoud V, Voizeux P, Bartamian L, Santangelo E, Bouhemad B, Nguyen M. Vasopressor-sparing strategies in patients with shock: a scoping-review and an evidence-based strategy proposition. J Clin Med 2021;10(14):3164.

[48] Gordon AC, Perkins GD, Singer M, McAuley DF, Orme RM, Santhakumaran S, Mason AJ, Cross M, Al-Beidh F, Best-Lane J, Brealey D, Nutt CL, McNamee JJ, Reschreiter H, Breen A, Liu KD, Ashby D. Levosimendan for the prevention of acute organ dysfunction in sepsis. N Engl J Med October 27, 2016;375(17):1638–48.

[49] Vincent JL, De Backer D, Wiedermann CJ. Fluid management in sepsis: the potential beneficial effects of albumin. J Crit Care October 2016;35:161–7.

[50] Caironi P, Tognoni G, Masson S, Fumagalli R, Pesenti A, Romero M, Fanizza C, Caspani L, Faenza S, Grasselli G, Iapichino G, Antonelli M, Parrini V, Fiore G, Latini R, Gattinoni L, ALBIOS Study Investigators. Albumin replacement in patients with severe sepsis or septic shock. N Engl J Med April 10, 2014;370(15):1412–21.

[51] Bertini P, Guarracino F. Septic shock and the heart. Curr Anesthesiol Rep 2019;9:165–73.

[52] Morelli A, Ertmer C, Westphal M, et al. Effect of heart rate control with esmolol on hemodynamic and clinical outcomes in patients with septic shock: a randomized clinical trial. JAMA 2013;310(16):1683–91.

[53] Schortgen F, Clabault K, Katsahian S, Devaquet J, Mercat A, Deye N, Dellamonica J, Bouadma L, Cook F, Beji O, Brun-Buisson C, Lemaire F, Brochard L. Fever control using external cooling in septic shock: a randomized controlled trial. Am J Respir Crit Care Med May 15, 2012; 185(10):1088–95.

FURTHER READING

[1] Glucocorticoid therapy in septic shock in adults. 2021. Accessed on 25th September 2021. UpToDate. Available at: https://www.uptodate.com/contents/glucocorticoid-therapy-in-septic-shock-in-adults.

CHAPTER 16

Mechanical Ventilation in Sepsis

CARLOS SÁNCHEZ • ORLANDO PÉREZ-NIETO • EDER ZAMARRÓN

Invasive mechanical ventilation (IMV) is a respiratory support therapy frequently used in the intensive care unit (ICU) [1]. Most patients in the ICU present with sepsis and septic shock as primary diagnoses and may require IMV during the course of their hospital stay. The most common infectious causes of acute respiratory distress syndrome (ARDS) include: viral pneumonias due to COVID-19, influenza viruses and other respiratory viruses, pneumonia of bacterial origin, and intraabdominal infections.

Indications for intubation and initiation of IMV in septic patients are varied, including: acute respiratory failure, neurological deterioration, increased work of breathing, and moderate-severe ARDS unresponsive to conventional oxygen therapy, high-flow oxygen therapy, or noninvasive ventilation (NIV) or when NIV is contraindicated. That is why it is not possible to talk about an exact moment to start mechanical ventilation (MV) in patients with sepsis or septic shock, but rather each decision must be individualized according to the condition of the patient and availability of resources [2]. IMV has also been proposed part of the sepsis treatment goals, by optimizing oxygen delivery to tissues (DO_2) [3], but this strategy has not been shown to improve survival [4].

Sepsis can cause lung injury. Prior to the COVID-19 pandemic, sepsis was the main cause of ARDS, associated with approximately >50% of cases [5]. MV may amplify the lung-specific inflammatory response in pre-injured lungs by elevating cytokine release and augmenting damage to the alveolar integrity; in addition, sepsis per se constitutes a risk factor for mechanical ventilator-induced lung injury (VILI). Inadequate ventilator setting can contribute to increased infection-induced organ failure and uncontrolled systemic inflammatory response [6].

For the diagnosis of ARDS, the Berlin criteria are used, which include (1) acute onset of the clinical picture, (2) bilateral involvement on chest X-ray or computed tomography, (3) noncardiac pulmonary edema, and (4) PaO_2/FiO_2 ratio <300 (with positive end-expiratory pressure [PEEP] >5 cm H_2O) [7]. In hospitals with limited resources, an SpO_2/FiO_2 ratio <315 and lung ultrasound can be used to diagnose [8].

Objectives of IMV are to maintain adequate gas exchange: maintain oxygenation goals and adequate ventilation; however, this therapy is not harmless, and the energy applied to the respiratory system (RS) can be associated with higher mortality. This energy, as a concept of mechanical power (MP), encompasses the VILI caused by the elastic component of the RS, which includes the tidal volume (TV), the plateau pressure (Pp) and the PEEP, plus the resistive component, which includes airflow, peak inspiratory pressure, and lastly, respiratory rate (RR). PM values > 17 j/L are associated with mortality (OR 1.70 [1.32−2.18]; $P < .001$) [9]. This can be easily measured in conventional ventilation modes with the following equations [10]:

$$MP = 0.098\ RR \cdot Vt \cdot [\text{Peak inspiratory pressure} - 1/2(\text{Plateau pressure} - PEEP)]$$

for volume control-continuous mandatory ventilation (VC-CMV) and

$$MP = VE(\text{Peak pressure} + PEEP + \text{Inspiratory flow}/6)/20$$

for pressure control-continuous mandatory ventilation (PC-CMV).

Regarding ventilatory modes, it has been proposed that VC-CMV may be more protective than PC-CMV, and it should be checked frequently if the patient with sepsis can tolerate spontaneous ventilation in pressure support ventilation mode [11].

TV has been shown to be frankly associated with mortality in patients with ARDS. A TV of ~6 mL/kg

The Sepsis Codex. https://doi.org/10.1016/B978-0-323-88271-2.00009-2

of predicted body weight (PBW) is associated with longer survival and fewer days on IMV compared to a VT of ~12 mL/kg of PBW (31.0% vs. 39.8%, $P = .007$) [12]. Moderate TV MV causes a more severe inflammatory response when compared to low TV MV in preinjured lungs, and this effect is more evident at a later phase (fourth day) of sepsis. Furthermore, low TV MV causes greater synergistic inflammatory effects at later period of sepsis [13].

The ARDSNet group protocol also implemented other notable ventilatory strategies: maintain $Pp < 30$ cm H_2O, lowering TV if necessary; maintain a $pH > 7.15$, increasing the RR or TV if the Pp allows it, and if not possible, with the use of intravenous sodium bicarbonate; establish a PEEP level through an easy-to-implement strategy with PEEP tables (see Table 16.1) according to the FiO_2 necessary to maintain a target peripheral oxygen saturation (SpO_2) of 88%–95%. The low PEEP/FiO_2 table shown here continues to show a survival benefit even today, when compared to other strategies for choosing the PEEP level (OR 4.10, 95% CI 1.68–9.99, $P = .002$) [14,15]. When using recruitment maneuvers, the surviving sepsis campaign guideline recommends against using incremental PEEP titration/strategy [16].

The ratio of VT to compliance of respiratory system compliance (CRS) is also associated with mortality and fits the rationale for the benefit of low VT. A low TV in a patient with a greatly decreased CRS may not be as beneficial as in a patient with a slightly decreased CRS. The driving pressure (DP) is the pressure necessary to distend the CRS with the VT implemented and can be calculated using the following formula:

$$DP = TV/CRS$$

or, in its simplified version:

$$DP = Plateau\ Preasure - PEEP$$

$DP > 15$ cm H_2O has been associated with mortality (relative risk, 1.41; 95% confidence interval [CI], 1.31–1.51; $P < .001$), even in patients with $PP < 30$ cm H_2O and TV of 6 mL/kg (relative risk, 1.36; 95% CI, 1.17–1.58; $P < .001$) [17].

Oxygenation should be constantly monitored; it may be reasonable to maintain a target arterial partial pressure of oxygen (paO_2) of 60–80 mm Hg [18], or an SpO_2 of 92%–96% for most patients. Hyperoxemia ($paO_2 > 150$ mm Hg or $SpO2 > 98\%$) has been associated with higher mortality in multiple scenarios due to oxygen toxicity, predisposition to the formation of free radicals, vasoregulatory disorders, and cell damage, so in theory is not recommended [19]. The policy of permissive hypoxia and hyperoxia avoidance for septic patients requiring MV had no significant association with reduced ICU mortality [20].

The prone position is a strategy that has reduced mortality in patients with moderate-severe ARDS when applied early and for >16 continuous hours per day versus the supine position (HR 0.44 [95% CI, 0.29–0.67]) [21]. It may be recommended to start this position <48 h after intubation and with a PaO_2/FiO_2 ratio <200 [22].

Caution should be exercised regarding the decision to initiate IMV in patients with sepsis and septic shock. A further analysis of the MIMIC-III study showed that when comparing patients who meet the criteria for Sepsis-3 versus patients without sepsis, IMV was associated with higher mortality at 30 days and more days of ICU stay (Odds Ratio 1.6, 95% interval confidence [1.49–1.75]) [23]. Adequate clinical judgment can help in the decision to intubate septic patients, and if IVM is necessary, lung protection goals should be pursued and consideration should be given to starting ventilator weaning as soon as possible. Carrying out daily awakening tests by withdrawing sedatives and spontaneous ventilation tests can help achieve this objective [24].

Sepsis-induced diaphragmatic dysfunction is a major risk factor of weaning failure during MV. Diaphragmatic ultrasound had been a useful tool for predicting successful liberation from MV. Both diaphragmatic ultrasound indices, namely diaphragmatic thickening fraction and diaphragmatic excursion, could be useful parameters for assessment of the success of liberation of patients on MV with sepsis [25]. Septic patients were associated with a more severe but reversible impaired diaphragm function as compared to nonseptic patients [26].

TABLE 16.1
Low PEEP/FiO_2 Table to Choose the Level of PEEP in ARDS

FiO_2	0.3	0.4	0.4	0.5	0.6	0.7	0.8	0.9	1.0
PEEP	5	5	8	8–10	10	10–14	14	14–18	18–24

Another important aspect of ventilation is the type of sedation to use, although we know that the majority of patients who need MV during a serious infection suffer from septic shock, and drugs should be sought that do not worsen the infection as far as possible. Hemodynamic status, so far there does not seem to be enough evidence to recommend one drug over another, mainly when comparing propofol versus dexmedetomidine regarding days alive without acute brain dysfunction, ventilator-free days, death at 90 days, or cognition at 6 months [27,28]. However, some small studies suggest that there was a trend toward decreased duration of MV with dexmedetomidine [29].

REFERENCES

[1] Esteban A, Anzueto A, Frutos F, Alía I, Brochard L, Stewart TE, et al. Characteristics and outcomes in adult patients receiving mechanical ventilation. JAMA 2002; 287(3):345–55.

[2] Darreau C, Martino F, Saint-Martin M, Jacquier S, Hamel JF, Nay MA, et al. Use, timing and factors associated with tracheal intubation in septic shock: a prospective multicentric observational study. Ann Intensive Care 2020;10:62. https://doi.org/10.1186/s13613-020-00668-6.

[3] Rivers E, Nguyen B, Havstad S, Ressler J, Muzzin A, Knoblich B, et al. Early goal-directed therapy in the treatment of severe sepsis and septic shock. N Engl J Med 2001;345(19):1368–77. https://doi.org/10.1056/NEJMoa010307.

[4] PRISM Investigators, Rowan KM, Angus DC, Bailey M, Barnato AE, Bellomo R, et al. Early, goal-directed therapy for septic shock—a patient-level meta-analysis. N Engl J Med 2017;376(23):2223–34. https://doi.org/10.1056/NEJMoa1701380.

[5] Sevransky JE, Levy MM, Marini JJ. Mechanical ventilation in sepsis-induced acute lung injury/acute respiratory distress syndrome: an evidence-based review. Crit Care Med 2004;32(11 Suppl. l):S548–53.

[6] Zampieri FG, Mazza B. Mechanical ventilation in sepsis: a reappraisal. Shock 2017;47(1S Suppl. 1):41–6. https://doi.org/10.1097/SHK.0000000000000702.

[7] ARDS Definition Task Force, Ranieri VM, Rubenfeld GD, Thompson BT, Ferguson ND, Caldwell E, et al. Acute respiratory distress syndrome: the Berlin definition. JAMA 2012;307(23):2526–33. https://doi.org/10.1001/jama.2012.5669.

[8] Riviello ED, Kiviri W, Twagirumugabe T, Mueller A, Banner-Goodspeed VM, Officer L, et al. Hospital incidence and outcomes of the acute respiratory distress syndrome using the kigali modification of the Berlin definition. Am J Respir Crit Care Med 2016;193(1):52–9. https://doi.org/10.1164/rccm.201503-0584OC.

[9] Serpa Neto A, Deliberato RO, Johnson AEW, Bos LD, Amorim P, Pereira SM, et al. Mechanical power of ventilation is associated with mortality in critically ill patients:

an analysis of patients in two observational cohorts. Intensive Care Med 2018;44(11):1914–22. https://doi.org/10.1007/s00134-018-5375-6.

[10] Chiumello D, Gotti M, Guanziroli M, Formenti P, Umbrello M, Pasticci I, et al. Bedside calculation of mechanical power during volume- and pressure-controlled mechanical ventilation. Crit Care 2020;24:417. https://doi.org/10.1186/s13054-020-03116-w.

[11] Neto AS, Schultz MJ, Festic E, Adhikari NK, Dondorp AM, Pattnaik R, et al. Ventilatory support of patients with sepsis or septic shock in resource-limited settings. In: Dondorp A, Dünser M, Schultz M, editors. Sepsis management in resource-limited settings. Cham: Springer; 2019. https://doi.org/10.1007/978-3-030-03143-5_6.

[12] Acute Respiratory Distress Syndrome Network, Brower RG, Matthay MA, Morris A, Schoenfeld D, Thompson BT, Wheeler A. Ventilation with lower tidal volumes as compared with traditional tidal volumes for acute lung injury and the acute respiratory distress syndrome. N Engl J Med 2000;342(18):1301–8.

[13] Xuan W, Zhou Q, Yao S, Deng Q, Wang T, Wu Q. Mechanical ventilation induces an inflammatory response in preinjured lungs in late phase of sepsis. Oxid Med Cell Longev 2015:8. https://doi.org/10.1155/2015/364020. Article ID 364020.

[14] See KC, Sahagun J, Taculod J. Patient characteristics and outcomes associated with adherence to the low PEEP/FIO2 table for acute respiratory distress syndrome. Sci Rep 2021;11(1):14619. https://doi.org/10.1038/s41598-021-94081-z. Published July 16, 2021.

[15] Writing Group for the Alveolar Recruitment for Acute Respiratory Distress Syndrome Trial (ART) Investigators, Cavalcanti AB, Suzumura ÉA, et al. Effect of lung recruitment and titrated positive end-expiratory pressure (PEEP) vs low PEEP on mortality in patients with acute respiratory distress syndrome: a randomized clinical trial. JAMA 2017;318(14):1335–45. https://doi.org/10.1001/jama.2017.14171.

[16] Evans L, Rhodes A, Alhazzani W, Antonelli M, Coopersmith CM, French C, et al. Surviving sepsis campaign: international guidelines for management of sepsis and septic shock 2021. Crit Care Med J November 2021;49(11).

[17] Amato MB, Meade MO, Slutsky AS, Brochard L, Costa EL, Schoenfeld DA, et al. Driving pressure and survival in the acute respiratory distress syndrome. N Engl J Med 2015;372(8):747–55. https://doi.org/10.1056/NEJMsa1410639.

[18] Young PJ, Hodgson CL, Rasmussen BS. Oxygen targets. Intensive Care Med 2022. https://doi.org/10.1007/s00134-022-06714-0.

[19] Singer M, Young PJ, Laffey JG, Asfar P, Taccone FS, Skrifvars MB, et al. Dangers of hyperoxia. Crit Care 2021;25(1):440. https://doi.org/10.1186/s13054-021-03815-y. December 19, 2021.

[20] Nishimoto K, Umegaki T, Ohira S, Soeda T, Anada N, Uba T, et al. Impact of permissive hypoxia and hyperoxia avoidance on clinical outcomes in septic patients receiving mechanical ventilation: a retrospective single-

center study. BioMed Res Int 2021:10. https://doi.org/10.1155/2021/7332027. Article ID 7332027.

[21] Guérin C, Reignier J, Richard JC, Beuret P, Gacouin A, Boulain T, et al. Prone positioning in severe acute respiratory distress syndrome. N Engl J Med 2013; 368(23):2159−68. https://doi.org/10.1056/NEJMoa1214103.

[22] Mathews KS, Soh H, Shaefi S, Wang W, Bose S, Coca S, et al. Prone positioning and survival in mechanically ventilated patients with coronavirus disease 2019-related respiratory failure. Crit Care Med 2021;49(7): 1026−37. https://doi.org/10.1097/CCM.0000000000004938.

[23] Liu N, Ren J, Yu L, Xie J. Mechanical ventilation associated with worse survival in septic patients: a retrospective analysis of MIMIC-III. J Emerg Crit Care Med 2020;4. https://doi.org/10.21037/jeccm.2020.01.01.

[24] Jung B, Vaschetto R, Jaber S. Ten tips to optimize weaning and extubation success in the critically ill. Intensive Care Med 2020;46(12):2461−3. https://doi.org/10.1007/s00134-020-06300-2.

[25] Eltrabili HH, Hasanin AM, Soliman MS, Lotfy AM, Hamimy WI, Mukhtar AM. Evaluation of diaphragmatic ultrasound indices as predictors of successful liberation from mechanical ventilation in subjects with abdominal sepsis. Respir Care May 2019;64(5). https://doi.org/10.4187/respcare.06391.

[26] Lecronier M, Jung B, Molinari N, Pinot J, Similowski T, Jaber S, et al. Severe but reversible impaired diaphragm function in septic mechanically ventilated patients. Ann Intensive Care 2022;12:34. https://doi.org/10.1186/s13613-022-01005-9.

[27] Hughes CG, Mailloux PT, Devlin JW, Swan JT, Sanders RD, Anzueto A, et al. Dexmedetomidine or propofol for sedation in mechanically ventilated adults with sepsis. N Engl J Med 2021;384:1424−36. https://doi.org/10.1056/NEJMoa2024922.

[28] Huang P, Zheng X, Liu Z, Fang X. Dexmedetomidine versus propofol for patients with sepsis requiring mechanical ventilation: a systematic review and meta-analysis. Front Pharmacol 2021;12:717023. https://doi.org/10.3389/fphar.2021.717023.

[29] Sigler MB, Islam E, Nugent K. Comparison of dexmedetomidine and propofol in mechanically ventilated patients with sepsis: a pilot study. Southwest Respir Crit Care Chron 2018;6(22):10−5.

CHAPTER 17

Extracorporeal Membrane Oxygenation for the Support of Patients with Refractory Septic Shock

JOSE ALFONSO RUBIO MATEO-SIDRÓN

INTRODUCTION

Appropriate and timely antimicrobial therapy, source control if indicated, fluid therapy, and targeted vasopressors have been the cornerstone of sepsis and sepsis shock treatment. A subset of these patients is unresponsive to standard resuscitation and deteriorates abruptly into refractory shock and progressive multiorgan failure with an associated mortality of up to 60%. However refractory septic shock (RSS) with microcirculatory failure and ischemic consequences is variably defined [1].

Alternative therapeutic strategies are desperately needed to improve outcomes in this small subgroup of critically ill patients. Extra corporeal membrane oxygenation (ECMO) has become an essential tool in the care of adults and children with severe cardiac and pulmonary dysfunction refractory to conventional management.

The encouraging outcomes of ECMO in pediatric sepsis with RSS means that it is potentially reversible and have led to it being recommended as a potential therapy in some societal guidelines [2,3].

However, the hemodynamic pattern of septic shock is markedly different across age groups and the use of ECMO, in particular, venoarterial (VA) ECMO, in adult with RSS remains controversial.

Nonetheless, single-center observational studies have shown that a subset of septic adults specifically those with septic cardiomyopathy (SCM) may benefit from VA ECMO for mechanical circulatory support [4].

We herein sought to summarize the hemodynamic status of patients with RSS and why might ECMO have such an apparent benefit in these patients. We then analyze the evidence on the use of ECMO in the adult patient with RSS. We conclude with the review of the current different configuration options to handle these critical issues.

HEMODYNAMICS OF SEPTIC SHOCK

Despite progress in treatment over the last decades, septic shock still has a high burden in terms of mortality and cost and continues to be a major challenge for health care systems.

Approximately, 15% of patients with sepsis develop septic shock, which accounts for about 10% of admissions to intensive care units and has a death rate close to 50% [5].

The incidence is rising, and in a recent analysis, the cost of septic shock care for inpatient admissions was more than 38.000 $ [6].

Recently, the sepsis-3 adult definition has refined the identification of septic shock patients [7]. In the last years, the use of sepsis bundles aiming a positive impact on sepsis evolution [8] and some studies have shown a reduction in hospital costs and lower mortality with the use of these tools. However, despite all these measures, a subset of patients deteriorates and presents progression toward multiorgan failure, essentially due to inadequate oxygen delivery. In this setting, ECMO has been routinely utilized for the neonatal and more recently in children population with reported survival rate of up to 70% [9,10]. Thus, neonatal and pediatric societal sepsis guidelines in their latest edition [2,3] recommend ECMO for RSS as last tier intervention when medical management has failed.

In adults, recent guideline recommends venovenous (VV) ECMO for adults with sepsis-induced severe ARDS [11]. Nevertheless, there is insufficient evidence for the effects on clinical outcomes of VA ECMO for cardiac dysfunction in RSS [12]. In fact, there are some case reports and observational studies of the use of VA ECMO for adult patients with RSS with a survival rate widely varied from 15% to 70% [4,13−16].

The Sepsis Codex. https://doi.org/10.1016/B978-0-323-88271-2.00024-9

This is partly explained by their different size, anatomy, and physiology between neonatal, children, and adults.

Different Clinical Features in Cardiovascular Physiology Between Neonatal, Children, and Adults

Severe hypovolemia is a hallmark of pediatric septic shock. However, almost 50% of children with septic shock present with cold, clamped down extremities, low cardiac output (CO), and elevated systemic vascular resistance (SVR), often referred to as "cold shock." This is due to children having limited cardiac reserve as compared to adults. The adult resting heart rate is 70; therefore, a twofold increase in heart rate from 70 to 140 beats per minute can be easily tolerated to maintain CO when stroke volume (SV) is decreased. Similar mechanisms are not possible in children. A resting heart rate of 140 beats per minute cannot be doubled to 280 beats per minute because there is not enough time for diastolic filling. Therefore, the predominant response to a decreasing CO in children is vasoconstriction. This continued increase in vasoconstriction is detrimental, as it further impairs CO leading to cardiac failure and death.

On the other hand, the presentation of septic shock is different in adults as compared to children. Almost 90% of the adult patients present with a "hyperdynamic shock syndrome" or warm shock. Clinical features of septic shock in adults are reduced SVR, standard or increased CI, tachycardia, and increased mixed venous saturations. This clinical presentation is also described as "warm shock" or distributive shock and is uncommon in children and very rare in neonates [17].

Despite the hyperdynamic state, these patients exhibit myocardial depression characterized by decreased ejection fraction (EF) and ventricular dilatation. Selected adults with RSS may present as well as cardiogenic shock due to cardiac dysfunction (SCM) characterized by persistently low CO refractory to inotrope. In this setting, the use of ECMO may also be recommended, while in septic patients with preserved CO, the use remains controversial [18].

Refractory Septic Shock

The subset of patients who are unresponsive to standard resuscitation are often labeled as having "RSS." RSS is typified by circulatory failure due to SCM with or without vasoplegia. RSS is potentially reversible with vasoactive agents and mechanical support. This is why an early identification of RSS is particularly relevant.

RSS has been defined as the association of: [1] evidence of organ hypoperfusion (extensive skin mottling, oliguria or altered mental status, blood lactate >8 mmol/L, or a 1 mmol/L lactate increase after 6 h of resuscitation) despite adequate intravascular volume, [2] the inability to maintain mean arterial pressure >65 mmHg despite infusion of very high-dose catecholamines (norepinephrine >1 μg/kg/min, vaso-inotrope dependency (vasoactive inotropic score [VIS] >200 mcg/kg min), and [3] myocardial dysfunction, defined with cardiac ultrasound findings with left ventricle ejection fraction (LVEF) < 25% or a CI < 2.2 L/min m^2 [19].

SCM may be an important component in the RSS scores and accounts for half of sepsis-related deaths in children within the first 24 h of hospital admission and can also occur in adult patients, albeit less commonly [20]. Although the pathogenesis of SCM is multifactorial, it is known to be reversible.

Septic Cardiomyopathy

From a practical perspective, the cardiovascular failure characterizing septic shock combines various and intricate alterations of both vascular (loss of vascular tone, microvascular shunts) and cardiac function (altered systolic and diastolic properties of both cardiac ventricles) so-called SCM. The combination of vasodilatation, depressed cardiac function, and compromised oxygen extraction results in tissue dysoxia and associated organ dysfunction.

The resulting hemodynamic profile depends on the degree of hypovolemia (absolute due to vascular leakage, relative due to vasoplegia), severity of cardiac failure, and potential ventriculo-arterial decoupling [21].

Importantly, the hemodynamic profile may greatly and rapidly vary according to the delay of sepsis diagnosis, the intensity of the host proinflammatory response, the presence of comorbidities (e.g., underlying cardiopathy), and initial management (volume of fluid resuscitation, vasopressor support). Accordingly, sequential evaluation of the hemodynamic status of patients with septic shock is currently suggested [5].

Pathophysiology of Sepsis Cardiomyopathy

SCM is an acute syndrome of cardiac dysfunction based on systemic infection and inflammation and lacks the ischemic component of coronary artery disease.

Cardiac dysfunction in sepsis may originate from three different mechanisms: right ventricle (RV) dysfunction and left ventricle (LV) diastolic and systolic dysfunction. These have been described to occur in association or alone and is reversible providing patients recover.

LV Systolic and Diastolic Disfunction. It is now known that cardiac dysfunction occurs "dynamically" and that it can be present much earlier than just in the late stage of septic shock.

Also, as intrinsic performance is always impaired, occurrence of LV systolic dysfunction is strongly associated with the level of LV afterload. For this reason, correction of LV afterload by norepinephrine infusion may unmask SCM. This is why serial evaluations have to be done along the evolution and treatment.

Furthermore, most studies using echocardiography report a slight increase in LV size in patients with decreased LVEF with an incidence of LV relaxation impairment of around 40%, independent of LV systolic dysfunction [22].

RV Systolic Dysfunction. Its incidence is difficult to determine since, as for the LV, it may depend on the coupling between the intrinsic contraction of the RV and its afterload.

By increasing right atrial pressure, RV systolic dysfunction leads to a decrease in systemic venous return, protects the pulmonary circulation, and thus explains in part why LV filling pressure remains in normal range despite LV systolic dysfunction when associated. Consequently, this may explain the difficulty in detecting LV systolic dysfunction by pulmonary artery catheter (PAC), which in this situation usually records low CO with nonelevated pulmonary artery occlusion pressure, not very suggestive of cardiac failure as usually expected. These discrepancies between PAC and echocardiography have been found in half of patients [23].

Interestingly, aside from SCM, sepsis may trigger stress cardiomyopathy (stress CM), also referred to as Takotsubo cardiomyopathy. In stress CM, the contractile function of the mid-to-apical segments of the LV is reduced with simultaneous hyperkinesis of the basal segments, resulting in a characteristic balloon-like appearance of the ventricle. In comparison, sepsis-induced cardiomyopathy is characterized by global ventricular dysfunction and dilation, and the absence of regional wall motion abnormalities [24].

Diagnosis of Sepsis Cardiomyopathy

Currently, the diagnostic criteria for adult SCM are not fully established, due to the complexity and variations in the cardiovascular response to infection [25]. Nonetheless, it is understood that transient and reversible

myocardial depression is common in septic patients, and early detection and intervention of SCM in patients with septic shock may reduce mortality.

First described by Parker et al. in 1984 [26], it is estimated an incidence of myocardial dysfunction in sepsis can vary from 18% to 29% in the first 6h and could be as high as 60% later on, during the course of the syndrome [27].

Despite standardization efforts at present, there are not enough data to support a precise definition of SCM and different authors propose the combination of various characteristics (Table 17.1).

Given that there is no definitive agreed upon definition or criteria, the diagnosis of SCM can be difficult.

Thus, estimating cardiac function during sepsis is particularly difficult without taking systemic hemodynamics, which can be significantly altered during the course of the infection. In fact, no singular monitoring strategy can determine both cardiac and systemic hemodynamics at the same time. Although an echocardiography in a hemodynamically unstable patient with sepsis is widely considered indispensable, its significance in estimating the degree of SCM is somewhat less clear. Even so, there is consensus and expert opinion that

TABLE 17.1
Main Characteristics of Septic Cardiomyopathy

L'Heureux M et al.	Martin L et al.
• Acute and reversible, within 7–10 days • Global biventricular dysfunction (systolic and Diastolic) with reduced contractility • Left ventricular dilatation • Diminished response to fluids resuscitation and catecholamines • Absence of acute coronary syndrome as etiology	Acute dysfunction unrelated to ischemia with one or more of the following: • Left ventricular dilatation with normal-filling or low-filling pressure • Reduced ventricular contractility • Right ventricular dysfunction or left ventricular (systolic or Diastolic) dysfunction with reduced response to volume

L'Heureux M, Sternberg M, Brath L, Turlington J, Kashiouris MG. Sepsis-induced cardiomyopathy: a comprehensive review. Curr Cardiol Rep. 2020 May 6; 22(5):35. 10.1007/s11886-020-01277-2. PMID: 32377972; PMCID: PMC7222131.

Martin L, Derwall M, Al Zoubi S, Zechendorf E, Reuter DA, Thiemermann C, Schuerholz T. The septic heart: current understanding of molecular mechanisms and clinical implications. Chest. 2019 Feb; 155(2):427–437. 10.1016/j.chest.2018.08.1037. Epub 2018 Aug 29. PMID: 30171861.

echocardiography is the cornerstone for the diagnosis of SCM and that every hemodynamically unstable patient should receive critical care echocardiography.

Echocardiographic Findings of SCM. Until recently, it was thought that diagnosis could be made based solely by a depressed LVEF. However, a major problem with the LVEF is that reduced afterload from the distributive shock may pseudo-normalize a depressed EF (coupling between contractility and afterload). This likely leads to underdiagnosis of SCM when LVEF is used alone.

SV and cardiac index (CI) can be also calculated, but the measurement of these indices is hard to interpret in SCM because of the profound variations in preload, afterload, and contractility intrinsic to septic shock.

RV systolic dysfunction is present in approximately two-thirds of patients with sepsis and septic shock. Measurements of RV function include the RV end-diastolic area in comparison to the LV, the RV fractional area change with tricuspid annular plane systolic excursion and tricuspid annulus tissue Doppler imaging (TDI), and the RV free wall TDI.

Diastolic dysfunction of LV is very common in septic shock. The septal relaxation in TDI (e′-wave, abnormal <8 cm/s) was a very strong predictor of mortality in septic shock patient. The peak early diastolic transmitral velocity during the passive filling of the heart (E)/peak early diastolic mitral annular TDI velocity (e′) have a significant and independent prediction of mortality.

A small pilot trial showed that myocardial impairment in sepsis can be detected by the global longitudinal strain (GLS). In patients with septic shock, GLS proved to be the most sensitive measurement of SCM with an average −14% (−17% to −23% more negative better) among patients with septic shock. Several trials have confirmed the benefit of the LV, and the RV GLS in diagnosing SCM with the additional advantage that it is not as susceptible to afterload reduction pseudo-normalization that plagues the LVEF [28−30]. However, although echocardiography has the potential for vastly improving the diagnosis of SCM, it also carries the disadvantage of being a discontinuous measurement [31].

Invasive and Noninvasive Devices for SCM Diagnosis. The PAC is not appropriate to rule out SCM since a low SVR may falsely elevate the measured CO, and CO does not necessarily reflect intrinsic cardiomyocyte function/contractility [32]. However, some authors consider a multimodal approach, including the use of a PAC in conjunction with echocardiography, in the setting of SCM [31] before starting ECMO support.

Other noninvasive devices such as pulse contour analysis, pulse pressure variation, and SV variation have not yet validated their use in the setting of SCM.

Taken all together, it becomes clear that only a multimodal (clinical, hemodynamic, and echocardiographic) approach allows for an adequate diagnosis, classification, and monitoring of SCM.

WHY MIGHT ECMO BE EFFECTIVE IN PATIENTS WITH REFRACTORY SEPTIC SHOCK?

VA ECMO may support decreased CO in patients with the cardiogenic form of septic shock that is unresponsive to very high doses of catecholamines and can potentially restore systemic perfusion pressure and increase oxygen delivery [19,33]. This corrects the cellular hypoxia and metabolic acidosis during SCM, ameliorating vasopressor dependence, and fluid overload, facilitating a reduction in ventilation and potentially improving the chances of survival [34].

Even though ECMO treatment per se does not restore microcirculation or cellular/mitochondrial oxygen uptake, it could increase the chances thereof by augmenting oxygen delivery and limiting the negative impact of generalized poor oxygenation [15].

On the other hand, in septic patients with vasoplegia and preserved cardiac function, it is hypothesized that VA ECMO may be contraindicated as it reduces preload and increases afterload, eventually decreasing CO. However, secondary beneficial effects from improved tissue oxygenation may play a role in stabilizing the circulation in this group of RSS.

Another point of interest is the use of VV ECMO in those patients with compromised hemodynamic status. In the early stages of hemodynamic compromise in the septic patient, right ventricular dysfunction plays an important role. VV ECMO could improve right ventricular function by contributing to correction of hypoxemia, acidosis, and pulmonary hyperinflation. After initiation of the support with this cannulation strategy, there is usually a notable hemodynamic improvement in which the reduction of pulmonary vascular resistance, better myocardial oxygenation, and a decrease in airway pressures all play a vital role [35].

Equally important is simply buying time. ECMO could provide extra time for recovery of the failing heart and support the perfusion of major organs until cardiac function spontaneously recovers and infection control can be achieved using antibiotics or drainage.

INDICATIONS

ECMO is considered a standard treatment for pediatric and neonatal patients with septic shock as opposed to the adult populations [36–38]. Even though ECMO has gained increased acceptance for the treatment of adult severe respiratory failure, the controversy remains concerning its usefulness in septic shock [34].

ECMO in Pediatric Septic Shock

According to recent guidelines for newborns with RSS related to PPHN-induced right ventricular failure, VV ECMO can unload the RV, reduce septal bowing, and improve LV output. However, for newborns with primary LV or biventricular failure refractory to inotropic and vasodilator support, VA ECMO is required to reverse shock [2].

For children with sepsis-induced ARDS and refractory hypoxia, VV ECMO may be useful. VA ECMO as a rescue therapy in children with septic shock only if refractory to all other treatments is suggested with weak recommendation and very low quality of evidence in recent guidelines [3].

ECMO in Adult Patients With Septic Shock

The number of reports of ECMO for adult patients with sepsis remains yet insufficient, and many of these are single-center retrospective observational studies. There have not been any RCTs investigating the treatment effectiveness, and thus its use remains with a weak recommendation within the sepsis guidelines [12].

However, patients with severe myocardial dysfunction receiving VA ECMO during the first four days of septic shock had significantly lower mortality than those without ECMO, with similar findings among observational case series reporting on VA ECMO for adult and pediatric SCM [16,20,33].

A recent review and metaanalysis of the current literature suggests that VA ECMO may be a viable salvage therapy among select adult patients with septic shock and concomitant myocardial depression, characterized by persistently low CO refractory to inotropes. By contrast, ECMO is associated with especially poor outcomes among patients with septic shock but without severe ventricular dysfunction. The analysis found that survival among patients with LVEF >35% was significantly lower than those with LVEF <20%. LVEF between 20% and 35% had intermediate survival (42.3%), suggesting a possible graded effect of LVEF on outcomes [39].

According to these studies, we can infer that adult patient with predominantly low flow secondary to SCM may be good candidates for VA ECMO support.

In contrast, in patients with a pattern of distributive shock with high CO and low SVR, VA ECMO is considered a controversial indication [15].

Simultaneously, in those septic patients with compromised hemodynamic status due to right ventricular dysfunction, VV ECMO could contribute to correct hypoxemia, acidosis, and pulmonary hyperinflation and improve right ventricular function.

Also, in the last edition of Surviving Sepsis Campaign guideline, the use of VV ECMO is suggested for adults with sepsis-induced severe ARDS, when conventional mechanical ventilation fails in experienced centers with the infrastructure in place to support its use [11].

In summary, clinicians should pay attention to the main mechanism of hemodynamic failure in RSS. If the condition is mainly secondary to SCM, a left ventricular failure, or vasoplegia, the VA ECMO strategy may be of interest. If the patient is not stabilized, clinicians should consider switching to a V-VA configuration. VV ECMO configuration is preferred in severe respiratory failure with ARDS and in the early stages of hemodynamic compromised septic patients when right ventricular dysfunction plays an important role. Some septic patients, mainly in cases of long VV ECMO runs, may suffer progression of the RV dysfunction and develop right backwards failure. In this situation, reversible causes must be ruled out. If the situation persists, conversion to other modes such as the VA or V-VA may be mandatory.

These patients are complex to treat not only from an experience point of view but also concerning resource demand, and they should only be treated at high-volume centers with experience and capability to perform all modes of ECMO according to patient's need. Therefore, as time might be an important predictor for survival, these patients should be transferred early to an experienced center whenever possible (Fig. 17.1).

WHEN INITIATING ECMO

There are no well-established criteria for initiating and managing ECMO support in adult patients with RSS. In any case, ECMO should be started only if the source of infection is controlled, adequate antibiotic treatment is initiated, and the conventional support measures are optimized.

From a practical point of view, an echocardiogram is essential to evaluate biventricular function before starting ECMO support. If the hemodynamic situation is attributed to right ventricular dysfunction, VV support

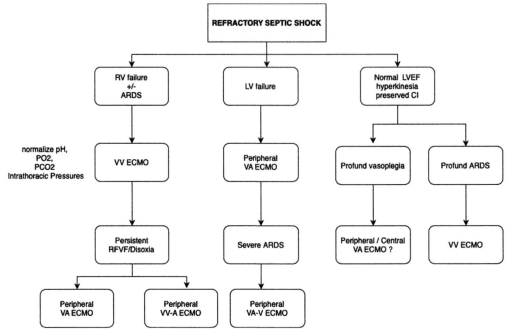

FIG. 17.1 Decision algorithm to set the ECMO configuration in adult patient with refractory septic shock. ARDS, acute respiratory distress syndrome; CI, cardiac index; LV, left ventricle; LVEF, left ventricular ejection fraction; RV, right ventricle; RVF, right ventricular failure; VA, venoarterial; VV, venovenous; V-VA, hybrid veno-venoarterial; VV-A, hybrid venovenous-arterial.

could be indicated, while if it is due to a clear left ventricular dysfunction, VA should be used.

MacLaren and Butt recommend considering the support if a child (a) receives doses of >1 μg/kg/min of epinephrine or equivalent, (b) has had resuscitation following the recommendations of the American College of Critical Care Medicine consensus statement, and (c) continues to deteriorate with worsening hypotension, rising lactates, or rapidly progressive multiorgan dysfunction in spite of treatment [40].

In adult patients, VA ECMO for cardiocirculatory support is considered in patient fulfillment of the "sepsis-3" definition, after adequate fluid resuscitation together with at least one of the following criteria of hypoperfusion and cardiovascular failure: persistent lactatemia greater than 5 mmol/L, mixed venous saturation (Svo2) less than 55%, or CI less than 2 L/min/m^2 (>1 h), rapidly deteriorating ventricular function, refractory arrhythmia, and VIS greater than 50 (>1 h), greater than 45 (>8 h), or greater than 40 if myocarditis.

Respiratory support (VV ECMO) is offered if the PaO$_2$-to-FiO$_2$ ratio is less than 60−80 (FiO$_2$ 1.0), with advanced respiratory critical care [15].

ECMO blood flow is usually maintained between 3.5 and 5.0 L/min to reach a preoxygenator oxygen saturation during VA ECMO of greater than 65% (VV >70%). Echocardiography is daily used to monitor cardiac function. Inopressors and/or inodilators are adjusted to maintain a mean arterial blood pressure greater than 65 mm Hg.

An important point in patient management is the early initiation of the adequate antibiotic [41]. To ensure its efficacy, its dose should be titrated adequately considering the altered drug pharmacokinetics in patients with ECMO support.

Importantly what is needed is a better understanding of the factors leading to poor outcomes that could lead to improvements in patient selection and development of adjuvant therapies [42].

PREDICTOR RISK FACTOR FOR ECMO IN SEPTIC SHOCK PATIENTS

No clear predictors of positive or negative outcome have been reported in RSS. However, a growing number of studies have identified factors associated with improved outcomes for patients with septic shock managed with ECMO. Previous studies to date have found age [4,13], severe cardiomyopathy [19], cardiac arrest prior to ECMO introduction, preexisting malignancy/immunosuppression [43], elevated arterial lactate levels pre- and post-ECMO [44], SOFA score before ECMO placement, shock-to-ECMO interval, and the number of cases who had the normal range of ScvO2% at 12, 18, and 24 h during ECMO [45] to be prognostic factors among adult patients with septic shock in which VA ECMO was introduced. The trend of SOFA score over time can facilitate decision-making regarding the appropriateness of organ support [45].

IN CONCLUSION

RSS is a complication of sepsis with high rates of morbidity and mortality. According to recent international guidelines, ECMO may be safely used to resuscitate and support neonates and children with sepsis and shock "refractory to all other treatments." There is, however, some controversy over its use in adult patients with RSS. So that, more evidence is needed before this technique can be universally recommended presently in this setting, although successful salvage cases have been published.

ECMO for SCM is an evolving field with several promising approaches being investigated. Despite this fact, randomization of ECMO in patients with septic shock refractory to conventional treatments is not possible and is unethical. Instead, a well-organized protocol outlining patient selection, monitoring of predictors, and management of ECMO will be needed to control this potential bias.

Furthermore, a multicenter registry study or prospective cohort study, however, is needed for a more complete assessment of the role of ECMO in RSS.

It is encouraging that in some countries, the survival rate of patients who received VV ECMO for ARDS in Japan has improved by over a factor of two from 36% (2009) to 79% (2016) [46], and future improvements in performance are expected even with the use of VA ECMO in adult patients with sepsis presenting with severe cardiac dysfunction.

Meanwhile, it is essential to consider three key points:

- ECMO should be considered early for stratified patients failing pharmacologic management of SCM in order to maximize ECMO benefits and hopefully improve survival.
- Patients with RSS should be transferred within hours of diagnosis to a referral ECMO center.

- Echocardiography is currently the gold standard of diagnosis of SCM, and evaluation of GLS is more sensitive and specific for SCM than LVEF or other common findings alone.

REFERENCES

[1] Morin L, Ray S, Wilson C, Remy S, et al. ESPNIC refractory septic shock definition taskforce the infection systemic inflammation sepsis section of ESPNIC. Refractory septic shock in children: a European society of paediatric and neonatal intensive care definition. Intensive Care Med December 2016;42(12):1948−57. https://doi.org/10.1007/s00134-016-4574-2. Epub 2016 Oct 5. PMID: 27709263; PMCID: PMC5106490.

[2] Davis AL, Carcillo JA, Aneja RK, et al. American College of critical care medicine clinical practice parameters for hemodynamic support of pediatric and neonatal septic shock. Crit Care Med June 2017;45(6):1061−93. https://doi.org/10.1097/CCM.0000000000002425. Erratum in: Crit Care Med. 2017 Sep;45(9):e993. Kissoon, Niranjan Tex [corrected to Kissoon, Niranjan]; Weingarten-Abrams, Jacki [corrected to Weingarten-Arams, Jacki]. PMID: 28509730.

[3] Weiss SL, Peters MJ, Alhazzani W, et al. Surviving sepsis campaign international guidelines for the management of septic shock and sepsis-associated organ dysfunction in children. Pediatr Crit Care Med February 2020;21(2): e52−106. https://doi.org/10.1097/PCC.000000000000 2198. PMID: 32032273.

[4] Bréchot N, Luyt CE, Schmidt M, et al. Venoarterial extracorporeal membrane oxygenation support for refractory cardiovascular dysfunction during severe bacterial septic shock. Crit Care Med July 2013;41(7):1616−26. https://doi.org/10.1097/CCM.0b013e31828a2370. PMID: 23563585.

[5] Cecconi M, De Backer D, Antonelli M, et al. Consensus on circulatory shock and hemodynamic monitoring. Task force of the European Society of Intensive Care Medicine. Intensive Care Med December 2014;40(12): 1795−815. https://doi.org/10.1007/s00134-014-3525-z. Epub 2014 Nov 13. PMID: 25392034; PMCID: PMC4239778.

[6] Paoli CJ, Reynolds MA, Sinha M, et al. Epidemiology and costs of sepsis in the United States-an analysis based on timing of diagnosis and severity level. Crit Care Med December 2018;46(12):1889−97. https://doi.org/10. 1097/CCM.0000000000003342. PMID: 30048332; PMCID: PMC6250243.

[7] Singer M, Deutschman CS, Seymour CW, et al. The third international consensus definitions for sepsis and septic shock (Sepsis-3). JAMA February 23, 2016;315(8): 801−10. https://doi.org/10.1001/jama.2016.0287. PMID: 26903338; PMCID: PMC4968574.

[8] Teles F, Rodrigues WG, Alves MGTC, et al. Impact of a sepsis bundle in wards of a tertiary hospital. J Intensive Care July 18, 2017;5:45. https://doi.org/10.1186/

s40560-017-0231-2. PMID: 28729904; PMCID: PMC55 16371.

[9] Reiterer F, Resch E, Haim M, et al. Neonatal extracorporeal membrane oxygenation due to respiratory failure: a single center experience over 28 years. Front Pediatr September 25, 2018;6:263. https://doi.org/10.3389/fped.2018.00263. PMID: 30320047; PMCID: PMC616 7543.

[10] MacLaren G, Butt W, Best D, Donath S. Central extracorporeal membrane oxygenation for refractory pediatric septic shock. Pediatr Crit Care Med March 2011;12(2):133–6. https://doi.org/10.1097/PCC.0b013e3181e2 a4a1. PMID: 20453704.

[11] Evans L, Rhodes A, Alhazzani W, et al. Surviving sepsis campaign: international guidelines for management of sepsis and septic shock 2021. Intensive Care Med October 2, 2021:1–67. https://doi.org/10.1007/s00134-021-065 06-y. Epub ahead of print. PMID: 34599691; PMCID: PMC8486643.

[12] Egi M, Ogura H, Yatabe T, et al. The Japanese clinical practice guidelines for management of sepsis and septic shock 2020 (J-SSCG 2020). J Intensive Care August 25, 2021; 9(1):53. https://doi.org/10.1186/s40560-021-00555-7. PMID: 34433491; PMCID: PMC8384927.

[13] Huang CT, Tsai YJ, Tsai PR, Ko WJ. Extracorporeal membrane oxygenation resuscitation in adult patients with refractory septic shock. J Thorac Cardiovasc Surg November 2013;146(5):1041–6. https://doi.org/10.1016/j.jtcvs. 2012.08.022. Epub 2012 Sep 7. PMID: 22959322.

[14] Cheng A, Sun HY, Tsai MS, et al. Predictors of survival in adults undergoing extracorporeal membrane oxygenation with severe infections. 1526-1536.e1 J Thorac Cardiovasc Surg December 2016;152(6). https://doi.org/10.1016/j.jtcvs.2016.08.038. Epub 2016 Aug 30. PMID: 27692951.

[15] Falk L, Hultman J, Broman LM. Extracorporeal membrane oxygenation for septic shock. Crit Care Med August 2019; 47(8):1097–105. https://doi.org/10.1097/CCM.0000000 000003819. PMID: 31162206.

[16] Vogel DJ, Murray J, Czapran AZ, et al. Veno-arteriovenous ECMO for septic cardiomyopathy: a single-centre experience. Perfusion May 2018;33(1_Suppl. l):57–64. https://doi.org/10.1177/0267659118766833. PMID: 29788842.

[17] Parker MM, Shelhamer JH, Natanson C, et al. Serial cardiovascular variables in survivors and nonsurvivors of human septic shock: heart rate as an early predictor of prognosis. Crit Care Med October 1987;15(10):923–9. https://doi.org/10.1097/00003246-198710000-00006. PMID: 3652707.

[18] Schmidt M, Bréchot N, Combes A. Ten situations in which ECMO is unlikely to be successful. Intensive Care Med May 2016;42(5):750–2. https://doi.org/10.1007/s00134-015-4013-9. Epub 2015 Aug 14. PMID: 26271905.

[19] Park TK, Yang JH, Jeon K, et al. Extracorporeal membrane oxygenation for refractory septic shock in adults. Eur J Cardio Thorac Surg February 2015;47(2):e68–74.

https://doi.org/10.1093/ejcts/ezu462. Epub 2014 Nov 25. PMID: 25425551.

[20] Bréchot N, Hajage D, Kimmoun A, , et al International ECMO Network. Venoarterial extracorporeal membrane oxygenation to rescue sepsis-induced cardiogenic shock: a retrospective, multicentre, international cohort study. Lancet August 22, 2020;396(10250):545–52. https://doi.org/10.1016/S0140-6736(20)30733-9. PMID: 32828186.

[21] Vignon P. Continuous cardiac output assessment or serial echocardiography during septic shock resuscitation? Ann Transl Med June 2020;8(12):797. https://doi.org/10.21037/atm.2020.04.11. PMID: 32647722; PMCID: PMC7333154.

[22] Bouhemad B, Nicolas-Robin A, Arbelot C, et al. Isolated and reversible impairment of ventricular relaxation in patients with septic shock. Crit Care Med March 2008; 36(3):766–74. https://doi.org/10.1097/CCM.0B013E 31816596BC. PMID: 18431265.

[23] Jardin F, Valtier B, Beauchet A, et al. Invasive monitoring combined with two-dimensional echocardiographic study in septic shock. Intensive Care Med November 1994;20(8):550–4. https://doi.org/10.1007/BF01705 720. PMID: 7706566.

[24] Sato R, Nasu M. A review of sepsis-induced cardiomyopathy. J Intensive Care November 11, 2015;3:48. https://doi.org/10.1186/s40560-015-0112-5. PMID: 26566443; PMCID: PMC4642671.

[25] Sanfilippo F, Orde S, Oliveri F, et al. The challenging diagnosis of septic cardiomyopathy. Chest September 2019; 156(3):635–6. https://doi.org/10.1016/j.chest.2019.04. 136. PMID: 31511158.

[26] Parker MM, Shelhamer JH, Bacharach SL, et al. Profound but reversible myocardial depression in patients with septic shock. Ann Intern Med April 1984;100(4):483–90. https://doi.org/10.7326/0003-4819-100-4-483. PMID: 6703540.

[27] Vieillard-Baron A. Septic cardiomyopathy. Ann Intensive Care April 13, 2011;1(1):6. https://doi.org/10.1186/2110-5820-1-6. PMID: 21906334; PMCID: PMC3159902.

[28] Orde SR, Pulido JN, Masaki M, et al. Outcome prediction in sepsis: speckle tracking echocardiography based assessment of myocardial function. Crit Care July 11, 2014; 18(4):R149. https://doi.org/10.1186/cc13987. PMID: 25015102; PMCID: PMC4227017.

[29] Sanfilippo F, Corredor C, Fletcher N, et al. Left ventricular systolic function evaluated by strain echocardiography and relationship with mortality in patients with severe sepsis or septic shock: a systematic review and meta-analysis. Crit Care August 4, 2018;22(1):183. https://doi.org/10.1186/s13054-018-2113-y. PMID: 30075792; PMCID: PMC6091069.

[30] Vallabhajosyula S, Rayes HA, Sakhuja A, et al. Global longitudinal strain using speckle-tracking echocardiography as a mortality predictor in sepsis: a systematic review. J Intensive Care Med February 2019;34(2):87–93. https://doi.org/10.1177/0885066618761750. Epub 2018 Mar 18. PMID: 29552957.

[31] Jozwiak M, Persichini R, Monnet X, et al. Management of myocardial dysfunction in severe sepsis. Semin Respir Crit Care Med April 2011;32(2):206–14. https://doi.org/10.1055/s-0031-1275533. Epub 2011 Apr 19. PMID: 21506057.

[32] Martin L, Derwall M, Al Zoubi S, et al. The septic heart: current understanding of molecular mechanisms and clinical Implications. Chest February 2019;155(2):427–37. https://doi.org/10.1016/j.chest.2018.08.1037. Epub 2018 Aug 29. PMID: 30171861.

[33] Maclaren G, Butt W. Extracorporeal membrane oxygenation and sepsis. Crit Care Resusc March 2007;9(1):76–80. PMID: 17352671.

[34] Bartlett RH. Extracorporeal support for septic shock. Pediatr Crit Care Med September 2007;8(5):498–9. https://doi.org/10.1097/01.PCC.0000282163.60836.2C. PMID: 17873786.

[35] Riera J, Argudo E, Ruiz-Rodríguez JC, Ferrer R. Extracorporeal membrane oxygenation for adults with refractory septic shock. Am Soc Artif Intern Organs J 2019 Nov/Dec;65(8):760–8. https://doi.org/10.1097/MAT.0000000000000905. PMID: 30325846.

[36] Chockalingam A, Mehra A, Dorairajan S, Dellsperger KC. Acute left ventricular dysfunction in the critically ill. Chest July 2010;138(1):198–207. https://doi.org/10.1378/chest.09-1996. PMID: 20605820.

[37] Dellinger RP, Levy MM, Rhodes A, et al. Surviving Sepsis Campaign Guidelines Committee including the Pediatric Subgroup. Surviving sepsis campaign: international guidelines for management of severe sepsis and septic shock: 2012. Crit Care Med February 2013;41(2):580–637. https://doi.org/10.1097/CCM.0b013e31827e83af. PMID: 23353941.

[38] Carcillo JA, Fields AI, American College of Critical Care Medicine Task Force Committee Members. Clinical practice parameters for hemodynamic support of pediatric and neonatal patients in septic shock. Crit Care Med June 2002;30(6):1365–78. https://doi.org/10.1097/00003246-200206000-00040. PMID: 12072696.

[39] Ling RR, Ramanathan K, Poon WH, et al. Venoarterial extracorporeal membrane oxygenation as mechanical circulatory support in adult septic shock: a systematic review and meta-analysis with individual participant data meta-regression analysis. Crit Care July 14, 2021;25(1):246. https://doi.org/10.1186/s13054-021-03668-5. PMID: 34261492; PMCID: PMC8278703.

[40] MacLaren G, Warwick B. ECMO for septic shock. In: Brogan TV, Lequier L, Lorusso R, MacLaren G, Peek G, editors. Extracorporeal life support: the ELSO red book. 5th ed. Ann Arbor: Extracorporeal Life Support Organization; 2017. p. 613–26.

[41] Park J, Shin DA, Lee S, et al. Investigation of key circuit constituents affecting drug sequestration during extracorporeal membrane oxygenation treatment. Am Soc Artif Intern Organs J 2017 May/Jun;63(3):293–8. https://doi.org/10.1097/MAT.0000000000000489. PMID: 2792 2880.

[42] Pagani FD. Extracorporeal membrane oxygenation for septic shock: heroic futility? J Thorac Cardiovasc Surg September 2018;156(3):1110–1. https://doi.org/10.1016/j.jtcvs.2018.04.076. Epub 2018 Apr 24. PMID: 29884486.

[43] Oberender F, Ganeshalingham A, Fortenberry JD, et al. Venoarterial extracorporeal membrane oxygenation versus conventional therapy in severe pediatric septic shock. Pediatr Crit Care Med October 2018;19(10):965–72. https://doi.org/10.1097/PCC.0000000000001660. PMID: 30048365.

[44] Ro SK, Kim WK, Lim JY, et al. Extracorporeal life support for adults with refractory septic shock. 1104-1109.e1 J Thorac Cardiovasc Surg September 2018;156(3). https://doi.org/10.1016/j.jtcvs.2018.03.123. Epub 2018 Apr 7. PMID: 29753504.

[45] Han L, Zhang Y, Zhang Y, et al. Risk factors for refractory septic shock treated with VA ECMO. Ann Transl Med September 2019;7(18):476. https://doi.org/10.21037/atm.2019.08.07. PMID: 31700912; PMCID: PMC6803222.

[46] Ohshimo S, Shime N, Nakagawa S, et al. Committee of the Japan ECMO project. Comparison of extracorporeal membrane oxygenation outcome for influenza-associated acute respiratory failure in Japan between 2009 and 2016. J Intensive Care July 11, 2018;6:38. https://doi.org/10.1186/s40560-018-0306-8. PMID: 30009033; PMCID: PMC6042359.

CHAPTER 18

Antimicrobials in the Management of Sepsis

JUDITH JACOBI

TIMELINESS OF THERAPY

Timeliness of sepsis recognition and therapy of an infection with antimicrobials and source control remain essential for patient outcome, especially in the most critically ill patients. Retrospective data from most studies indicate that each hour of delay to administration of the correct antimicrobial is associated with an increased in-hospital mortality for septic shock per hour of delay, depending on the population and trial. Other factors that influence mortality risk include high severity of illness, site of infection, longer time to correct hypotension, and significant comorbidities [1,2]. For patients with septic shock or a high likelihood of sepsis, all delays should be eliminated through efficient assessment, utilization of protocols, drug delivery systems that ensure rapid availability, and engaged personnel. The Surviving Sepsis Campaign (SSC) Guidelines recommend immediate antibiotic administration, ideally within 1 h of recognition [1]. While there may be more flexibility to allow for greater use of diagnostics in less critical patients (possible sepsis without shock), standardization for quality will remain essential and the SSC suggests rapid investigation for infection and a three-hour therapy window when concern for infection persists.

ANTIMICROBIAL STEWARDSHIP

Important components of antimicrobial stewardship regarding therapeutic interventions are to control the source of infection, prescribe antimicrobials when they are truly needed, with adequate doses, reassess treatment when culture results are available, and use the shortest duration, based on evidence. Empiric use of broad-spectrum antimicrobials is important to increase the likelihood that the potential pathogen is treated but may lead to inappropriate use in patients when infection is suspected but other diagnoses were ultimately made. A substantial proportion of patients hospitalized in 2015 with community-acquired pneumonia (CAP) or urinary tract infection were found to have received antimicrobial therapy that was not supported by data 55.9% overall and as high as 79.5% for CAP because of inappropriate initiation, duration of therapy, or choice of agent [3]. For patients with suspected bacterial infections, a post hoc diagnosis of viral infection, fluid overload, or heart failure, drug effects and hypovolemia were reported in one-third of patients [4]. Similar results have been reported worldwide, although with the complex nature of sepsis diagnosis and delays to receipt of definitive data, it is not surprising that the diagnosis would change in hindsight.

Risks of antimicrobial misuse include treatment failures, worsening resistance, secondary infections such as *Clostridium difficile* or fungemia, adverse effects (e.g., kidney injury, neurologic dysfunction, vascular injury), excessive cost of care, etc.

Clinicians can optimize antimicrobial utilization with adjunctive testing (e.g., appropriate cultures, rapid testing for pathogen identification and presence of resistance markers, utilization of biomarkers, etc.), discontinuing or narrowing treatment in response to testing or when an alternative diagnosis is made, by following evidence-based protocols, and using the shortest effective duration of therapy. Antimicrobial Stewardship Programs (ASPs) utilize multiprofessional teams that are accountable for the core elements for their size and location and should educate, measure, track, and report progress in optimizing antimicrobial utilization [5]. Established protocols for empiric antimicrobial use should be established to ensure that agents are chosen appropriately, and stewardship principles should be followed to ensure timely de-escalation.

CHOICE OF ANTIMICROBIAL THERAPY

As discussed in other chapters, clinicians are challenged to consider several variables when faced with a patient with sepsis to make the proper diagnosis, initiate diagnostics, and treat in a timely manner, and to reassess response. Clinical practice guidelines and governmental quality indicators provide a general framework, and local protocols are important for efficient and consistent care. However, it remains essential that the care team members understand antimicrobial advantages and disadvantages to optimally treat individual patients [1,6]. Broad-spectrum coverage is initiated to increase the likelihood of effective coverage in sepsis, preferably with an initial loading dose for most agents, and with doses maximized at the start, anticipating reductions to avoid accumulation as the degree of organ dysfunction is quantified over the next 24–36 h. Factors such as the treatment of infections in the previous six months and especially within 30 days should lead to the consideration of potential multidrug-resistant (MDR) pathogens such as *Pseudomonas aeruginosa*, Enterobacterales, Methicillin-resistant *Staphylococcus aureus* (MRSa), or *Acinetobacter baumannii* and addition of appropriate therapy [1,7]. More detailed discussion of the mechanisms of antimicrobial resistance and therapies can be found in Chapter 27. Many other factors influence the choice of drug or the dosing including patient-related factors, drug-specific factors, organ function, and disease state (Table 18.1). The SSC suggests against addition of empiric therapy for *S. aureus* or *P. aeruginosa* for patients at a low risk for these infections but do suggest the use of empiric antifungal therapy in high-risk patients [1].

Pharmacokinetics and Pharmacodynamics

Clinical pharmacists are experts in drug dosing and the principles of pharmacokinetics (PK) and pharmacodynamics (PD), but not every site has this valuable resource. Intensive care unit (ICU) and emergency department (ED) clinicians should understand how these parameters impact antimicrobial dosing and the role of serum concentration monitoring (Fig. 18.1). Most antimicrobials are hydrophilic with low protein binding and distribute readily in the serum and interstitial fluid. They have a low volume of distribution (Vd) that is comparable to the extracellular volume. However, with initial crystalloid resuscitation approaching or

Patient Factors	Pathogen Factors	Drug Factors
BMI	Site of infection	Hydrophilic versus lipophilic
GFR	Resistance patterns	Time versus concentration dependent
Fluid balance	Cell wall mediated killing	Ability to penetrate to site of infection
Severity of illness	Bactericidal versus inhibitory	Mechanism of action
IV access options	Potential synergy	Mixed with an enzyme inhibitor
Time-sensitive goals	Actual MIC	Ability to monitor concentration
Immunosuppression		Dose and frequency
Neutropenia		Protein binding
Albumin level		

TABLE 18.1
Factors to Consider when Selecting and Antimicrobial Agent

BMI, body mass index; *GFR*, glomerular filtration rate; *IV*, intravenous; *MIC*, minimum inhibitory concentration.

sometimes exceeding 30 mL/kg, acute expansion of the Vd has a dilutional effect on the peak drug concentration. A larger, loading dose of these agents is essential to exceed the minimum inhibitory concentration (MIC) of the bacterial pathogen, achieve a rapid bactericidal effect, and sustain concentrations above the MIC until the ongoing/maintenance regimen can be initiated. Piperacillin 8 gm or cefepime/ceftazidime 4 gm over 3 h or meropenem 2 gm over 30 min has been proposed based on modeling, but not tested clinically and a range of doses have been suggested elsewhere [8]. In the ED setting, a loading dose may be administered as an intravenous (IV) push dose over 3–5 min for efficient and timely drug delivery and increased likelihood of achieving the 1-h target with minimal risk, other than infiltration of a more concentrated and potentially irritating infusate [9,10]. A review of agents with data on rapid administration has been published and summarized in Table 18.2, but updated guidance should be sought when designing sepsis therapy protocols [11]. Alternatively, having premixed antimicrobial

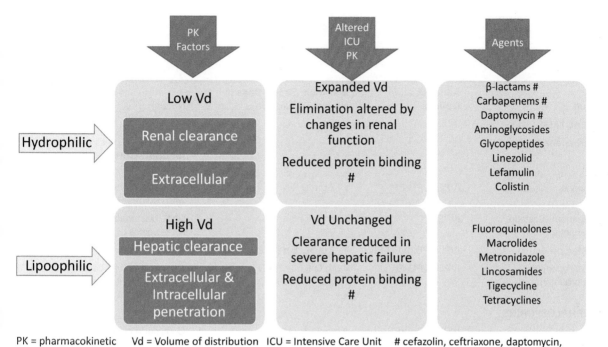

PK Factors	Altered ICU PK	Agents

Hydrophilic

Low Vd
- Renal clearance
- Extracellular

Expanded Vd
Elimination altered by changes in renal function
Reduced protein binding #

β-lactams #
Carbapenems #
Daptomycin #
Aminoglycosides
Glycopeptides
Linezolid
Lefamulin
Colistin

Lipoophilic

High Vd
- Hepatic clearance
- Extracellular & Intracellular penetration

Vd Unchanged
Clearance reduced in severe hepatic failure
Reduced protein binding #

Fluoroquinolones
Macrolides
Metronidazole
Lincosamides
Tigecycline
Tetracyclines

PK = pharmacokinetic   Vd = Volume of distribution   ICU = Intensive Care Unit   # cefazolin, ceftriaxone, daptomycin, ertapenem, tigecycline

FIG. 18.1 Consideration of pharmacokinetic factors for antimicrobial agents used in intensive care unit patients based on affinity for hydrous or lipid spaces, site of organ elimination, and protein binding [24]. (Adapted from Póvoa P, Moniz P, Pereira JG, Coelho L. Optimizing antimicrobial drug dosing in critically ill patients. Microorganisms 2021;9:1401. https://doi.org/10.3390/microorganisms9071401. Copyright: 2021 by the authors. Licensee MDPI, Basel, Switzerland. This article is an open access article distributed under the terms and conditions of the Creative Commons Attribution (CC BY) license (https://creativecommons.org/licenses/by/4.0/).)

minibags available and ready to infuse has been shown to reduce treatment delays [12].

In sepsis, there is ongoing expansion of the Vd related to positive fluid balance, damage to the glycocalyx (inflammatory, shear injury) with capillary "leakage" and expanded interstitial volume, and reduced albumin levels related to both volume and reduced production. For hydrophilic agents, a persistently expanded Vd contributes to slower elimination rate (ke), despite consistent clearance (Cl). The mathematical relationship is $CL = ke \times Vd$. The ke is inversely related to half-life (the time it takes to eliminate 50% of the drug), thus half-life may be longer in the face of volume expansion. This may translate into the need for a longer interval (>24 h) with agents such as aminoglycosides, where a low/undetectable concentration is desired prior to redosing to reduce accumulation in the tubules and the risk for nephrotoxicity.

The selected group of lipophilic agents shown in Fig. 18.1 can penetrate to the intracellular space more readily and are less altered by volume expansion, and hepatic elimination contributes more to elimination. Alterations in protein binding may impact free drug concentrations, with a subsequent increase in free fraction. Free drug has greater renal elimination and larger Vd, risking subtherapeutic concentrations. Highly protein-bound agents include cefazolin, ceftriaxone, daptomycin, and ertapenem, but clinical impact of these PK changes has not been well characterized [13].

The site of infection may influence antimicrobial penetration. The cerebral spinal fluid and bronchoalveolar lavage fluid have been sampled and lower concentrations are found with many agents [14]. The MIC of the organism will be important, as adequate drug concentrations will be difficult to achieve with more resistant pathogens (higher MIC). Some unusual factors that prevent the use of some antibiotics include daptomycin inactivation by pulmonary surfactant making it inadequate for pneumonia treatment and colistin (Polymyxin E) failure to penetrate lung tissue from systemic doses.

TABLE 18.2

Special Considerations for Individual Agents with Potential Use for Sepsis and Septic Shock (Does Not Include Every Potential Antimicrobial Agent and All Information Needed to Prescribe, Clinicians Should Consult a Complete Drug Information Source)

Drug	Administration Options	Maximum Sepsis Dose If Normal Elimination	Notes
β-LACTAMS			
Carbapenems			Carbapenem class preferred for ESBL-GNR empiric therapy
Imipenem-cilastatin	IVPB, IVPB-EI	1–2 gm Q 6 h	GNR, resistance rates higher with new breakpoint 1 mcg/mL
Imipenem-cilastatin-relebactam	IVPB	1.25 gm Q 6 h	GNR, *Bacteroides* spp., *P. aeruginosa*
Meropenem	IVP, IVPB, IVPB-EI	1–2 gm Q 8 h IVPB-EI	GNR, *Streptococcal* spp.
Meropenem-vaborbactam	IVPB, IVPB-EI	4 gm Q 8 h IVPB-EI	Combo improves coverage of most ESBL but does not increase activity versus DTR
CEPHALOSPORINS			
Cefazolin	IVP, IVPB, IVPB-EI, CI	2 gm IVPB Q 8 h	Consider a higher dose for weight ≥120 kg, 80% protein bound, low cross-allergenicity with other β-lactams
Cefepime	IVP, IVPB, IVPB-EI, CI	2 gm IVPB-EI Q 8 h	Neurologic adverse effects possible
Ceftaroline	IVP, IVPB	600 mg Q 8 h	Active against MRSa, MRSe, and GNR
Ceftazidime	IVP, IVPB, IVPB-EI, CI	2 gm IVPB-EI Q 8 h	Covers GNR, but not ESBL
Ceftazidime-avibactam	IVPB-EI (2 h)	2.5 gm Q 8 h	Combo covers *P. aeruginosa*, most ESBL-GNR
Ceftriaxone	IVP, IVPB, CI	2 gm IVPB Q 24 h	Q 12 h in meningitis
Ceftolozane-tazobactam	IVPB, IVPB-EI, CI	3 gm IVPB-EI Q 8 h	Combo covers *P. aeruginosa*, most ESBL-GNR
Ceftobiprole	IVPB-EI (2 h)	500 mg Q 8 h	GPC, GNR, MRSa
Cefiderocol	IVPB-EI	2 gm IVPB-EI Q 8 h	No GPC coverage
PENICILLINS			
Nafcillin	IVP-slow, IVPB, CI	2 gm IVPB Q 4 h	High protein binding (90%–94%), no dose change in renal failure, neutropenia
Oxacillin	IVP-slow, IVPB, CI	2 gm IVPB Q 4 h	High protein binding (90%), hepatic dysfunction risk, eosinophilia
Piperacillin-tazobactam	IVP, IVPB, IVPB-EI	4.5 gm IVPB-EI Q 8 h	Avoid use for ESBL-GNR
MONOBACTAM			
Aztreonam	IVP, IVPB, IVPB-EI, CI	2 gm IVPB Q 6 h	Cross-allergenicity possible with ceftazidime and cefiderocol

TABLE 18.2

Special Considerations for Individual Agents with Potential Use for Sepsis and Septic Shock (Does Not Include Every Potential Antimicrobial Agent and All Information Needed to Prescribe, Clinicians Should Consult a Complete Drug Information Source)—cont'd

FLUOROQUINOLONES

Ciprofloxacin	IVPB	400 mg IVPB Q 8 h	Neurologic adverse effects with high doses
Levofloxacin	IVPB	750 mg IVPB Q 24 h	Adequate concentrations unlikely if MIC $\geq$2 mcg/mL

GLYCOPEPTIDES

Daptomycin	IVP, IVPB	12 mg/kg IVPB Q 24 h	Do not use for pneumonia, myopathy associated with high doses, adjusted weight in obesity
Telavancin	IVPB	10 mg/kg IVPB	QT prolongation, dysgeusia
Vancomycin	IVPB, CI	20–35 mg/kg IVPB then 15 –20 mg/kg Q 8 h	Load up to 3000 mg maximum. AUC guided dosing, with Bayesian software preferred

TETRACYCLINES

Eravacycline	IVPB	1 mg/kg IVPB Q 12 h	Increase dose with strong CYP3A4 inducer. For complicated intraabdominal infections, only, especially for ESBL-GNR. Not for pregnancy/lactation.
Tigecycline	IVPB	150–200 mg IVPB then 75 –100 mg Q 12 h	High dose of last resort only, associated with GI side effects

AMINOGLYCOSIDES

Amikacin	IVPB	25–30 mg/kg IVPB Q 24 h	Measure two levels after first dose to achieve peak 10 $\times$ MIC and trough <1 mg/L
Gentamicin or tobramycin	IVPB	7–10 mg/kg IVPB Q 24 h	Measure two levels after first dose to achieve peak 10 $\times$ MIC and trough <0.5 mg/L

MISCELLANEOUS ANTIBACTERIAL

Colistimethate (CMS)	IVP, IVPB, CI	Initial dose 4 mg CBA/kg IVPB	Doses adjusted for renal function, see ColistinDose calculator (Table 18.3) then $\leq$360 mg CBA/day divided Q 8 –12 h
Polymyxin B	IVPB	25,000 IU/kg (2.5 mg/kg) over 2 h then 1.5 mg/kg IVPB Q 12 h	Preferred over CMS, no dose adjustment for renal function, use actual weight in obesity
Linezolid	IVPB	600 mg IVPB Q 12 h	Thrombocytopenia with prolonged use
Tedizolid	IVPB	200 mg IVPB daily	Prodrug, bacteriostatic vs. MRSa and MRSe and enterococci. Labeled for skin infection.

Continued

TABLE 18.2

Special Considerations for Individual Agents with Potential Use for Sepsis and Septic Shock (Does Not Include Every Potential Antimicrobial Agent and All Information Needed to Prescribe, Clinicians Should Consult a Complete Drug Information Source)—cont'd

Drug	Administration Options	Maximum Sepsis Dose If Normal Elimination	Notes
ANTIFUNGALS			
Amphotericins	IVPB, CI	Various, depends on form use	For *Histoplasma, Candida* sp. except not for *C. lusitaniae, Aspergillus* sp, and others. Nephrotoxicity, infusion-related rigors, fever.
Azoles			**Assess for drug interactions**
Fluconazole	IVPB	400 mg Q 24 h	*Candida krusei and glabrata* are resistant
Isavuconazonium	IVPB	372 mg Q 8 h × 6 then daily	For *Aspergillus* sp. and mucormycosis, prodrug converted to isavuconazole
Posaconazole	IVPB	Primarily for prophylaxis	Oral formulations not interchangeable
Voriconazole	IVPB	6 mg/kg Q 12 h then 4 mg/kg Q 12 h	For *Aspergillus* sp. and *Candida* sp.
Echinocandins			**For *Candida* sp., *Aspergillus***
Anidulafungin	IVPB	200 mg × 1 then 100 mg Q 24 h	Histamine release with rapid infusion
Caspofungin	IVPB	70 mg × 1 then 50 mg Q 24 h	Reduce dose in moderate to severe hepatic insufficiency
Micafungin	IVPB	100 mg Q 24 h	Increase dose in CRRT

AUC, area under the concentration-time curse; *CBA*, colistin base activity; *CI*, continuous infusion; *CRRT*, continuous renal replacement therapy; *CYP*, cytochrome; *dd*, divided doses; *DTR*, Acinetobacter baumannii, Pseudomonas aeruginosa, Stenotrophomonas maltophilia; *EI*, extended infusion over 2–4 h; *ESBL-GNR*, Extended-spectrum β-lactamase producing gran negative rods (Bacilli), *GI*, gastrointestinal; *gm*, gram; *GNR*, gram negative bacilli; *GPC*, gram positive cocci; *h*, hours; *IU*, international units; *IVP*, IV push over 3–5 min; *IVPB*, intermittent infusion over 30–60 min; *IVPB-EI*, IVPB over 3–4 h; *mg*, milligram; *MIC*, minimum inhibitory concentration; *MRSa/e*, methicillin resistant Staphylococcus aureus/epidermidis; *Q*, every.

Impact of renal function

The loading dose or initial dose of antimicrobials can be standardized without regard to renal function and may be based on weight. An early dose reduction for acute creatinine elevation is not advised in most settings, as half of patients will respond to resuscitation with resolution of acute kidney injury (AKI) markers and improved urine output. With ongoing therapy, there is time to assess renal function and consider dose adjustments for worsening renal function based on the presence of oliguria or rising creatinine or cystatin C. Formulas to estimate glomerular filtration rate (GFR) from creatinine assume a steady state, and that is rarely true in septic shock [15]. Incorporating cystatin C into the predictive formula for Clcr appears to improve results, may be a better measure

of declining GFR in AKI, and is associated with improved vancomycin dosing [16–19]. Collection of urine for Clcr over at least 8 h has been proposed to identify clearance more accurately than standard equations based on serum creatinine [20]. Creatinine clearance measurement is particularly important for patients with augmented renal clearance (ARC) (Clcr generally greater than 130 mL/min) who are at risk for underdosing [21]. Independent risk factors for ARC include trauma, young age, and male sex, especially when serum creatinine is normal.

Dose adjustments for reduced Clcr in product labeling have been developed for patients with chronic kidney disease, but elimination may be higher in a patient in the initial phases of AKI, thus a delay in dose reduction may be appropriate to maximize early and adequate

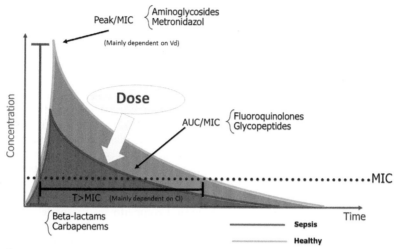

FIG. 18.2 Pharmacokinetics and pharmacodynamics: After an antibiotic infusion, a ratio between the peak concentration and the minimal inhibitory concentration, the area under the concentration—time curve and the minimal inhibitory concentration, and the time the antibiotic concentration is above the minimal inhibitory concentration can be defined. These three parameters all decreased in septic patients, with an increased volume of distribution and clearance. The only secure way to achieve effective antibiotic concentration is to adjust the dose. [24] *Cl*, Clearance; *MIC*, minimal inhibitory concentration; *T > MIC*, time that the antibiotic concentration is above the minimal inhibitory concentration; *Vd*, vole of distribution. (Adapted from: Póvoa P, Moniz P, Pereira AG, Coelho L. Optimizing antimicrobial dosing in critically ill patients. *Microorganisms*. 2021; 9(7): 1401. https://doi.org/10.3390/microorganisms9071401). This article is an open access article distributed under the terms and conditions of the Creative Commons Attribution (CC BY) license (https:// creativecommons.org/licenses/by/4.0/).)

treatment [22,23]. At the same time, there is also a greater risk of adverse drug events when serum concentrations are maximized, so close follow-up is needed.

Time-dependent agents

Antimicrobial agents can be characterized by the PK and PD—essentially the relationship between concentration and killing. The β-lactam agents and carbapenems exhibit time-dependent killing, such that achieving and maintaining an adequate concentration is needed for efficient bactericidal effect throughout the dosing interval (Fig. 18.2) [24]. The antibacterial effect for these agents is best predicted by the percentage of the dosing interval that the free or unbound (*f*) concentration is above MIC (*f*MIC). Targets in non-ICU patients are penicillins 50%, cephalosporins 60%—70%, and carbapenems 40% of time above MIC. Patients who are overweight, have ARC, and more resistant pathogens (higher MIC) commonly fail to achieve an adequate *f*MIC, have variability in β-lactam levels and lower odds for a positive clinical outcome [25]. Most clinicians do not have access to actual drug concentrations, so population-based dosing with Bayesian modeling is suggested [26]. It has been suggested that critically ill

patients may benefit from *f*MIC for 100% of the dosing interval to compensate for the many potential physiologic and PK changes in septic shock (Fig. 18.1), requiring a continuous infusion, more frequent dosing, or higher doses at the usual interval.

Following rapid administration of the loading dose (5—30 min), the concentration may rapidly fall below the MIC with dilution/distribution and rapid elimination. The first dose of a maintenance regimen may be initiated earlier than the usual interval (e.g., first dose in 4 h for a regimen of every 6-h dosing), especially if a loading dose was not given. Assessment of barriers to timely continuation of therapy should be done to eliminate inappropriate gaps, such as during transition between ED and ICU orders. The optimal frequency of subsequent doses is related to the PK/PD and may be different from what is in the product label.

While a continuous infusion is most effective at maintaining time above MIC, logistical challenges make this an infrequent option. Instead, prolonged infusions of intermittent doses over 3—4 h increase the time above MIC and allow for other therapies to be administered in the same access site [27]. This strategy is suggested in the SSC 2021 guidelines [1].

Concentration-dependent agents

Aminoglycosides, colistin, and daptomycin demonstrate a concentration-dependent effect such that a high initial peak is needed for optimal bactericidal effect. The PK−PD relationship is described as peak:MIC ratio (Fig. 18.2). Doses in septic shock patients are often much higher than in the product label and will be discussed with the individual agents.

A postantibiotic effect has been suggested as a component of concentration-dependent killing with an in vitro model where bacteria are exposed to a high drug concentration and then drug removed but continues to provide an inhibitory effect. In vivo, the drug concentration falls more slowly, so the clinical significance of the postantibiotic effect is unproven. Nevertheless, a large dose given at a longer interval (e.g., every 24 h) has been used to maximize efficacy and minimize nephrotoxicity of aminoglycosides.

Mixed concentration and time-dependent agents

A combination of concentration and time-dependent effects are observed for fluoroquinolones, tigecycline, linezolid, colistin, and glycopeptides. The ratio of 24-h area under the concentration-time curve (AUC_{24}) to the MIC is the target and is the best measure of fluoroquinolone effectiveness (>125 or >250, depending on organism) [28]. Similarly, the vancomycin endpoint of AUC_{24}:MIC $\geq 400-600$ is now the accepted measure of effectiveness, based on retrospective data in patients with MRSa bacteremia to maximize effectiveness and especially to minimize the risk of nephrotoxicity [29]. The trough vancomycin concentration was previously used as a surrogate but is not adequately descriptive of the AUC_{24} especially in complex or critically ill patients. A modified linear model for dose adjustment was proposed using two concentrations at steady state [30]. The first postdose level is postdistribution (1.75−3 h after end of infusion) followed by a level prior to the next dose with extrapolated values used to calculate the AUC using the formula: $AUC_{interval}$ = (extrapolated level at start of infusion − extrapolated trough)/ke and multiplied by the number of doses per day. The calculation process is available in detail and in medical calculators [30,31]. The simplicity must be balanced with the need for two levels and a slight overprediction of the AUC. Current guidelines prefer the use of Bayesian modeling, especially with complex critically ill patients as they may be used in the first 24−48 h with a single trough or random concentration, although using two levels improves Bayesian accuracy and is preferred [29]. Software programs are available [32].

Repeated trough or random concentrations are suggested when clinical changes occur or for those at high risk of nephrotoxicity, changing renal function, more than five days of therapy, and weekly when stable [29].

The PK−PD measure for colistimethate (CMS, polymyxin E) is also based on AUC and time, with an endpoint of free (f) $fAUC_{24}$:MIC >25 or total drug AUC_{24}:MIC >50, although drug concentrations are not readily available in the clinical setting [33−36]. Colistimethate is a prodrug which is rapidly renally cleared with a linear two-compartment PK model [36]. Only 25% of CMS is converted to colistin, the active moiety, which has nonrenal clearance and a linear 1-compartment PK model, potentially delaying the time to achieve adequate colistin concentrations. The clearance of CMS with high/normal Clcr (>80 mL/min) may be faster than its conversion to active colistin and increases the likelihood that standard doses will fail to achieve adequate concentrations (Fig. 18.3). While adequate bladder colistin concentrations may occur with local transformation, pulmonary tissue acquires minimal colistin with systemic therapy [37]. Procedures to standardize ordering are needed as

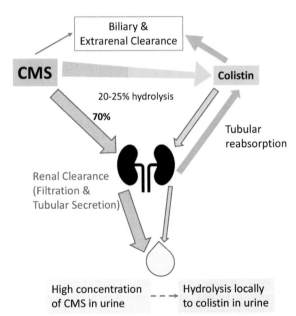

FIG. 18.3 Colistin and colistimethate (CMS) elimination pathways with normal renal function. Standard doses of CMS may be eliminated faster than conversion to colistin, the active moiety, potentially resulting in low systemic and lung tissue levels.

1 mg colistin-base activity (CBA) is equivalent to CMS 30,000 units or approximately 2.4 mg CMS.

Polymyxin B is less well studied but has more optimal PK characteristics [36,38]. It is administered as active drug, so it achieves therapeutic concentrations rapidly, provides more predictable serum concentrations, does not require renal dose adjustment and may not require a loading dose, but does not achieve adequate urine concentrations. A target AUC, 24 h 50−100 or average concentration of 2−4 mCg/mL may be acceptable from a toxicity perspective [39].

ANTIMICROBIAL SELECTION

Prior to initiation, the appropriate laboratory workup should be ordered, and although blood cultures will capture a 12% (95% CI 5.4%−18.6%) higher positive return if collected prior to antimicrobial initiation [40]. Treatment should not be excessively delayed (>45 min) in critically ill patients with septic shock [1]. As discussed in Chapter 9, a variety of other diagnostic tools can assist with the identification of sepsis and causative pathogens. Treatment for sepsis and septic shock must be initiated with broad-spectrum coverage prior to culture results, although new tools for early detection may accelerate that process [41,42].

The optimal antimicrobial for empiric therapy depends on the site of infection, severity of illness, comorbidities, prior antimicrobial use, and known or potential resistance issues.

Using excessively broad coverage may be suboptimal as well, by exposing the patient to unnecessary therapy. The challenge of antimicrobial resistance is so fluid that the European Society of Clinical Microbiology and Infectious Diseases (ESCMID), Infectious Diseases Society of America (IDSA) guidelines may be updated on their website regularly and hospitals should reevaluate their protocols when new options are available [7]. See Chapter 27 for more discussion of resistance mechanisms. Clinical decision support tools, machine learning, and artificial intelligence analysis should improve decision-making for empiric coverage by incorporating broad data from the patient and combination therapy antibiograms that are syndromic (based on site of infection) as discussed in Chapter 38 [43,44].

Combination Therapy

Clinicians typically approach the topic of empiric therapy based on the site of infection but should consider alternative treatments or combinations when MDR is highly likely. While the use of multiple agents (such as aminoglycoside with a β-lactam) for empiric

P. aeruginosa coverage has been traditional, most studies have failed to demonstrate a broad benefit compared with monotherapy when evaluating mortality [45]. However, in patients with septic shock, the SSC and IDSA support combination therapy to increase the chance of providing an effective therapy [1,46]. Discordant coverage is more common when patients with bloodstream infections have antibiotic-resistant pathogens. [47] The most common gram-negative pathogens associated with discordant therapy are Stenotrophomonas maltophilia, A. baumannii, and P. aeruginosa, but the Enterobacterales such as Morganella morganii, Serratia spp., Enterobacter spp., and Klebsiella oxytoca are also prevalent. Gram-positive organisms leading to discordant therapy are Enterococcus faecium, S. aureus, and Streptococcus pneumoniae.

Despite the use of a variety of combinations, the clinical outcomes for GNR pneumonia maybe inadequate related to inadequate drug doses, ineffective agents, MDR organisms, or failure to penetrate to the lung [48].

De-escalation

De-escalation of antimicrobials is a basic tenant of ASP with a goal to reduce both resistance and adverse events relative to antimicrobial overuse and cost while maintaining microbiologic outcomes. The regimen should be reassessed daily to be more focused or to eliminate unneeded therapies based on culture results or clinical improvement [1]. A task force has recommended antibiotic de-escalation be done within 24 h of definitive culture result availability [49,50]. Clinically, it is challenging to trust culture results, especially those without a pathogen due to fear of what may be present but was not captured due to the site of infection, culture technique, adequacy of source control, or prior acute dose of antibiotic. A consistent process with the assistance of the ASP team and infectious diseases specialists improves effectiveness (Chapters 33 and 35).

Duration

The suggested duration of antimicrobial therapy in many cases was developed anecdotally, and longer courses were intended to prevent relapse and reinfection. It is now recognized that prolonged antimicrobials may contribute to secondary infections such as C. difficile overgrowth with colitis or lead to infections with resistant pathogens such as Stenotrophomonas or Acinetobacter. Prospective trials comparing shorter to longer treatments have generally shown noninferiority leading to a "shorter is better" approach and many have been reviewed [51]. Unfortunately, critically ill patients with sepsis are underrepresented in most trials, but investigations are underway by the Canadian Clinical Trial Group to assess 7 versus 14 days of therapy for bacteremia in various severity of illness groups, including ICU patients [52,53]. The SHORTEN trial from Spain found that a seven-day course for Enterobacterales bacteremia (*Escherichia coli* in 66%, from a urinary source in 5%−60%) was noninferior to a 14-day course, but only 13% presented with septic shock [54]. Similarly, short courses of ventilator-associated pneumonia (VAP) therapy (3−5 days) are being compared with ≥8 days for ICU patients [55].

Important factors to consider when selecting a duration of treatment include the complexity factors such as pathogen virulence and persistence, host factors such as neutropenia or immunosuppression, the severity of infection, and severity of host response (severity of sepsis syndrome). While there is no clear association between severity of illness and the need for a longer course of therapy, the expectation that a patient will show signs of improvement prior to de-escalation may have influence on duration. The SSC suggests that clinicians reassess daily for de-escalation opportunities, over the use of a fixed duration [1].

Difficult to treat resistance (DTR) is a term that has been applied to gram-negative pathogens that are resistant to first-line antimicrobials, although this term may still not adequately describe multidrug and extremely drug-resistant organisms [56]. Infection with a DTR gram-negative bacteremia is associated with lower survival, likely related to delayed onset of optimal therapy, but it is unclear if a longer course of therapy can influence that outcome. Organisms such as *P. aeruginosa*, *A. baumannii*, and *S. maltophilia* may have the defining DTR characteristics, outlined as resistance to β-lactams (±β-lactamase inhibitors), carbapenems, and fluoroquinolones [56].

Infection with *S. aureus* poses a challenge for defining optimal duration due to its invasive nature and risk of endovascular and satellite infections, but the subset of uncomplicated bacteremia (rapid improvement, bacterial clearance, and no metastatic infection or prosthetic devices) seems to be distinct in successful treatment with shorter courses than apparently needed for a complicated infection [57].

Neutropenia makes determination of a specific duration of empiric therapy challenging. Empiric antimicrobials are traditionally continued for 72 h but may stop if there is no documented infection, the patient is afebrile, and the absolute neutrophil count is >500 cells/mm^3 or ANC recovery is imminent. Unfortunately, noninfectious causes (neoplastic, paraneoplastic, drug-induced, thrombosis) or nonbacterial infections (fungal) can complicate the clinical assessment of fever. Persistent fever despite antibiotics may indicate the need for empiric antifungal therapy.

Thus, while the shortest effective course is needed, appropriate individualization, potential use of biomarkers (PCT), and clinical assessment of response to therapy will need to be considered, although this remains a suggestion with a low level of evidence in the SSC [1]. Additionally, the PK characteristics of the therapy may be a factor if the agent has a long tissue half-life, such as azithromycin.

ROUTE OF ADMINISTRATION

Intravenous

As discussed in the section on initiation, most antimicrobial therapy will be via the IV route. Giving the first dose IV push improves timeline of the first dose, especially in septic shock, although intermittent infusions of varying duration are used to maintain optimal concentrations, and a continuous infusion is used in some settings [10].

Oral/Enteral

Selected agents are well absorbed from a functioning gastrointestinal (GI) tract and after initial IV therapy may be given enterally. Examples include doxycycline, azithromycin, levofloxacin, moxifloxacin, linezolid, fluconazole, trimethoprim-sulfamethoxazole, and metronidazole. A systematic and programmatic approach to route conversion may reduce expenditures.

Inhalation

Selected agents are used as inhalation therapy due to inadequate drug delivery to the pulmonary tissue or epithelial lining fluid. Challenges to efficient therapy are related to the mode of delivery, as particle size and velocity influence depth of penetration, with larger droplets remaining in large airways [58]. Aerosolization of antimicrobials also raises concern for environmental effects on the local microbiota and promotion of resistance.

The aminoglycosides can all be delivered via inhalation, with amikacin available as an approved product for *Mycobacterium avium* complex with a proprietary delivery system for a liposomal suspension and tobramycin solution or powder via proprietary delivery systems for cystic fibrosis. However, the injectable products have been used via inhalation for many years for mechanically ventilated patients. Debate on the effectiveness and safety continues, as injectables may contain preservatives or other chemicals that influence tolerability [59]. A recent prospective study was inconclusive, but metaanalyses found that while aerosolized amikacin, tobramycin, and colistin are variably associated with clinical recovery, definitive recommendations are not possible [59–63]. The decision to use this route should be based on the risks and benefits in individual patients, and generally not used as routine treatment, except for colistin aerosol adjunctive treatment of *Acinetobacter* [64].

Aerosolized injectable colistin has shown at least equivalent results compared with systemic colistin alone with MDR-GNR, likely related to failure of systemic colistin to penetrate lung tissue and noninferior when combined with systemic imipenem-cilastatin [62,65]. Treatment of *A. baumannii* with an effective systemic antimicrobial and inhaled colistin was suggested in the IDSA guidelines for hospital-or ventilator-associated pneumonia for its potential benefit and relatively low risk of harm, but others have suggested that inhaled colistin with 1 dose of IV colistin may be adequate for pneumonia, in conjunction with other systemic antimicrobials [64,66]. A colistin dry powder inhalation is approved by the European Medicines Agency. Newer agents such as cefiderocol may reduce the need for aerosol colistin.

Comments on Specific Agents for ICU Patients

Specific information on choice of antimicrobial, dosing, and adverse effects should be evaluated prior to the use of any antimicrobial. Dosing information is summarized for agents likely to be used in ICU patients with sepsis in Table 18.2. The β-lactam agents (penicillins, cephalosporins, monobactam, and carbapenem) should be administered with a loading dose in septic shock followed by intermittent, prolonged infusions for maintenance, based on moderate evidence in the SSC [1].

Aminoglycosides: Aminoglycosides are a standard second agent for serious infections where more resistant GNR are likely (including *P. aeruginosa*), specifically when antibiotics have been used in prior 90 days, neutropenia, or other conditions associated with GNR colonization. Inadequate dosing in septic shock may reduce effectiveness, as volume resuscitation will have a dilutional effect. Amikacin 30 mg/kg or gentamicin/tobramycin 8–10 mg/kg loading doses reduce the frequency of suboptimal concentrations but also increases the risk of overexposure and adverse outcomes [67,68]. Intermittent dosing (extended interval also called once-daily) with an interval long enough to achieve near complete elimination is advised with therapeutic drug monitoring and PK individualization. Inhalation therapy is an option for selected patients.

De-escalation should be prompt if a resistant GNR is not detected. Renal tubular necrosis, cochlear injury, and vertigo are potential adverse effects that may be dose (elevated trough, or duration [>3 days]) related but may also be related to genetic susceptibility or concurrent therapy.

The dose in obese patients (BMI >30 mg/kg/m^2) should be based on an adjusted body weight equal to ideal BW + 0.4 × (actual BW − ideal BW).

Carbapenems: These agents have broad spectrum of activity and are drug of choice for extended-spectrum β-lactamase (ESBL) GNR organisms but also have antianaerobic activity. Higher doses may be required for *Pseudomonas* sp. treatment. Increasing resistance from carbapenemase production (serine-based; *Klebsiella pneumoniae* carbapenemase, New Delhi metallo-β-lactamase, Verona integron-encoded, oxallinase-type, etc.) is reported. Addition of β-lactamase inhibitors (relebactam or vaborbactam) increases coverage of hospital-acquired GNR including ESBL and serine-based carbapenemases and *P. aeruginosa*.

High concentrations of all carbapenems can cause seizures, although risk appears higher with imipenem agents. Carbapenems have cross-allergenicity potential with other β-lactams, but despite patient-declared allergy, few have clinically significant reactions [69]. Ertapenem does not have activity against *P. aeruginosa*. Doripenem is not approved for pneumonia treatment.

Cephalosporins: These β-lactam agents are grouped by spectrum of activity. Third and fourth generation agents with *P. aeruginosa* coverage are ceftazidime, cefoperazone-sulbactam, and cefepime and are used empirically for their broad spectrum of coverage against gram-negative organisms and many gram-positive species (methicillin susceptible *S. aureus* (MSSa), *Streptococcus,* but not anaerobic organisms or enterococcus). Cefiderocol and ceftazidime-avibactam have activity against metallo-carbapenemase producing GNR and other DTR GNR.

Coverage of *MSSa* bacteremia (not meningitis) with older cephalosporins such as cefazolin has been shown noninferior and to cause less nephrotoxicity than nafcillin or oxacillin [70,71]. Combination therapy with vancomycin or daptomycin may increase bacteremia clearance rate but did not reduce a composite endpoint of mortality, bacteremia, relapse, or treatment failure in a prospective trial, although it was stopped early for increased nephrotoxicity [72]. Ceftaroline is approved for *MRSa* skin infections but not for pneumonia. Ceftobiprole has activity against *MRSa* but is not approved for use in all large countries.

Seizures are possible with high concentrations, and cefepime-induced neurologic effects are widely reported and electroencephalographic monitoring may be needed to detect occult injury [73]. Cross-allergenicity with other β-lactam agents is possible, most often with similar R-1 side chain structures but is infrequent with carbapenem or monobactam agents [74]. Widespread use of cephalosporins has been associated with an increased risk of *C. difficile* infections compared with more heterogenous use from different classes [75].

Higher doses are suggested in obesity for older agents in this class (cefazolin, cefepime) but may be true of newer agents with more experience.

Fluoroquinolones: These agents are highly utilized in many settings due to perceived ease of use and broad coverage. Use for double gram-negative coverage produced comparable outcomes to a β-lactam and aminoglycoside combination in nosocomial bacteremia or pneumonia in a retrospective review [76]. Nosocomial infections may require a higher dose, but adverse effects are potentially limiting, especially with renal insufficiency.

Fluoroquinolone overuse has contributed to resistance (both chromosomal and plasmid-mediated) and serious side effects, including tendon and muscle injury potentially leading to rupture and aneurysm development. Drug interactions have the potential to cause additive electrocardiographic changes (QTc prolongation and torsades de pointes).

Dosing guidance in obesity is still evolving, but higher doses may be needed to achieve adequate drug exposure.

Glycopeptides and glycolipopeptides: This is a group of antimicrobial agents with activity against gram-positive organisms, including *MRSa* and enterococcus, with variable effectiveness against more resistant strains.

Vancomycin is the commonly used agent due to familiarity and effectiveness, starting with a loading dose infused at 10–15 mg/min. Maintenance doses are given intermittently or as continuous infusion and adjusted for renal function. Resistance is increasingly common, indicated by a MIC ≥ 4 mCg/mL, but clinically it may be difficult to treat an organism effectively and safely if the MIC ≥ 2 mCg/mL. Dosing with an AUC_{24} strategy (goal concentration 400–600 mCg/mL $\times$ h) is recommended for severe but susceptible *S. aureus* infections, regardless of MIC [29].

Adverse effects are related to the rate of infusion, with an anaphylactoid reaction to early dose given rapidly. Vascular irritation is also likely with repeated doses at a peripheral site of infusion.

Vancomycin doses in obesity are calculated for actual body weight but with lower mg/kg targets

(loading 20–25 and maintenance 15–20 mg/kg) with a maximum of 3000 mg per dose and 4500 mg total per day.

Oral vancomycin doses are not absorbed, so are not appropriate for a systemic infection but is an alternative to fidaxomicin for *C. difficile* enteritis [77].

Daptomycin: This agent is an alternative to vancomycin for gram-positive infections and vancomycin-resistant enterococcal infection. It is not used for pulmonary infections due to a unique issue of surfactant inactivation. Resistance has been reported, but typically the MIC to other antimicrobial options improves when this occurs and has been called a seesaw effect [78]. High doses may lead to myopathy, so a weekly creatine phosphokinase level is suggested as a monitoring tool along with the elimination of concurrent statin therapy. Daptomycin may cause a laboratory interference and factitious prolongation of the prothrombin time.

Patients with morbid obesity may benefit from a dose based on actual body weight, but some have suggested that an adjusted weight, as is used for aminoglycosides, may be acceptable [79].

Televancin: This lipoglycopeptide is noninferior to vancomycin for *MRSa* pneumonia and effective for complicated staphylococcal skin/structure infections and *MSSa* pneumonia. It has concentration-dependent bactericidal activity. It is a potential teratogen for women of childbearing potential. Weight-based dosing is used, but a fixed dose of 750 mg every 24 h is proposed for obese patients for fewer toxic adverse effects [80].

Monobactam: Aztreonam is a monobactam considered for patients with a β-lactam allergy, but the structure is similar to ceftazidime, and cefiderocol adds potential for cross-allergenicity. It is active against gram-negative organisms (spectrum similar to ceftazidime) but not gram-positive or anaerobes. An inhaled version is available for selected cystic fibrosis patients.

Oxazolidinones: Linezolid and tedizolid have similar activity against gram-positive cocci such as *S. aureus*, *E. faecium*, and *S. pneumoniae*. Linezolid has emerged as a more effective agent for *MRSa* pneumonia than vancomycin (based on traditional dosing/monitoring) in metaanalyses comparing clinical or microbiological cure but not mortality, but the most recent IDSA guidelines for severe CAP suggest that either agent may be used when there is a high suspicion for *MRSa*, such as prior presence on cultures and/or recent hospitalization with antimicrobial exposure [81,82]. Linezolid may be a preferred alternative to vancomycin when also using piperacillin-tazobactam if nephrotoxicity risk is high.

Linezolid inhibits toxin production in toxic-shock syndromes with *S. aureus* or *Streptococcus pyogenes*. Both may inhibit monoamine oxidase and may lead to serotonin syndrome symptoms, especially when used with an agent that increases serotonin levels. Prolonged use is associated with thrombocytopenia, anemia, or leukopenia due to myelosuppression.

In obese patients, a standard linezolid dose may be inadequate, based on emerging data from case reports.

Penicillins: Broad-spectrum coverage in sepsis usually dictates the use of an agent such as piperacillin-tazobactam, but other agents may be used for de-escalation to more focused therapies, as dictated by susceptibility testing. While piperacillin-tazobactam is often a workhorse agent, it should not be used for empiric coverage of organisms producing ESBL (ceftriaxone-resistant) due to higher mortality [83]. Combination therapy with piperacillin-tazobactam and vancomycin has been associated with higher rates of creatinine elevation in retrospective studies compared with vancomycin alone or vancomycin plus other gram-negative agents, leading to avoidance of this combination [84]. Unfortunately, these retrospective data are associated with significant heterogeneity of population, definition of renal failure, and outcomes. Thus, prospective studies need to establish the clinical significance of this controversy [85].

As discussed with cephalosporins, the oxacillin and nafcillin are effective alone for *MSSa* and may increase vancomycin effectiveness against *MRsa* [72]. Nafcillin does not need dose adjustment for renal failure, and both may cause neutropenia with more than three weeks of therapy. Oxacillin may cause dose-related hepatic dysfunction. Cross-allergenicity with other β-lactams is most dependent on the R-1 side chain [74].

Higher doses may be needed in obese patients with piperacillin-tazobactam 6.75 gm over 4 h and dosed every 8 h suggested to achieve concentration targets if normal renal function.

Polymyxins: These agents are used for the treatment of MDR-GNR, especially *Acinetobacter baumanii*, *P. aeruginosa*, etc. Polymyxin E (Colistimethate or colistin) has been the most studied of this class but is a prodrug and onset of effect is delayed, so a loading dose is needed. It is the preferred choice from this class for resistant GNR urinary infection treatment. There are dosing guidelines proposed for colistin based on the mg of CBA and Clcr, but these have not been tested prospectively, vary by region, and continue to evolve (Table 18.3) [36,37]. Many authors prefer the PK regimen using the ColistinDose calculator [86]. A

TABLE 18.3

Polymyxin E (Colistin) Colistin-Base Activity (CBA) Maximum Daily Dosing. Loading Dose 4 × Weight in kg (Use Lower of Ideal or Actual Weight). Maintenance Dose Started 12 h After Loading Dose (As Either 2–3 Doses Per Day) up to 360 mg Per Day [36,37]

Clcr (mL/min)	PK study group Doses 2/day[a]	EMA Doses 2–3/day[a]	US FDA[a] (Use ideal body weight)
≥90	360 mg	300 mg	2.5–5 mg/kg/day doses 2–4/day
80–89	340 mg	300 mg	2.5–5 mg/kg/day doses 2–4/day
70–79	300 mg	300 mg	2.5–3.8 mg/kg/day doses 2/day
60–69	275 mg	300 mg	2.5–3.8 mg/kg/day doses 2/day
50–59	245 mg	300 mg	2.5–3.8 mg/kg/day doses 2/day
40–49	220 mg	183–250 mg	2.5 mg/kg/day doses 1–2/day
30–39	195 mg	183–250 mg	2.5 mg/kg/day doses 1–2/day
20–29	175 mg	150–183 mg	1.5 mg/kg every 36 h
10–19	160 mg	150–183 mg	1.5 mg/kg every 36 h
5–9	145 mg	117 mg	Not recommended
<5	130 mg	117 mg	Not recommended
CRRT		400 mg (doses 2/day)[b]	

Clcr, Creatinine clearance; *EMA*, European Medicines Agency; *PK*, Pharmacokinetic; *US FDA*, United States Food and Drug Agency.
[a] All doses as colistin-base activity (CBA). CBA 300 mg = colistimethate sodium (CMS) 9,000,000 units and adjusted for renal function calculated using the Cockcroft-Gault equation with an adjusted body weight (ideal body weight [IBW] + 0.4 [total body weight − IBW])
[b] CRRT = Continuous renal replacement therapy − dosing for dialysate or ultrafiltration rate of 1–2 L/h.
Adapted with permission from Lexi-Drugs/Colistimethate. UpToDate Inc. Accessed July 4, 2022.

mobile application is available to clinicians. A maintenance regimen is initiated within 12 h of the loading dose [37]. Systemic therapy may be insufficient for severe pneumonia therapy, and concurrent inhalation is suggested using 50—75 mg CBA in 3—4 mL saline and administered via a vibrating mesh nebulizer with 2—3 doses/day to achieve effective lung tissue levels [37,38].

Colistin systemic therapy is associated with AKI in retrospective cohort studies although not in and prospective cohorts or randomized studies requiring consideration of risk versus benefit. AKI is not only related to concurrent nephrotoxins and comorbidities but also to dose and duration of therapy [37,87]. A variety of antioxidants have been studied to reduce AKI risk, with variable results, including ascorbic acid 2 g every 12 h. Neurotoxicity may present as vertigo, paresthesia, visual changes, and confusion.

Polymyxin B has different pharmacology and dosing, although a similar spectrum of activity. It is not renally eliminated and will not treat a urinary infection. It is not a prodrug, so has a faster onset. Adverse effects are similar to colistin, and infusion-related effects are reported, including thoracic pain, paresthesia, and hypoxemia.

Colistimethate (CBA) doses in obese patients may be calculated as 4 × body weight in kilogram, with the lower of actual versus ideal weight. Polymyxin B is dosed on actual weight but may evolve with addition utilization and research [36].

Tetracyclines

Eravacycline is a synthetic fluocycline tetracycline for complex intraabdominal infections. MICs are often lower than with tigecycline. Dosing adjustment is not required in renal insufficiency or obesity (use actual weight). Higher doses are needed with concurrent use of strong Cytochrome P450 (CYP3A4) inducer such as carbamazepine, phenytoin, or rifampin. Like others in this class should, it is not used after the first trimester of pregnancy to avoid tooth discoloration. Nausea/vomiting may not be as frequent as tigecycline.

Tigecycline: This is a derivative of minocycline, has greater ability to overcome resistance improving effectiveness over some strains of *A. baumannii* and carbapenemase-producing gram-negative organisms, also for intraabdominal infections, skin infections, and CAP. It is not active against Pseudomonal isolates. It is an alternative to more traditional agents such as β-lactams due to higher potential mortality and adverse events. Nausea and vomiting are frequent and may be dose-related. Maltose is present in some formulations and may cause factitious blood glucose measurements.

ANTIFUNGAL AGENTS

Patients with septic shock may present with multiple potential pathogens, including fungus. While bacteria are more common, risk factors for invasive *Candida* sepsis include prior colonization, invasive central lines, neutropenia, immunosuppression, GI surgery or perforation, parenteral nutrition, burn injury, or prior broad-spectrum antibiotics. Elevation of a biomarker such as serum beta-D-glucan may be helpful to select patients at risk. Similar risk factors for endemic yeast and mold include neutropenia, transplantation, high-dose corticosteroids/immunosuppressive agents, viral infections (human immunodeficiency virus and SARS-CoV-2), and elevated biomarkers such as histoplasma, blastomyces, or cryptococcal antigens or galactomannan [1].

An invasive fungal infection has a higher mortality rate than bacterial sepsis, likely related to delays in therapy. Mediators of the sepsis syndrome include gliotoxin, a fungal metabolite that is damaging to the gut tissue and other toxins and trigger release of mediators such as interleukin-17 [88]. The SSC suggests the use of empiric antifungal treatment for patients with sepsis or septic shock who are at a high risk of fungal infection [1].

While most fungal infections are nosocomial, early recognition is difficult and a high sense of suspicion is needed when patients fail to respond to antibacterial therapies. Early empiric use of antifungal therapy has not changed fungal infection-free survival in nonneutropenic, nontransplant critically ill patients with ICU-acquired sepsis [89]. Diagnosis is difficult with disseminated *Candida* infections as blood cultures are positive in less than half of patients. Newer diagnostic testing methods that detect biomarkers of fungal infection, cellular components, or antibody response should improve the ability to identify fungal infection if used in the proper population and at the right time [90]. Guidelines for application of these methods focus on clinical scenarios and risk patterns [91].

Susceptibility testing of fungal pathogens has become important with increased azole resistance and highly resistant strains such as *Candida auris*. An echinocandin such as micafungin, caspofungin, or anidulafungin are generally used empirically to treat *Candida* spp. for patients with unstable hemodynamics, especially when patients have previously received an azole such as fluconazole. Highly immunosuppressed patients are at greater risk of mold infections, and starting an amphotericin product should be considered [92]. Newer azole agents, such as voriconazole and isavuconazole are alternatives for candidiasis and invasive aspergillosis, although adverse effects and drug interactions may be significant. Stewardship principles that include de-escalation of empiric antifungal agents should be followed, and azole agents can be used when susceptible with a treatment duration of 14 days after the first negative blood culture in the absence of metastatic fungal disease [92]. Inadequate source control (e.g., failure to remove an infected IV catheter) may lead to longer courses, based on individual risks and response.

Pharmacokinetic alterations related to organ dysfunction, reduced protein binding, altered Vd, and supportive technologies such as continuous renal replacement therapy (CRRT), extracorporeal membrane oxygenation (ECMO), and drug interactions make dosing more complex and ICU patients are at risk for inadequate treatment [93]. See Table 18.2 for details on dosing.

Amphotericin: These agents are effective versus a broad group of yeasts and molds. The product selected within this class will determine the dosing and administration requirements. Standard amphotericin is a colloidal suspension that must be prepared in a dextrose solution and may cause infusion-related adverse effects due to the release of cytokines and chemokines. While rapid infusions may be used, infusion over 4–24 h may improve tolerance, along with pretreatment with acetaminophen and antihistamine.

Amphotericin metabolic fate is not well characterized but have a long half-life >15 days with 33% urine excretion and 45% fecal excretion as unchanged drug [94]. The lipid complex has a larger distribution volume and lower serum levels, but higher lung levels than the other products. Clinically, although comparative data are limited, an efficacy difference is not apparent.

The lipid vehicle products (lipid complex and liposomal) may be more well tolerated. A fixed dose of liposomal amphotericin B has been suggested in patients weighing ≥100 kg.

Azole antifungals: The azole group of antifungals are well tolerated and available for both IV and enteral administration, although conversion may not be straightforward when dosing is considered with different formulations. Prophylactic use increases the risk of resistance and diminishes their therapeutic potential. All have drug interaction potential through the inhibition of CYP enzymes, although CYP enzyme inducers such as carbamazepine, phenobarbital, phenytoin, rifampin, and rifabutin should not be combined with voriconazole or isavuconazole due to low antifungal levels. Others in this class may be affected and require monitoring. Most of the interactions impact the other agent.

Azole dosing in obese patients may be improved with the use of higher doses (fluconazole, posaconazole) and monitor serum concentrations (voriconazole) to individualize dosing [95].

Echinocandins: These antifungals are remarkably well tolerated and treat a variety of *Candida* sp. and *Aspergillus* sp. Micafungin was studied as an empiric agent for patients with ICU-acquired sepsis who were suspected of having a fungal infection based on presence of risk factors (not including neutropenia or transplant), prior antibacterial therapy, and with new organ dysfunction [89]. There was no difference in fungal infection-free survival, although there was a reduction in occurrence of new fungal infection.

Dosing should be increased for all three agents to improve effectiveness in obese patients.

Summary: This overview of important considerations of various antimicrobial agents used in sepsis patients is a starting point for clinicians to appreciate key characteristics of individual agents and classes. Additional resources should be utilized to individual dosing based on organ dysfunction, use of supportive therapies such as CRRT or ECMO, and local knowledge of susceptibility patterns and concurrent drug therapy.

REFERENCES

[1] Evans L, Rhodes A, Alhazzani W, et al. Surviving Sepsis Campaign: international guidelines for the management of sepsis and septic shock 2021. Crit Care Med 2021; 49(11):e1063–143.

[2] Asner SA, Desgranges F, Schrijver IT, et al. Impact of the timeliness of antibiotic therapy on the outcome of patients with sepsis and septic shock. J Infect 2021;82: 125–34.

[3] Magill SS, O'Leary E, Ray SM, et al. Assessment of the appropriateness of antimicrobial use in US hospitals. JAMA Netw Open 2021;4(3):e212007. https://doi.org/10.1001/jamanetworkopen.2021.2007.

[4] Shappell CN, Klompas M, Ochoa A, et al. Likelihood of bacterial infection in patients treated with broad-spectrum IV antibiotics in the emergency department. Crit Care Med 2021;49(11):1144–e1150.

[5] Centers for Disease Control and Prevention. National center for emerging and zoonotic infectious diseases (NCEZID). In: Division of healthcare quality promotion (DHQP); April 28, 2021. www.cdc.gov/antibiotic-use/core-elements/hospital.html#anchor_1573591750074. [Accessed 10 September 2021].

[6] Bassetti M, Rello J, Blasi F, et al. Systematic review of the impact of appropriate versus inappropriate initial antibiotic therapy on outcomes of patients with severe bacterial infections. Int J Antimicrob Agents 2020;56(6):106184.

[7] Tamma PD, Aitken SL, Bonomo RA, et al. Infectious diseases society of America guidance on the treatment of extended-spectrum β-lactamase producing enterobacterales (CRE), carbapenem-resistant enterobacterales (CRE), and *Pseudomonas aeruginosa* with difficult-to-treat resistance. Clin Infect Dis 2021;72(7):1109–16.

[8] Delattre IK, Hites M, Laterre PF, et al. What is the optimal loading dose of broad-spectrum β-lactam antibiotics in septic patients? Results from a pharmacokinetic simulation modelling. Int J Antimicrob Agents 2020;56(4):106113.

[9] Gregorowicz AJ, Costello PG, Gajdosik DA, et al. Effect of IV push antibiotic administration on antibiotic delays in sepsis. Crit Care Med 2020;48(8):1175–9.

[10] Rech MA, Gottlieb M. Intravenous push antibiotics should be administered in the emergency department. Ann Emerg Med 2021;78(3):384–5.

[11] Spencer S, Ipema H, Hartke P, et al. Intravenous push administration of antibiotics: literature and considerations. Hosp Pharm 2018;53(3):157–69.

[12] Kufel WD, Seabury RW, Meola GM, et al. Impact of premix antimicrobial preparation and time to administration in septic patients. CJEM 2018;20(4):565–71.

[13] Ulldemolins M, Roberts JA, Rello J, et al. The effects of hypoalbuminaemia on optimizing antibacterial dosing in critically ill patients. Clin Pharmacokinet 2011;50:99–110.

[14] Veiga RP, Paiva JA. Pharmacokinetics-pharmacodynamics issues relevant for the clinical use of beta-lactam antibiotics in critically ill patients. Crit Care 2018;22:233.

[15] Bragadottir G, Redfors B, Ricksten S-E. Assessing glomerular filtration rate (GFR) in critically ill patients with acute kidney injury—true GFR versus urinary creatinine clearance (Clcr) and estimating equations. Crit Care 2013;17:R108.

[16] Inker LA, Eneanya ND, Coresh J, et al. New creatinine- and cystatin c-based equations to estimate GFR without race. N Engl J Med 2021. https://doi.org/10.1056/NEJMoa2102953.

[17] Murty MSN, Sharma UK, Kankare SB. Serum cystatin C as a marker of renal function in detection of early acute kidney injury. Indian J Nephrol 2013 ;23(3):180–3.

[18] Teaford HR, Stevens RW, Rule AD, et al. Prediction of vancomycin levels using cystatin c in overweight and obese patients: a retrospective cohort study of hospitalized patients. Antimicrob Agents Chemother 2021;65(1):e01487–20.

[19] Frazee E, Rule AD, Lieske JC, et al. Cystatin C-guided vancomycin dosing in critically ill patients: a quality improvement project. Am J Kidney Dis 2017;69:658–66.

[20] Cherry RA, Eachempati SR, Hydo L, Barie PS. Accuracy of short-duration creatinine clearance determinations in predicting 24-hour creatinine clearance in critically ill and injured patients. J Trauma 2002;53:267–71.

[21] Baptista JP, Martins PJ, Marques M, Pimentel JM. Prevalence and risk factors for augmented renal clearance in a population of critically ill patients. J Intensive Care Med 2020;35(10):1044–52.

[22] Crass RL, Rodvold KA, Mueller BA, Pai MP. Renal dosing of antibiotics: are we jumping the gun? Clin Infect Dis 2019;68(9):1596–602.

[23] González de Molina FJ, Ferrer R. Appropriate antibiotic dosing in severe sepsis and acute renal failure factors to consider. Crit Care 2011;15(4):175.

[24] Póvoa P, Moniz P, Pereira AG, Coelho L. Optimizing antimicrobial dosing in critically ill patients. Microorganisms 2021;9(7):1401. https://doi.org/10.3390/microorganisms9071401.

[25] Roberts JA, Paul SK, Akova M, et al. DALI: defining antibiotic levels in intensive care unit patients: are current beta-lactam antibiotic doses sufficient for critically ill patients? Clin Infect Dis 2014;8:1072–83.

[26] Fratoni AJ, Nicolau DP, Kuti JL. A guide to therapeutic drug monitoring of β-lactam antibiotics. Pharmacotherapy 2021;41(2):220–33.

[27] Grupper M, Kuti JL, Nicolau DP. Continuous and prolonged intravenous beta-lactam dosing: implications for the clinical laboratory. Clin Microbiol Rev 2016;4:759–72.

[28] Zelenitsky SA, Ariano RE. Support for higher ciprofloxacin AUC 24/MIC targets in treating Enterobacteriaceae bloodstream infection. J Antimicrob Chemother 2010;65:1725–32.

[29] Rybak M, Le J, Lodise TP, et al. Therapeutic drug monitoring of vancomycin for serious methicillin-resistant *Staphylococcus aureus* infections: a revised consensus guideline and review by the American society of health-system pharmacists, the infectious diseases society of America, the pediatric infectious diseases society, and the society of infectious diseases pharmacists. Am J Health Syst Pharm 2020;77(11):835–64.

[30] Pai MP, Neely M, Rodvold KA, Lodise TP. Innovative approaches to optimizing the delivery of vancomycin in individual patients. Adv Drug Deliv Rev 2014;77:50–7.

[31] Black D. Vancomycin AUC24 Explained | Guide to Vancomycin AUC24. www.sanfordguide.com, Sanford Guide, Accessed November 15, 2021.

[32] Turner RB, Kojiro K, Shephard EA, et al. Review and validation of Bayesian dose-optimizing software and equations for calculation of the vancomycin area under the curve in critically ill patients. Pharmacotherapy 2019;38(12):1174–8.

[33] Fage D, Deprez G, Wolff F, et al. Investigation of unbound colistin A and B in clinical samples using a mass spectrometry method. Int J Antimicrob Agents 2019;53:330–6.

[34] Heffernan AJ, Sime FB, Lipman J, Roberts JA. Individualizing therapy to minimize bacterial multidrug resistance. Drugs 2018;78:621–41.

[35] Tsala M, Vourli S, Georgiou PC, et al. Exploring colistin pharmacodynamics against *Klebsiella pneumoniae*: a need to revise current susceptibility breakpoints. J Antimicrob Chemother 2018;73:953–61.

[36] Tsuji BT, Pogue JM, Zavascki AP, et al. International consensus guidelines for the optimal use of the polymixins: endorsed by the American college of clinical pharmacy (ACCP), European society of clinical microbiology and infectious diseases (ESCMID), infectious diseases society of America (IDSA), international society for anti-infective pharmacology (ISAP), society of critical care medicine (SCCM), and society of infectious diseases pharmacists (SIDP). Pharmacotherapy 2019; 39(1):10–39.

[37] Nation RL, Garonzik SM, Thamlikitkul V, Giamarellos-Bourboulis EJ, Forrest A, Paterson DL, et al. Dosing guidance for intravenous colistin in critically-ill patients. Clin Infect Dis 2017;64(5):565–71.

[38] Lin YW, Aye SM, Rao G, et al. Treatment of infections caused by gram-negative pathogens: current status on the pharmacokinetics/pharmacodynamics of parenteral and inhaled polymyxins in patients. Int J Antimicrob Agents 2020;56:106199.

[39] Ahiskali A, Gens K. The great debate: polymyxin B versus polymyxin E. ContagionLive 2017;2(1). www.contagionlive.com/view/the-great-debate-polymyxin-b-versus-polymyxin-e. [Accessed 20 August 2021].

[40] Cheng MP, Stenstrom R, Paquette K, et al. Blood culture results before and after antimicrobial administration in patient surviving with severe manifestations of sepsis. Ann Intern Med 2019;171:547–54.

[41] Tsalik EL, Henao R, Montgomery JL, et al. Discriminating bacterial and viral infection using a rapid host gene expression test. Crit Care Med 2021. https://doi.org/10.1097/CCM.0000000000005085.

[42] Schenz J, Weigand MA, Uhle F. Molecular and biomarker-based diagnostics in early sepsis: current challenges and future perspectives. Expert Rev Mol Diagn 2019;19(12): 1069–78.

[43] Klinker KP, Hidayat LK, DeRyke CA, et al. Antimicrobial stewardship and antibiograms: importance of moving beyond traditional antibiograms. Therap Adv Infect Dis 2021;8:1–9.

[44] Van der Werf TS. Artificial intelligence to guide empirical antimicrobial therapy-ready for prime time? Clin Infect Dis 2021;72:e856–8.

[45] Paul M, Lador A, Grozinsky-Glasberg S, et al. Beta lactam antibiotic monotherapy versus beta lactam-aminoglycoside antibiotic combination therapy for sepsis. Cochrane Database Syst Rev 2014;1:CD003344.

[46] Septimus EJ, Coopersmith CM, Whittle J, et al. Sepsis national hospital inpatient quality measure (SEP-1): multi-stakeholder work group recommendations for appropriate antibiotics for the treatment of sepsis. Clin Infect Dis 2017;65(9):1565–9.

[47] Kadri SS, Lai YL, Warner S, et al. Inappropriate empirical antibiotic therapy for bloodstream infections based on discordant in-vitro susceptibilities: a retrospective cohort analysis of prevalence, predictors, and mortality risk in US hospitals. Lancet Infect Dis 2021;21:241–5.

[48] Wunderink RG. POINT: should inhaled antibiotic therapy be used routinely for the treatment of bacterial lower respiratory tract infections in the ICU setting? Yes Chest 2017;151(4):737–9.

[49] Tabah A, Bassetti M, Kollef MH, et al. Antimicrobial de-escalation in critically ill patients: a position statement from a task force of the European society of intensive care medicine (ESICM) and European society of clinical microbiology and infectious diseases (ESCMID) critically ill patient study group. Intensive Care Med 2020;46: 245–65.

[50] De Waele JJ, Schouten J, Beovic B, et al. Antimicrobial de-escalation as part of antimicrobial stewardship in intensive care: no simple answers to simple questions—a viewpoint of experts. Intensive Care Med 2020;46:236–44.

[51] Busch LM, Kadri SS. Antimicrobial treatment duration in sepsis and serious infections. J Infect Dis 2020;222(S2): S142–5.

[52] Daneman N, Rishu AH, Pinto R, et al. Canadian critical care trials group. 7 versus 14 days of antibiotic treatment for critically ill patients with bloodstream infection: a pilot randomized clinical trial. Trials 2018;19:111.

[53] Daneman N, Rishu AH, Pinto RL. On behalf of the Canadian clinical trials group et al. Bacteremia antibiotic length actually needed for clinical effectiveness (BALANCE) randomized clinical trial: study protocol. BMJ Open 2020;10(5):e038300.

[54] Molina J, Montero-Mateos E, Praena-Segovia J, et al. Seven-versus 14-day course of antibiotics for the treatment of bloodstream infections by Enterobacterales: a randomized, controlled trial. Clin Microbiol Infect 2022;28(4):550–7. https://doi.org/10.1016/j.cmi.2021.09.001.

[55] Mo Y, West TE, MacLaren G, et al. Reducing antibiotic treatment duration for ventilator-associated pneumonia (REGARD-VAP): a trial protocol for an randomised clinical trial. BMJ Open 2021;11:e050105.

[56] Kadri SS, Adjemian J, Lai YL, et al. Difficult- to- treat resistance in gram-negative bacteremia at 173 US hospitals: retrospective cohort analysis of prevalence, predictors, and outcome of resistance to all first-line agents. Clin Infect Dis 2018;67(12):1803–14.

[57] Liu C, Bayer A, Cosgrove SE, , et alInfectious Diseases Society of America. Clinical practice guidelines by the

infectious diseases society of America for the treatment of methicillin-resistant *Staphylococcus aureus* infections in adults and children. Clin Infect Dis 2011;52:e18–55.

[58] Restrrepo MI, Keyt H, Reyes LF. Aerosolized antibiotics. Respir Care 2015;60(6):762–73.

[59] Stokker J, Karami M, Hoek R, et al. Effect of adjunctive tobramycin inhalation versus placebo on early clinical response int the treatment of ventilator-associated pneumonia: the VAPORISE randomized-controlled trial. Intensive Care Med 2020;46:546–8.

[60] Daniels LM, Juliano J, Marx A, Weber DJ. Inhaled antibiotics for hospital-acquired and ventilator-associated pneumonia. Clin Infect Dis 2017;64(3):386–7.

[61] Kollef MH. Should inhaled antibiotic therapy be used routinely for the treatment of bacterial lower respiratory tract infections in the ICU setting? No Chest 2017; 151(4):740–3.

[62] Xu F, Che LQ, Li W, et al. Aerosolized antibiotics for ventilator-associated pneumonia: a pairwise and Bayesian network meta-analysis. Crit Care 2018;22:301.

[63] Qin JP, Huang HB, Zhou H, et al. Amikacin nebulization for the adjunctive therapy of gram-negative pneumonia in mechanically ventilated patients: a systematic review and meta-analysis of randomized controlled trials. Sci Rep 2021;11:6969.

[64] Kalil AC, Metersky ML, Klompas M, et al. Hospital-acquired and ventilator-associated pneumonia: 2016 clinical practice guidelines by the infectious diseases society of America and the American thoracic society. Clin Infect Dis 2016;63(5):e61–111.

[65] Abdellatif SA, Trifi A, Daly F, et al. Efficacy and toxicity of aerosolized colistin in ventilator-associated pneumonia: a prospective, randomized trial. Ann Intensive Care 2016;6:26.

[66] Choe J, Sohn YM, Jeong SH, et al. Inhalation with intravenous loading dose of colistin in critically ill patients with pneumonia caused by carbapenem-resistant gram-negative bacteria. Ther Adv Respir Dis 2019;13:1–12.

[67] Allou N, Bouteau A, Allyn J, et al. Impact of a high loading dose of amikacin in patients with severe sepsis or septic shock. Ann Intenaive Care 2016;6:106.

[68] Roger C, Nucci B, Louart B, et al. Impact of 30 mg/kg amikacin and 8 mg/kg gentamicin on serum concentrations in critically ill patients with severe sepsis. J Antimicrob Chemother 2016;71(1):208–12.

[69] Shenoy ES, Macy E, Rowe T, Blumenthal KG. Evaluation and management of penicillin allergy: a review. JAMA 2019;321(2):188–9.

[70] Monogue ML, Ortwine JK, Wei W, et al. Nafcillin versus cefazolin for the treatment of methicillin-susceptible *Staphylococcus aureus* bacteremia. J Infect Public Health 2018;11(5):727–31.

[71] Li J, et al. Beta-lactam therapy for methicillin-susceptible *Staphylococcus aureus* bacteremia: a comparative review of cefazolin versus anti staphylococcal penicillins. Pharmacotherapy 2017;37(3):346–60.

[72] Tong SYC, Lye DC, Yahav D, et al. Effect of vancomycin or daptomycin with or without an antistaphylococcal β-lactam on mortality, bacteremia, relapse, or treatment failure in patients with MRSa bacteremia. JAMA 2020; 323(6):527–37.

[73] Payne LE, Gagnon DJ, Riker RR, et al. Cefepime-induced neurotoxicity: a systematic review. Crit Care 2017;21:276.

[74] Chaudhry SB, Veve MP, Wagner JL. Cephalosporins: a focus on side chains and β-lactam cross reactivity. Pharmacy 2019;7:103.

[75] Wilcox MH, Chalmers JD, Nord CE, et al. Role of cephalosporins in the rea of *Clostridium difficile* infection. J Antimicrob Chemother 2017;72(1):1–18.

[76] Ereshefsky BJ, Al-Hasan MN, Gokun Y, Martin CA. Comparison of β-lactam plus aminoglycoside versus β-lactam plus fluoroquinolone empirical therapy in serious nosocomial infections due to gram-negative bacilli. J Chemother 2017;29(1):30–7.

[77] Johnson S, Lavergne V, Skinner AM, et al. Clinical practice guideline by the infectious diseases society of America (IDSA) and society for healthcare epidemiology of America (SHEA): 2021 focused update guidelines on management of clostridioides difficile infection in adults. Clin Infect Dis 2021;73(5):e1029–44.

[78] Molina KC, Morrisette T, Miller MA, et al. The emerging role of β-lactams in the treatment of methicillin-resistant *Staphylococcus aureus* bloodstream infections. Antimicrob Agents Chemother 2020;64(7):e00468–20.

[79] Fox AN, Smith WJ, Kupiec KE, et al. Daptomycin dosing in obese patients: analysis of the use of adjusted body weight versus actual body weight. Ther Adv Infect Dis 2019;6. 2049936118820230.

[80] Bunnell KL, Pai MP, Sikka M, et al. Pharmacokinetics of telavancin at fixed doses in normal-body-weight and obese (classes I, II, and III) adult subjects. Antimicrob Agents Chemother 2018;62(40):e02475–17.

[81] Kato H, Hagihara M, Asai N, et al. Meta-analysis of vancomycin versus linezolid in pneumonia with proven methicillin-resistant *Staphylococcu aureus*. J Global Antimicrob Resist 2021;24:98–105.

[82] Metlay JP, Waterer GW, Long AC, et al. Diagnosis and treatment of adults with community-acquired pneumonia. An official clinical practice guideline of the American thoracic society and infectious diseases society of America. Am J Respir Crit Care Med 2019;200(7):e45–67.

[83] Harris PNA, Tambyah PA, Lye DC, et al. Effect of piperacillin-tazobactam vs meropenem on 30-day mortality for patients with *E. coli* or *Klebsiella pneumoniae* bloodstream infection and ceftriaxone resistance. A randomized clinical trial. JAMA 2018;320(10):984–94.

[84] Ciarambino T, Giannico OV, Campanile A, et al. Acute kidney injury and vancomycin/piperacillin/tazobactam in adult patients: a systematic review. Internal Emerg Med 2020;15:327–31.

[85] Avedissian SN, Pais GM, Liu J, et al. Piperacillin-tazobactam added to vancomycin increases risk for acute

kidney injury: fact or fiction. Clin Infect Dis 2020;71(2): 426–32.

[86] Hua X, Li C, Pogue JM, et al. ColistinDose, a mobile app for determining intravenous dosage regimens of colistimethate in critically ill adult patients: clinician-centered design and development study. JMIR Mhealth Uhealth 2020;8(12):e20525.

[87] Chien HT, Lin YC, Sheu CC, et al. Is colistin-associated acute kidney injury clinically important in adults? A systematic review and meta-analysis. Int J Antimicrob Agents 2020;55:105889.

[88] Huang J, Meng S, Hong S, Lin X, Jin W, Dong C. IL-17C is required for lethal inflammation during systemic fungal infection. Cell Mol Immunol 2016;13:474–83.

[89] Timsit JF, Azoulay E, Schwebel C, et al. Empirical micafungin treatment and survival without invasive fungal infection in adults with ICU-acquired sepsis, *Candida* colonization, and multiple organ failure. The EMPIRICUS randomized clinical trial. JAMA 2016;316(15): 1555–64.

[90] Clancy CJ, Nguyen MH. Non-culture diagnostics for invasive candidiasis: promise and unintended consequences. J Fungi 2018;4(1):27.

[91] Hage CA, Carmona EM, Epelbaum O, et al. Microbiological laboratory testing in the diagnosis of fungal infections in pulmonary and critical care practice. An official American thoracic society clinical practice guideline. Am J Respir Crit Care Med 2019;200(5):535–50.

[92] Martin-Loeches I, Antonelli M, Cuenca-Estrella M, et al. ESICM/ESCMID task force on practical management of invasive candidiasis in critically ill patients. Intensive Care Med 2019;45:789–805.

[93] Sinnollareddy MG, Roberts JA, Lipman J, et al. Pharmacokinetic variability and exposures of fluconazole, anidulafungin, and caspofungin in intensive care unit patients: data from multinational defining antibiotic levels in Intensive care unit (DALI) patients study. Crit Care 2015;19:33.

[94] Hamill RJ. Amphotericin B formulations: a comparative review of efficacy and toxicity. Drugs 2013;73(9): 919–34.

[95] Klatt ME, Eschenauer GA. Review of pharmacologic considerations in the use of azole antifungals in lung transplant recipients. J Fungi 2021;7(2):76.

CHAPTER 19

Kidney Support in Sepsis

JAVIER MAYNAR • HELENA BARRASA • ALEX MARTIN • ELENA USÓN • FERNANDO FONSECA

INTRODUCTION

Sepsis-associated acute kidney injury (S-AKI) is a frequent complication of the critically ill patient and is associated with unacceptable morbidity and mortality [1]. For septic patients in the intensive care unit (ICU), several studies reported a 40%–50% incidence of acute kidney injury (AKI) with increased risk of death [2,3]. In S-AKI, 15%–20% of patients develop severe stages of renal insufficiency and need renal replacement therapy (RRT) [4]. Although sepsis is the most common contributing factor for developing AKI, AKI of any origin is associated with higher risk of developing sepsis [5].

Sepsis is a life-threatening clinical syndrome characterized by organ dysfunction caused by a patient's dysregulated response to infection. Once a vasopressor is needed to maintain mean arterial pressure (MAP) ≥65 mmHg and serum lactate increases to >2 mmol/L despite adequate volume resuscitation, we speak of septic shock [6].

Sepsis is the most common cause of AKI in critically ill patients. Despite this, the pathophysiologic mechanisms of S-AKI are not well understood and, therefore, therapy remains reactive and nonspecific [1]. The prevailing pathophysiologic mechanism attributes S-AKI to the decreased global renal blood flow associated with hypoperfusion and shock; however, it is becoming increasingly clear that ischemia injury is not the only mechanism involved. S-AKI may develop in the absence of renal hypoperfusion or clinical signs of hemodynamic instability and in the presence of normal or increased global renal blood flow [7,8]. Regardless of the organ involved, three mechanisms are consistent with sepsis organ injury: inflammation, microcirculatory dysfunction, and metabolic reprogramming [1].

Currently, the strategies to prevent AKI are three: treat its cause, correct hemodynamic alterations (even when the exact MAP and perfusion targets to prevent AKI in individual patients are not known [9]), and be careful with the use of nephrotoxic substances.

We must carry out an early recognition of AKI. Ideally, renal function should be measured and monitored in real time, so that AKI is diagnosed as soon as it occurs, allowing for adjustments of clinical management and drug dosing. However, the diagnosis of AKI is based on serum creatinine increase and/or a fall in urine output, two markers that are not renal-specific and have serious limitations. Some researchers have called for further refinement of AKI diagnosis adding to these traditional functional markers, new kidney damage and stress biomarkers [10,11].

Once detected, care of patients with established AKI involves a correction of volume status, individualized hemodynamic resuscitation, avoidance of further nephrotoxic insults, and use of RRT.

Correctly treating sepsis will be beneficial in improving the prognosis of AKI, and correctly treating AKI will be beneficial in improving the prognosis of the septic patient.

Avoidance of nephrotoxic insults must be the other arm for AKI management.

FLUID MANAGEMENT IN AKI

Fluid resuscitation is one the cornerstone of sepsis therapy [12]. However, after initial resuscitation, excessive fluid administration may contribute to edema and organ dysfunction [13].

Although intravascular fluid administration is important in volume-depleted patients, it can be counterproductive and harmful once intravascular volume has been restored [14].

Focusing on kidney function, although it is true that fluid administration may be beneficial if AKI is precipitated by circulatory shock or intravascular volume depletion, as is the case in initial stages of sepsis, there is increasing evidence that excessive fluid administration after hypovolemia correction leads to adverse outcomes including worsening of renal function [15].

The Sepsis Codex. https://doi.org/10.1016/B978-0-323-88271-2.00014-6

Some mechanisms involved are renal interstitial edema, increasing in renal venous pressure, interstitial pressure, and salt and water retention besides a decrease in renal blood flow [16]. In addition, there are some kinds of fluids that are considered nephrotoxic, as hydroxyethyl starches [17].

In the resuscitation from sepsis-induced hypoperfusion, the "Surviving Sepsis Campaign" guidelines [12] recommend at least 30 mL/kg of fluids within the first three hours, preferably of crystalloid solutions. Although there is no firm recommendation to prioritize balanced solutions over saline, it is well known that the administration of large amounts of saline carries the risk of hypernatremic hyperchloremic metabolic acidosis and AKI [18]. Chloride restrictive strategies could be beneficial in reducing the risk of developing acute kidney failure [19–21] or the composite outcome of death, new RRT or persistent renal dysfunction [22], although current evidence is still scarce. Albumin may be beneficial in septic shock, but other colloids such as starches, dextrans, and gelatins appear to increase the risk of death and AKI [13].

After that initial phase, the risks and benefits of further fluid administration should be carefully considered, guiding it by frequent reassessment of hemodynamic status. In that sense, dynamic variables (better than static ones as central venous pressure) should be used to predict fluid responsiveness (passive leg raising test [23], variables related to heart–lung interactions [24], etc.) in order to identify those patients that could benefit from a volume load, as long as hypoperfusion is present (hypotension, lactate levels >2 mmol/L, etc.). The reason for fluid administration should be to restore sepsis induced hypovolemia, to increase cardiac output and to opimize renal blood flow; with the aim to prevent or to reverse AKI. Whether the volume load has a positive effect on renal flow will depend on at which point of the ventricular function curve (Frank–Starling curve) [25] the heart is operating at, the arterial system status (dynamic arterial elastance) [26], and on glomerular autoregulation, among other factors. Thus, it is important to highlight that although oliguria may be hypoperfusion data and therefore a trigger to assess the volume status, it is not an absolute indication for the administration of fluids nor should be diuresis, the target of resuscitation.

Given the large amount of fluids administered during sepsis treatment (resuscitation, maintenance and nutritional fluids, blood products, medication, etc.) and the increased permeability syndrome due to capillary leak, septic patients tend to present significant fluid overload. In septic patients, a positive fluid balance has been identified among the strongest prognostic factor for death [2], and in patients with AKI, a higher degree of fluid overload at RRT initiation predicts worse renal recovery [27]. Bedside the measurement of intra-abdominal pressure, extravascular lung water index, fluid balance, and capillary leak index could help to evaluate fluid overload [28].

According to the conceptual fluid management strategies named SOSD (salvage, optimization, stabilization, and de-escalation), suggested by Vincent [29] and ROSE (resuscitation, optimization, stabilization, and evacuation), proposed by Malbrain [30], once hemodynamic stability has been restored and hypoperfusion evidence has disappeared, "de-resuscitation" should be started as soon as possible, and treatment focus should shift toward the prevention of further fluid overload and the active removal of accumulated excess salt and water [31]. To achieve "euvolemic status," there are two major options available: diuretics or extracorporeal ultrafiltration. Choice of diuretic therapy over mechanical fluid removal will be dependent on renal function, urine output, electrolyte status, and severity of fluid overload.

Although the use of diuretics in the treatment and prevention of the development of AKI has been controversial [32], and KDIGO guidelines recommend against it except in the management of fluid overload [33], its use for management fluid balance may be logical and clinically supportable, as long as response is adequately assessed [34]. These drugs can achieve effective diuresis in the majority of patients, but their use may be limited because of adverse effects such as electrolyte abnormalities, neurohormonal stimulation, and worsening of renal function [35]. When this happens and/or in the presence of an established kidney failure, RRT can be an option for fluid removal. It is important to note that during extracorporeal fluid removal, fluid is primarily removed from the intravascular compartment and is the rate of plasma refilling from the interstitial compartment what determines the change of the intravascular blood volume [36]. In this sense, continuous hemodynamic monitoring tools or intermittent evaluation using ultrasound guided protocols [37] can be useful to achieve a safe and efficient dehydration.

RRT PRINCIPLES

The performance of the RRT actions is unable to manage the myriad abnormalities that occur during AKI. Nevertheless the ability to eliminate water and solutes, give them the opportunity to balance some disorders related with renal function impairment: fluid overload and electrolytes alterations. The mechanisms are diffusion (dialysis) and/or convection (hemofiltration) and adsorption, this in a less significant proportion.

With dialysis, diffusive mechanism, RRT is able to transport solutes trough RRT membranes based on Fick's law [38]. This is a nonselective process that could imply movement of the molecule from plasma to dialysate due to concentration gradient and membrane permeability. The amount of material removed due to Fick's law will increase if the magnitude of the concentration gradient, the area through which diffusion takes place, and the time of work increase. In addition, it will diminish if the distance for the molecule travel (membrane thickness) increases. This nonselective mechanism could also transport molecules from the dialysate to the plasma based on the same law. These two transports will achieve the desired plasma composition with the aim to decrease bad molecules and to equalize good molecules in plasma. The main target type of molecules for this mechanism are endproducts of nitrogen metabolism (urea, creatinine, uric acid). From the dialysate, the repletion of the bicarbonate deficit is easy. This is the reason why diffusion is the favorite mechanism to treat AKI disorders. The amount of dialysate per hour and the blood flow will decide the final clearance.

Other valuable molecules are also affected by diffusion: antimicrobials, vitamins, ions trace elements, etc. It implies that doctors applying these therapies must bear in mind to balance these losses properly minimizing the possibility to develop Dialytrauma [39] (see specific section).

With hemofiltration (convection), RRT is able to tackle the other main problem in AKI syndrome: fluid management [40]. Thanks to the hydrostatic force, through the semipermeable membrane, convection will remove body water from patients. The amount of this water will be controlled by the RRT machine. The user could select from zero hemofiltration up to many liters. The amount of the reposition fluid will get the final fluid balance and also will affect the total clearance.

In anuric patients, these RRT is commonly used to eliminate fluid overload and/or daily mandatory fluid intake. Nevertheless, the water that RRT eliminate by convection will be accompanied by dissolved substances from blood to the dialysate compartment. In that way, convection will share the clearance of endproducts of nitrogen metabolism and the other listed molecules.

We must highlight that the prescription of fluid loss during RRT implies an intimate knowledge of the patient underlying condition and a close monitoring of the hemodynamic response to fluid removal (see specific section).

Adsorption is a mechanism with an insignificant effect in AKI management. Capillary architecture is not the best in terms of quantity for adsorption and it is self-limited.

Diffusion and convection will work together for the transport of molecules. However, the ultrafiltration fluid has molecules that imply a reduction in the osmotic transmembrane gradient. The assessment of the final clearance of a molecule will need to analyze the final mix of dialysate and filtrate (effluent) following the equation:

$$\text{Clearance of } x = ([x]\text{effluent} / [x]\text{blood})$$

$$\times (\text{Volume of effluent} / \text{period of time}).$$

The clearance of molecules and the fluid balance could be reached in few hours with intermittent renal replacement therapy (IRRT) or in 24 h with CRRT, and IRRT could extend the time as the sustained low-efficiency dialysis (SLED) therapy do. Logistic determinants and patient hemodynamic status will determine the RRT-type selection (see specific sections). Interestingly, the clearance obtained in a day of CRRT could be equivalent to that achieved in a session of IRRT [40].

The loss of heat is also related with RRT, mainly with CRRT. It is due to the warming of the fluids by blood [39]. This loss is a part of the possible Dialytrauma and must be avoided with heaters in the CRRT machines or with external devices.

RENAL REPLACEMENT THERAPY

There are clinical practice guidelines for AKI and RRT [33]. We must start RRT emergently in patients with AKI when life-threatening changes in fluid, electrolyte, and acid−base balance exist. Continuous RRT is the predominant form in critically ill patients with hemodynamic instability and in neurocritical patients. We must establish a starting dose, but this must be related to the therapeutic objective that we set for ourselves. There are controversies regarding timing of treatment initiation and cessation, therapy mode, dose, type of anticoagulation, and management of fluid overload [41]. Currently, there are authors who defend a personalized and dynamic approach to RRT in patients with AKI [39,42,43]. This means that RRT:

1. Is prescribed based on the clinical situation of the patient.
2. Is always prescribed with specific treatment goals.
3. We must avoid fixed-dose treatment. Treating severe hyperkalemia is not the same as treating fluid overload.
4. We must decide when to start net ultrafiltration (UF_{net}) and at what speed to do it without deteriorating the patient's hemodynamics. UF_{net} may be initiated during the stabilization and deresuscitation phases in patients who are administered stable dose of a vasopressor with careful monitoring [36]. In this sense, the assessment of systolic volume and on-line volemia systems can help us.
5. Monitorization of the patient and the extracorporeal circuit to detect early changes must be maintained.
6. The rest of the patient's treatment must be adapted to the modality and dose prescribed.

INTERMITTENT RENAL REPLACEMENT THERAPY

CRRT is the predominant modality for RRT in ICU. It seems to be the most suitable modality for unstable patients due to its longer operating time, allows greater fluid removal and more hemodynamical stability, mainly in S-AKI.

Nevertheless, there are situations when other strategies as hybrid intermittent modalities between CRRT and conventional ischemic heart disease (IHD) should be considered. This consists of prolonged sessions of intermittent hemodialysis. The most common terms are extended daily dialysis, SLED, or prolonged IRRT [44].

All of them have in common the use of conventional heart disease machines but with blood and dialyzing fluid flow rates between the usual rates in IHD and CRRT, blood pump speeds rates between 100 and 200 mL/min, and dialyzing fluid flow rates between 200 and 300 mL/min. Treatment duration and frequency are greater than in IHD (6−10 h approximately), so hemodynamic tolerance and fluid removal are not a problem [4].

Other advantage is anticoagulation: SLED could be safely and efficiently performed without anticoagulation using saline flushes [15].

Intermittent modalities have obvious contraindications as hemodynamic instability, neurotrauma patients, exuberant inflammatory response, or hypercoagulability [45], but the ideal modality remains controversial and randomized controlled trials have not shown a survival advantage [46]. Nevertheless, there are patients where alternative treatment schedules as hybrid

modalities have been suggested: using SLED as a step between CRRT and IHD in the dialysis weaning phase.

In conclusion, although CRRT is the most accepted therapy in critical patients, there are other feasible options and intermittent modalities should be considered [45]. Therefore, with any RRT modality (whether continuous, hybrid, or intermittent), prescribing should be an individualized therapy. Intensivist must know each technique in order to personalize and adapt treatment to each patient according to their clinical evolution [47].

CONTINUOUS RENAL REPLACEMENT THERAPY

In acute renal failure associated with sepsis (S-AKI), 15%−20% of the critically ill patients develop severe renal insufficiency and if it is not treated, it is associated with high mortality. As in other causes of AKI, in the case S-AKI, there is controversy regarding RRTs. The three main questions are: Which? When? and How much? [4,41].

Although there is no clear evidence of superiority between CRRT and IRRT, and accepting that they are two complementary therapies in AKI patients, CRRT appears to be the indicated technique in certain groups of patients requiring personalized treatment [33,47,48]. CRRT is indicated in critically ill patients at risk of hemodynamic instability and in neurocritical patients [33]. In S-AKI, the effectiveness of CRRT is mainly due to its accurate volume control, pH and electrolyte correction, and achievement of hemodynamic stability [15,44,46,48]. The most widely used CRRT modalities in critically ill patients are continuous venovenous hemofiltration, continuous venovenous hemodialysis, and continuous venovenous hemodiafiltration [4,44,49].

Regarding the timing to start CRRT in S-AKI, there is no consensus since no benefit has been demonstrated regarding early onset compared to conventional onset [33,41,50−53]. It seems clear that CRRT must be initiated emergently when life-threatening changes in fluid, electrolyte, and acid−base balance exist [33] (refractory hyperkalemia with $K^+ > 6.5$ mmol/L or rapidly increasing or with cardiac toxicity, refractory metabolic acidosis with pH $< 7.1−7.2$ despite normal or low arterial pCO_2, or bicarbonate level $< 12−15$ mmol/L, clear symptoms of fluid overload with acute lung edema or heart failure or intestinal congestion or refractory edema despite the use of diuretics, symptoms or complications attributable to uremia with bleeding or pericarditis or encephalopathy) [41,51]. Apart from these, there is no broad consensus to guide clinicians. In critically ill patients with S-AKI and non-S-AKI, CRRT should be assessed to start, at least, with AKIN III stage [41]. An earlier onset could be evaluated and assessed by individualizing the clinical context of the patient either as a preventive measure before the development of advanced complications or to help the removal of inflammatory mediators [4,51]. On the other hand, although early initiation could have advantages, it may be associated with the increase of adverse effects such as vascular access complications (hemorrhage, thrombosis, vascular injury or infection), ionic alterations (hypocalcemia, hypophosphatemia, or hypokalemia), undesired loss of antibiotics, immunosuppressant drugs, or other solutes [47]. The timing to stop CRRT is defined when no longer it is required because kidney function has been recovered sufficiently or the goals that motivated its initiation have been achieved. Diuretics are not recommended to achieve recovery of kidney function [33,41]. There are clinical indicators such as a urinary output greater than 500 mL/24h (without diuretics), hemodynamic stability, and the correction of water overload, which can help us in making decisions to suspend CRRT and assess the need or not to complement with IRRT [4].

In CRRT, the recommended dose is 20–25 mL/kg/h. In order to achieve this dose, it is generally necessary to prescribe higher doses and minimize interruptions in CRRT [33,41]. Dose above 20–25 mL/kg/h has been studied in AKI patients without evidence of differences in survival rates. Even higher convection doses for S-AKI patients have been evaluated without finding differences in mortality [1,4,15,41,44,46–48]. Anyway, it should be a dynamic approach to achieve the goals of care, in the same way that we do in the management of other pathologies in critically ill patients [39].

Complementing the answers to the above questions, it is necessary to prevent dialyzer/hemofilter clotting and ensure the delivery of the required dose while maintaining the continuity of treatment. Filtration fraction should not exceed 20%–25%. The system requires anticoagulation during CRRT if the patient is not at risk of bleeding or coagulopathy or is not receiving systemic anticoagulation. Regional citrate anticoagulation should be the chosen modality in patients who do not have contraindications for citrate. If there are contraindications for citrate, unfractionated or low-molecular-weight heparin is recommended [4,33,46,47]. The vascular location of the catheter, to ensure the correct functioning of the CRRT, should be the right internal jugular vein, followed by the femoral vein and the left internal jugular vein [4,33].

RENAL DOSAGE ADJUSTMENT FOR ANTIMICROBIALS

In the treatment of sepsis, selecting not only the antibiotic but also the most appropriate dosing regimen is mandatory. Traditionally, renal function in critically ill patients has been assessed to identify renal dysfunction, and dose adjustment is generally accepted in such a context to avoid toxicity. However, antibiotic renal dose adjustments are determined in patients with stable chronic kidney disease, and there are increasing evidence that those recommendations may not be applicable to patients with acute renal failure in whom the need for dose reduction may be overestimated. Therefore, some authors suggest deferred renal dose adjustment during the first 48h of acute infection [54]. On the other hand, augmented renal clearance (ARC), defined as a creatinine clearance (CrCl) ≥ 130 mL/min/1.73 m^2, is a less well-studied phenomenon that could lead to faster elimination of drugs [55], resulting in subtherapeutic concentrations and poorer clinical outcomes when standard dosage guidelines are followed [56]. ARC can influence the pharmacokinetic profile of antimicrobial drugs that are renally cleared and known to have a direct correlation between their renal clearance and CrCl, such as beta-lactams, vancomycin, aminoglycosides, or linezolid [57–60]. In antibiotics with time-dependent activity, the use of extended/continuous perfusions may be useful in this context [60]. Further studies are needed to define the appropriate dosing regimen in this group of patients.

In addition, as previously mentioned, RRT may result in a significant loss of antibiotics. Therefore, it is important to identify which drugs are potentially and/or significantly removed by RRT in order to avoid or, at least, reduce the risk of insufficient dosing. The profile of antimicrobials at risk of RRT elimination includes low volume of distribution, low protein binding, and a predominant renal clearance. General principles for antibiotic dosing in patients during CRRT are summarized in Table 19.1.

Summarizing, the main recommendations are to administer a loading dose unchanged (when indicated) to adjust the dose upwards to avoid subtherapeutic concentrations and to establish the dosing regimen according to pharmacokinetic/pharmacodynamic criteria (prioritize maintaining short intervals/extended perfusions in time-dependent antibiotics versus maintaining the proposed dosage by adjusting the dosing interval in concentration-dependent ones).

TABLE 19.1
Recommendations to Guide Drug Dosing During CRRT [39].

Loading dose does not require adaptation for extracorporeal removal but for differences in volume distribution

Adapt maintenance dose to the reduced renal function according to drug information

Increase maintenance dose in patients with AKI receiving RRT when extracorporeal clearance is clinically significant (i.e. ≥25%)

- Select dose based on published data
- Select dose based on current creatinine clearance (i.e. residual and extracorporeal). This does not apply for drugs with tubular secretion or reabsorption (e.g. fluconazole dose must be increased because tubular reabsorption is absent in AKI and RRT)
- Calculate empirical dose as normal dose multiplied by current clearance fraction
- Calculate the dose from dose used in anuria

Compare different methods of rule 3 and select the maximum dose. In case of nontoxic drugs, mainly antimicrobials, a 30% dose increase is acceptable

Select dose or modify dosing interval depending on drug pharmacodynamic profile: time dependant vs concentration dependent

- For time dependent antibiotics (beta-lactams): PK/PD* index: time above minimal inhibitory concentration (MIC). Action: the interval will be maintained with the calculated dose
- For concentration dependent antibiotics (aminoglycosides, daptomycin etc.). PK/PD index: peak/MIC. Action: the highest dose must be administered to reach the highest peak concentration which provides a postantibiotic effect and less toxicity, adjusting the interval.
- In case drug plasma levels can be monitored, recorded levels must guide the dose accordingly

If possible, select drugs with doses unaffected by renal impairment

Bear in mind that the higher the dose, the higher the need to counterbalance drug losses

PK/PD, pharmacokinetic/pharmacodynamic.

REFERENCES

[1] Peerapornratana S, et al. Acute kidney injury from sepsis: current concepts, epidemiology, pathophysiology, prevention and treatment. Kidney Int 2019;96(5):1083−99.

[2] Vincent JL, et al. Sepsis in European intensive care units: results of the SOAP study. Crit Care Med 2006;34(2):344−53.

[3] Xu X, et al. Epidemiology and clinical correlates of AKI in Chinese hospitalized adults. Clin J Am Soc Nephrol 2015;10(9):1510−8.

[4] Karkar A, Ronco C. Prescription of CRRT: a pathway to optimize therapy. Ann Intensive Care 2020;10(1):32.

[5] Mehta RL, et al. Sepsis as a cause and consequence of acute kidney injury: program to improve care in acute renal disease. Intensive Care Med 2011;37(2):241−8.

[6] Singer M, et al. The third international consensus definitions for sepsis and septic shock (Sepsis-3). JAMA 2016;315(8):801−10.

[7] Langenberg C, et al. Renal blood flow in experimental septic acute renal failure. Kidney Int 2006;69(11):1996−2002.

[8] Langenberg C, et al. Renal blood flow in sepsis. Crit Care 2005;9(4):R363—74.

[9] Pickkers P, et al. The intensive care medicine agenda on acute kidney injury. Intensive Care Med 2017;43(9): 1198—209.

[10] Endre ZH, et al. Differential diagnosis of AKI in clinical practice by functional and damage biomarkers: workgroup statements from the tenth Acute Dialysis Quality Initiative Consensus Conference. Contrib Nephrol 2013;182:30—44.

[11] Katz NM, Kellum JA, Ronco C. Acute kidney stress and prevention of acute kidney injury. Crit Care Med 2019; 47(7):993—6.

[12] Rhodes A, et al. Surviving sepsis campaign: international guidelines for management of sepsis and septic shock: 2016. Intensive Care Med 2017;43(3):304—77.

[13] Brown RM, Semler MW. Fluid management in sepsis. J Intensive Care Med 2019;34(5):364—73.

[14] Hjortrup PB, et al. Restricting volumes of resuscitation fluid in adults with septic shock after initial management: the CLASSIC randomised, parallel-group, multicentre feasibility trial. Intensive Care Med 2016;42(11):1695—705.

[15] Poston JT, Koyner JL. Sepsis associated acute kidney injury. BMJ 2019;364:k4891.

[16] Malbrain M, et al. Principles of fluid management and stewardship in septic shock: it is time to consider the four D's and the four phases of fluid therapy. Ann Intensive Care 2018;8(1):66.

[17] Bagshaw SM, Chawla LS. Hydroxyethyl starch for fluid resuscitation in critically ill patients. Can J Anaesth 2013;60(7):709—13.

[18] Yunos NM, et al. Association between a chloride-liberal vs chloride-restrictive intravenous fluid administration strategy and kidney injury in critically ill adults. JAMA 2012; 308(15):1566—72.

[19] Chowdhury AH, et al. A randomized, controlled, double-blind crossover study on the effects of 2-L infusions of 0.9% saline and plasma-lyte® 148 on renal blood flow velocity and renal cortical tissue perfusion in healthy volunteers. Ann Surg 2012;256(1):18—24.

[20] Van Regenmortel N, Jorens PG. Effect of isotonic vs hypotonic maintenance fluid therapy on urine output, fluid balance, and electrolyte homeostasis: a crossover study in fasting adult volunteers. Reply from the authors. Br J Anaesth 2017;119(5):1065—7.

[21] Van Regenmortel N, et al. Effect of isotonic versus hypotonic maintenance fluid therapy on urine output, fluid balance, and electrolyte homeostasis: a crossover study in fasting adult volunteers. Br J Anaesth 2017;118(6): 892—900.

[22] Semler MW, et al. Balanced crystalloids versus saline in critically ill adults. N Engl J Med 2018;378(9):829—39.

[23] Monnet X, Marik P, Teboul JL. Passive leg raising for predicting fluid responsiveness: a systematic review and meta-analysis. Intensive Care Med 2016;42:1935—47.

[24] Teboul FMaJ-L. Predicting fluid responsiveness in ICU patients. Chest; 2002.

[25] Marik PE, Monnet X, Teboul J-L. Hemodynamic parameters to guide fluid therapy. Ann Intensive Care 2011;1: 1—9.

[26] Monge García MI, Barrasa González H. Why did arterial pressure not increase after fluid administration?,?Por qué la presión arterial no aumentó después de la administración de líquidos? Med Intensiva 2017;41(9):546—9.

[27] Heung M, et al. Fluid overload at initiation of renal replacement therapy is associated with lack of renal recovery in patients with acute kidney injury. Nephrol Dial Transplant 2012;27(3):956—61.

[28] Cordemans C, et al. Fluid management in critically ill patients: the role of extravascular lung water, abdominal hypertension, capillary leak, and fluid balance. Ann Intensive Care 2012;2(Suppl. 1 Diagnosis and management of intra-abdominal hyperten):S1.

[29] Vincent JL, De Backer D. Circulatory shock. N Engl J Med 2013;369(18):1726—34.

[30] Malbrain ML, et al. Fluid overload, de-resuscitation, and outcomes in critically ill or injured patients: a systematic review with suggestions for clinical practice. Anaesthesiol Intensive Ther 2014;46(5):361—80.

[31] Perner A, et al. Fluid management in acute kidney injury. Intensive Care Med 2017;43(6):807—15.

[32] Ho KM, Sheridan DJ. Meta-analysis of frusemide to prevent or treat acute renal failure. BMJ 2006;333(7565): 420.

[33] Khwaja A. KDIGO clinical practice guidelines for acute kidney injury. Nephron Clin Pract 2012;120(4): c179—84.

[34] Goldstein S, et al. Pharmacological management of fluid overload. Br J Anaesth 2014;113(5):756—63.

[35] Uri Elkayam PH, Janmohamed M. The challenge of correcting volume overload in hospitalized patients with decompensated heart failure. J Am Coll Cardiol 2007; 49:684—6.

[36] Balakumar V, Murugan R. Kidney replacement therapy for fluid management. Crit Care Clin 2021;37(2):433—52.

[37] Wang L, et al. Fluid removal with ultrasound guided protocol improves the efficacy and safety of dehydration in post-resuscitated critically ill patients: a quasi-experimental, before and after study. Shock 2018;50(4): 401—7.

[38] Clayton JA, Shelly MP. Atlas of hemofiltration. Br J Anaesth 2002;89(1):191.

[39] Maynar Moliner J, et al. Handling continuous renal replacement therapy-related adverse effects in intensive care unit patients: the dialytrauma concept. Blood Purif 2012;34(2):177—85.

[40] Ronco C, Ricci Z. Renal replacement therapies: physiological review. Intensive Care Med 2008;34(12):2139—46.

[41] Romagnoli S, et al. Renal replacement therapy for AKI: when? How much? When to stop? Best Pract Res Clin Anaesthesiol 2017;31(3):371—85.

[42] Forni LG, Chawla L, Ronco C. Precision and improving outcomes in acute kidney injury: personalizing the approach. J Crit Care 2017;37:244—5.

[43] Bagshaw SM, et al. Precision continuous renal replacement therapy and solute control. Blood Purif 2016; 42(3):238−47.

[44] Ronco C, Bellomo R, Kellum JA. Acute kidney injury. Lancet 2019;394(10212):1949−64.

[45] Ramirez-Sandoval JC, et al. Prolonged intermittent renal replacement therapy for acute kidney injury in COVID-19 patients with acute respiratory distress syndrome. Blood Purif 2021;50(3):355−63.

46. Boongird SS, Kananuraks S, Nongnuch A. Sepsis and renal replacement therapy. J Clin Nephrol Renal Care 2017;3(2):030.

[47] Valdenebro M, et al. Renal replacement therapy in critically ill patients with acute kidney injury: 2020 nephrologist's perspective. Nefrologia 2021;41(2):102−14.

[48] Bellomo R, et al. Acute kidney injury in sepsis. Intensive Care Med 2017;43(6):816−28.

[49] Negi S, et al. Renal replacement therapy for acute kidney injury. Renal Replacement Therapy 2016;2(1):31.

[50] Zarbock A, et al. Effect of early vs delayed initiation of renal replacement therapy on mortality in critically ill patients with acute kidney injury: the ELAIN randomized clinical trial. JAMA 2016;315(20):2190−9.

[51] Bagshaw SM, Wald R. Strategies for the optimal timing to start renal replacement therapy in critically ill patients with acute kidney injury. Kidney Int 2017;91(5): 1022−32.

[52] Gaudry S, et al. Delayed versus early initiation of renal replacement therapy for severe acute kidney injury: a systematic review and individual patient data meta-analysis of randomised clinical trials. Lancet 2020; 395(10235):1506−15.

[53] Bagshaw SM, et al. Timing of initiation of renal-replacement therapy in acute kidney injury. N Engl J Med 2020;383(3):240−51.

[54] Crass RL, et al. Renal dosing of antibiotics: are we jumping the gun? Clin Infect Dis 2019;68(9):1596−602.

[55] Udy AA, et al. Augmented renal clearance: implications for antibacterial dosing in the critically ill. Clin Pharmacokinet 2010;49(1):1−16.

[56] Bilbao-Meseguer I, et al. Augmented renal clearance in critically ill patients: a systematic review57. Clin Pharmacokinet; 2018. p. 1107−21.

[57] Gastmeier P, et al. Risk factors for death due to nosocomial infection in intensive care unit patients: findings from the Krankenhaus Infektions Surveillance System. Infect Control Hosp Epidemiol 2007;28(4):466−72.

[58] Damas P, et al. Intensive care unit acquired infection and organ failure. Intensive Care Med 2008;34(5):856−64.

[59] Petrosillo N, et al. Some current issues in the pharmacokinetics/pharmacodynamics of antimicrobials in intensive care. Minerva Anestesiol 2010;76(7):509−24.

[60] Barrasa H, et al. Impact of augmented renal clearance on the pharmacokinetics of linezolid: advantages of continuous infusion from a pharmacokinetic/pharmacodynamic perspective. Int J Infect Dis 2020;93:329−38.

CHAPTER 20

Hematological Support in Sepsis

ZULMI ARANDA • GERHALDINE MORAZAN • ALLYSON HIDALGO

INTRODUCTION

Sepsis induces an important systemic inflammation, and its sequalae represent a continuum of clinical and pathological severity [1]. The sepsis has well-defined phases that characterize the population at risk of developing complications. The ability of the host to respond to an infection is the most important determinant of mortality, not the pathogen itself [2]. The progression to multiple organ dysfunction in a patient with sepsis represents the extreme of the clinical scenario in sepsis and carries an increased risk of death [2]. Therefore, health care providers treating septic patients must be familiar with organ dysfunction's signs and symptoms and potential complications.

The hematology system plays a critical role in oxygen delivery, carbon dioxide disposal, hemostasis, and defense against pathogens. As a result of its widespread distribution and disparate functions, the hematology system is often overlooked as an organ in the work-up of the patients with sepsis [2]. This is critical for several reasons:

First, hematology changes are present in virtually every patient with severe sepsis (see Table 20.1 Hematologic Changes in Sepsis). Second, patients with hematology dysfunction have increased morbidity and mortality. Third, rapid identification and treatment of a hematology dysfunction may lead to improved survival [2].

THE ENDOTHELIUM

Endothelial cell function is tightly integrated with the physiology of the hematologic system, and dysfunction plays a crucial role in many hematologic manifestations of sepsis. The endothelium is considered the largest organ in the body and surpasses the skin [3]. Most of the endothelium is located in the microvasculature, where the endothelial surface area per unit of blood volume is 2−3000 times greater than in the larger blood vessels. Endothelial dysfunction is a crucial element in the pathogenesis of severe sepsis. This may be secondary to the effects of endotoxins—proinflammatory cytokines reactive oxygen species and other inflammatory mediators. Severe endothelial injury from various etiologies can produce microvascular coagulopathy and acute organ dysfunction. In patients with severe sepsis, endothelial cell apoptosis may produce abnormalities in the trafficking of blood cells into an infected focus [3]. Vasoregulation and the antithrombosis—thrombosis balance may contribute to the pathogenesis of septic manifestations such as multiple organ dysfunction, impaired microvascular blood flow, and the inability of the body to restore homeostasis [3].

The mechanism that leads to microcirculatory dysfunction: the presence of the damaged molecular patterns, pathogen-associated molecular patterns, the presence of oxidative stress, along with alterations in nitric oxide production, all of them contribute to endothelial dysfunction [4,5]. An inducible nitric oxide synthase—dependent decrease in endothelial nitric oxide synthase—derived nitric oxide production with the consequential results of the loss of endothelial protection vias loss of direct vasodilation and loss of platelet aggregation and leukocyte activation inhibition and platelet adhesion and coagulation cascade activation in the setting of endothelial dysfunction [4,5]. As a result, the glycocalyx denudation alters the colloid osmotic gradient between the lumen of the capillaries and the protein-rich area protected by the glycocalyx layer, which leads to an increase in the capillary leak and increased adhesion of platelets and neutrophils. The continuum of these events leads to: and alteration on the red blood cells (RBCs) deformability, increased in blood viscosity, platelet activation, leukocyte adhesion and rolling, and finally activation of the coagulation systems and the complement [4,5].

THE WHITE BLOOD CELLS IN SEPSIS

In patients suffering from sepsis, the white blood cell (WBC) is normally elevated (leukocytosis) with an increased number of neutrophils (neutrophilia). In

The Sepsis Codex. https://doi.org/10.1016/B978-0-323-88271-2.00028-6

TABLE 20.1
Hematologic Changes in Sepsis

WBC	**Most commonly Leukocytosis, will see a left shift deviation and we can see changes in the morphology as: toxic granulation, vacuolization, and/or the presence of Dohle bodies.**
RBC	Will see anemia (decreased oxygen-carrying capacity), decreased platelet–endothelial interaction, decreased deformability, an increased viscosity, and decreased tissue perfusion. Rarely, pathogens (e.g., *Clostridium perfringens*) interact directly with red blood to induce hemolytic anemia. Some patients may present to the intensive care unit with a preexisting anemia: Examples shown are Cancer, autoimmune hemolytic anemia, anemia of chronic disease, and hemorrhage.
PLT	Sepsis is more commonly associated with thrombocytopenia that increase the risk of bleeding, excessive PLT activation (proinflammatory/coagulant), and microparticle formation (proinflammatory/coagulant). The blood film will show: clumping, (pseudo) schistocytes (disseminated intravascular coagulation).
Activation of Coagulation	Sepsis results in the induction of tissue factor (TF) on the surface of monocytes and some possible subsets of endothelial cells. TF initiates the clotting cascade, decreased Protein C (proinflammatory/coagulant), consumption coagulopathy bleeding (disseminated intravascular coagulation), and excessive thrombin and fibrin generation.

PLT, platelet; *RBC*, red blood cell; *TF*, tissue factor; *WBC*, white blood cell.

some cases, the patients may present with neutropenia, in particular, we see that in the pediatric population [2,3].

WBC alterations are commonly seen in patients with sepsis. In the acute phase response, we see a demargination of neutrophils from the endothelial surface, release and increased production of neutrophils and/or monocytes from the bone marrow, and activation of circulating leukocytes. Occasionally, neutropenia or leukemoid reaction is reported in patients with sepsis. An increase or a decrease in the number of the WBC can be seen and can be related with patient medical background. Occasionally, neutropenia or leukemoid reaction is reported in patients with sepsis. An increase or a decrease in the number of WBC can be seen and can be related to the patient with a medical background, such as cancer or associated with chemotherapy or corticosteroids [2,3].

The presence of leukocytosis or leukopenia is diagnosed on the basis of a complete blood cell count. On the blood film will see toxic granulations, vacuolization, and the presence of Dohle bodies in polymorphonuclear cells.

THE RED BLOOD CELLS IN SEPSIS

One of the most common findings in sepsis-related RBC changes is anemia (common to see in the critically ill patients regardless of the presence of sepsis, which results from the iron sequestration in monocytes and macrophages, a reduction in erythropoietin production, and a blunt bone marrow response) [2,3]. How an anemia will impact the patient with sepsis is the reflection of the high transfusion requirements in this particular group of patients. Sepsis is complicated with disseminated intravascular coagulation (DIC); secondary hemolysis is more likely responsible for anemia. Some pathogens like *Clostridium perfringens* have direct interaction with RBC and have the potential to induce hemolytic anemia. On the other hand, some patients admitted to the intensive care unit have anemia related to preexisting medical conditions: cancer, autoimmune hemolytic anemia, anemia of chronic disease, and bleeding [2,3].

One of other signs we observe in patients with sepsis is hemoconcentration, more likely due to the extravascular leak of fluids. This can lead to a relative erythrocytosis. However, one of the most common changes in the erythron in patients with sepsis is anemia, which results in a decrease in the oxygen-carrying capacity of the blood [6].

The membrane properties as well as the mechanics of the RBC can change during sepsis and lead to reduced deformability (an important determinant of the blood flow, particularly at the microcirculation level) [5]. This translates into a reduced flow and increased transit time. That will affect tissue oxygen delivery and contribute to organ dysfunction. Sepsis also can favor aggregation of the RBCs and can be responsible for an elevated erythrocyte sedimentation rate. Another phenomenon we see when sepsis presents with critical destruction of the RBC is the release of free hemoglobin into the circulation. The critically ill patients lose blood through a continuous collection of blood samples. Also, these patients can experience gastrointestinal bleeding and surgical procedures. The exact inflammation process can produce anemia, and we can see this occur within days of the initial insult. The complex mechanism involves decreased erythropoietin production, the bone marrow's response to the erythropoietin is altered, and the survival of the RBC is reduced [5].

THE PLATELETS IN SEPSIS

The most common finding associated with platelets (activated during sepsis, and their activation provides the release of proinflammatory mediators, phospholipid-rich surface for coagulation complexes, and interaction with endothelial cells and leukocytes) in sepsis is thrombocytopenia. Some of the most common mechanisms implicated are the binding of platelets to the activation of endothelium, which results in destruction and sequestration within the small vessels [2,3]. Consumption of platelets is reported in sepsis complicated with DIC. On infrequent occasions, platelet-specific autoantibodies (immunoglobulin G) may play a role in immune-mediated platelet destruction. And some patients probably have a medical history of related platelets dysfunction, for example: cancer, thrombotic thrombocytopenic purpura (TTP), hemolytic uremic syndrome (UHS), idiopathic thrombocytopenic purpura, and thermal injury [2,3,6,7].

PLATELETS INVOLVEMENT

Clinical sepsis management remains a difficult challenge, and pathophysiological advances have not yet been translated into effective therapeutic protocols. Notably, strategies to counteract the runaway proinflammatory state in sepsis, such as inhibiting specific inflammatory mediators, have given disappointing results. What is known on the pathophysiology stress on cellular and humoral factors, altered inflammation response to infectious events, suggests that therapies targeting a single mediator will not demonstrate effectiveness. Medical comorbidities and some individual diseases add additional complexity that would necessitate unique therapies.

Platelets' (drive multiple inflammatory pathways) participation in several immune response pathways is leading to the assumption that platelets and platelets-derived effectors represent a treatment target [8].

Some of the positive effects of the antiplatelet agents: aspirin, clopidogrel, platelet P2Y12 inhibitor, or GPIIb/IIIa antagonists are the reduction of morbidity and mortality in critically ill patients, according to some observational and retrospective clinical studies [8].

Some of this to have in consideration is the heterogeneity of the patient with sepsis, such as the causal germ, severity, site, age, and genetic background, among others.

An inadequate response to clopidogrel or aspirin treatment may concern up to 30% or 40% of individuals. Also, antiplatelet therapies have differential effects on platelet functions. Therefore, proinflammatory/procoagulant condition as met in sepsis, it remains to be determined whether antiplatelet treatments efficiently inhibit platelet activation. Platelets are an essential blood reservoir of proinflammatory cytokines that may participate in the sepsis-related cytokine storm [8]. The understanding the mechanisms of thrombocytopenia in sepsis is essential concerning transfusion. Platelet transfusion is mainly used to prevent/treat bleeding. The severity and persistence of thrombocytopenia, immature platelet fractions, and platelet microvesicle composition are strong predictors of mortality in sepsis [9]. (See Table 20.2. Platelets as a diagnostic tool).

COAGULATION FACTORS IN SEPSIS

The loss of the blood's ability to clot is defined as coagulopathy, and the hemostatic pathway is very complex. A disruption of the normal anticoagulative state within the vasculature is seen in sepsis and septic shock. Sepsis results in a hypercoagulable condition characterized by microvascular thrombi, fibrin deposition, neutrophil extracellular trap formation, and endothelial injury. Inflammatory cytokines and other mediators, such as platelet-activating factor and cathepsin G, target the endothelium and platelets. Platelet activation can propagate coagulation and the inflammatory response by forming aggregates that can activate thrombin release.

Tissue factor (TF) is essentially expressed in the extravascular matrix to activate clotting at the site of

TABLE 20.2
At the Intensive Care Unit, We Need To Take A Complete Medical History and A Physical Exam, Since Several Conditions can Produce Similar Laboratory Findings

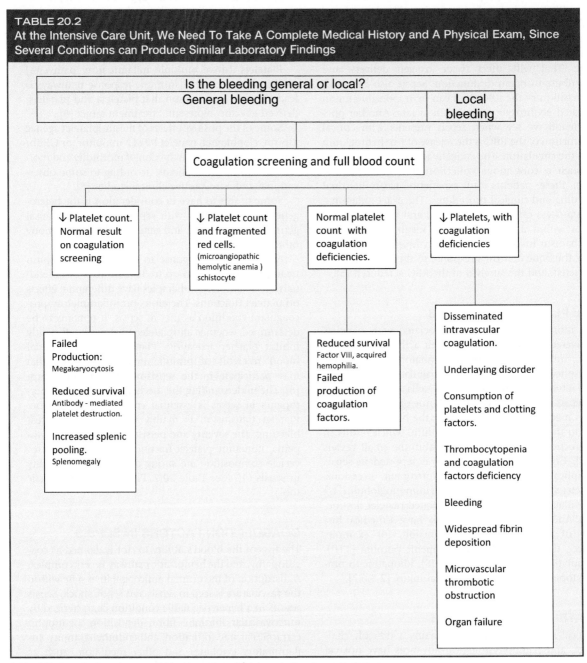

A blood film is a simple and very useful tool to analyze platelets and other diagnostic features.

disruption of endothelial continuity, and the primary initiator of coagulation in sepsis as well. In a systemic infection, activated monocytes, endothelial cells, and circulating microvesicles express TF. TF is activated during sepsis on the monocytes' surface and in some subsets of endothelial cells. The TF is in charge of initiating the coagulation cascade with the ultimate formation of fibrin and thrombin generation.

Three major proteins control the formation of clots (blood clotting): antithrombin, tissue factor pathway inhibitor (TFPI), and activated protein C (APC). Thrombin, factor IXa, and factor VIIa: TF complex [10,11]. TFPI is an endothelial cell-derived serine protease inhibitor that blocks factor Xa activity bound to factor VIIa: TF complex. Protein C and protein S attenuate coagulation by the capacity of APC to proteolytically inactivate the acceleration factors Va and VIIIa. The fibrinolytic system by plasmin generation further controls hemostasis. A major inhibitor of fibrinolysis is plasminogen activator inhibitor type I (PAI-1). In cases of severe sepsis, the activities of antithrombin, TFPI, the protein S-APC system, and fibrinolysis are all impaired, resulting in a net procoagulant state. PAI-1 is a highly effective inhibitor of fibrinolysis, and elevated circulating levels of PAI-1 are highly predictive of an unfavorable outcome in sepsis [10,11].

The clotting cascade is typically inhibited by several natural anticoagulants mechanism, including TFPI, antithrombin III (ATIII), thrombomodulin, protein C, protein S, and fibrinolysis. In the patient with sepsis, the circulating levels of APC and ATIII are decreased. Additionally, there is an attenuation of thrombomodulin expression on the surface of the endothelial cells. Finally, the fibrinolytic pathway is inhibited [2,3]. The endothelium may express a procoagulant phenotype, with increased expression of TF, plasminogen activator inhibitor, von Willebrand factor, and decreased expression of TM. Activation of endothelial cells and platelet membranes, as well as the formation of microparticles, results in the acceleration of clotting reactions. Once activated, the clotting factors may interact with protease-activated receptors on the surface of endothelial cells, monocytes, and platelets, amplifying the proinflammatory response [2,3,6,7]. To date, no single biological response modifier is available that is currently approved for use in sepsis.

The major pathways that lead to DIC and sepsis-induced coagulopathy involve the activation of coagulation inflammatory cell like neutrophils, lymphocytes, platelets, and injury to the endothelium. TF, a critical component of the extrinsic coagulation pathway, expressed on macrophages and monocytes, was thought to play a central role coagulation initiation.

The expression of the TF is by extracellular residue and phosphatidylserine, an initiator of the contact pathway expressed by cell membranes and know to activate hemostasis and the formation of clot.

GENERAL APPROACH OF SEPSIS-INDUCED COAGULOPATHY

The last Surviving Sepsis Campaign recommendation addresses the utilization of red blood cell transfusion for adults with sepsis or septic shock using a restrictive over-the-liberal transfusion strategy. We need to consider the overall clinical assessment of the patient scenario, and we should not be guided by the hemoglobin concentration alone. We need special consideration for patients with acute myocardial infarction, severe hypoxemia, or acute hemorrhage [12].

Critical to the management of sepsis-induced coagulopathy is the rapid and timely treatment of the underlying infection. Other strategies that have been extensively studied are directed at suppressing the prothrombotic effects. Heparin and heparinoids are the most popularly used anticoagulants for a variety of thromboembolic diseases; however, their effectiveness for treating sepsis-induced coagulopathy or DIC still is debated and generally limited to the prevention of deep vein thrombosis [13].

There is no globally approved therapeutic agent at present for the specific treatment of sepsis-induced coagulopathy. The effectiveness of natural anticoagulants, such as antithrombin, APC, and TF pathway inhibitors, has been studied in large-scale controlled trials in the early 21st century. Unfortunately, the primary goal could not be achieved in any of these trials, although it must be remembered that all of these trials targeted sepsis and not sepsis-associated coagulopathy and DIC. In contrast, post hoc analyses performed to examine the effects in the DIC patient subgroup showed favorable effects of antithrombin and recombinant APC [13].

Although recombinant APC has been withdrawn from the world market, the efficacy of antithrombin for septic DIC has been extensively studied in Japan, and nationwide-database studies have repeatedly demonstrated a potential survival benefit of supplemental doses of antithrombin supplementation [13].

In addition, a metaanalysis demonstrated a trend toward better survival associated with antithrombin use in septic patients with DIC. However, the use of antithrombin has not been recommended in the international sepsis guidelines. The important lesson to learn from these studies is that anticoagulant therapy may be expected to be beneficial for sepsis patients who developed coagulopathy but not in those without a coagulation disorder [6].

Although the role of fresh frozen plasma as a therapeutic approach in patients with sepsis-induced DIC may have potential theoretical benefits, there are no data supporting its application unless there is a specific therapy to treat including bleeding or factor depletion beyond antithrombin [13].

Based on this consideration, the effect of recombinant thrombomodulin was recently examined in a multinational, randomized controlled phase III trial in sepsis patients with coagulopathy (with a platelet count less than 150 Å~ 109/L and a prothrombin time ratio of more than 1.4). The 28-day mortality improved by 2.6% in a total of 800 sepsis patients, although this result was not found to reach statistical significance [13].

Reports say that more than 20% of the patients recovered even before the initiation of the treatment, and a subgroup analysis performed in the patients who fulfilled the entry criteria at baseline (approximately 600 cases) revealed a reduction of the 28-day all-cause mortality by 5.4%. In summary, the effectiveness of natural anticoagulants has not yet been proven, and continued research is warranted [13].

Coagulopathy is an important and common complication in patients with sepsis and contributes to the development of organ dysfunction. Sepsis is associated with vascular injury and thrombocytopenia and can progress to DIC, which is synonymous with sepsis-induced coagulopathy. DIC is a laboratory-based diagnosis representing changes in the coagulation also seen in other conditions like trauma-related injury, cardiogenic shock, and multiorgan failure. The diagnosis of coagulopathy disorder in sepsis is a challenge. The other condition that we also need to look like UHS and TTP conditions that should be differentiated for the therapeutic approach is different. Although the diagnosis of sepsis-induced coagulopathy is made based on the combination of hemostatic biomarkers, new candidates that would allow simpler diagnosis could emerge in the future. Continued efforts to develop new therapeutics to treat these complicated disorders and a more target-specific approach are needed [13].

REFERENCES

[1] Venet F, Rimmele T, Monneret G. Management of sepsis-induced immunosuppression. Crit Care Clin 2018;34: 79—106.

[2] Aird W. The hematologic system as a maker of organ dysfunction in sepsis. Mayo Clin Proc 2003;78:869—81.

[3] Goyette RE, Key NS, Ely EW. Hematologic changes in sepsis and their therapeutic implications. Semin Respir Crit Care Med 2004;25(6):645—59. Thieme Medical Publishers.

[4] Gomez H, Kellum JA. Sepsis-induced acute kidney injury. Curr Opin Crit Care 2016;22(6):546—53. https://doi.org/10.3389/fimmu.2019.01687.

[5] Pool R, Gomez H, Kellum J. Mechanism of organ dysfunction in sepsis. Crit Care Clin 2018;34:63—80.

[6] Goyette R, Key N, Ely E. Hematologic changes in sepsis and their therapeutic implications. Semin Respir Crit Care Med 2005;25:645—59. https://doi.org/10.1055/s-2004-860979.

[7] Hunt B. Bleding and coagulopathies in critical care. N Engl J Med 2014;370:847—59. https://doi.org/10.1056/NEJMra1208626.

[8] Dewitte A, Lepreux S, Villeneuve J, Rigothier C, Combe C, Ouattara A, Ripoche J. Blood platelets and sepsis pathophysiology: a new therapeutic prospect in critical ill patients? Ann Intensive Care 2017;7:115. https://doi.org/10.1186/s13613-017-0337-7.

[9] Alice A, Schrottmaier WC, Salzmann M, Julie R. Platelets in sepsis: an update on experimental models and clinical data. Front Immunol 2019;10. https://doi.org/10.3389/fimmu.2019.01687. ISSN:1664-3224.

[10] Levi M, Van Der Poll T. Two-way interaction between inflammation and coagulation. Trends Cardiovasc Med 2005;15(7):254—9.

[11] Esmon CT. The interaction between inflammation and coagulation. Br J Hematol 2005;131(4):417—30.

[12] Evans L, Rhodes A, Alhazzani W, Antonelli M, Coopersmith CM, French C, et al. Surviving sepsis campaign: international guidelines for management of sepsis and septic shock 2021. Crit Care Med November 2021;49(11):e1063—143. https://doi.org/10.1097/CCM.0000000000005337.

[13] Iba T, Levy JH. Sepsis-induced coagulopathy and disseminated intravascular coagulation. http://pubs.asahq.org/anesthesiology/article-pdf/132/5/1238/517774/20200500_0-00040.pdf. By Guest on June 13, 2022.

CHAPTER 21

Specific Treatment of Focus Control in Sepsis

XAVIER GUIRAO • MONTSERRAT JUVANY • CLARA CENTENO • JOSEP M. BADIA

INTRODUCTION

Although relevant improvements in perioperative care and empirical antibiotic treatment have promoted an increased survival in patients with sepsis, significant adverse events are still present highlighting the complexity of the adequate treatment of such patients. Among risk factors associated with sepsis-related poor outcome are those related with previous patients' comorbidities and inadequate sepsis management. Also, we must highlight that, because of its specific pathogeny, some source of sepsis deserves coadjuvant treatment with additional interventional/surgical procedures to mechanically remove the excessive burden of microbiological and host's defensive products. Then, the concept of sepsis focus control arises, and it is known that such technique is needed when we must deal with a patient with secondary peritonitis, postoperative intraabdominal abscess, obstructive cholangitis or pyelonephritis, or severe necrotizing fasciitis (NF). Consequently, besides initial fluids and vasopressor resuscitation and early adequate antibiotic treatment, adequate sepsis focus control is an additional variable that should be included into the final equation of the adequate management of patients with sepsis.

Relevant efforts have been done to improve septic patients' outcome. For instance, automatized protocols for early detection of sepsis have decreased pitfalls and late detection and treatment of sepsis, making empirically early antibiotic treatment more feasible. Nevertheless, on time, type and extension of source focus control have still some misbalances that might be related with the complexity of the process because of different healthcare scenarios and professionals/specialists are simultaneous or consecutively involved.

This chapter wants to clarify those aspects related with the adequate focus control in septic patients that might eventually benefit from such additional maneuver at different settings such as emergency department or in the intensive care unit (ICU).

EDUCATIONAL GOALS OF THE CHAPTER

- To state the relevance of patients with severe sepsis with a potentially drainable source of sepsis admitted to the ICU.
- To clarify how focus control fits into the general management of septic patients.
- To approach the focus control maneuver in a very comprehensive manner.
- To clarify general concepts of focus control.
- To delineate specific focus control treatments for the most frequent types of drainable source of sepsis.

EPIDEMIOLOGY AND SHORT-TERM OUTCOME OF PATIENTS WITH DRAINABLE SOURCE OF SEPSIS

We can infer the relevance of the specific source of sepsis site by reviewing the published rates of the different types of patients admitted to the ICUs. Nevertheless, such rate is highly dependent on the type of ICU (medical, surgical, or mixed units) and the health system where these patients are treated. Overall, in mixed ICU units, respiratory source of infection is leading the site-specific severe sepsis cases deserving admittance to the ICU, ranging from 61.8% to 20.5% from the overall sites of infection [1–5], even in nonwestern countries [3,5]. Nevertheless, drainable source type of sepsis encompasses a relevant number of patients requiring intensive care either before or after performing focus control. Then, intraabdominal infections (IAIs) account for the second cause of sepsis sites treated at the mixed units [2–6] being the leading site at the surgical ICU [7]. Severe IAI is the second cause of admission to the ICU just after complicated pneumonia [1] and 77% percent of these complained diffuse secondary peritonitis [8] presenting a mortality rate ranging from 10% to 50% [1,8,9]. Morbidity and mortality are highly depending on the initial severity, the associated comorbidity, and the source of infection. Then, gastroduodenal, hepato-bilio-pancreatic, small bowel, and colorectal focus correlated with the highest mortality rate [10,11]. Contrary to the previous century, it has been observed an increased number (roughly 50% of admitted patients) [2] of nosocomial acquired peritonitis. This is a matter of some concern as 60% of these intrahospital IAI are postoperative peritonitis [12].

Although IAI is the mainstay of sepsis sites and efforts should be directed to understand this type of process, additional infection sites should not be disregarded and full attention to this less frequent source of sepsis should also be paid. Accordingly, severe skin and soft tissue infections (SSTIs) are also able to induce severe sepsis requiring early identification and surgical debridement. It has been documented a variable rate of SSTI at the different ICU from 4.3% to 7.2% at the mixed-medical ICU (1−5) being much higher (14%) when reviewed patients admitted to the surgical ICU [7]. Also, thoracic and urinary tract infections (UTIs) are a quite relevant sources of infection deserving focus control. Rates of either urinary tract or genitourinary infections severe enough to be admitted to the ICU range from 7.2% to 18.7% [1−5] of the overall sites of infection.

FOCUS CONTROL INTO THE CONTEXT OF THE GENERAL PRINCIPLES OF SEPSIS MANAGEMENT

Indications of Source Control

Source control of infection should be considered whether the site of infection is amenable to mechanically decrease the elicited products of sepsis. The most frequent foci of infection that may benefit from source control are related with IAIs. Then, beside resuscitation and antibiotic treatment, solid viscera or peritoneal abscesses, peritonitis secondary to gastrointestinal perforation, ischemic bowel or volvulus, cholangitis and cholecystitis, deserve on time percutaneous or surgical drainage.

Less frequent source of sepsis but critically relevant are those patients with obstructive pyelonephritis, severe skin-soft tissue infection, empyema, deep neck infections, septic arthritis, and implanted device-related infections. Such smorgasbord of different anatomical

septic compartments may also deserve focus control at some point by applying specific surgical specialties-related techniques. Such less frequent type of drainable sepsis is associated with additional logistic complexity regarding the adequate coordination of the main stakeholders involved into the process.

In critically ill patients, especially those on septic shock, it is mandatory to achieve source control as soon as possible along with concurrent medical treatment. In other words, without adequate source control, those patients with severe sepsis will not stabilize or improve despite adequate resuscitation and appropriate antibiotic treatment [13].

In general, optimal source control methods should reach the best risk−benefit ratio. Radiological-guided percutaneous drainages and endoscopic approach must be prioritized when judiciously feasible. However, specific septic focus such as generalized peritonitis, bowel ischemia, and soft tissue NF with hemodynamic instability often will require an expeditious open-source control [14].

Preparing the Patient: Resuscitation, Antibiotic Treatment, and Timing of Focus Control

There are two critical factors at the initial steps of sepsis that may have influence on survival: Delay in definitive intervention more than 24 h after symptoms started and the inability to obtain an adequate source control at surgery [15].

Timing of source control may change considering two different clinical scenarios: patients with clinical stability and localized IAI (uncomplicated appendicitis) and patients with sepsis and organ failure with/without hemodynamic repercussion.

In the first situation, antibiotic treatment and close monitorization must be started. Although source control should ideally be performed as soon as possible, consensus statements agree that logistic delay up to 24 h may be acceptable [16]. Nevertheless, close follow-up is warranted as the first goal in the management of patients with initially localized low-grade sepsis is to avoid running to the operating room (OR) in a patient with nonanticipated severe sepsis or septic shock. For instance, in patients with diffuse peritonitis, when comparing patients that were operated early on, it has been substantiated a significant lower Mannheim Peritonitis Index score than those who were taken to the OR after 24 h [17].

Nonintended delays in patients with source control amenable sepsis are multifaceted in origin. Structural and logistic system derangements may combine with insufficient staffed and/or crowded OR emergency departments. It has been observed in patients with surgical sepsis firstly attended in a regional hospital who ultimately were transferred to the tertiary center for a definitive treatment, those patients with a much delayed transfer presented a higher nosocomial infections and mortality [7]. More specifically, prolonged intervals between symptoms initiation and source control [18] in-hospital delay and time of admission [19,20] have been associated with a higher rate of perforated appendicitis.

Also, evidence reinforce the concept that source control is a priority in those patients with an impending organ failure and/or hemodynamic instability [21]. Patients in septic shock with gastrointestinal perforation submitted to a structured hemodynamic reanimation, comparing those who were operated on within the first two hours versus more than six hours delay, 60-day survival was 98% versus 0%, respectively [22]. Also, patients with endoscopic retrograde cholangio-pancreatography—related duodenal perforation showed an increased mortality when focus control was performed after 24 h [23]. Then, in these situations, to avoid preventable mortality, close follow-up and precise radiological assessment of type of periduodenal perforations should be done [24]. Otherwise, early intervention in a patient with infected pancreatic necrosis may produce severe uncontrolled adverse events, and delayed step-up approach with antibiotic, percutaneous, or video-assisted retroperitoneal drainage has been associated with a significant lower morbidity when compared with a regular laparotomy [21,25].

Overall, as De Waele nicely suggested, we might deal with three different scenarios: 1—Severe septic patient that medical treatment concomitantly done both at the emergency department (or at surgical ward) and the OR should not delay immediate source control; 2—Septic but otherwise stable patient that by judiciously deferring for some hours surgical focus control allows to correct physiological derangements; and 3—Planned delay of surgical intervention to improve both systemic and local conditions. This is the case for infected pancreatic necrosis and intraabdominal abscess in formation, keeping on mind that we must find an adequate balance between improving patient's condition without delay of source control when necessary [20].

If timely source control seems critical for adequate treatment of septic patients with IAI, when facing severe skin soft tissue infections as NF, urgent surgical diagnosis and immediate debridement are mandatory. Low threshold for surgical exploration is needed in a patient with alarming clinical and biological signs before a clear and well-stablished skin and subcutaneous disseminated necrosis is clinically apparent. Then, it has been observed that both time of initial symptoms to diagnosis more than 72 h and diagnosis to surgical treatment more than 14 [26] or 24 h [27] delay have been independently associated with an increased mortality.

USEFULNESS OF ANCILLARY TEST FOR GENERAL ASSESSMENT IN PATIENTS WITH POTENTIALLY FOCUS CONTROL OF SEPSIS
Blood Test and Biomarkers

If timely source control seems critical to avoid protracted and consolidated sepsis, early diagnosis of an impending infectious process is also paramount. Then, laboratory test may be extremely helpful to understand how the inflammatory response is doing and at which stage septic process is.

White blood cells (WBCs): In the diagnosis of acute appendicitis, WBC cut-off value of higher than 10,000—12,000 cell/mm yielded sensitivity and specificity values between 65% and 85% and 32% and 82%, respectively. Nevertheless, WBC should not be relied upon to change the diagnosis workup on its own due to its nonspecific role in inflammatory responses [28]. Also, WBC could neither be used in order to predict severity nor need for surgery in acute diverticulitis [29]. In the diagnosis of postoperative infections, WBC performs poorly because of response to a recent surgical stressful stimulus [30]; consequently, another biological marker must be considered in this field.

Lactate: In severe sepsis, lactate has been used as a marker of occult septic shock. High values of serum lactate are associated with mortality independently of organ failure and shock. Then, when lactate levels are increased before hypotension starts, *goal-directed therapy* must be initiated in order to reduce mortality in patients with suspected infection [31,32]. On high-risk surgical patients after cardiac and abdominal surgery, postoperative levels of serum lactate have correlated with postoperative mortality [33,34]. Also, immediately postoperative serum lactate values are associated with anastomotic leakage in patients operated on abdominal surgery [35—37]. Such findings suggest that patients with postoperative high levels of serum lactate should be strictly scrutinized and resuscitation guided by hemodynamics and lactate levels, as a strategy to "protect" surgical anastomosis [38].

Procalcitonin (PCT) and C-reactive protein (CRP): PCT can be useful in differentiating bacterial infections from other causes of inflammation. However, there is not enough scientific evidence to recommend its use on IAI diagnosis [39]. Also, PCT-relevant alarming postoperative elevations occur when intrabdominal and systemic sepsis is still consolidated.

CRP has been recognized as a good biomarker in appendicitis diagnosis (CRP >10 mg/L doubles the probabilities) [28] as well as in cholecystitis (CRP >30 mg/L has been included as diagnostic criteria in Tokyo Guidelines [TG]) [40] and in diverticulitis (CRP >50 mg/L increases by two the probabilities) [41]. CRP has also been studied to assess the usefulness in diagnosing early postoperative complications after abdominal surgery [42]. Also, in colorectal [43,44] and in bariatric surgery [45,46], several metaanalysis conclude that CRP values could be helpful for discarding anastomotic dehiscence and intraabdominal septic complications.

Imaging Diagnosis Test

Classically, it was stated that patients with signs of diffuse peritonitis without criteria of primary spontaneous peritonitis, imaging diagnosis is not essential, and the surgical procedure may be performed right away. However, radiological tests allow for the precise diagnosis and targeted surgical treatment. Nowadays, patients with sepsis seldomly undergo surgery without an image-based test.

Plain chest or abdominal X-rays are nonspecific but can be useful in certain cases, such as the presence of pneumoperitoneum after hollow viscus perforation. In perforated gastroduodenal ulcer, 50%–70% of patients will present visible subdiaphragmatic pneumoperitoneum.

Although the USA literature focuses diagnostic imaging tests on computed tomography (CT), in Europe, ultrasound (US) exam prevails as first step in image diagnosis. US provides valuable information in cases of acute cholecystitis, appendicitis, and diverticulitis. In doubtful cases or in diffuse peritonitis, the most sensitive test is CT. Abdominal CT provides information on the entire abdominal cavity as well as on the retroperitoneum and can also assess visceral blood perfusion when performed with intravenous contrast [14].

A multicenter Dutch study clearly demonstrated that CT sensitivity was significantly higher than US (89% and 70% for CT and US, respectively). Also, the best sensitivity was obtained with a conditional strategy, where CT was performed when US was negative or inconclusive (only 6% missed urgent conditions). Selective CT scan exam strategy reduced such image test by 49%, allowing for unnecessary exposure to radiation [47].

Microbiological Assessment

There is some controversy on whether peritoneal fluid should be sampled and cultured. Severe septic patients and nosocomial IAI should always be sampled as there is an increased risk for multiresistant bacteria and fungi. Nevertheless, when sampling fecal peritonitis, nonspecific microbiological diagnosis will be given confirming a mixed flora infection. Otherwise, in those cases with no such overwhelming peritoneal contamination, Gram stain and oriented microbiological identification (asking for gram-negative resistant bacteria, Enterococcus sp. or Candida sp.) might be useful to readequate empirical antibiotic treatment in those patients with risk factors such as postoperative peritonitis, previous antibiotic treatment, or patients with purulent fluid in severe sepsis or septic shock [48]. If this is the case, adequate sampling should be done by inoculating relevant peritoneal fluid in an adequate vial transport for both aerobic anerobic cultures. Inoculating intraabdominal fluid into blood culture bottles is an option and may increase microbiological sensitivity in those cases where low bacterial load is suspected. In any case, sampling by simple swabbing should be avoided [49].

ORGAN SYSTEM-SPECIFIC FOCUS CONTROL OF SEPSIS

Intraabdominal

Image test-guided percutaneous drainage

Intraabdominal abscess is a well-defined purulent fluid collection isolated from the peritoneal cavity by a fibrous capsule. Abscesses can be classified as community-acquired or nosocomial, most of which are postsurgical. The most common causes are appendicitis, diverticulitis, cholecystitis, cholangitis, pancreatitis, colon neoplasia, intestinal ischemia, inflammatory bowel disease, pelvic inflammatory disease, abdominal trauma, and postoperative abdominal surgery.

Source control can currently be achieved through percutaneous or surgical drainage. Image-guided percutaneous aspiration is defined as the evacuation of a sample of the fluid from a collection using a needle or catheter during a single session, with removal of the catheter or needle immediately after aspiration. Entry routes of percutaneous drainage [50] can be through natural orifice (transrectal, transvaginal) or transcutaneous. The overall process includes the location of the collection and the placement of one or more catheters, as well as their maintenance, monitoring, and eventual replacement. Nowadays, peritoneal dialysis (PD) may be placed in multiple or multiloculated abscesses, in those with difficult access or associated with intestinal fistulae and in critically ill patients.

Percutaneous drainage achieves resolution rates of 95% in single and well-defined abscesses, accessible without going through parenchyma or hollow viscera, dropping to 70% in multiloculated, complex, septate, and with high-density fluids abscesses. In these cases, fibrinolytic therapy with tissue plasminogen activator through the drain can be tested [51–53]. Percutaneous drainage allows microbiology samples (including Gram stain) and may be useful for adequacy of the formerly empirical antibiotic treatment. Drain should be adequately secured and saline flushed every 8–12 h. Image test elicited assessment should be done and mobilized if necessary. It is not advisable to remove the drain without having verified its resolution by imaging tests. Risk factors for PD failure are: age >60 years, gastric surgery, pancreatic abscess, size of the abscess, absence of antibiotic treatment, severity of the illness and late diagnosis in the overall abscess and cardiovascular disease, and cancer surgery in gastrointestinal leaks–related collections [54].

Even though most abdominal abscesses or pelvic collections can be drained percutaneously, there is a small number that may seem nonaccessible to drainage [55]. Abscesses located in the pelvic areas, low presacral space, perirectal or perineal, subphrenic spaces, epigastric, peripancreatic, and retroperitoneal space are usually difficult to access. In deep collections, access can be difficult by US and CT is the alternative.

The access routes that are considered to be safe in case of not having a route without crossing any adjacent organ are: transhepatic, transgastric, transvaginal, and transrectal. Both the liver and the stomach are examples of organs that are considered safe to pass through to place drains in difficult-to-access collections (mainly those in the epigastric region) when there are no other options. The organs that must be avoided are: pancreas, spleen, gallbladder, small and large intestine, urinary bladder, uterus, and ovaries. Abscesses or collections located in most of these organs (pancreas, spleen, gallbladder, and ovaries) can be drained, but these organs should not be used as an access route to deeper collections. Collections at pelvic level are especially difficult to drain, given the interposition of structures such as pelvic bones, large vessels, nerve structures, intestine, and urinary bladder. Multiple drainage routes have been used such as the transvaginal, transrectal, and transgluteal routes [56,57]. Abscesses located in the presacral or low perirectal space or at the perineal level may require a transperineal access that can be guided by both US or CT. Drainage of subphrenic collections is especially difficult when they are small due to the risk

of complications such as pneumothorax, pleural effusion, or empyema. Postsplenectomy abscess may be difficult to drain because of the interposition of intestinal loops. Collections at the retroperitoneal space are also difficult to approach due to their deep location. Because these abscesses frequently cross the midline, we can approach from the contralateral side, mainly when the aorta, the inferior vena cava, or the duodenum have to be avoided.

Surgical management of intraabdominal infections

Minimally invasive versus open surgery. Laparoscopy plays an important role, both in the diagnosis and treatment of IAI, although the potential use of the endoscopic approach is highly depending on the type of infection, the hemodynamic status of the patient, and the complexity of the planned operation [14]. The use of laparoscopic technique in well-selected patients allows a less invasive approach, with a reduction in postoperative pain, wound-related complications (such as superficial infection and incisional hernia), and a reduction in hospital stay. Some of the accepted scenarios for the laparoscopic approach are the diagnosis and treatment of peritonitis of uncertain etiology, cholecystectomy in acute cholecystitis, the treatment of pelvic infection of gynecological origin, or gastroduodenal ulcer perforation. Absolute contraindications to laparoscopy are hemodynamic instability, severe abdominal distention with signs of intraabdominal hypertension, fecal peritonitis, and abdominal sepsis of vascular origin that requires wide bowel resection. Also, previous laparotomy constitutes a relative contraindication for endoscopic approach of nonpreviously localized IAI as bowel adhesions may difficult to assess the abdominal cavity and there is a high risk of unnoticed bowel injury during the surgical process. The increase in abdominal pressure due to the pneumoperitoneum and the prolongation of the surgical intervention in this group of patients who are already seriously ill can compromise the perfusion of the abdominal organs and alter the venous return and cardiac output. Furthermore, although there is clear evidence that endoscopic approach significantly alleviates surgical trauma elicited inflammatory response in elective surgery [36,42], complex and inadequately prolonged endoscopic surgical procedures may overshadow such beneficial effect [58].

Damage control, open abdomen, and second-look treatment. Severe complicated intraabdominal sepsis still has a relevant incidence with documented mortality rates ranging from 11.4% [9] to 45% [59] and may go up to 80% when more than five organ systems are involved [60]. Mortality results from disruption of previously performed anastomosis and/or residual infection collections, progressive and self-perpetuating inflammatory response leading to multiple organ failure. In order to reduce mortality in such severe situations, close follow-up is needed to figure it out whether source control has failed or inadequate antibiotic treatment (or both) is behind the persistent/recurrent IAI. Although, on demand relaparotomy has proved superior to planned second look in those patients with high-risk IAI who have been treated with primary abdominal wall closure [61], more aggressive approach by employing open abdomen (OA) technique has been advocated to decrease the still high rate of IAI mortality.

OA is mandatory in front of an impending abdominal compartment syndrome and after open-source control of infected pancreatic necrosis. Additional potential indications for OA and delayed abdominal wall closure have been suggested after dealing with bowel resection and risky anastomosis in front of either local or systemic dismal conditions [62]. Nevertheless, OA has been associated with severe adverse events such as enteroatmospheric fistula and the impossibility of achieving delayed adequate fascial closure [63]. Metaanalysis of OA techniques showed that negative pressure wound therapy combined with fascial traction had the lowest fistula risk (5.7%), achieving acceptable fascial

closure rates (73.1%) [64]. Hopefully, ongoing randomized controlled trial (RCT) will further provide new insights regarding the benefits and clear indications of OA in treating patients with IAI [65]. Additional comments regarding OA when discussing organ-specific focus control follows. Fig. 21.1 depicts a potential useful algorithm of decision.

General management of open treatment in secondary peritonitis. In secondary peritonitis, adequate focus control (on time and the best surgical approach for the patient's condition and the disease) has proven critical. Nevertheless, we think that a structured approach should be delineated to achieve the best outcome (Table 21.1).

Organ-based treatment of patients with peritonitis: focus control

The main surgical procedures directed to contain and eventually restore physiological conditions entitled the concept of focus control. Because this is a multifaceted process, the quality of focus control in diffuse peritonitis is difficult to evaluate [66]. Nevertheless, there are several clinical and surgical conditions precluding for an adequate focus control that will be briefly discussed.

A. Appendix. Exclusive treatment with antibiotics of acute appendicitis has been controversial since it was first mentioned in 1959 [67]. More recently,

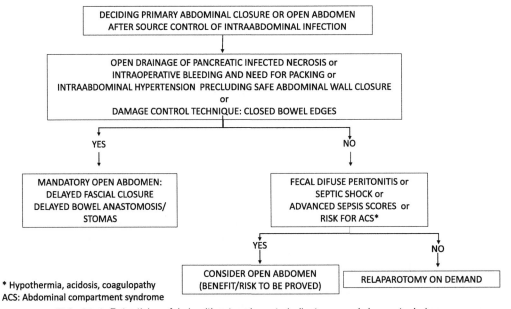

FIG. 21.1 Potential useful algorithm to adequate indicate open abdomen technique.

TABLE 21.1
Step-By-Step Approach for the Open Treatment of Patient With Secondary Peritonitis

Phase	Goal	Maneuver
Initial	Severity assessment	Applying score of sepsis
	Sepsis containment and restore homeostasis	Adequate and early empirical antibiotic treatment
		Early goal-directed therapy-guided resuscitation
	Preparing for surgery	Assure hemostasis and normothermia
FOCUS CONTROL		
First	SSI prevention (incisional)	Antibiotic prophylaxis[a]
		Wound protection
		Normothermia
	Microbiological diagnosis	Peritoneal cultures
	Decrease peritoneal inoculum	Initial abdominal cleansing
	Peritonitis assessment	Looking for the source of the infection
Second	Focus control	Simple closure
		Resection ± intestinal anastomosis
		Stoma
		Damage control management: Leaving closed intestinal edges
	Decrease peritoneal inoculum	Final abdominal cleansing
Third	Abdominal wall management	Primary or open abdomen technique
Final	Treatment of residual inoculum and peri-operative resuscitation	Adequate empirical antibiotic treatment
		Endorsement to Survival Sepsis campaign principles
		Postoperative resuscitation

[a] Although septic patients are under the antibiotic treatment, additional dose is needed to achieve adequate antibiotic concentrations by the time of surgical wound is created and potentially contamination occurs.

improvements in diagnostic imaging and antibiotics have facilitated a more selective approach. Abdominal CT imaging very reliably establishes a diagnosis of complicated appendicitis. Some randomized clinical trials with short and incomplete follow-up have proved the feasibility of antibiotic-only treatment for appendicitis [68,69]. However, a study with longer follow-up demonstrates that appendectomy is needed in 40% of the nonoperated patients at five years [70]. Consequently, appendectomy still remains the gold standard treatment for acute appendicitis [71–73].

Laparoscopic appendectomy has also been disputable. In earlier studies, complication rates were comparable between the two approaches, except for a higher wound infection rate for the open approach and a higher intraabdominal abscesses rate for the laparoscopic procedure [74,75]. Systematic reviews including a relevant number of perforated appendicitis showed little difference of organ space surgical site infection (SSI), suggesting that with added experience, surgeons can reduce the rate of abscess formation [76,77]. Laparoscopic appendectomy is recommended as a good

alternative to open technique at SAGES guidelines, especially on fertile women and obese patients [78]. Then, in hemodynamic stable patients, laparoscopic approach of appendicitis elicited peritonitis is feasible. In these cases, neither peritoneal irrigation after pus suction nor intraabdominal drains confers additional advantages and are not justified [79].

B. Biliary tree and gallbladder. Cholecystitis and appendicitis embody the paradigm of IAI with a surgical amenable focus.

Cholecystectomy. Clinical results of early cholecystectomy are clearly superior to those of delayed surgery (antibiotic treatment and surgery in a second admission after six weeks). The appropriate time frame for early surgery has been extended to the first 7–10 days from the onset of symptoms [80]. Several metaanalyses comparing early and delayed surgery found neither differences in morbidity or mortality [81,82] nor in the rate of injury to the bile duct, both with open and laparoscopic techniques. Financial studies show lower healthcare costs and better quality of life for patients when a policy of early laparoscopic surgery for acute cholecystitis is applied [83].

The indication for early surgery is one of the points of discrepancy between Western practice and the TG recommendations. The treatment algorithms of the latter use the level of inflammation of the gallbladder and its classification of severity to operate [84]. Otherwise, in Western world, the most common recommendation is to indicate surgery regardless of the degree of inflammation of the gallbladder, providing the baseline condition of the patient does not preclude it [85,86]. Nevertheless, recent published systematic review reinforces the concept that early cholecystectomy is safer than delayed procedure as long surgery may be carried within the 72 h of the onset of symptoms [87].

Percutaneous cholecystostomy. The insertion of a percutaneous drainage catheter into the gallbladder directed by US or CT scan is a good alternative in cases of severe inflammation, septic shock, or patients at high risk for general anesthesia achieving a success rate in calculous cholecystitis of 90.7% [88]. The main issue regarding its indication is the definition of a high-risk patient. TG contraindicate early cholecystectomy in "high surgical risk" Grade III cholecystitis (with associated organ dysfunction) or patients with ASA ≥ III or a Charlson comorbidity index ≥6 [84].

These limits seem too strict in Western practice [89], where it is considered that, apart from septic shock, there are no validated risk criteria to identify patients as high surgical risk [80]. There are also no studies comparing emergency cholecystectomy and cholecystostomy in elderly or high-risk patients. Even in critical patients, a systematic review of 53 studies and 1918 patients [88] did not find enough evidence to support the recommendation of TG in favor of percutaneous drainage instead of urgent surgery. In fact, reported mortality from urgent cholecystectomy for cholecystitis is between 0% and 1.5% in studies with patients over 65–70 years in the last decade [90]. Cholecystostomy is the definitive treatment for acalculous cholecystitis, but patients with gallstones should be assessed for cholecystectomy, as the risk of readmission for biliary causes is 49% in the first year [91]. Patients who are definitely not suitable for surgery may be offered nonsurgical treatments for gallstones or stone removal through the cholecystostomy route after six weeks of the acute process.

Acute acalculous cholecystitis (AAC): AAC has a high incidence of gallbladder gangrene (50%) and perforation (10%–15%). Two forms of presentation are distinguished: primary AAC complicating another serious disease and secondary infection of the gallbladder from a systemic infection. It has been described as a postoperative complication of aortic aneurysms, trauma, burns, heart transplantation, and conventional heart surgery. Secondary AAC appears during systemic bacterial, fungal, or viral infections, *Salmonella typhi*, brucellosis, disseminated candidiasis, systemic leptospirosis and cytomegalovirus, hepatitis, or Ebstein–Barr virus infections [92].

The pathogenesis differs from calculous cholecystitis, and ischemia has been suggested as the main cause, which may explain the high percentage of mucosal necrosis, arteriolar thrombosis, gangrene, and perforation. Other factors that may interact are increased intraluminal pressure, biliary stasis secondary to fasting and gastrointestinal hypomotility, compression of the cystic duct, and spasm of the sphincter Oddi secondary to opioid analgesics. As in calculous AC, bacterial infection is a secondary phenomenon [93]. Diagnosis can be difficult in critically ill patients with nonspecific signs of systemic inflammatory response syndrome (SIRS) or sepsis admitted to ICU and unable to express their symptoms [94]. Cholecystectomy offers the best therapeutic results, but in unstable patient, cholecystostomy is an excellent alternative in more than 85% of cases [88]. If there is no rapid improvement in symptoms after cholecystostomy, surgery should be performed without delay. Open cholecystostomy allows limited vision to the right upper quadrant, while laparoscopic cholecystostomy allows evaluation of the rest of the abdomen. Both operations have the same limitations: the presence of a gangrenous or perforated vesicular wall, which forces a cholecystectomy [95,96].

Cholangitis. According to the TG, early diagnosis, antibiotic treatment, and drainage of the bile duct are deemed critical in the management of acute cholangitis [97]. For source control, minimally invasive techniques (Endoscopic retrograde cholangio-pancreatography (ERCP) or Percutaneous transhepatic cholangiography (PTC)) are the first option. In unstable patients or patients in septic shock, bile decompression should be performed within 6 h [98]. A recent metaanalysis regarding the timing of ERCP found a 20% reduced mortality when ERCP is performed <24 h compared with ≥24 h [99]. Early ERCP with sphincterotomy and biliary drainage provides less morbidity and mortality than surgical or percutaneous decompression [100].

In very severe patients, nasobiliary drainage or stenting may be the first step before definitive treatment. Emergency surgical intervention should be reserved for episodes of acute cholangitis that cannot be satisfactorily treated by less aggressive means. In the presence of risk factors, the postoperative morbidity and mortality rates are 91% and 55%, respectively [101].

C. ColoRectal. After complicated appendicitis, colorectal is probably the most frequent abdominal focus that surgeon should deal with when treating patients with IAI [66]. Complicated diverticulitis is right now the first cause of colonic peritonitis. Recent guidelines [102] point out the most relevant aspects of acute diverticulitis. Surgical source control is advised in CT scan diagnosis of Hinchey III—IV acute diverticulitis (generalized purulent-fecaloid peritonitis), nonresponse initially treated with antibiotics diverticulitis with distant gas from inflamed bowel segment, and Hinchey II with an abscess of more than 4 cm that could not be percutaneously drained. Nevertheless, in such situations, conservative treatment might also be tested as long close follow-up is performed to anticipate dismal ongoing sepsis. In any other situations, antibiotic treatment and radiological-guided percutaneous drainage should be the first option.

Laparoscopic peritoneal lavage and drainage has been advocated as a quick and less aggressive focus control in patients with acute diverticulitis elicited peritonitis, trying to avoiding colostomy or a highly technically demanding colorectal anastomosis. RCT (LOLA and SCANDIV) [103,104] and observational studies [105] clearly demonstrated significant treatment failure with laparoscopic washout comparing with colonic resection both at early and late follow-up [106]. Although this effect is not universal (DILALA study) [107], we cannot advise such approach as the first-line treatment in these patients and may be considered as inadequate focus control in most cases.

Although Hartmann's procedure is still an accepted procedure for an adequate focus control in patients with diverticular peritonitis, in clinically stable and relatively young patients with no comorbidities, primary resection with anastomosis with or without a diverting stoma should be considered. Two RCTs (DIVERTI [108] and LADIES [109]) have shown 12-month stoma-free survival was significantly better for patients undergoing primary anastomosis with comparable results in terms of morbidity and mortality. Nevertheless, observational studies reinforce the concept that primary anastomosis should be performed when the assistance of colorectal surgeons is available [110]. Furthermore, laparoscopic approach in patients with diffuse peritonitis should be considered only if colorectal unit team is available by the time that focus control is needed.

Damage control surgery with staged laparotomies can be taken into consideration in selected unstable patients with diffuse peritonitis due to diverticular perforation. The aim of this strategy is to achieve rapid source control, stabilization of the patient, and reconstruction of bowel continuity in the planned second-look operation in order to improve mortality and reduce stoma formation. Quality of evidence is low [111—115], and the only RCT [116] stopped the recruitment of patients prior to achieve the calculated sample size because an interim analysis revealed much longer time that previewed to complete patient recruitment and because minimal invasive surgery technique was incorporated into the daily practice. Overall, further controlled trials are warranted to clarify which patients may benefit from OA and planed second look. Such strategy should clearly overcome potential adverse events associated with prolonged mechanical ventilation and exposed intestinal viscera. Otherwise, in view that associated adverse events with OA are not negligible [117], the decision to leave the abdomen open must be based on clinical and peritoneal patient's condition and prognosis rather than to avoid Hartmann procedure at any price.

In the management of colorectal postoperative infection, it is mandatory to achieve an early diagnosis, especially in patients enrolled to an ERAS and early hospital discharge protocol. Biological markers could play an important role as adjuvant diagnostic method along with clinical and hemodynamic assessment [36,42]. IAI is mainly related to anastomotic leakage, and it must be treated with the most conservative treatment: wide-spectrum antibiotics and radiological percutaneous drainage if possible. Endoscopically placed sponge-negative pressure-based new devices have been recently reviewed. Low-quality reviewed studies show that such endoscopic technique might be useful in those patients with localized IAI without severe sepsis or septic shock and further controlled studies are warranted [118]. However, in cases of clinical instability and peritonitis, surgical approach is required. The decision to dismantle or preserve colorectal anastomosis (with temporary ostomy) should be taken at the time of focus control procedure being highly depending on patient's and local peritoneal and anastomosis conditions.

D. Esophageal. Sepsis originated from esophageal source is a much less frequent event that intensivists and emergency department surgeons have to deal with. Nevertheless, esophageal elicited sepsis after spontaneous esophageal perforation (Boerhaave syndrome), postoperative leak, foreign body, or endoscopic perforation are of great concern with a relevant morbidity and mortality. Contained esophageal perforations or leaks are better managed conservatively with antibiotics, antifungals, and pleural drains as needed as long patients are stable without impending signs or biological parameters of sepsis [119]. Otherwise, overt and clinically relevant esophageal perforations, open surgical control of focus through left thoracotomy is the best judicious approach [119,120]. The usefulness of plastic/metallic covered stents in an otherwise stable patient without mediastinal or pleural involvement is a still debatable measure. Low quality of evidence substantiates that mainly plastic stents, present migration and a relatively high repositioning needs [121]. Such adverse events associated with the stents have fueled additional research to find alternative and less-invasive methods to contain esophageal leaks such as endoscopic vacuum system [122].

E. Gastroduodenal. Peritonitis from gastroduodenal origin has still its own spot early in the morning at the surgical meeting. Fresh and small perforated duodenal ulcer is best treated by laparoscopic-assisted intracorporeal suture closure. Nevertheless, postoperative morbidity has been associated when such procedure is made in a protracted peritonitis from large, chronic and/or friable peptic ulcers in an unstable patient. In these circumstances, quick and safe open repair through a conservative midline incision may suffice [66]. More difficult focus to deal with from gastroduodenal origin are periampullar post-ERCP perforation (mortality rate of 16%–18% [123]) and early leaking from duodenal stump after gastrectomy. Adequate severity assessment and a clear identification of the type of injury are critical to delineate the best treatment. Although conservative treatment may be suitable in a post-ERCP pneumoperitoneum in an otherwise stable patient, quick open laparotomy should be done in front of the evidence of acute abdomen or progression of SIRS (24, 25). Leaking from duodenal stump deserves early source control by an effective, large caliber draining device [124]. Because the consequences of a protracted IAI after bariatric surgery may be dismal, much attention has been paid recently to early detect and treat (either laparoscopic or endoscopically) any initial form of leaking [125].

F. Pancreatic. *Infected pancreatic necrosis*: The entity that probably better represents the evolution that has occurred during the recent years in the nonsurgical drainage of abdominal and retroperitoneal sepsis approach is infected pancreatic necrosis. Early surgical debridement, by means of laparotomy and wide necrosectomy, has traditionally been associated with high morbidity and mortality, digestive fistulas, ostomies, incisional hernias, and endocrine and exocrine pancreatic insufficiency [126,127]. Nowadays, it is recommended to delay the surgical control of the focus for at least four weeks if possible by performing the least aggressive approach, to allow a hemodynamic and nutritional stabilization and an adequate demarcation (walled-off) of the necrotic tissue. The step-up approach is proposed as the first alternative when there is suspicion of infected necrosis. Such planned delay also applies for percutaneous and or endoscopic focus control as recently published RCT clearly demonstrated that early placement of catheter drainage was associated with a significantly increased need of additional drainage interventions [128].

The first step is antibiotic treatment, followed by percutaneous drainage [25,129], and if the septic condition is not controlled, a retroperitoneal necrosectomy should be performed. This lately approach can be done by video-assisted retroperitoneoscopy [130,131], transgastric endoscopy [126], or transabdominal laparoscopy [132], leaving open necrosectomy for the rare cases of previous steps failure [130]. With such minimally invasive approach, a 30% reduction in the number of laparotomies and classic complications such as perforation of the hollow viscus, enterocutaneous fistula, hemorrhage, and multiorgan failure has been described [129].

G. Small bowel. Peritonitis due to small bowel focus is not uncommon. The main entities related are those associated with bowel obstruction, blunt trauma, injuries for foreign bodies, diverticular perforation, protracted mesenteric ischemia, and intraoperative undetected bowel injury, mainly during laparoscopic procedure or aesthetic liposuction [133].

It is a universal belief that segmental resection and primary anastomosis are the best focus controls once the peritoneal cavity has firstly cleared from purulent liquid. Nevertheless, in some circumstances, primary anastomosis should be withheld until peritoneal compartment, bowel edema, and general patient's condition improve. In such circumstances, the principles of damage control-OA technique should prevail [62] (Table 21.2).

Severe Skin and Soft Tissue Infections

Although seldomly represented at the ICU, patients with severe SSTIs deserve a brief discussion regarding the general management and the specific tactics of

TABLE 21.2

Degree of Quality of Peritonitis Focus Control From Different Organ-specific Infection Source

| Type | Quality | | |
	Accepted or Adequate	Risky or Inadequate	Difficult
Gastroduodenal	Perforated duodenal ulcus: OPEN: Simple closure LAP: Simple closure in fresh, small, and nonfriable ulcus	Perforated duodenal ulcus: LAP: Simple closure in protracted, large and friable ulcus	Postoperative leak of duodenal stump
Hepato-bilio-pancreatic	Perforated cholecystitis: OPEN or LAP cholecystectomy in stable patient OPEN partial cholecystectomy in patient with shock and/or sepsis related intraoperative coagulopathy	Perforated cholecystitis: LAP complete cholecystectomy in patient with shock and/or sepsis-related intraoperative coagulopathy	Infected pancreatic necrosis
Appendix	Perforated appendicitis: OPEN appendectomy LAP appendectomy	Perforated appendicitis: LAP long duration, diffuse peritonitis in patient in septic shock	Perforated appendix with diffuse peritonitis in a patient with previous abdominal surgery and peritoneal adhesions
Small bowel	Resection and primary anastomosis in stable patient Temporary stoma or damage control OA in an edematous intestine with ACS	Resection and primary anastomosis in patient with septic shock or in a long-standing perforation with edematous intestine and abdominal hypertension	Mesenteric ischemia
Colorectal	OPEN hartmann procedure OPEN/LAP resection and primary anastomosis in stable patient	LAP washout in perforated hinchey III diverticulitis OPEN resection and primary anastomosis in fecaloid peritonitis and/or in septic shock	Mesenteric ischemia. Fecaloid peritonitis

source control. The percentage of patients with severe SSTI admitted to the ICU ranges from 4.3% to 14.7% [1,2,7]. The most frequently involved entities are necrotizing cellulitis and necrotizing fasciitis and myonecrosis. Different types of classifications have been proposed although none of them have been universally accepted. Nevertheless, we can empirically classify such potentially severe infections taking into account both the anatomical space involved and the main responsible microorganisms (Table 21.3). Characteristically, necrotizing infections encompass different entities usually seen in a previously debilitated patients (although healthy patients may also be infected). Poly-monomicrobial [134] and fungal infections [135] have been described. Also, more specific professional-related pathogens have been involved [136–138]. NF

use to progress rapidly. Initial nonspecific signs and symptoms include disproportionate pain over a skin area with initially middle inflammatory signs and a worrisome hematological and biological laboratory profile. The key point of treatment (along with an early and adequate antibiotic treatment) is to perform an early surgical exploration to anticipate an obvious disseminated necrotic infection. Multidisciplinary approach is also mandatory, and coordinated actions between emergency physicians (early recognition and empirical antibiotic treatment), intensivists/anesthesiologists (pre- and postoperative treatment and resuscitation), and consultation to different surgical specialties (orthopedic, vascular, general, or head and neck surgeons depending on the anatomical region involved) are needed [134].

TABLE 21.3

Main Severe Skin and Soft Tissue Infections: Characteristics, Microbiology and Challenges of Focus Control

Type of SSTI	Characteristics	Microbiology	FOCUS Control Challenge
Necrotizing cellulitis	Necrotizing cellulitis: Postoperative or posttraumatic injury. Skin and subcutaneous tissue necrosis, deeper fascia, and muscle are preserved	Mixed flora: *Bacteroides* spp., gram-positive bacteria, enterobacteriaceae, *Clostridium* spp.	Wide surgical excision beyond the necrotic area. Be prepared for planned reexcision
	Cracking cellulitis: Mainly incisional abdominal wound infections and in diabetic foot. Usually no evidence of skin infections	*Clostridium* spp. and *E. coli*.	
	Synergistic Meleney's gangrene	Synergistic infections with streptococcus and *Staphylococcus* ± gram-negative bacteria	
Fascia and muscle necrotizing infections			
Polymicrobial	Fournier's gangrene: Protracted perineal infection from anal abscess or prostate infections	Anaerobes (*Bacteroides* spp., *Streptococcus* spp ± *Enterobacteriacea* ± *Enterococcus* spp.) *Clostridium* spp.	Early diagnosis is critical Disproportionate pain and systemic derangement with initial skin benign appearance Rapid progression High index of suspicion should elicit rapid surgical exploration, before clinically apparent necrotizing infection. Early and effective surgical debridement may be both diagnostic and therapeutic. Planned redebridement is always needed Negative pressure wound therapy has proved useful. Nevertheless, such therapy should not interfere with daily wound assessment. Graft and reconstructive surgery may be also needed.
	Wound infection in dirty surgery, inadequate focus control of peritonitis, and posttraumatic unnoticed bowel injury		
	Cervicofacial infections	*Peptostreptococcus* spp.	

TABLE 21.3

Main Severe Skin and Soft Tissue Infections: Characteristics, Microbiology and Challenges of Focus Control—cont'd

Type of SSTI	Characteristics	Microbiology	FOCUS Control Challenge
Monomicrobial	Limb and thoracic infections in both fragile and in otherwise previously healthy patients	*Streptococcus pyogenes* alone or associated with *Staphylococcus aureus*	
	Wound contaminated with brackish water or shellfish ingestion More frequent in fragile with immunosuppression diseases but also in previously healthy patients. Cirrhosis as a predisposing factor	*Vibrio* spp. or *Aeromonas* spp.	
Invasive fungal infections	Invasive and angioinvasive fungal infections mostly in a previously debilitated and/or immunocompromised/ immunosuppressed patients	*Mucor* spp.	Early tissue biopsy and cultures are critical First wide debridement is needed Deep seated protracted invasion may include neural and vessel involvement precluding limb salvage surgery

Urinary Tract Infections

Urosepsis represents 9%—31% [139] of the total cases of sepsis and may be community-acquired or healthcare-associated infections. Mortality rates associated with sepsis are highly dependent on the source of infection. In general, elicited UTI sepsis shows a relative lower mortality (from 20% to 40%) compared with other focus of sepsis [140].

Although sepsis is more common in men than in women, UTI (and therefore urosepsis) is more frequent in women. However, all UTI in male patients should be listed as complicated UTI (cUTI) and should be ultimately treated according to the risk that entails.

Type of severe urinary tract infections: obstructive pyelonephritis

Severity of urosepsis depends on both the host response and local factors. Elderly as well immunocompromised patients are more likely to develop urosepsis than young immunocompetent ones. Also, the presence of calculi, urinary obstruction, and congenital urinary tract defects are common risk factors associated with urosepsis.

Although all patients may be susceptible to acquire UTI, there are different risk factors associated with cUTI [141]. Given its high mortality rate, subsequent neurological and cognitive sequelae, and the costs of increased hospitalization [142], patients with risk for cUTI—and further progression to urosepsis—should be promptly and rigorously recognized (Table 21.4) [141].

Escherichia coli, Proteus spp., *Klebsiella* spp., *Pseudomonas* spp., *Serratia* spp., *and Enterococcus* spp. are the most common species involved [141]. Organisms isolated from patients with cUTI and urosepsis tend to be more resistant to antibiotics than strains isolated in uncomplicated UTI [143].

Appropriate management of the underlying complicating factor is mandatory. Optimal antimicrobial therapy for cUTI depends on local resistance patterns and specific host factors (allergies, kidney function). Urine culture and susceptibility testing should be performed and initial empirical therapy should be tailored on the basis of the host's risk factors and predominant flora and the antibiotic resistance pattern of the area.

Management of obstructive pyelonephritis: from the adequate early diagnosis to on-time focus control

It is important to reinforce the concept that patients with an initially stable UTI may develop a severe urosepsis in a relatively short period of time [144].

TABLE 21.4
Common Risk Factors for Complicated Urinary Tract Infection and Potential Preventive Measures

Generic Factors	Preventive Measures
Male sex	Urinary tract infection in men is considered complicated by definition, thus short courses of antimicrobial therapy should be avoided
Pregnancy	Treatment of asymptomatic bacteriuria
Diabetes mellitus	Adequate blood glucose control
Immunosuppression	Anticipate to overt UTI
Multiple resistant bacteria colonization	Adherence to the antibiotic stewardship programs
Healthcare-associated infections	Proper guidelines for preventive measures of hospital-acquired infections
URINARY TRACT—RELATED INFECTIONS	
Obstruction of urinary tract Upper urinary tract: Obstructive pyelonephritis Lower urinary tract: Acute prostatitis	Proper management of benign prostate hyperplasia and neurogenic bladder at the primary care or urologist office setting
Incomplete voiding	
Congenital or functional malformations	Early detection, follow-up in specialized units if necessary
Neurogenic bladder	
Foreign body (indwelling catheter, nephrostomy, bladder calculi)	Assessment of indication and on time removal of bladder catheter
Recent history of instrumentation/urologic or gynecologic operations (whangehermer, 2008)	Adequate follow-up after instrumentation or surgical procedure

Initial assessment is critical to clearly identify patients at risk. Then, pragmatic and easy to run sepsis scores should be employed at the emergency department. Although SIRS has been recently criticized and

is no longer included in the grading of sepsis in some guidelines, alerting symptoms such as fever-hypothermia, leukocytosis-leukopenia, tachycardia, and tachypnea are sensitive enough to anticipate an impending sepsis and should always be taken into consideration. Although quick-SOFA score is easy to apply, some parameters (hypotension) may appear later on in a fully consolidated process. More complex scores such as SOFA are also useful once the patient has been admitted and fully evaluated [141,142]. A SOFA score of 2 or higher has an overall mortality risk of approximately 10% [145].

Urine, blood cultures, and if appropriate, drainage fluids microbiological cultures should be taken right away.

As the most common cause of urosepsis is obstruction (78% of men and 54% of women [Hotchkiss, 2003 #118]), US or CT scan should be performed early on. US of kidney, bladder, and prostate is the fastest method for examining the urogenital tract. In 93% of cases, US is able to detect kidney dilation and prostatic abscesses, among other urosepsis causes. However, US sensitivity is highly operator-dependent and is not always available (24 h/day, 7 d/week) in all centers [146]. Then, if urosepsis is suspected and US is not available—or unable to show a reasonable cause—a CT scan should be carried out (Fig. 21.2).

Once diagnosis is established, treatment should be expeditiously initiated, including vital support, empirical antibiotic therapy [142], taking into account the principles of antibiotic treatment adequacy. In parallel, without additional delay, surgical management of the associated urological pathology should be initiated as soon as possible. Surgical treatment is a priority, and it has to be done fast and as minimally invasive as possible. That means that the treatment of the underlying cause is not recommended (lithiasis or tumor) in order to avoid prolonged operative time, anesthesia, secondary bacteremia, bleeding, and possible intraoperative incidents [142].

Drainage of upper urinary tract obstruction can be done externally (percutaneous nephrostomy) or internally (double ureteral stent J) at the urologist criteria [142]. Urologists used to avoid internal drainage (ureteral stent) when the obstruction is caused by a neoplasm of the urinary tract in order to avoid further spreading of infection. Otherwise, percutaneous nephrostomy can be a wise option as long as the coagulation status of the patient allows it.

It is sensible to consider that a septic patient with any kind of dilatation in the urinary tract (without other reasonable cause of sepsis) has a unilateral (more

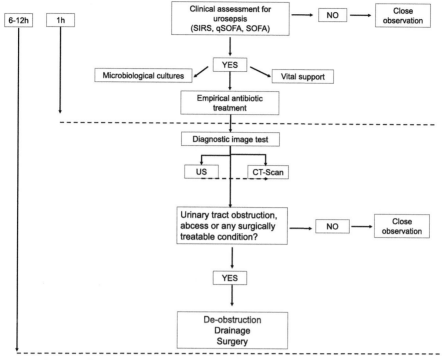

FIG. 21.2 Decision algorithm to manage potential serious urinary tract infections.

common in obstructive pyelonephritis) or bilateral urinary tract obstruction (suggesting lower urinary tract obstruction secondary to acute prostatitis, for instance) being these patients able to benefit from adequate drainage.

The degree of urinary tract dilatation is not proportional to the severity of the sepsis. However, if the clinicians are in front of a critically septic patient and the imaging study, usually a US, shows little to no dilatation; it is prudent both to reconsider the cause of the sepsis and to order further imaging studies (CT scan). In the absence of an alternative cause, when dealing with a scarcely urinary tract dilatation, drainage of urinary tract usually improves patient's condition. Additionally, in patients with acute prostatitis (lower urinary tract obstruction), it might be adequate to perform a cystostomy to avoid urethral manipulation [142]. Fig. 21.2 depicts comprehensive management of patients with urosepsis.

Thoracic Infections

Empyema is a common thoracic surgery presentation defined as pus in the pleural space. The most common precursor of empyema is bacterial pneumonia and subsequent parapneumonic effusion. Out of 20%–40% of hospitalized patients with pneumonia have parapneumonic effusion, and 5%–10% of these parapneumonic effusions will progress to empyema. Despite the commonality of empyema, consensus on initial management remains ambiguous. Two standard treatment options include inserting a chest tube and the administration of intrapleural fibrinolytics or an initial surgical approach, with surgical decortication. Because of the complexity of pleural space infection, repeated procedures are often required in order to achieve adequate source control.

Ideally, tube thoracostomy must be placed by image-guided US. Such guides insertion decreases the complication rate (pneumothorax, infection, procedure failure, and intercostal bleeding), compared with a blind chest tube insertion [147]. Intrapleural fibrinolytics agents are also required on empyema management. An RCT demonstrated the usefulness of intrapleural fibrinolytics for the treatment of pleural empyema, establishing the combination for t-PA and DNase as the gold standard therapy when fibrinolytics are employed [148].

Surgical decortication is another commonly accepted standard of practice. This includes the removal of the thick fibrous peel of an empyema, suctioning of pus, washout of the pleural space, and chest tube placement. Typically, this can be accomplished with a minimally invasive approach using small intercostal incisions (video-assisted thoracoscopic surgery, VATS). A Cochrane Systematic Review of eight trials examining treatment methods for empyema demonstrated similar complication rates between VATS decortication and chest tube drainage with a decreased length of hospital stay in VATS-treated patients [149]. Additionally, a recent study from the United States using the New York State Inpatient Database examined 4095 patients with a diagnosis of empyema. Patients who received a chest tube compared with those who underwent an initial surgical approach had higher mortality and higher readmission rate, lending support that an initial surgical approach for empyema is warranted [150].

Ongoing RCT comparing VATS with thoracostomy as an initial treatment of empyema will provide further insights on empyema management [151].

REFERENCES

[1] Kumar A, Roberts D, Wood KE, Light B, Parrillo JE, Sharma S, et al. Duration of hypotension before initiation of effective antimicrobial therapy is the critical determinant of survival in human septic shock. Crit Care Med 2006;34(6):1589–96.

[2] Alberti C, Brun-Buisson C, Burchardi H, Martin C, Goodman S, Artigas A, et al. Epidemiology of sepsis and infection in ICU patients from an international multicentre cohort study. Intensive Care Med 2002; 28(2):108–21.

[3] Paary TT, Kalaiselvan MS, Renuka MK, Arunkumar AS. Clinical profile and outcome of patients with severe sepsis treated in an intensive care unit in India. Ceylon Med J 2016;61(4):181–4.

[4] Jeganathan N, Yau S, Ahuja N, Otu D, Stein B, Fogg L, et al. The characteristics and impact of source of infection on sepsis-related ICU outcomes. J Crit Care 2017; 41:170–6.

[5] Ullah AR, Hussain A, Ali I, Samad A, Ali Shah ST, Yousef M, et al. A prospective observational study assessing the outcome of Sepsis in intensive care unit of a tertiary care hospital. Peshawar. Pak J Med Sci. 2016;32(3):688–93.

[6] Kumar A, Ellis P, Arabi Y, Roberts D, Light B, Parrillo JE, et al. Initiation of inappropriate antimicrobial therapy results in a fivefold reduction of survival in human septic shock. Chest 2009;136(5):1237–48.

[7] Loftus TJ, Wu Q, Wang Z, Lysak N, Moore FA, Bihorac A, et al. Delayed interhospital transfer of critically ill patients with surgical sepsis. J Trauma Acute Care Surg 2020;88(1):169–75.

[8] Barie P, Hydo L, Eachempati S. Longitudinal outcomes of intra-abdominal infection complicated by critical illness. Surg Infect 2004;5(4):365–73.

[9] Montravers P, Lepape A, Dubreuil L, Gauzit R, Pean Y, Benchimol D, Dupont H. Clinical and microbiolocal profiles and community-acquired and nosocomial intra-abdominal infections:reults of the French prospective, observational EBIIA study. J Antimicrob Chemother 2009;63(4):785–94.

[10] Farthmann E, Schöffel U. Epidemiology and pathophysiology of IAI. Infection 1998;26(5):329–34.

[11] Biondo S, Ramos E, Deiros M, Rague JM, De Oca J, Moreno P, et al. Prognostic factors for mortality in left colonic peritonitis: a new scoring system. J Am Coll Surg 2000;191(6):635–42.

[12] Inui T, Haridas M, Claridge JA, Malangoni MA. Mortality for intra-abdominal infection is associated with intrinsic risk factors rather than the source of infection. Surgery 2009;146(4):654–61. discussion 61-2.

[13] Rhodes A, Evans LE, Alhazzani W, Levy MM, Antonelli M, Ferrer R, et al. Surviving sepsis campaign: international guidelines for management of sepsis and septic shock: 2016. Intensive Care Med 2017;43(3): 304–77.

[14] Sartelli M, Chichom-Mefire A, Labricciosa FM, Hardcastle T, Abu-Zidan FM, Adesunkanmi AK, et al. The management of intra-abdominal infections from a global perspective: 2017 WSES guidelines for management of intra-abdominal infections. World J Emerg Surg 2017;12:29.

[15] Leppaniemi A, Kimball EJ, De Laet I, Malbrain ML, Balogh ZJ, De Waele JJ. Management of abdominal sepsis—a paradigm shift? Anaesthesiol Intensive Ther 2015;47(4):400–8.

[16] Solomkin JS, Mazuski JE, Bradley JS, Rodvold KA, Goldstein EJ, Baron EJ, et al. Diagnosis and management of complicated intra-abdominal infection in adults and children: guidelines by the Surgical Infection Society and the Infectious Diseases Society of America. Clin Infect Dis 2010;50(2):133–64.

[17] Seiler CA, Brugger L, Forssmann U, Baer HU, Buchler MW. Conservative surgical treatment of diffuse peritonitis. Surgery 2000;127(2):178–84.

[18] Ditillo MF, Dziura JD, Rabinovici R. Is it safe to delay appendectomy in adults with acute appendicitis? Ann Surg 2006;244(5):656–60.

[19] Busch M, Gutzwiller FS, Aellig S, Kuettel R, Metzger U, Zingg U. In-hospital delay increases the risk of perforation in adults with appendicitis. World J Surg 2011; 35(7):1626–33.

[20] De Waele JJ. Early source control in sepsis. Langenbeck's Arch Surg 2010;395(5):489–94.

[21] Marshall JC, Maier RV, Jimenez M, Dellinger EP. Source control in the management of severe sepsis and septic shock: an evidence-based review. Crit Care Med 2004; 32(11 Suppl. l):S513–26.

[22] Azuhata T, Kinoshita K, Kawano D, Komatsu T, Sakurai A, Chiba Y, et al. Time from admission to initiation of surgery for source control is a critical determinant of survival in patients with gastrointestinal

perforation with associated septic shock. Crit Care 2014; 18(3):R87.

[23] Avgerinos DV, Llaguna OH, Lo AY, Voli J, Leitman IM. Management of endoscopic retrograde cholangiopancreatography: related duodenal perforations. Surg Endosc 2009;23(4):833–8.

[24] Stapfer M, Selby RR, Stain SC, Katkhouda N, Parekh D, Jabbour N, et al. Management of duodenal perforation after endoscopic retrograde cholangiopancreatography and sphincterotomy. Ann Surg 2000;232(2):191–8.

[25] van Santvoort HC, Besselink MG, Bakker OJ, Hofker HS, Boermeester MA, Dejong CH, et al. A step-up approach or open necrosectomy for necrotizing pancreatitis. N Engl J Med 2010;362(16):1491–502.

[26] Boyer A, Vargas F, Coste F, Saubusse E, Castaing Y, Gbikpi-Benissan G, et al. Influence of surgical treatment timing on mortality from necrotizing soft tissue infections requiring intensive care management. Intensive Care Med 2009;35(5):847–53.

[27] Wong CH, Chang HC, Pasupathy S, Khin LW, Tan JL, Low CO. Necrotizing fasciitis: clinical presentation, microbiology, and determinants of mortality. J Bone Joint Surg Am 2003;85(8):1454–60.

[28] Kabir SA, Kabir SI, Sun R, Jafferbhoy S, Karim A. How to diagnose an acutely inflamed appendix; a systematic review of the latest evidence. Int J Surg 2017;40:155–62.

[29] Tang B, Eslick G, Craig J, McLean A. Accuracy of procalcitonin for sepsis diagnosis in critically ill patients: systematic review and meta-analysis. Lancet Infect Dis 2007;7:210–7.

[30] Kaukonen KM, Bailey M, Bellomo R. Systemic inflammatory response syndrome criteria for severe sepsis. N Engl J Med 2015;373(9):881.

[31] Howell MD, Donnino M, Clardy P, Talmor D, Shapiro NI. Occult hypoperfusion and mortality in patients with suspected infection. Intensive Care Med 2007;33(11):1892–9.

[32] Mikkelsen ME, Miltiades AN, Gaieski DF, Goyal M, Fuchs BD, Shah CV, et al. Serum lactate is associated with mortality in severe sepsis independent of organ failure and shock. Crit Care Med 2009;37(5):1670–7.

[33] Haanschoten MC, Kreeftenberg HG, Arthur Bouwman R, van Straten AH, Buhre WF, Soliman Hamad MA. Use of postoperative peak arterial lactate level to predict outcome after cardiac surgery. J Cardiothorac Vasc Anesth 2017;31(1):45–53.

[34] Creagh-Brown BC, De Silva AP, Ferrando-Vivas P, Harrison DA. Relationship between peak lactate and patient outcome following high-risk gastrointestinal surgery: influence of the nature of their surgery: elective versus emergency. Crit Care Med 2016;44(5):918–25.

[35] Ip B, Ng KT, Packer S, Paterson-Brown S, Couper GW. High serum lactate as an adjunct in the early prediction of anastomotic leak following oesophagectomy. Int J Surg 2017;46:7–10.

[36] Juvany M, Guirao X, Oliva JC, Badia Perez JM. Role of combined post-operative venous lactate and 48 hours C-reactive protein values on the etiology and predictive

capacity of organ-space surgical site infection after elective colorectal operation. Surg Infect 2017;18(3):311–8.

[37] Velickovic J, Palibrk I, Milicic B, Velickovic D, Jovanovic B, Rakic G, et al. The association of early postoperative lactate levels with morbidity after elective major abdominal surgery. Bosn J Basic Med Sci 2019;19(1):72–80.

[38] Giglio MT, Marucci M, Testini M, Brienza N. Goal-directed haemodynamic therapy and gastrointestinal complications in major surgery: a meta-analysis of randomized controlled trials. Br J Anaesth 2009;103(5):637–46.

[39] Claeys R, Vinken S, Spapen H, ver Elst K, Decochez K, Huyghens L, et al. Plasma procalcitonin and C-reactive protein in acute septic shock: clinical and biological correlates. Crit Care Med 2002;30(4):757–62.

[40] Beliaev AM, Marshall RJ, Booth M. C-reactive protein has a better discriminative power than white cell count in the diagnosis of acute cholecystitis. J Surg Res 2015; 198(1):66–72.

[41] Lameris W, van Randen A, van Gulik TM, Busch OR, Winkelhagen J, Bossuyt PM, et al. A clinical decision rule to establish the diagnosis of acute diverticulitis at the emergency department. Dis Colon Rectum 2010; 53(6):896–904.

[42] Guirao X, Juvany M, Franch G, Navinés J, Amador S, Badia J. Value of C-reactive protein in the assessment of organ-space surgical site infections after elective oepn and laparoscopic colorectal surgery. Surg Infect 2013;14(2):209–15.

[43] Singh PP, Zeng IS, Srinivasa S, Lemanu DP, Connolly AB, Hill AG. Systematic review and meta-analysis of use of serum C-reactive protein levels to predict anastomotic leak after colorectal surgery. Br J Surg 2014;101(4):339–46.

[44] Cousin F, Ortega-Deballon P, Bourredjem A, Doussot A, Giaccaglia V, Fournel I. Diagnostic accuracy of procalcitonin and C-reactive protein for the early diagnosis of intra-abdominal infection after elective colorectal surgery: a meta-analysis. Ann Surg 2016;264(2):252–6.

[45] Bona D, Micheletto G, Bonitta G, Panizzo V, Cavalli M, Rausa E, et al. Does C-reactive protein have a predictive role in the early diagnosis of postoperative complications after bariatric surgery? Systematic review and bayesian meta-analysis. Obes Surg 2019;29(11):3448–56.

[46] Lee Y, McKechnie T, Doumouras AG, Handler C, Eskicioglu C, Gmora S, et al. Diagnostic value of C-reactive protein levels in postoperative infectious complications after bariatric surgery: a systematic review and meta-analysis. Obes Surg 2019;29(7):2022–9.

[47] Lameris W, van Randen A, van Es HW, van Heesewijk JP, van Ramshorst B, Bouma WH, et al. Imaging strategies for detection of urgent conditions in patients with acute abdominal pain: diagnostic accuracy study. BMJ 2009; 338:b2431.

[48] Mazuski JE, Tessier JM, May AK, Sawyer RG, Nadler EP, Rosengart MR, et al. The surgical infection society

revised guidelines on the management of intra-abdominal infection. Surg Infect 2017;18(1):1–76.

[49] Baron EJ, Miller JM, Weinstein MP, Richter SS, Gilligan PH, Thomson Jr RB, et al. A guide to utilization of the microbiology laboratory for diagnosis of infectious diseases: 2013 recommendations by the Infectious Diseases Society of America (IDSA) and the American Society for Microbiology (ASM)(a). Clin Infect Dis 2013;57(4):e22–121.

[50] Bohmer R, Byrne P, Maddern G. A peeling mesh. Hernia 2002;6:86–7.

[51] Akinci D, Akhan O, Ozmen MN, Karabulut N, Ozkan O, Cil BE, et al. Percutaneous drainage of 300 intraperitoneal abscesses with long-term follow-up. Cardiovasc Intervent Radiol 2005;28(6):744–50.

[52] Theisen J, Bartels H, Weiss W, Berger H, Stein HJ, Siewert JR. Current concepts of percutaneous abscess drainage in postoperative retention. J Gastrointest Surg 2005;9(2):280–3.

[53] Mehendiratta V, McCarty BC, Gomez L, Graviss EA, Musher DM. Computerized tomography (CT)-guided aspiration of abscesses: outcome of therapy at a tertiary care hospital. J Infect 2007;54(2):122–8.

[54] Felder SI, Barmparas G, Murrell Z, Fleshner P. Risk factors for failure of percutaneous drainage and need for reoperation following symptomatic gastrointestinal anastomotic leak. Am J Surg 2014;208(1):58–64.

[55] Maher MM, Gervais DA, Kalra MK, Lucey B, Sahani DV, Arellano R, et al. The inaccessible or undrainable abscess: how to drain it. Radiographics 2004;24(3):717–35.

[56] Harisinghani MG, Gervais DA, Hahn PF, Cho CH, Jhaveri K, Varghese J, et al. CT-guided transgluteal drainage of deep pelvic abscesses: indications, technique, procedure-related complications, and clinical outcome. Radiographics 2002;22(6):1353–67.

[57] Robert B, Chivot C, Rebibo L, Sabbagh C, Regimbeau JM, Yzet T. Percutaneous transgluteal drainage of pelvic abscesses in interventional radiology: a safe alternative to surgery. J Vis Surg 2016;153(1):3–7.

[58] Maca J, Peteja M, Reimer P, Jor O, Sedenkova V, Panackova L, et al. Surgical injury: comparing open surgery and laparoscopy by markers of tissue damage. Therapeut Clin Risk Manag 2018;14:999–1006.

[59] Biondo S, Pares D, Marti Rague J, De Oca J, Toral D, Borobia FG, et al. Emergency operations for nondiverticular perforation of the left colon. Am J Surg 2002;183(3):256–60.

[60] Anaya DA, Nathens AB. Risk factors for severe sepsis in secondary peritonitis. Surg Infect 2003;4(4):355–62.

[61] van Ruler O, Mahler CW, Boer KR, Reuland EA, Gooszen HG, Opmeer BC, et al. Comparison of on-demand vs planned relaparotomy strategy in patients with severe peritonitis: a randomized trial. JAMA 2007;298(8):865–72.

[62] Sartelli M, Abu-Zidan FM, Ansaloni L, Bala M, Beltran MA, Biffl WL, et al. The role of the open abdomen procedure in managing severe abdominal

sepsis: WSES position paper. World J Emerg Surg 2015;10:35.

[63] Adkins AL, Robbins J, Villalba M, Bendick P, Shanley CJ. Open abdomen management of intra-abdominal sepsis. Am Surg 2004;70(2):137–40. discussion 40.

[64] Atema JJ, Gans SL, Boermeester MA. Systematic review and meta-analysis of the open abdomen and temporary abdominal closure techniques in non-trauma patients. World J Surg 2015;39(4):912–25.

[65] Kirkpatrick AW, Coccolini F, Ansaloni L, Roberts DJ, Tolonen M, McKee JL, et al. Closed or open after source control laparotomy for severe complicated intra-abdominal sepsis (the COOL trial): study protocol for a randomized controlled trial. World J Emerg Surg 2018;13:26.

[66] Soreide K, Thorsen K, Soreide JA. Strategies to improve the outcome of emergency surgery for perforated peptic ulcer. Br J Surg 2014;101(1):e51–64.

[67] Coldrey E. Five years of conservative treatment of acute appendicitis. J Int Coll Surg 1959;32:255–61.

[68] Hansson J, Korner U, Khorram-Manesh A, Solberg A, Lundholm K. Randomized clinical trial of antibiotic therapy versus appendicectomy as primary treatment of acute appendicitis in unselected patients. Br J Surg 2009;96(5):473–81.

[69] Vons C, Barry C, Maitre S, Pautrat K, Leconte M, Costaglioli B, et al. Amoxicillin plus clavulanic acid versus appendicectomy for treatment of acute uncomplicated appendicitis: an open-label, non-inferiority, randomised controlled trial. Lancet 2011;377(9777):1573–9.

[70] Salminen P, Tuominen R, Paajanen H, Rautio T, Nordstrom P, Aarnio M, et al. Five-year follow-up of antibiotic therapy for uncomplicated acute appendicitis in the APPAC randomized clinical trial. JAMA 2018;320(12):1259–65.

[71] Huston JM, Kao LS, Chang PK, Sanders JM, Buckman S, Adams CA, et al. Antibiotics vs. Appendectomy for acute uncomplicated appendicitis in adults: review of the evidence and future directions. Surg Infect 2017;18(5):527–35.

[72] Sakran JV, Mylonas KS, Gryparis A, Stawicki SP, Burns CJ, Matar MM, et al. Operation versus antibiotics–The "appendicitis conundrum" continues: a meta-analysis. J Trauma Acute Care Surg 2017;82(6):1129–37.

[73] Podda M, Cillara N, Di Saverio S, Lai A, Feroci F, Luridiana G, et al. Antibiotics-first strategy for uncomplicated acute appendicitis in adults is associated with increased rates of peritonitis at surgery. A systematic review with meta-analysis of randomized controlled trials comparing appendectomy and non-operative management with antibiotics. Surgeon 2017;15(5):303–14.

[74] Sauerland S, Jaschinski T, Neugebauer EA. Laparoscopic versus open surgery for suspected appendicitis. Cochrane Database Syst Rev 2010;10:CD001546.

[75] Tuggle KR, Ortega G, Bolorunduro OB, Oyetunji TA, Alexander R, Turner PL, et al. Laparoscopic versus

open appendectomy in complicated appendicitis: a review of the NSQIP database. J Surg Res 2010;163(2): 225—8.

[76] Athanasiou C, Lockwood S, Markides GA. Systematic review and meta-analysis of laparoscopic versus open appendicectomy in adults with complicated appendicitis: an update of the literature. World J Surg 2017;41(12): 3083—99.

[77] Yu MC, Feng YJ, Wang W, Fan W, Cheng HT, Xu J. Is laparoscopic appendectomy feasible for complicated appendicitis ?A systematic review and meta-analysis. Int J Surg 2017;40:187—97.

[78] Korndorffer Jr JR, Fellinger E, Reed W. SAGES guideline for laparoscopic appendectomy. Surg Endosc 2010; 24(4):757—61.

[79] Di Saverio S, Podda M, De Simone B, Ceresoli M, Augustin G, Gori A, et al. Diagnosis and treatment of acute appendicitis: 2020 update of the WSES Jerusalem guidelines. World J Emerg Surg 2020;15(1):27.

[80] Ansaloni L, Pisano M, Coccolini F, Peitzmann AB, Fingerhut A, Catena F, et al. 2016 WSES guidelines on acute calculous cholecystitis. World J Emerg Surg 2016; 11:25.

[81] Papi C, Catarci M, D'Ambrosio L, Gili L, Koch M, Grassi GB, et al. Timing of cholecystectomy for acute calculous cholecystitis: a meta-analysis. Am J Gastroenterol 2004;99(1):147—55.

[82] Gurusamy KS, Davidson C, Gluud C, Davidson BR. Early versus delayed laparoscopic cholecystectomy for people with acute cholecystitis. Cochrane Database Syst Rev 2013;(6):CD005440.

[83] Wilson E, Gurusamy K, Gluud C, Davidson BR. Cost-utility and value-of-information analysis of early versus delayed laparoscopic cholecystectomy for acute cholecystitis. Br J Surg 2010;97(2):210—9.

[84] Okamoto K, Suzuki K, Takada T, Strasberg SM, Asbun HJ, Endo I, et al. Tokyo Guidelines 2018: flowchart for the management of acute cholecystitis. J Hepatobiliary Pancreat Sci 2018;25(1):55—72.

[85] Bingener J, Richards ML, Schwesinger WH, Strodel WE, Sirinek KR. Laparoscopic cholecystectomy for elderly patients: gold standard for golden years? Arch Surg 2003; 138(5):531—5. discussion 5-6.

[86] Gomes CA, Junior CS, Di Saverio S, Sartelli M, Kelly MD, Gomes CC, et al. Acute calculous cholecystitis: review of current best practices. World J Gastrointest Surg 2017; 9(5):118—26.

[87] Borzellino G, Khuri S, Pisano M, Mansour S, Allievi N, Ansaloni L, et al. Timing of early laparoscopic cholecystectomy for acute calculous cholecystitis: a meta-analysis of randomized clinical trials. World J Emerg Surg 2021; 16(1):16.

[88] Winbladh A, Gullstrand P, Svanvik J, Sandstrom P. Systematic review of cholecystostomy as a treatment option in acute cholecystitis. HPB 2009;11(3):183—93.

[89] Campanile FC, Catena F, Coccolini F, Lotti M, Piazzalunga D, Pisano M, et al. The need for new

"patient-related" guidelines for the treatment of acute cholecystitis. World J Emerg Surg 2011;6(1):44.

[90] Persson G. GallRiks. In: The Swedish register for gallstone surgery and ERCP; 2008 [Available from: http:// www.ucr.uu.se/gallriks/.

[91] de Mestral C, Rotstein OD, Laupacis A, Hoch JS, Zagorski B, Alali AS, et al. Comparative operative outcomes of early and delayed cholecystectomy for acute cholecystitis: a population-based propensity score analysis. Ann Surg 2014;259(1):10—5.

[92] Ganpathi IS, Diddapur RK, Eugene H, Karim M. Acute acalculous cholecystitis: challenging the myths. HPB 2007;9(2):131—4.

[93] Soria Aledo V, Galindo Iniguez L, Flores Funes D, Carrasco Prats M, Aguayo Albasini JL. Is cholecystectomy the treatment of choice for acute acalculous cholecystitis? A systematic review of the literature. Rev Esp Enferm Dig 2017;109(10):708—18.

[94] Rehman T, deBoisblanc BP. Persistent fever in the ICU. Chest 2014;145(1):158—65.

[95] Barie PS, Eachempati SR. Acute acalculous cholecystitis. Gastroenterol Clin N Am 2010;39(2):343—57 [x].

[96] Huffman JL, Schenker S. Acute acalculous cholecystitis: a review. Clin Gastroenterol Hepatol 2010;8(1):15—22.

[97] Kiriyama S, Kozaka K, Takada T, Strasberg SM, Pitt HA, Gabata T, et al. Tokyo Guidelines 2018: diagnostic criteria and severity grading of acute cholangitis (with videos). J Hepatobiliary Pancreat Sci 2018;25(1):17—30.

[98] Karvellas CJ, Abraldes JG, Zepeda-Gomez S, Moffat DC, Mirzanejad Y, Vazquez-Grande G, et al. The impact of delayed biliary decompression and anti-microbial therapy in 260 patients with cholangitis-associated septic shock. Aliment Pharmacol Ther 2016;44(7):755—66.

[99] Du L, Cen M, Zheng X, Luo L, Siddiqui A, Kim JJ. Timing of performing endoscopic retrograde cholangiopancreatography and inpatient mortality in acute cholangitis: a systematic review and meta-analysis. Clin Transl Gastroenterol 2020;11(3):e00158.

[100] Lai EC, Mok FP, Tan ES, Lo CM, Fan ST, You KT, et al. Endoscopic biliary drainage for severe acute cholangitis. N Engl J Med 1992;326(24):1582—6.

[101] Gigot JF, Leese T, Dereme T, Coutinho J, Castaing D, Bismuth H. Acute cholangitis. Multivariate analysis of risk factors. Ann Surg 1989;209(4):435—8.

[102] Sartelli M, Weber DG, Kluger Y, Ansaloni L, Coccolini F, Abu-Zidan F, et al. 2020 update of the WSES guidelines for the management of acute colonic diverticulitis in the emergency setting. World J Emerg Surg 2020;15(1):32.

[103] Vennix S, Musters GD, Mulder IM, Swank HA, Consten EC, Belgers EH, et al. Laparoscopic peritoneal lavage or sigmoidectomy for perforated diverticulitis with purulent peritonitis: a multicentre, parallel-group, randomised, open-label trial. Lancet 2015; 386(10000):1269—77.

[104] Schultz JK, Yaqub S, Wallon C, Blecic L, Forsmo HM, Folkesson J, et al. Laparoscopic lavage vs primary resection for acute perforated diverticulitis: the SCANDIV

randomized clinical trial. JAMA 2015;314(13): 1364–75.

[105] O'Leary DP, Myers E, O'Brien O, Andrews E, McCourt M, Redmond HP. Persistent perforation in non-faeculant diverticular peritonitis–incidence and clinical significance. J Gastrointest Surg 2013;17(2):369–73.

[106] Sneiders D, Lambrichts DPV, Swank HA, Blanken-Peeters C, Nienhuijs SW, Govaert M, et al. Long-term follow-up of a multicentre cohort study on laparoscopic peritoneal lavage for perforated diverticulitis. Colorectal Dis 2019;21(6):705–14.

[107] Angenete E, Thornell A, Burcharth J, Pommergaard HC, Skullman S, Bisgaard T, et al. Laparoscopic lavage is feasible and safe for the treatment of perforated diverticulitis with purulent peritonitis: the first results from the randomized controlled trial DILALA. Ann Surg 2016; 263(1):117–22.

[108] Bridoux V, Regimbeau JM, Ouaissi M, Mathonnet M, Mauvais F, Houivet E, et al. Hartmann's procedure or primary anastomosis for generalized peritonitis due to perforated diverticulitis: a prospective multicenter randomized trial (DIVERTI). J Am Coll Surg 2017;225(6): 798–805.

[109] Lambrichts DPV, Vennix S, Musters GD, Mulder IM, Swank HA, Hoofwijk AGM, et al. Hartmann's procedure versus sigmoidectomy with primary anastomosis for perforated diverticulitis with purulent or faecal peritonitis (LADIES): a multicentre, parallel-group, randomised, open-label, superiority trial. Lancet Gastroenterol Hepatol 2019;4(8):599–610.

[110] Trenti L, Biondo S, Golda T, Monica M, Kreisler E, Fraccalvieri D, et al. Generalized peritonitis due to perforated diverticulitis: hartmann's procedure or primary anastomosis? Int J Colorectal Dis 2011;26(3):377–84.

[111] Gasser E, Alexander P, Reich-Weinberger S, Buchner S, Kogler P, Zitt M, et al. Damage control surgery for perforated diverticulitis: a two center experience with two different abdominal negative pressure therapy devices. Acta Chir Belg 2019;119(6):370–5.

[112] Tartaglia D, Costa G, Camillo A, Castriconi M, Andreano M, Lanza M, et al. Damage control surgery for perforated diverticulitis with diffuse peritonitis: saves lives and reduces ostomy. World J Emerg Surg 2019;14:19.

[113] Sohn M, Iesalnieks I, Agha A, Steiner P, Hochrein A, Pratschke J, et al. Perforated diverticulitis with generalized peritonitis: low stoma rate using a "damage control strategy. World J Surg 2018;42(10):3189–95.

[114] Kafka-Ritsch R, Birkfellner F, Perathoner A, Raab H, Nehoda H, Pratschke J, et al. Damage control surgery with abdominal vacuum and delayed bowel reconstruction in patients with perforated diverticulitis Hinchey III/IV. J Gastrointest Surg 2012;16(10):1915–22.

[115] Perathoner A, Klaus A, Muhlmann G, Oberwalder M, Margreiter R, Kafka-Ritsch R. Damage control with abdominal vacuum therapy (VAC) to manage perforated diverticulitis with advanced generalized

peritonitis–a proof of concept. Int J Colorectal Dis 2010;25(6):767–74.

[116] Kafka-Ritsch R, Zitt M, Perathoner A, Gasser E, Kaufman C, Czipin S, et al. Prospectively randomized controlled trial on damage control surgery for perforated diverticulitis with generalized peritonitis. World J Surg 2020;44(12):4098–105.

[117] Waibel BH, Rotondo MF. Damage control for intra-abdominal sepsis. Surg Clin 2012;92(2):243–57 [viii].

[118] Dhindsa BS, Naga Y, Saghir SM, Daid SGS, Chandan S, Mashiana H, et al. Endo-sponge in management of anastomotic colorectal leaks: a systematic review and meta-analysis. Endosc Int Open 2021;9(9):E1342–9.

[119] Dent B, Griffin SM, Jones R, Wahed S, Immanuel A, Hayes N. Management and outcomes of anastomotic leaks after oesophagectomy. Br J Surg 2016;103(8):1033–8.

[120] Schweigert M, Beattie R, Solymosi N, Booth K, Dubecz A, Muir A, et al. Endoscopic stent insertion versus primary operative management for spontaneous rupture of the esophagus (Boerhaave syndrome): an international study comparing the outcome. Am Surg 2013;79(6):634–40.

[121] Kamarajah SK, Bundred J, Spence G, Kennedy A, Dasari BVM, Griffiths EA. Critical appraisal of the impact of oesophageal stents in the management of oesophageal anastomotic leaks and benign oesophageal perforations: an updated systematic review. World J Surg 2020; 44(4):1173–89.

[122] Thompson SK, Watson DI. We asked the experts: "to stent or not to stent... What is the best management of an esophageal leak or benign perforation? World J Surg 2020;44(4):1190–1.

[123] Sarli L, Porrini C, Costi R, Regina G, Violi V, Ferro M, et al. Operative treatment of periampullary retroperitoneal perforation complicating endoscopic sphincterotomy. Surgery 2007;142(1):26–32.

[124] Degremont R, Brehant O, Fucks D, Sabbagh C, Dhari A, Browert F, et al. Management of supras-mesocolic peritonitis using the Levy helicoid drain (Hélisonde). J Vis Surg 2011;148:e291.

[125] Nguyen N, Amstrong C. Management of gastrointestinal leaks and fistula. In: Nguyen N, Blakstone R, Morton J, Ponce J, Rosenthal R, editors. The ASMBS textbook of bariatric surgery, vol. 1. Springer; 2015. p. 221–7.

[126] Chang YC. Is necrosectomy obsolete for infected necrotizing pancreatitis? Is a paradigm shift needed? World J Gastroenterol 2014;20(45):16925–34.

[127] Wei AL, Guo Q, Wang MJ, Hu WM, Zhang ZD. Early complications after interventions in patients with acute pancreatitis. World J Gastroenterol 2016;22(9): 2828–36.

[128] Boxhoorn L, van Dijk SM, van Grinsven J, Verdonk RC, Boermeester MA, Bollen TL, et al. Immediate versus postponed intervention for infected necrotizing pancreatitis. N Engl J Med 2021;385(15):1372–81.

[129] van Grinsven J, van Santvoort HC, Boermeester MA, Dejong CH, van Eijck CH, Fockens P, et al. Timing of

catheter drainage in infected necrotizing pancreatitis. Nat Rev Gastroenterol Hepatol 2016;13(5):306–12.

[130] Raraty MG, Halloran CM, Dodd S, Ghaneh P, Connor S, Evans J, et al. Minimal access retroperitoneal pancreatic necrosectomy: improvement in morbidity and mortality with a less invasive approach. Ann Surg 2010;251(5): 787–93.

[131] Castellanos G, Pinero A, Serrano A, Llamas C, Fuster M, Fernandez JA, et al. Translumbar retroperitoneal endoscopy: an alternative in the follow-up and management of drained infected pancreatic necrosis. Arch Surg 2005;140(10):952–5.

[132] Mathew MJ, Parmar AK, Sahu D, Reddy PK. Laparoscopic necrosectomy in acute necrotizing pancreatitis: our experience. J Minimal Access Surg 2014;10(3): 126–31.

[133] Talmor M, Hoffman LA, Lieberman M. Intestinal perforation after suction lipoplasty: a case report and review of the literature. Ann Plast Surg 1997;38(2):169–72.

[134] Sartelli M, Guirao X, Hardcastle TC, Kluger Y, Boermeester MA, Rasa K, et al. WSES/SIS-E consensus conference: recommendations for the management of skin and soft-tissue infections. World J Emerg Surg 2018;13:58.

[135] Bloch D, Gonzalez MD, Haight A, Abramowsky C, Yildirim I. Necrotizing fasciitis caused by Mucor indicus in a pediatric bone marrow transplant recipient. Pediatr Transplant 2018;22(8):e13294.

[136] Cheung JP, Fung B, Tang WM, Ip WY. A review of necrotising fasciitis in the extremities. Hong Kong Med J 2009; 15(1):44–52.

[137] Goodell KH, Jordan MR, Graham R, Cassidy C, Nasraway SA. Rapidly advancing necrotizing fasciitis caused by Photobacterium (Vibrio) damsela: a hyperaggressive variant. Crit Care Med 2004;32(1):278–81.

[138] Huang TY, Peng KT, Hsu WH, Hung CH, Chuang FY, Tsai YH. Independent predictors of mortality for aeromonas necrotizing fasciitis of limbs: an 18-year retrospective study. Sci Rep 2020;10(1):7716.

[139] Levy MM, Artigas A, Phillips GS, Rhodes A, Beale R, Osborn T, et al. Outcomes of the Surviving Sepsis Campaign in intensive care units in the USA and Europe: a prospective cohort study. Lancet Infect Dis 2012;12(12):919–24.

[140] Wagenlehner FM, Pilatz A, Naber KG, Weidner W. Therapeutic challenges of urosepsis. Eur J Clin Invest 2008; 38(Suppl. 2):45–9.

[141] EAU. EAU guidelines office arnhem. The Nehterlands. 2021. Available from: http://uroweb.org/guidelines/ compilations-of-all-guidelines/.

[142] Guliciuc M, Maier AC, Maier IM, Kraft A, Cucuruzac RR, Marinescu M, et al. The urosepsis-A literature review. Medicina (Kaunas) 2021;57(9).

[143] Kalra OP, Raizada A. Approach to a patient with urosepsis. J Global Infect Dis 2009;1(1):57–63.

[144] Peach BC, Li Y, Cimiotti JP. The weekend effect in older adult urosepsis admissions. Med Care 2020;58(1): 65–9.

[145] Seymour CW, Liu VX, Iwashyna TJ, Brunkhorst FM, Rea TD, Scherag A, et al. Assessment of clinical criteria for sepsis: for the third international consensus definitions for sepsis and septic shock (Sepsis-3). JAMA 2016;315(8):762–74.

[146] Porat A, Bhutta BS, Kesler S. Urosepsis. Treasure Island (FL): StatPearls; 2021.

[147] Shen KR, Bribriesco A, Crabtree T, Denlinger C, Eby J, Eiken P, et al. The American Association for Thoracic Surgery consensus guidelines for the management of empyema. J Thorac Cardiovasc Surg 2017;153(6): e129–46.

[148] Rahman NM, Maskell NA, West A, Teoh R, Arnold A, Mackinlay C, et al. Intrapleural use of tissue plasminogen activator and DNase in pleural infection. N Engl J Med 2011;365(6):518–26.

[149] Redden MD, Chin TY, van Driel ML. Surgical versus nonsurgical management for pleural empyema. Cochrane Database Syst Rev 2017;3:CD010651.

[150] Semenkovich TR, Olsen MA, Puri V, Meyers BF, Kozower BD. Current state of empyema management. Ann Thorac Surg 2018;105(6):1589–96.

[151] Williams E, Hanna N, Menard A, Mussari B, Nasirzadeh R, Tarulli E, et al. Study protocol for DICE trial: video-assisted thoracoscopic surgery decortication versus interventional radiology guided chest tube insertion for the management of empyema. Contemp Clin Trials Commun 2021;22:100777.

CHAPTER 22

Sepsis Adjunctive Therapies

JAVIER PEREZ-FERNANDEZ • PAOLA PEREZ

INTRODUCTION

Sepsis is a multifaceted clinical entity proved to have high levels of morbidity and mortality worldwide. Yet, for over 20 years, scientists and clinicians around the globe have placed many efforts in defining, clarifying, and better managing the disease. Despite the overwhelming expansion in knowledge regarding the pathophysiology of sepsis, a lot remains unknown. Howbeit, patient populations suffering from sepsis or septic shock benefit from the utilization of treatment and managing strategies pointed toward abetting a robust immune response.

As patients with severe sepsis and septic shock are critically ill and universally require supportive therapies, the need for adjunctive treatments on many occasions is an independent process itself that responds to the general condition of the patient. Thus, it is difficult to entirely establish if there is a benefit provided by those therapies or whether that benefit can be applied independently to the sepsis process or rather to the status of the patient.

In this chapter, we will spotlight on the reasoning and the clinical information accessible on practiced adjunctive therapies, including pharmacological approaches and hormonal interventions.

GLYCEMIC CONTROL

From all aspects related to patient support in critical care, it is glycemic control that has likely called the most attention in the last several years. Since hyperglycemia has been associated to worse outcomes in critical care as well as in infectious processes, attention to blood sugar control in the intensive care unit (ICU) has been the subject of multiple investigations [1]. Stress hyperglycemia has been found in injuries, burns, serious medical procedures, myocardial ischemia, and sepsis, among others. In some of those conditions, the presence of uncontrolled glycemic levels has been strongly associated with worse clinical outcomes [2].

Stress hyperglycemia seems, by all accounts, to be caused transcendently by elevating the liver's glucose stores. Cortisol and catecholamines, elevated during stress situations, have metabolic effects that lead to an increase in glucose in the blood by activating catalytic enzymes responsible for the hepatic glycogenolysis and gluconeogenesis. Inflammatory markers also work to increase insulin resistance at the cellular level.

Attempts have been made to achieve tight blood sugar control in patients with sepsis, mostly after the publication of sentinel trials demonstrating better outcomes in critically ill surgical patients [3]. However, the results of those could not be translated into septic patients or even general critical care population [1,4]. Currently, for adult patients with sepsis or septic shock, it is recommended to maintain blood sugar levels <180 mg/dL, considering early use of insulin to achieve the goal (moderate level of evidence). Special attention should be given to avoid hypoglycemia as the detrimental effects of such are broadly demonstrated [1,5]. The mechanisms for which hypoglycemia can be harmful to the patient are beyond the intrinsic low blood sugar level and include the disruption of the possible protective role of stress hyperglycemia and its value in increasing survival in periods of stress [6]. In regard to the glycemic level needed to initiate insulin, there is no definitive number, but the lower the threshold is, the higher the risk of provoking hypoglycemic episodes. Therefore, maintaining glycemic levels between 108 mg/d and 180 mg/dL should be the standard of care.

VTE PROPHYLAXIS

Sepsis induces the initiation of the coagulation cascade, further affecting organ function. Coagulation abnormalities have been postulated as one of the principal mechanisms for injury in sepsis. Thrombin and fibrin, in exaggerated levels during the sepsis response are considered inflammatory elements, heightening the complex state.

The Sepsis Codex. https://doi.org/10.1016/B978-0-323-88271-2.00029-8

Following that rationale, there have been attempts to modify this response and target survival in sepsis [7]. Perhaps, the most important from those trials was the one that investigated recombinant human activated protein C and its use as an adjunctive treatment for sepsis, initially noting to provide improvement in survival [8,9]. Unfortunately, there was later refuting evidence and eventually its use was discontinued [10].

What is accepted in regards with the abnormal coagulation response in sepsis is the need to provide with venous thromboembolism (VTE) prophylaxis to patients admitted to the ICU.

The prevalence of deep vein thrombosis occurring in patients hospitalized in the ICU has been reported to be as high as 10%, while the incidence of pulmonary embolism in the same patient population can oscillate between 2% and 4% [11,12]. Initial studies were demonstrative of the benefit of applying VTE prophylaxis in specific populations in the ICU [13]. The benefits were also demonstrated in patients with sepsis [14].

Regarding the choice of anticoagulation, low-molecular-weight heparins (LMWHs) have exhibited lower incidences of DVT compared to unfractionated heparin, though studies were never powered to show statistical differences in bleeding, mortality, or pulmonary embolism (CITE). The decision to use LMWH over UFH is entirely arbitrary or based on trending supporting evidence favoring LMWH as more feasible and advantageous. Among the features advocating for LMWH is it facility to concord compliance, only requiring one injection per day in most circumstances as well as its clinical profile [5].

The use of mechanical prophylaxis with intermitting pneumatic compression devices when pharmacologic prophylaxis cannot be attained is standard of practice and recommended by expert panels, although with a low degree of evidence [15]. More recent data have been published showing that the use of mechanical devices alone could be as effective in preventing VTEs than when used in combination with pharmacologic prophylaxis [16]. The most recent surviving sepsis campaign guidelines suggest against the use of mechanical prophylaxis concertedly with pharmacological agents in patients with sepsis or septic shock, over pharmacologic prophylaxis alone [5]. In individuals in whom pharmacologic prophylaxis is contraindicated, the use of mechanical prophylaxis is indicated and preferred to none.

NUTRITION

As a complete chapter of this book is dedicated to nutritional support in septic patients, we will only mention the need for nutritional support in septic patients along with every critically ill patient. Enteral nutrition is preferred over parenteral nutrition when there is feasibility and tolerance.

The use of targeted formulas, immunomodulators, and specific supplements is covered in the nutrition chapter.

STRESS ULCER PROPHYLAXIS

Along nutritional support, the role of stress ulcer prophylaxis will be extensively discussed in another chapter of this book.

LONG-TERM OUTCOMES

The recovery process for patients with sepsis and septic shock could be long and rough. In addition to physical consequences of the disease, the psychological impact of the complicated course over the patient and the family members could be sometimes painful and uncertain. Modern ICU care calls for a more active patient and family participation in the development of the plan of care and recommends a thorough discussion and to include all interested parties in order to establish realistic expectations and plans [5].

The discussions with patients, families, and members of the healthcare team must encompass different aspects of the delivery of healthcare such as the individual differences among patients, levels of care available, treatment plan including dosages of medications, and alternative options. In addition, it is important to plan the discharge moment (both from the ICU and potentially form the hospital) and explain the process as well as the possibility of negative outcomes. Addressing goals of care early seems to be best practice. Although the right timing for those discussions has not been established, the best evidence and expert opinion suggest that these conversations should occur within 72 h of the patient's admission to ICU [5,17].

Albeit these measures can provide relief and support to patients and families and create a more friendly and collaborative atmosphere in the ICU, they have not demonstrated impact in hospital mortality or length of stay, or as stated in some studies, no changes in family satisfaction [18].

Involving the patient and the families in the decision-making process is also a recommendation by the current expert panels and guidelines. The process is more likely to result in goals in accordance with the patient's preferences and expressions [5].

PALLIATIVE CARE

Given the challenge of determining prognosis and life expectancy among critically ill patients with sepsis in the ICU, palliative care should be offered during the patient's hospital course regardless of survival status. There are misconceptions among clinicians that critical care and palliative care are sequential or even separate excellent practices. However, these processes are complementary to one another and both approaches should be taken simultaneously in order to better provide medical care for a septic patient.

Palliative care is patient-focused and enhances satisfaction by preparing, expecting, forestalling, and treating ailments and associated symptoms regardless of the intent to cure. Since mortality in ICU remains relatively high contributing to nearly a quarter of a million deaths each year in the United States alone, it is not surprising that once a patient is admitted to the ICU, there might be an onerous prognosis implied and such impression can be certainly extended to the family and patients themselves [19]. The complex nature and history of these patients complicates their care and chance of survival as many suffer a myriad of illnesses apart from sepsis. The goal of intensive care is to maintain or regain patients' organ functionality to reduce mortality and prevent future morbidity. Palliative care aims to improve the quality of life and comfort during treatment without regard to prognosis. Thus, both entities are not mutually exclusive and can be approached concurrently.

For this to function well, intensivists should involve families, given that patients are unable to fend for themselves, early on to set plans, goals of care and expectations. The goals should be patient-centered and thus should be directed according to expressions or preferences the patient themselves had shared. If patients have already written an advanced directive, it would be crucial during this time to rely on those documents for guidance. If not, the medical team and the patient's spokespeople should do their utmost to try and reflect the patients' values, desires, and needs.

Ideally, critically care doctors should obtain some level of competency in palliative care. Previous national surveys have suggested intensivists be trained in palliation and its fundamentals concepts to have the tools necessary to apply them in practice [20]. Requiring such training globally could become a prodigious task and isslikely unattainable. As an alternative, hospitals and institutions can offer programs aimed to teach and review palliative care principles for medical teams. When available, intensivists can consult palliative care physicians in their institutions.

Proactive palliative involvement during ICU rounds and frequent family engagment in patients who were considered high risk was related with more expeditious and reduced length of hospital stays [21].

All in all, evidence suggests that proactively offering palliation for ICU patients, whether it be through consultive services or integrative programs, or practices from intensivists, forsooth reduced hospital, and ICU length of stay. Even more worthy of note is that such interventions did not affect mortality rates [22].

It remains hard to assess which specific palliative care interventions are best, due in great part to the ambiguous nature of the term, which in brief, encompasses providing comfort for the ill. Nevertheless, it is evidently and consistently supported and established by literature that palliative care is of great benefit to critically ill patients.

MUSIC THERAPY

The benefit of music therapy in patients in critical conditions has been postulated for over a century [23]. Since then, multiple publications have appeared showing benefits in different aspects of the care, including decreasing the need of sedatives during mechanical ventilation, reducing the length of stay or even restituting mental equilibrium among others [24]. The benefits of music therapy in facilitating relaxation and reducing anxiety have also been subject of different publications [25,26].

The literature is abundant in references of the usefulness and benefits of music therapy in neonates and premature children [27,28]. The benefit of music could be attributable to brain stimulation and bioregulatory effects that can be carried out through multiple conditions. It is then reasonable to think that music therapy could translate and be part of the adjuvant therapies for patients with sepsis and septic shock, although further studies might be needed to establish a stronger casual relation.

SLEEP THERAPY

No argument could be made against the beneficial effect of sleep in healing the body and the mind. However, our ICUs are not precisely a resting field for our patients. Full of noises, alarms, and lights, in addition to the continuous invasion of the privacy required by the nature of the "intensive treatment," makes the ICU a far-enough place for resting. The use of sedatives and pain medication, enhanced by the breakage of the intrinsic circadian cycle is a major disruption in the sleep architecture.

Few trials have attempted to address the issue of sleep as treatment or even its association with better outcomes. Specifically, in sepsis, melatonin has been a subject of investigation [29]. However, the intrinsic benefits of such are not well demonstrated.

It seems at least prudent to state that an adequate sleep time will help the well-being of the patients and that ICUs must create a more peaceful and comfortable environment for our patients and their families. Patient-centered care should be the motive of our modern ICUs.

REFERENCES

[1] Finfer S, Chittock DR, Su SY, et al. The NICE-SUGAR Study Investigators: intensive versus conventional glucose control in critically ill patients. N Engl J Med 2009;360: 1283–97.

[2] Badawi O, Waite MD, Fuhrman SA, Zuckerman IH. Association between intensive care unit-acquired dysglycemia and in-hospital mortality. Crit Care Med 2012; 40:3180–8. https://doi.org/10.1097/CCM.0b013e3182 656ae5.

[3] Carr JM, Sellke FW, Fey M, et al. Implementing tight glucose control after coronary artery bypass surgery. Ann Thorac Surg 2005;80:902–9.

[4] Fahy BG, Sheehy AM, Coursin DB. Glucose control in the intensive care unit. Crit Care Med 2009;37(5):1769–76. https://doi.org/10.1097/CCM.0b013e3181a19ceb.

[5] Evans L, Rhodes A, Alhazzani W, et al. Surviving sepsis campaign: international guidelines for the management of sepsis and septic shock 2021. Intensive Care Med 2021;47:1181–247.

[6] Marik PE, Bellomo R. Stress hyperglycemia: an essential survival response. Crit Care March 6, 2013;17(2):305. https://doi.org/10.1186/cc12514. PMID: 23470218; PMCID: PMC3672537.

[7] Vincent JL, Francois B, Zabolototskikh I, et al. Effect of a recombinant human soluble thrombomodulin on mortality in patients with sepsis-associated coagulopathy. The SCARLET randomized clinical trial. JAMA 2019; 321(20):1993–2002.

[8] McCoy C, Matthews SJ. Drotrecogin alfa (recombinant human activated protein C) for the treatment of severe sepsis. Clin Therapeut February 2003;25(2):396–421. https://doi.org/10.1016/s0149-2918(03)80086-3. PMID: 12749504.

[9] Dhainaut J-F, Yan SB, Joyce DE, et al. Treatment effects of drotrecogin alfa (activated) in patients with severe sepsis with or without overt disseminated intravascular coagulation. J Thromb Haemostasis 2004;2(11): 1924–33.

[10] Ranieri VM, Thompson BT, Dhainaut J-F, et al. Drotrecogin alfa (activated) in adults with septic shock. N Engl J Med 2012;366(22):2055–64.

[11] Fan Y, Jiang M, Gong D, Zou C. Efficacy and safety of low-molecular-weight heparin in patients with sepsis: a meta-analysis of randomized controlled trials. Sci Rep May 16, 2016;6:25984. https://doi.org/10.1038/srep25984. PMID: 27181297; PMCID: PMC4867648.

[12] Alhazzani W, Lim W, Jaeschke RZ, et al. Heparin thromboprophylaxis in medical-surgical critically ill patients: a systematic review and meta-analysis of randomized trials. Crit Care Med 2013;41(9):2088–98.

[13] Hirsh J, Hoak J. Management of deep vein thrombosis and pulmonary embolism. Circulation 1996;93:2212–45.

[14] Cook D, Crowther M, Meade M, et al. Deep venous thrombosis in medical-surgical critically ill patients: prevalence, incidence and risk factors. Crit Care Med 2005; 33(7):1565–71.

[15] Kwok M, Tan JA. Stratified meta-analysis of intermittent pneumatic compression of the lower limbs to prevent venous thromboembolism in hospitalized patients. Circulation 2013;128:1003–20.

[16] Arabi YM, Al-Hameed F, Burns KEA, et al. Adjunctive intermittent pneumatic compression for venous thromboprophylaxis. N Engl J Med 2019;380(14): 1305–15.

[17] White DB, Angus DC, Shields AM, et al. A randomized trial of a family-support intervention in intensive care units. N Engl J Med 2018;378(25):2365–75.

[18] Andereck WS, McGaughey JW, Scheneiderman LJ, et al. Seeking to reduce nonbeneficial treatment in the ICU: an exploratory trial of preactive ethics intervention. Crit Care Med 2014;42(4):824–30.

[19] Rhee C, Dantes R, Epstein L, et al. CDC Prevention Epicenter Program. Incidence and trends of sepsis in US hospitals using clinical vs claims data, 2009–2014. JAMA 2017;318(13):1241–9. https://doi.org/10.1001/jama.2017.13836.

[20] Cortegiani A, Russotto V, Raineri SM, Gregoretti C, Giarratano A, Mercadante S. Attitudes towards end-of-life issues in intensive care unit among Italian anesthesiologists: a nation-wide survey. Support Care Cancer 2017;26:1773–80.

[21] Braus N, Campbell TC, Kwekkeboom KL, et al. Prospective study of a proactive palliative care rounding intervention in a medical ICU. Intensive Care Med January 2016; 42(1):54–62. https://doi.org/10.1007/s00134-015-4098-1. Epub 2015 Nov 10. PMID: 26556622; PMCID: PMC4945103.

[22] Aslakson R, Cheng J, Vollenweider D, et al. Evidence-based palliative care in the intensive care unit: a systematic review of interventions. J Palliat Med February 2014;17(2): 219–35. https://doi.org/10.1089/jpm.2013.0409. PMID: 24517300; PMCID: PMC3924791.

[23] Kane EON. Phonograph in operating room. JAMA 1914; 62:1829.

[24] Hetland B, Lindquist R, Chlan LL. The influence of music during mechanical ventilation: a review. Heart Lung 2015;44:416–25.

[25] Chlan L. Effectiveness of a music therapy intervention on relaxation and anxiety for patients receiving ventilatory assistance. Heart Lung 1998;27(3):169–76.

[26] Watson H, Marshall P. Rapid realist review: anxiolytic effects of music therapy on mechanically ventilated patients. medRxiv 2021.09.11.21263390. https://doi.org/10.1101/2021.09.11.21263390.

[27] Costa VS, Bündchen DC, Sousa H, et al. Clinical benefits of music-based interventions on preterm infants' health: a systematic review of randomised trials. Acta Paediatr 2022;111(3):478–89. https://doi.org/10.1111/apa.16222.

[28] Loewy J, Stewart K, Dassler AM, et al. The effects of music therapy on vital signs, feeding, and sleep in premature infants. Pediatrics 2013;131(5):902–18. https://doi.org/10.1542/peds.2012-1367.

[29] Galley HF, Lowes DA, Allen L, et al. Melatonin as a potential therapy for sepsis: a phase I dose escalation study and an ex vivo whole blood model under conditions of sepsis. J Pineal Res 2014;56:427–38.

CHAPTER 23

Glycemic Control and Stress Ulcer Prophylaxis

DEEPA GOTUR • JANICE L. ZIMMERMAN

The molecular and metabolic pathophysiology unleashed by sepsis is complex and dynamic and related to a proinflammatory state [1]. Organ dysfunction exacerbated by sepsis occurs at the tissue level affecting specialized functions of the gastrointestinal (GI) tract as a defense barrier and secretory organ as well as affecting insulin sensitivity and gluconeogenesis predisposing to stress ulcers and hyperglycemia, respectively. In this section, we review the disturbances of glycemia in sepsis, management, and outcomes related to glucose control. We also review indications and complications related to stress ulcer prophylaxis (SUP).

GLYCEMIC CONTROL

Introduction

The glycemic state in sepsis is a complex interplay of multiple factors: cytokine-mediated suppression of gluconeogenesis, stress hormone—induced glucose utilization and gluconeogenesis, steroid therapy—related hyperglycemia, drug-related hypoglycemia, hepatic organ dysfunction—related glycogen depletion, and baseline comorbidities such as diabetes, obesity, and metabolic syndrome. All these factors have dynamic effects on glucose response and should be considered in treating sepsis.

Glucose Metabolism in Sepsis

In sepsis, inflammatory cytokines particularly interleukin-6 (IL-6), tumor necrosis factor α (TNF-α), and interleukin-1 (IL-1) stimulate the hypothalamic-pituitary-adrenal axis to increase cortisol production. In addition, the impaired clearance of glucocorticoids due to suppressed cortisol metabolism in the liver and kidneys sustains elevated cortisol levels in later phases of sepsis [2]. Hepatic dysfunction in septic shock causes reduced production of corticosteroid-binding globulin as well as enhanced activity of elastase which result in increased free cortisol. There is also loss of diurnal variation in cortisol levels. Glucocorticoid receptors (GRs) are amplified by an increase in number and sensitivity to cortisol. Cortisol promotes not only the maintenance of fluid homeostasis and vascular tone but also gluconeogenesis causing hyperglycemia [3]. The hyperglycemia resulting from increased cortisol effects and decreased insulin activity may counter the effects of hypoperfusion in sepsis. Hypoperfusion causes reduced blood flow and glucose delivery to poorly perfused cells in a bed of increased interstitial fluid space. Thus, hyperglycemia may be an adaptive mechanism to increase glucose delivery [4]. In late phases of septic shock, GR suppression is reported leading to cortisol resistance, hypoglycemia, and lethal shock [5].

Glucose dysregulation due to stress hormone release can be easily measured in relation to the baseline glycemic index. There is no universal definition or threshold for stress-induced hyperglycemia. Stress hyperglycemia ratio has been recently proposed as a ratio of glucose level at the time of hospital admission to the estimated average glucose derived from glycated hemoglobin [6]. While this ratio is calculated to control for chronic hyperglycemia, stress hyperglycemia can also occur in the absence of preexisting glucose intolerance and typically resolves with the resolution of acute illness. The prevalence of stress hyperglycemia in sepsis is unknown, but in critically ill patients, it is estimated to be 20%—75% depending on the threshold used for its estimation [7,8]. Stress hyperglycemia is a significant risk factor for poor outcome. A stress hyperglycemia index above 1.14 also has excellent discriminant capacity for case fatality prediction [8,9].

The liver usually increases plasma glucose through gluconeogenesis. Sepsis can cause hepatic injury from pathogens, toxins, or inflammatory mediators, and hypoperfusion. Preexisting liver disease may also contribute to liver dysfunction. Liver dysfunction commonly causes hypoglycemia rather than hyperglycemia. The hepatic SOFA score is significantly higher in patients with hypoglycemia than those with euglycemia or hyperglycemia [10]. Hepatic dysfunction in patients with sepsis is a specific and independent risk factor for poor outcome [11].

Insulin Resistance in Sepsis

Tissue glucose utilization is low due to high levels of insulin resistance in patients with sepsis and organ dysfunction [12]. Insulin resistance can be measured using homeostasis model assessment method first described in 1985 [13]. This method evaluates pancreatic β-cell function and insulin resistance from basal glucose and insulin or C-peptide concentrations which reflects the balance between hepatic glucose output and insulin secretion. This balance is maintained by a feedback loop between the liver and β-cells. The predictions used in the model arise from experimental data in humans and animals. In patients with sepsis and septic shock, the levels are much higher in nonsurvivors and both stress-induced hyperglycemia and insulin resistance are associated with mortality [12].

Innate Immune Response and Glucose Milieu

Acute hyperglycemia has also been associated with adverse outcomes due to its profound effects on innate immune responses including cellular defenses, complement activation, and cytokine release. In the clinical sepsis phenotypes described by Seymour and colleagues, the δ phenotype which is the most proinflammatory phenotype with the risk of highest mortality was associated with higher glucose levels [14].

Effects of hyperglycemia are most noted on neutrophils which have pivotal phagocytic property needed for innate immunity. Hyperglycemia attenuates neutrophil activation, decreases chemotaxis, impairs neutrophil respiratory burst capacity, inhibits phagocytosis, reduces extracellular trap formation, and affects bactericidal capacity. These effects are thought to be secondary to the inhibition of G6PD or activation of protein kinase C and direct cellular effects through protein glycosylation and membrane perturbation from increased osmolality [15].

Other cellular host defense mechanisms of innate immunity such as vascular endothelial function are also inhibited in hyperglycemia. Bradykinin-dependent increase in nitric oxide synthesis promotes vasodilation and increased vascular permeability increasing the blood flow at the site of infection during early sepsis. Elevated glucose concentrations significantly augment vascular hyperpermeability by dysregulation of the nitric oxide pathway which can cause multisystem organ dysfunction and shock [16].

Complement system activation functions as an integral part of innate immunity by promoting opsonization and phagocytosis of microorganisms by macrophages. Hyperglycemia can inhibit complement-mediated phagocytosis [17]. Hyperglycemia also appears to have divergent effects in cytokine release and alters the balance of proinflammatory and antiinflammatory cytokine responses increasing mortality [18].

Glycemic Variability

Several factors that cause hyperglycemia and variability in blood glucose levels are common in septic critically ill patients (Table 23.1). One measure of glucose variability, the mean amplitude of glycemic excursions (MAGE), is calculated as the average of differences between consecutive peaks and nadirs greater than the standard deviation of the mean glucose value during continuous glucose monitoring. Glycemic variability leads to oxidative stress due to imbalance of free radicals and reactive oxygen and reactive nitrogen species and hence can worsen sepsis-related outcomes. MAGE in septic patients is higher in nonsurvivors compared to survivors [19]. In one study, a MAGE cut off of 65 mg/dL was used to discriminate high versus low

TABLE 23.1 Factors Affecting Glycemia in Sepsis	
Internal factors	**External factors**
Cortisol	Intermittent infusions of glucose containing solutions
Inflammatory cytokines (e.g., IL-6, TNF-α, IL-1)	Paralytic ileus
Insulin resistance	Steroid therapy
Hepatic injury	Enteral and parenteral nutrition

levels, and patients with high MAGE tended to have higher HbA1C (6.7 ± 1.8% vs. 5.9 ± 0.9%, $P < .01$) and were more likely to have diabetes mellitus (50.0% vs. 23.4%, $P < .01$) compared with the low MAGE group [20]. This study also found that high glycemic variability within the first 24 h of onset of sepsis was associated with increased mortality, and this association was stronger in the nondiabetic group compared with the diabetic group [20]. High glycemic variability was also associated with increased major adverse events such as stroke, heart failure, myocardial infarction, acute renal failure, and death in the postoperative period following surgery for endocarditis [21].

Diabetic Septic Patients

Van Vught and colleagues investigated the relation of admission hyperglycemia in patients with sepsis and found that severe hyperglycemia (>200 mg/dL, >11.1 mmol/L) but not mild hyperglycemia (141−199 mg/dL, 7.8−11 mmol/L) at admission was associated with increased 30-day mortality (HR 1.66; 95% confidence interval [CI]: 1.24−2.23) among patients with diabetes and without diabetes [22]. This observation contrasts with previous findings by Stegenga et al. who reported an association of hyperglycemia and mortality only in patients without diabetes [23]. There have been several theories about the protective effects of diabetic therapies such as insulin and metformin. However, plasma biomarkers for systemic inflammation, activation of the coagulation cascade, and vascular endothelial damage were not significantly different between patients on chronic insulin therapy and those who were not. Similarly, plasma protein markers for host inflammatory response to sepsis and the whole genome transcriptome in blood leukocytes did not differ between patients with diabetes mellitus who had and had not received prior metformin therapy [24].

Obesity and Glycemia in Sepsis

Obese patients have alterations of innate and adaptive immune responses, and obesity is a proinflammatory disease that has been linked in preclinical studies to cytokine storm during infection [25]. Adipose tissue secretes inflammatory substances such as IL-6 and TNF-α that promote insulin resistance. Ectopic lipid also accumulates in the liver and muscles that can contribute to insulin resistance through the production of toxic lipid metabolites, including diacylglycerol or ceramides [26,27].

Management for Glycemic Control

Hyperglycemia, hypoglycemia, and increased glycemic variability are associated with increased mortality in critically ill patients [8,28,29]. A more intensive glucose control approach in a single center study, targeting blood glucose to 80−110 mg/dL (4.4−6.1 mmol/L) noted reduced intensive care unit (ICU) mortality [7]; however, this finding was unable to be reproduced in subsequent multicenter randomized controlled trials [30,31]. Metaanalyses also report a higher incidence of hypoglycemia (glucose <40 mg/dL [2.2 mmol/L]) in critical patients where blood glucose was targeted to 80−110 mg/dL (4.4−6.1 mmol/L) [32,33]. The relationship of hypoglycemia and increased risk of mortality is more evident in nondiabetic patients than those with diabetes [10].

The 2016 Surviving Sepsis Campaign (SSC) guidelines strongly recommended a protocolized approach to blood glucose management in ICU patients with sepsis, commencing regular insulin infusion when two consecutive blood glucose levels are >180 mg/dL (10 mmol/L) and maintaining upper blood glucose level ≤180 mg/dL rather than ≤110 mg/dL (6.1 mmol/L) [34]. This recommendation was derived from the NICE-SUGAR trial [35]. In the recent SSC 2021 guidelines, initiation of insulin therapy for levels >180 mg/dL (10 mmol/L) is strongly recommended with a typical target blood glucose range of 144−180 (8−10 mmol/L) mg/dL [36]. Similarly, the American Diabetes Association, in its most recent recommendations for glycemic control of critically ill patients, recommended the initiation of insulin therapy for persistent hyperglycemia >180 mg/dL with a target glucose range of 140−180 mg/dL [37].

In a recent metaanalysis of 35 randomized controlled trials [38] that compared four different blood glucose targets (<110, 110−144, 144−180, and >180 mg/dL), no significant difference in the risk of hospital mortality was observed between the blood glucose ranges. Target glucose levels of <110 (6.1 mmol/L) and 110−144 mg/dL (6.1−8 mmol/L) were associated with a four to ninefold increase in the risk of hypoglycemia compared with the higher glucose ranges. No significant difference in the risk of hypoglycemia comparing a target of 144−180 and > 180 mg/dL was demonstrated.

Continuous insulin infusion therapy is the preferred regimen for ICU patients with hyperglycemia regardless of underlying diagnosis of diabetes. Once the patient's condition has improved, transition to subcutaneous insulin regimens is appropriate if glucose measurements are stable for at least 4–6 h. Insulin requirements are estimated from the average amount of insulin infused during the 12 h before transition considering also the basal and nutritional insulin needs [39].

Subcutaneous sliding scale insulin protocols treat hyperglycemia after it has already occurred and should be discouraged. Findings from randomized trials have consistently shown better glycemic control with a basal–bolus approach than with sliding scale insulin alone [40].

More research needs to be conducted to identify the optimal range of glycemia in specific ICU populations such as diabetics, medical patients, and surgical patients.

STRESS ULCER PROPHYLAXIS

Ulcers caused from physiological stress in critically ill sepsis patients may affect the esophagus, stomach, or duodenum. It is a multifactorial disease with multiple complex mechanisms that lead to mucosal breakdown. Factors such as low cardiac output, hypotension, vasoconstriction, and inflammation can cause splanchnic and mucosal hypoperfusion. In addition to low mucosal blood flow, stress-triggered vagal stimulation, reduced bicarbonate secretion, acid back-diffusion, and lower GI motility can converge to impair the integrity of the mucosal lining [41]. The immune system and brain–immune interactions have also been implicated in the genesis of stress ulcer lesions [42].

Risk Factors

Some of the many risk factors associated with stress ulcers are listed in Table 23.2. Additional risk factors include shock, sepsis, history of peptic ulcer disease, history of GI bleeding, three or more coexisting illnesses, extracorporeal life support, trauma, traumatic brain injury, spinal cord injury, thermal injury >35% body surface area, partial hepatectomy, organ transplantation, alcohol abuse, long ICU stay, and therapies such as antiplatelets agents, nonsteroidal antiinflammatory drugs, high dose glucocorticoids, etc. Assessment of risk factors when determining whether to initiate SUP is important to prevent possible adverse effects of acid suppression. In one study, stress ulcers resulting in overt bleeding led to half of affected patients requiring

TABLE 23.2
Risk Factors Associated With Stress Ulcer Bleeding

Risk factor	OR (95% CI or P value)
Mechanical ventilation for >48 h [43]	15.6 (P < .001)
Coagulopathy (platelet count <50,000/mL^3, INR>1.5 or PTT > two times control value) [44,45]	4.3 (P < .001)
Maximum serum creatinine level [46]	1.16 (1.02–1.32)
Acute kidney injury [47]	1.21 (1.02–1.43)
Acute respiratory failure [47]	1.31 (1.10–1.56)[a]
Age >50 y (vs. < 40 y) [47] 50–59 y 60–69 y 70–79 y >80 y	1.46 (1.18–1.83)[a] 1.66 (1.26–2.19)[a] 1.72 (1.27–2.34)[a] 2.04 (1.48–2.83)[a]
Acute hepatic injury [47]	1.56 (1.29–1.88)[a]
Chronic hepatic injury [47]	1.85 (1.47–2.33)[a]
Male gender versus female [47]	1.17 (1.03–1.33)[a]

[a] Propensity score odds ratio.
Table adapted from Bardou M, et al. Stress-related mucosal disease in the critically ill patient. Nat Rev. Gastroenterol Hepatol 2015;12(2): 98–107.

endoscopy or surgery, and approximately half of patients requiring blood transfusion [48].

GI bleeding from stress ulcers is categorized into four groups of graded severity as noted in Table 23.3 [49]. The risk factors identified in a recent metaanalysis for clinically important GI bleeding were acute kidney injury, male gender, coagulopathy, shock, and chronic liver disease [50]. The effect of mechanical ventilation as a risk factor was unclear in this metaanalysis.

Treatment

SUP is suggested by the SSC guidelines for patients with sepsis or septic shock who have risk factors for GI bleeding [36]. The 2021 SSC recommendation was based on a moderate quality of evidence; the administration of SUP probably has a favorable outcome of a modest reduction in GI hemorrhage. This recommendation was downgraded from the strong recommendation made in 2016 SSC guidelines for the use of SUP in at-risk patients [34].

TABLE 23.3
Categories of Stress Ulcer Bleeding

Category	Definition
Mucosal or submucosal ulceration	Endoscopically documented gastroduodenal mucosal or submucosal erosions or ulcerations
Occult bleeding	Gastric or fecal occult samples positive for guaiac testing
Overt bleeding	Hematemesis, frank blood or coffee-grounds findings in nasogastric aspirate or melena
Clinically important bleeding	Overt bleeding in addition to one or more of the following 1. Spontaneous drop in systolic or diastolic blood pressure of ≥20 mm Hg within 24 h before or after bleeding 2. Orthostatic increase in pulse of ≥20 beats/min and decrease in systolic blood pressure of 10 mm Hg 3. Decrease in hemoglobin of ≥2 g/dL over a 24-h period or transfusion of ≥2 units of packed red cells within 24 h after the start of bleeding 4. Invasive interventions (e.g., therapeutic endoscopy or vasopressor initiation or increase)

An additional new randomized controlled study resulted after the 2016 guidelines did not demonstrate mortality or clinically relevant composite endpoints [48]. These results changed the metaanalysis for SCC prompting use of SUP as a weak recommendation in the 2021 guidelines. A metaanalysis of randomized clinical trials comparing SUP using proton pump inhibitors (PPIs) or histamine H2 receptor antagonists (H2Ras) with placebo or no prophylaxis found no difference in all-cause mortality (Table 23.4) [51].

However, multiple methodological limitations in the included trials limit the robustness of the conclusion. This metaanalysis also found that SUP reduced the occurrence of any GI bleeding but not clinically significant GI bleeding [51]. In another large randomized study comparing pantoprazole and placebo, a predefined subgroup analysis of ICU patients suggested that there was no difference in the 90-day mortality in surgical ICU patients receiving SUP compared to medical ICU patients [48].

A clinical decision on the use of PPIs or H2Ras is a challenging one, and there are many studies comparing them head-to-head. PPIs are the most used agents, followed by H2RAs for SUP. PPIs have been shown to have a higher risk of nosocomial pneumonia [51–53], *Clostridium difficile* infection [54,55], and myocardial infarction [56] in some studies. There are a multitude of studies on cost-effectiveness of PPIs with higher estimated costs for PPI usage [57,58].

In one of the largest randomized cluster crossover trials to compare two approaches for SUP among adults in the ICU requiring invasive mechanical ventilation, there was no significant difference in 90-day mortality rates (18.3% in PPI strategy vs. 17.5% in H2RAs). Very few sepsis patients were included in the study, rates of pneumonia were not measured, and *C. difficile* infection was rarely reported; however, they had fewer patients with GI bleeding in the PPI group [59]. A recent propensity matched retrospective study of ICU patients with data extracted from the MIMIC-III database concluded that PPIs were associated with higher in-hospital mortality and higher risk of GI bleeding and pneumonia than H2RAs [53]. Given the variable trial and metaanalyses results, either class of agents can be used, and selection may be dependent on risk of GI bleeding, pneumonia, *C. difficile* infection, and available resources.

Sucralfate has been studied in relation to reducing ICU-acquired pneumonia and clinically important GI bleeding. A systematic review and metaanalysis suggest that there was no impact on GI bleeding in comparison to H2RAs and moderate quality of evidence for reduction in ICU-acquired pneumonias. Sucralfate is not recommended for SUP in septic patients.

Other Considerations
Duration of SUP therapy depends on the continued presence of risk for stress ulceration. Although there are no specific criteria to indicate safe discontinuation of SUP, most clinicians consider discontinuing prophylaxis at discharge from the ICU unless other major risk factors persist.

TABLE 23.4
Meta analysis of RCTs Comparing Stress Ulcer Prophylaxis and No Prophylaxis on Clinically Relevant Outcomes

QUALITY ASSESSMENT							EFFECT		
No, of studies	Risk of bias	Inconsistency	Indirectness	Imprecision	Stress ulcer prophylaxis	No prophylaxis	Relative (95% CI)	Absolute (95% CI)	Certainty of evidence
MORTALITY (5656 PARTICIPANTS)									
28	Serious	Not serious	Not serious	Not serious	769/2942 (26.1%)	725/2714 (26.7%)	RR 1.01 (0.93 –1.10)	3 more per 1000 (from 19 fewer to 27 more)	Moderate
GASTROINTESTINAL HEMORRHAGE (6627 PARTICIPANTS)									
39	Serious	Serious	Not serious	Not serious	218/3404 (6.4%)	395/3223 (12.3%)	RR 0.52 (0.45 –0.61)	59 fewer per 1000 (from 48 fewer to 67 fewer)	Low
***CLOSTRIDIOIDES DIFFICILE* COLITIS (3698 PARTICIPANTS)**									
4	Serious	Not serious	Not serious	Very serious	23/1854 (1.2%)	29/1844 (1.6%)	RR 0.78 (0.46 –1.34)	3 fewer per 1000 (from 8 fewer to 5 more)	Very low
PNEUMONIA (4951 PARTICIPANTS)									
16	Serious	Not serious	Not serious	Serious	400/2250 (15.7%)	358/2401 (14.9%)	RR 1.07 (0.94 –1.21)	10 more per 1000 (from 9 fewer to 31 more)	Low

CI, confidence interval; *RR*, risk ratio.
Adapted from Barbateskovic M. Intensive Care Med 2019;45:143–58.

REFERENCES

[1] Moine P, Abraham E. Immunomodulation and sepsis: impact of the pathogen. Shock 2004;22(4):297−308.

[2] Van den Berghe G, Boonen E, Walker BR. Reduced cortisol metabolism during critical illness. N Engl J Med 2013;369(5):481.

[3] Ingels C, Gunst J, Van den Berghe G. Endocrine and metabolic alterations in sepsis and implications for treatment. Crit Care Clin 2018;34(1):81−96.

[4] Losser MR, Damoisel C, Payen D. Bench-to-bedside review: glucose and stress conditions in the intensive care unit. Crit Care 2010;14(4):231.

[5] Vandewalle J, Timmermans S, Paakinaho V, Vancraeynest L, Dewyse L, Vanderhaeghen T, Wallaeys C, Van Wyngene L, Van Looveren K, Nuyttens L, et al. Combined glucocorticoid resistance and hyperlactatemia contributes to lethal shock in sepsis. Cell Metab 2021;33(9). 1763-1776 e1765.

[6] Roberts GW, Quinn SJ, Valentine N, Alhawassi T, O'Dea H, Stranks SN, Burt MG, Doogue MP. Relative hyperglycemia, a marker of critical illness: introducing the stress hyperglycemia ratio. J Clin Endocrinol Metab 2015;100(12):4490−7.

[7] van den Berghe G, Wouters P, Weekers F, Verwaest C, Bruyninckx F, Schetz M, Vlasselaers D, Ferdinande P, Lauwers P, Bouillon R. Intensive insulin therapy in critically ill patients. N Engl J Med 2001;345(19):1359−67.

[8] Siegelaar SE, Hermanides J, Oudemans-van Straaten HM, van der Voort PH, Bosman RJ, Zandstra DF, DeVries JH. Mean glucose during ICU admission is related to mortality by a U-shaped curve in surgical and medical patients: a retrospective cohort study. Crit Care 2010;14(6):R224.

[9] Fabbri A, Marchesini G, Benazzi B, Morelli A, Montesi D, Bini C, Rizzo SG. Stress hyperglycemia and mortality in subjects with diabetes and sepsis. Crit Care Explor 2020;2(7):e0152.

[10] Kushimoto S, Abe T, Ogura H, Shiraishi A, Saitoh D, Fujishima S, Mayumi T, Hifumi T, Shiino Y, Nakada TA, et al. Impact of blood glucose abnormalities on outcomes and disease severity in patients with severe sepsis: an analysis from a multicenter, prospective survey of severe sepsis. PLoS One 2020;15(3):e0229919.

[11] Kramer L, Jordan B, Druml W, Bauer P, Metnitz PG. Austrian Epidemiologic Study on Intensive Care ASG: incidence and prognosis of early hepatic dysfunction in critically ill patients—a prospective multicenter study. Crit Care Med 2007;35(4):1099−104.

[12] Pretty CG, Le Compte AJ, Chase JG, Shaw GM, Preiser JC, Penning S, Desaive T. Variability of insulin sensitivity during the first 4 days of critical illness: implications for tight glycemic control. Ann Intensive Care 2012;2(1):17.

[13] Matthews DR, Hosker JP, Rudenski AS, Naylor BA, Treacher DF, Turner RC. Homeostasis model assessment: insulin resistance and beta-cell function from fasting plasma glucose and insulin concentrations in man. Diabetologia 1985;28(7):412−9.

[14] Seymour CW, Kennedy JN, Wang S, Chang CH, Elliott CF, Xu Z, Berry S, Clermont G, Cooper G, Gomez H, et al. Derivation, validation, and potential treatment implications of novel clinical phenotypes for sepsis. JAMA 2019;321(20):2003−17.

[15] Alba-Loureiro TC, Munhoz CD, Martins JO, Cerchiaro GA, Scavone C, Curi R, Sannomiya P. Neutrophil function and metabolism in individuals with diabetes mellitus. Braz J Med Biol Res 2007;40(8):1037−44.

[16] Liu XJ, Zhang ZD, Ma XC. High glucose enhances LPS-stimulated human PMVEC hyperpermeability via the NO pathway. Exp Ther Med 2013;6(2):361−7.

[17] Saiepour D, Sehlin J, Oldenborg PA. Hyperglycemia-induced protein kinase C activation inhibits phagocytosis of C3b- and immunoglobulin g-opsonized yeast particles in normal human neutrophils. Exp Diabesity Res 2003;4(2):125−32.

[18] Leonidou L, Mouzaki A, Michalaki M, DeLastic AL, Kyriazopoulou V, Bassaris HP, Gogos CA. Cytokine production and hospital mortality in patients with sepsis-induced stress hyperglycemia. J Infect 2007;55(4):340−6.

[19] Furushima N, Egi M, Obata N, Sato H, Mizobuchi S. Mean amplitude of glycemic excursions in septic patients and its association with outcomes: a prospective observational study using continuous glucose monitoring. J Crit Care 2021;63:218−22.

[20] Chao WC, Tseng CH, Wu CL, Shih SJ, Yi CY, Chan MC. Higher glycemic variability within the first day of ICU admission is associated with increased 30-day mortality in ICU patients with sepsis. Ann Intensive Care 2020;10(1):17.

[21] Liang M, Xiong M, Zhang Y, Chen J, Feng K, Huang S, Wu Z. Increased glucose variability is associated with major adverse events in patients with infective endocarditis undergo surgical treatment. J Thorac Dis 2021;13(2):653−63.

[22] van Vught LA, Wiewel MA, Klein Klouwenberg PM, Hoogendijk AJ, Scicluna BP, Ong DS, Cremer OL, Horn J, Bonten MM, Schultz MJ, et al. Admission hyperglycemia in critically ill sepsis patients: association with outcome and host response. Crit Care Med 2016;44(7):1338−46.

[23] Stegenga ME, Vincent JL, Vail GM, Xie J, Haney DJ, Williams MD, Bernard GR, van der Poll T. Diabetes does not alter mortality or hemostatic and inflammatory responses in patients with severe sepsis. Crit Care Med 2010;38(2):539−45.

[24] van Vught LA, Scicluna BP, Hoogendijk AJ, Wiewel MA, Klein Klouwenberg PM, Cremer OL, Horn J, Nurnberg P, Bonten MM, Schultz MJ, et al. Association of diabetes and diabetes treatment with the host response in critically ill sepsis patients. Crit Care 2016;20(1):252.

[25] Ramos Muniz MG, Palfreeman M, Setzu N, Sanchez MA, Saenz Portillo P, Garza KM, Gosselink KL, Spencer CT. Obesity exacerbates the cytokine storm elicited by francisella tularensis infection of females and is associated with increased mortality. BioMed Res Int 2018;2018:3412732.

[26] Hardy OT, Czech MP, Corvera S. What causes the insulin resistance underlying obesity? Curr Opin Endocrinol Diabetes Obes 2012;19(2):81–7.

[27] Kong LC, Wuillemin PH, Bastard JP, Sokolovska N, Gougis S, Fellahi S, Darakhshan F, Bonnefont-Rousselot D, Bittar R, Dore J, et al. Insulin resistance and inflammation predict kinetic body weight changes in response to dietary weight loss and maintenance in overweight and obese subjects by using a Bayesian network approach. Am J Clin Nutr 2013;98(6):1385–94.

[28] Badawi O, Waite MD, Fuhrman SA, Zuckerman IH. Association between intensive care unit-acquired dysglycemia and in-hospital mortality. Crit Care Med 2012;40(12):3180–8.

[29] Krinsley JS. Glycemic variability: a strong independent predictor of mortality in critically ill patients. Crit Care Med 2008;36(11):3008–13.

[30] Brunkhorst FM, Engel C, Bloos F, Meier-Hellmann A, Ragaller M, Weiler N, Moerer O, Gruendling M, Oppert M, Grond S, et al. Intensive insulin therapy and pentastarch resuscitation in severe sepsis. N Engl J Med 2008;358(2):125–39.

[31] Preiser JC, Devos P, Ruiz-Santana S, Mélot C, Annane D, Groeneveld J, Iapichino G, Leverve X, Nitenberg G, Singer P, et al. A prospective randomised multi-centre controlled trial on tight glucose control by intensive insulin therapy in adult intensive care units: the Glucontrol study. Intensive Care Med 2009;35(10):1738–48.

[32] Griesdale DE, de Souza RJ, van Dam RM, Heyland DK, Cook DJ, Malhotra A, Dhaliwal R, Henderson WR, Chittock DR, Finfer S, et al. Intensive insulin therapy and mortality among critically ill patients: a meta-analysis including NICE-SUGAR study data. CMAJ (Can Med Assoc J) 2009;180(8):821–7.

[33] Song F, Zhong LJ, Han L, Xie GH, Xiao C, Zhao B, Hu YQ, Wang SY, Qin CJ, Zhang Y, et al. Intensive insulin therapy for septic patients: a meta-analysis of randomized controlled trials. BioMed Res Int 2014;2014:698265.

[34] Rhodes A, Evans LE, Alhazzani W, Levy MM, Antonelli M, Ferrer R, Kumar A, Sevransky JE, Sprung CL, Nunnally ME, et al. Surviving sepsis campaign: international guidelines for management of sepsis and septic shock. Intensive Care Med 2017;43(3):304–77.

[35] Intensive versus conventional glucose control in critically ill patients. N Engl J Med 2009;360(13):1283–97.

[36] Evans L, Rhodes A, Alhazzani W, Antonelli M, Coopersmith CM, French C, et al. Surviving sepsis Campaign: international guidelines for management of sepsis and septic shock 2021. Crit Care Med 2021;49:e1063–143.

[37] Diabetes care in the hospital: Standards of medical care in diabetes—2018. Diabetes Care 2018;41(Suppl. 1):S144–51.

[38] Yatabe T, Inoue S, Sakaguchi M, Egi M. The optimal target for acute glycemic control in critically ill patients: a network meta-analysis. Intensive Care Med 2017;43(1):16–28.

[39] Pasquel FJ, Lansang MC, Dhatariya K, Umpierrez GE. Management of diabetes and hyperglycaemia in the hospital. Lancet Diabetes Endocrinol 2021;9(3):174–88.

[40] Lee YY, Lin YM, Leu WJ, Wu MY, Tseng JH, Hsu MT, Tsai CS, Hsieh AT, Tam KW. Sliding-scale insulin used for blood glucose control: a meta-analysis of randomized controlled trials. Metabolism 2015;64(9):1183–92.

[41] Bardou M, Quenot JP, Barkun A. Stress-related mucosal disease in the critically ill patient. Nat Rev Gastroenterol Hepatol 2015;12(2):98–107.

[42] Ray A, Gulati K, Henke P. Stress gastric ulcers and cytoprotective strategies: perspectives and trends. Curr Pharm Des 2020;26(25):2982–90.

[43] Cook DJ, Fuller HD, Guyatt GH, Marshall JC, Leasa D, Hall R, Winton TL, Rutledge F, Todd TJ, Roy P, et al. Risk factors for gastrointestinal bleeding in critically ill patients. Canadian Critical Care Trials Group. N Engl J Med 1994;330(6):377–81.

[44] Gururangan K, Holubar MK. A case of postoperative methicillin-resistant staphylococcus aureus enterocolitis in an 81-Year-old man and review of the literature. Am J Case Rep 2020;21:e922521.

[45] Laine L, Curtis SP, Langman M, Jensen DM, Cryer B, Kaur A, Cannon CP. Lower gastrointestinal events in a double-blind trial of the cyclo-oxygenase-2 selective inhibitor etoricoxib and the traditional nonsteroidal anti-inflammatory drug diclofenac. Gastroenterology 2008;135(5):1517–25.

[46] Cook D, Heyland D, Griffith L, Cook R, Marshall J, Pagliarello J. Risk factors for clinically important upper gastrointestinal bleeding in patients requiring mechanical ventilation. Canadian Critical Care Trials Group. Crit Care Med 1999;27(12):2812–7.

[47] Frandah W, Colmer-Hamood J, Nugent K, Raj R. Patterns of use of prophylaxis for stress-related mucosal disease in patients admitted to the intensive care unit. J Intensive Care Med 2014;29(2):96–103.

[48] Krag M, Marker S, Perner A, Wetterslev J, Wise MP, Schefold JC, Keus F, Guttormsen AB, Bendel S, Borthwick M, et al. Pantoprazole in patients at risk for gastrointestinal bleeding in the ICU. N Engl J Med 2018;379(23):2199–208.

[49] Cook D, Guyatt G. Prophylaxis against upper gastrointestinal bleeding in hospitalized patients. N Engl J Med 2018;378(26):2506–16.

[50] Granholm A, Zeng L, Dionne JC, Perner A, Marker S, Krag M, MacLaren R, Ye Z, Moller MH, Alhazzani W, et al. Predictors of gastrointestinal bleeding in adult ICU patients: a systematic review and meta-analysis. Intensive Care Med 2019;45(10):1347–59.

[51] Barbateskovic M, Marker S, Granholm A, Anthon CT, Krag M, Jakobsen JC, Perner A, Wetterslev J, Moller MH. Stress ulcer prophylaxis with proton pump inhibitors or histamin-2 receptor antagonists in adult intensive care patients: a systematic review with meta-analysis and trial sequential analysis. Intensive Care Med 2019;45(2):143–58.

[52] Lewis SC, Li L, Murphy MV, Klompas M, Epicenters CDCP. Risk factors for ventilator-associated events: a case-control multivariable analysis. Crit Care Med 2014;42(8):1839–48.

[53] Huang M, Han M, Han W, Kuang L. Proton pump inhibitors versus histamine-2 receptor blockers for stress ulcer prophylaxis in patients with sepsis: a retrospective cohort study. J Int Med Res 2021;49(6). 3000605211025130.

[54] Selvanderan SP, Summers MJ, Finnis ME, Plummer MP, Ali Abdelhamid Y, Anderson MB, Chapman MJ, Rayner CK, Deane AM. Pantoprazole or placebo for stress ulcer prophylaxis (POP-UP): randomized double-blind exploratory study. Crit Care Med 2016; 44(10):1842–50.

[55] D'Silva KM, Mehta R, Mitchell M, Lee TC, Singhal V, Wilson MG, et al. Proton pump inhibitor use and risk for recurrent Clostridioides difficile infection: a systematic review and meta-analysis. Clin Microbiol Infect 2021:S1198–743X(21)00035-5.

[56] Charlot M, Ahlehoff O, Norgaard ML, Jorgensen CH, Sorensen R, Abildstrom SZ, Hansen PR, Madsen JK, Kober L, Torp-Pedersen C, et al. Proton-pump inhibitors are associated with increased cardiovascular risk independent of clopidogrel use: a nationwide cohort study. Ann Intern Med 2010;153(6):378–86.

[57] Bischoff LM, Faraco LSM, Machado LV, Bialecki AVS, Almeida GM, Becker SCC. Inappropriate usage of intravenous proton pump inhibitors and associated factors in a high complexity hospital in Brazil. Arq Gastroenterol 2021;58(1):32–8.

[58] Hammond DA, Kathe N, Shah A, Martin BC. Cost-effectiveness of Histamine2 receptor antagonists versus proton pump inhibitors for stress ulcer prophylaxis in critically ill patients. Pharmacotherapy 2017;37(1): 43–53.

[59] PEPTIC Investigators for the Australian and New Zealand Intensive Care Society Clinical Trials Group, Alberta Health Services Critical Care Strategic Clinical Network, and the Irish Critical Care Trials Group, Young PJ, Bagshaw SM, Forbes AB, Nichol AD, Wright SE, Bailey M et al. Effect of stress ulcer prophylaxis with proton pump inhibitors vs histamine-2 receptor blockers on in-hospital mortality among ICU patients receiving invasive mechanical ventilation: the PEPTIC randomized clinical trial. JAMA 2020;323(7):616–26.

CHAPTER 24

Nutrition in Sepsis

VICTOR MANUEL SANCHEZ NAVA • HECTOR ALEJANDRO RAMIREZ GARCIA

INTRODUCTION

Sepsis is a potentially life-threatening organ dysfunction that is caused by an unregulated host response to infection [1]. Despite multiple advances in the areas of diagnosis, monitoring, and treatment, mortality remains high [2] The patient in sepsis represents a challenge from the nutritional point of view, since it has several differences from general critical patients of intensive therapy, including significant limitation of metabolic function with mitochondrial dysfunction [3]. There are multiple guidelines and recommendations regarding optimal nutritional management in critically ill patients, but there is still an important limitation of the available evidence in the context of sepsis [4,5]. This chapter will focus on an overview of the pathophysiological aspects of sepsis, as well as its impact on nutrition, and a review of the options available in both its enteral and parenteral forms.

PATHOPHYSIOLOGY OF SEPSIS AND ITS IMPACT ON METABOLISM

The word "metabolism" refers to the totality of chemical reactions that occur in an organism. It consists of catabolic and anabolic processes that are in a state of equilibrium or homeostasis. This balance can be disturbed by multiple pathological conditions, among which is sepsis [6].

Sepsis has multiple components within the umbrella definition of an unregulated host response to infection, including inflammation, the main focus in clinical research, but also includes elements of hemostasis, microbiota, thermoregulation, and circadian rhythm disturbances [7]. Traditionally, sepsis has been considered a syndrome that evolves from an initial state of hypermetabolism and systemic inflammation, and which ends in a phase of prolonged immunosuppression. Crucial to this view are cytokines, both proinflammatory, including interleukin 1 (IL-1), interleukin 6 (IL-6), and tumor necrosis factor alpha (TNF-a), along with their antiinflammatory counterparts (IL-4, IL-1,

IL-10 and IL-13). Within the traditional view, the initial inflammatory phase is characterized by the creation of a procoagulant environment, as well as an increase in the production of reactive oxygen species and nitric oxide, to later move on to a phase of immunosuppression when the production pathways are exhausted of the proinflammatory markers [8].

More recent paradigms suggest, rather, that the response of the immune system to the septic insult is in two different directions at the same time, with data that support both inflammation and excessive immunosuppression, and that cellular metabolic processes undergo fundamental changes, without being able to return for a long time to its state prior to the septic episode [3]. Target organ damage is the end result of a complex mix of endothelial activation, coagulopathy, disturbances in the immunocirculation, altered mitochondrial function, increased apoptosis, increased permeability of the intestine, and alterations in the protein and glucose metabolism [9].

Changes in the metabolism of the septic patient have been described according to a typical pattern. The initial symptoms of fever, increased heart rate, and activation of the immune system lead to an increase in energy consumption secondary to the neuroendocrine reaction, produced by proinflammatory cytokines [10]. The initial phase is associated with an increase in catabolic processes, with a suppression of anabolic ones. The increase in insulin resistance and the release of anterior pituitary hormones contribute to the availability of substrates for energy production [11]. Later in the phase of hypometabolism, the cells reach a state of adaptive and functional metabolic suppression, similar to hibernation, as protection against adenosine triphosphate depletion and that enables long-term survival if the organism survives the initial insult [12].

The end result of these changes is a derangement in the metabolism of all macronutrients. When the body enters a state of stress, it activates multiple compensatory responses, including an activation of hepatic gluconeogenesis and glycogenolysis, together with an

The Sepsis Codex. https://doi.org/10.1016/B978-0-323-88271-2.00025-0

increase in systemic resistance to insulin, which leads to hyperglycemia. The liver also increases lipolysis, with an increase in plasma free fatty acid concentration, and proteolysis, with the release of amino acids from multiple sources including skeletal muscle [6]. This phenomenon has come to be called "septic autocannibalism," since the body consumes not only its reserves but also involves proteins that play a structural or motor role [9].

The consequences of the septic self-consumption condition, if prolonged, are associated with multiple complications seen in patients who survive the initial septic insult in intensive care, including loss of muscle mass with protein catabolism, persistent organ failure, neuromuscular weakness, cachexia, poor wound healing, recurrent infections, and cognitive impairment. This state has been called: "Persistent inflammation-immunosuppression syndrome and catabolism" [13] and brings with it multiple consequences, including prolonged functional dependence and poor long-term survival [14].

The metabolic response within sepsis significantly depletes the patient's nutritional stores and generates large amounts of cellular debris. Nutrient supplementation during the acute phase is generally neglected in daily clinical practice, giving greater priority to hemodynamic stabilization and reestablishment of perfusion at the macrovascular level [3]. Although it makes sense to think that in the face of such profound changes in metabolism, it is necessary to start an aggressive and early nutritional therapy, the studies in this regard have not been conclusive. The ASPEN and ESPEN guidelines recognize a lack of evidence in the field of nutrition in sepsis, especially in patients with septic shock, and research in the underfeeding concept has yielded interesting results, which could explain some of these phenomena.

Permissive underfeeding emerged as a natural extension regarding the phenomenon of "disease-related anorexia" (sickness-associated anorexia), a set of behaviors preserved in an evolutionary way which favor the decrease in intake and function of the digestive system mediated by inflammatory markers of deliberate manner, including intestinal motility, bilirubin transport and synthesis, exocrine function of the pancreas, and central appetite [15]. The suppression of the digestive system seems to be guided toward the promotion of autophagy as a cell survival mechanism [16]. The guided destruction of intracellular structures releases resources that can then be spent on more urgent processes. Other multiple benefits include: offering an additional barrier against proteins with defects in the folding process [17], remodeling of the proteasome

toward a configuration more apt to survive in an inflammatory environment [18], a possible protection against alterations in the mitochondrial function given in febrile temperature ranges [19], and a mechanism of destruction of invasive pathogenic organisms, together with a more efficient processing and presentation of antigens in MHC 1 and MHC 2 [20]. These theoretical benefits, however, must be confirmed using clinical studies, in order to see if there is any role for permissive underfeeding in the septic patient population as a management strategy.

NUTRITION IN SEPSIS

Much of the research and evidence regarding nutritional therapy in septic patients have been extrapolated from the general critically ill patient population, secondary to a lack of high-quality studies conducted in the field. Even so, it can be useful to compare the general recommendations and contrast them with specific concrete evidence when it becomes available.

Calories

The estimation of energy expenditure in critically ill patients must be carried out through objective methods and preferably not through predictive equations, which tend to underestimate or overestimate caloric needs [21,22]. The gold standard for estimating energy expenditure at rest is indirect calorimetry (IC), and it is on this foundation that we must base ourselves to individualize the nutritional objective of each patient [23]. According to measurements made by IC in septic patients, there is an increase in resting energy expenditure after the onset of sepsis, which reaches its peak during the second week of stay in intensive care, up to 1.7 times the basal metabolism [24]. Even with all the efforts made in the last years, access to IC remains far from universal, and in the places where it is not available, using either VO_2 (oxygen consumption) from pulmonary artery catheter or VCO_2 (carbon dioxide production) derived from the ventilator can give an adequate evaluation of energy expenditure. If neither of these are available, a calculation tool can be used instead, such as the Weir formula, taking into account its limitations and using clinical judgment [5].

The large studies reviewed in the ASPEN 2022 guidelines did not show a significant difference in prognosis, mortality, or any other clinical outcome in adult critically ill patients who received higher or lower calorie nutrition within the range of current recommendations, so they were unable to make a precise recommendation regarding the energy intake recommended as a baseline in critically ill patients. The range of 12−25 kcal/kg was given within the first 7−10 days of stay in intensive care, taking into account the additional contribution provided by lipids in the medications and gastrointestinal tolerance [4]. Research focused on the caloric intake of the septic patient showed that insufficient nutrition in patients with immune dysfunction did not have a synergistic role in mortality, but it did in patients without immune dysfunction [25]. The patients enrolled in the TARGET study were subjected to two different levels of caloric intake, with an average intake of 1863 +- 478 kcal/day in the group with the highest caloric density compared to an intake of 1262 kcal +- 313 kcal/day in the group with the lowest caloric density. The study did not demonstrate any significant difference between the different clinical measures at the end of the intervention [26].

Glucose

In the initial phase of sepsis, there is a massive mobilization of the caloric reserves in the human body [27]. Muscle, glycogen, and lipids are broken down to generate endogenous glucose, which can cover up to 75% of the metabolic needs during the first days of illness, without significant suppression by feeding or intravenous glucose infusion. This exposes the patient to a significant risk of hyperglycemia during the first days of illness, which is associated with both a higher production or expression of proinflammatory cytokines, adherence of leukocytes, and alterations in endothelial integrity [28].

Some recommendations have been issued about the importance of gradually increasing caloric intake, in order to reach specific nutritional goals as the shock situation is resolved and to avoid the deleterious effects of overfeeding early in the course of illness. The amount of glucose (in parenteral nutrition) or carbohydrates (enteral nutrition) should not exceed 5 mg/kg/min in any moment of nutritional therapy, and early full enteral and parenteral nutrition should not be used in critically ill patients at least during the first 48 h, but should be prescribed within the first 3−7 days of stay in the intensive care unit (ICU) (5) [27].

Proteins

The evidence regarding protein supplementation in the different phases of sepsis is limited [29]. Protein losses increase fourfold in the first 24 h of critical illness [28], which supports feeding a high proportion of protein-derived calories early in the course of sepsis. Protein underfeeding is a recognized problem in ICU care, with large international surveys indicating that ICU

practitioners deliver an average of 0.6 g/kg/day of protein for the first two weeks following ICU admission, for a total of 33%−50% of the recommended delivery [27]. According to the recommendations for critical patients issued by ASPEN in 2022, based on a limited database, the administration of protein in greater or lesser amounts in the quantities previously recommended in adult critical patients did not lead to any difference in clinical results [4]. The previous recommendation of 1.2−2.0 g/kg/day of the ASPEN 2016 guidelines was upheld [30], with additional measures such as measurement of the nitrogen balance, the monitoring of the relationship between nonprotein calories with the total amount of nitrogen provided, and the total percentage of carbon and lipid calories being part of a comprehensive bundle in adjusting the nutritional input [5].

The retrospective studies that have been carried out, including PROTIVENT [31,32], seem to support the conclusion that medium-term mortality in critical patients is lower if the protein is increased gradually from the first days in the ICU until higher levels can be achieved from day 5 onwards, but it must be considered that these studies have a low proportion of septic patients (approximately 20%), so their applicability may be limited. Prospective studies such as EFFORT will be useful in the future to resolve this question [33].

Lipids

Lipids play an essential role in multiple functions of cell metabolism, including cell wall formation, gene expression, and as precursors of lipid metabolites, such as prostaglandins [4]. When considering the contribution of lipids to the septic patient, it is necessary to take into account the amount provided by medications and sedatives, since otherwise the patient may be exposed to ranges of toxicity or overfeeding.

Lipids should generally be part of parenteral nutrition. Lipids (including those provided by nonnutritional sources) should not exceed 1.5 gr/kg/day and soybean oil, fish oil, and mixed oils can be considered [5].

Immunonutrition

Immunonutrition emerged in the 1980s as a result of research conducted by Eric Newsholme at the University of Oxford [34] on the concept of immunometabolism. During the following years, multiple compounds with a profound involvement in the function of immune cells were identified, creating the idea that their supplementation could carry out an improvement in their function and an improvement in the prognosis of patients subjected to stress, including patients with burns, trauma, and sepsis [35]. Although the role of immunonutrition is currently the subject of intense debate, the ASPEN 2022 guidelines decided not to make a statement for or against, but to publish a specified review of this extensive topic in the near future.

Glutamine

Glutamine is the most abundant and versatile amino acid in the body and is of fundamental importance for intermediary metabolism, interorgan nitrogen exchange, and pH homeostasis. It is also used in all cells for the synthesis of nucleotides, antioxidants, and multiple functions related to cell integrity and function [36]. Immune system cells must normally function in nutrient-restricted microenvironments, with glutamine being used as an alternative source in amounts equal to or greater than glucose in certain contexts such as sepsis [37].

Excessive consumption of glutamine during periods of stress in the human body, both by the immune system and by the liver, can lead to a deficit, especially by reducing the contribution of skeletal muscle, the main source in mammals [36]. This can conditionally convert glutamine to an essential amino acid. Prolonged glutamine deficiency can lead to worsening of active disease and an increased risk of subsequent superinfection [38].

Although theory dictates that glutamine supplementation should provide some clinical benefit to a patient in a hypercatabolic state such as early sepsis, evidence has not shown superiority over usual management. Glutamine supplementation even increased in-hospital and six-month mortality in the REDOXS study, especially in patients with kidney failure [39,40]. In the ESPEN guideline, regular glutamine supplementation was not recommended except in patients with trauma or burns [5]. In the 2016 ASPEN guideline, it was not recommended to use it routinely in the general critical patient [30].

Omega-3 Fatty Acids

Fish oil contains multiple fatty acids that have been experimentally shown to modulate metabolic processes and decrease inflammation; these have been generally called omega-3 fatty acids [41]. The evidence regarding supplementation with omega-3 fatty acids in critically ill patients has not shown a significant difference in clinical outcomes, either in its exclusive modality with fish oil or with a mixture of varied oils when compared to using only soybean oil [4].

Vitamin C

Septic patients have very low levels of vitamin C during the inflammatory process despite adequate supplementation [42]. Vitamin C is an essential cofactor for the endogenous production of epinephrine, norepinephrine, and vasopressin [43]. Although initially there were promising results based on supraphysiological supplementation in septic patients [44,45], more recent and higher quality studies have shown that the effect of vitamin C in the septic patient appears to be negligible when compared against usual management [46,47].

ENTERAL AND PARENTERAL FEEDING

Enteral feeding is the most economical and physiological way to provide nutrition to the critical septic patient, including among its benefits: improve and maintain immune function, improve nitrogen balance, improve wound healing, improve protein synthesis, increase the antioxidant system intracellular, decrease the hypermetabolic response, and preserve the integrity of the intestinal barrier [48]. In septic patients specifically, it could prevent bacterial translocation and stress ulcerations [3], but it has its own risks that must be taken into account when selecting a feeding modality. Enteral feeding may not be delivered in the required dose due to irregular absorption or slow gastric emptying, defined as a gastric aspirate >500 mL/6 h, with increased risk of aspiration. Likewise, it can present transit problems, with vomiting and diarrhea and is frankly contraindicated when there is bowel injury, ischemia, obstruction, uncontrolled shock, uncontrolled hypoxemia and acidosis, uncontrolled upper GI bleeding, abdominal compartment syndrome, and high output fistula without distal feeding access [5]. Complications with glycemic control, respiratory acidosis, or hypertriglyceridemia may also lead to decreased feeding [4].

Multiple measures have been proposed in order to counteract the complications of enteral feeding in the septic critical patient: The monitoring of gastric residual volume in established enteral nutrition may not be necessary and could be done mainly to identify intolerance during initiation or progression [5]. In case there is significant gastric residue, prokinetics may be considered, including metoclopramide and erythromycin [1]. If significant residual gastric volume remains, one may consider postpyloric feeding over withholding EN, and in patients with high risk of aspiration, jejunal feeding may be performed [5].

In order to clarify whether there was any difference between the two feeding routes in the context of critically ill patients, two clinical trials were carried out: CALORIES and NUTRIREA-2. CALORIES did not specify what percentage of their patients were in septic shock, but more than 80% of their patients had some type of vasopressor support, with no significant difference in outcomes when comparing parenteral versus enteral feeding, and a nonsignificant increase in gastrointestinal complications in enterally fed patients [49]. NUTRIREA-2 assigned patients on vasopressors and invasive mechanical ventilation support to receive either parenteral or enteral nutrition and included a large proportion of patients in septic shock, greater than 66% of patients in both comparison arms. Neither of the two groups presented significant differences in most of the results, other than an increase in the enteral feeding group of intestinal complications, including vomiting, diarrhea, intestinal ischemia, and acute colonic pseudo-obstruction [50]. With this, we can specifically state that in patients with septic shock, early enteral feeding prior to resolution of shock can increase the risk of gastrointestinal complications [51].

In adult critically ill patients who were candidates for enteral nutrition and received parenteral nutrition as their primary feeding modality in the first week, there were no differences in clinical outcomes. There is no significant difference when a similar amount of energy is given for short periods of time either enterally or parenterally. The main factors to take into account when selecting a modality are the cost and convenience of providing either of the two modes of feeding, with the most important considerations being avoiding overfeeding, glycemic control, and catheter care. No solid evidence was found in favor of supplementation with parenteral nutrition in patients who did not reach goals with enteral nutrition alone during the first seven days, it being preferable to wait until tolerance is achieved. There are specific recommendations in this regard which mention the possibility of starting parenteral feeding specifically in the context of patients with severe malnutrition with no tolerance of enteral feedings [4].

SCREENING FOR NUTRITIONAL RISK IN SEPTIC PATIENTS

The general critical patient is at significant risk for malnutrition, and multiple screening tools exist to give an assessment, due to the difficulty of evaluating both weight changes and wasting of lean tissues in the ICU. The ESPEN 2019 guidelines states that MNA-SF (mini nutrition assessment) had the highest specificity, while NRS 2002 (nutritional risk screening) had the highest sensitivity when subjective global assessment was the gold standard [5]. There is no recent universally accepted tool to define the at-risk patient, but the ASPEN 2016 guidelines suggested categorizing patients according to NRS 2002 or NUTRIC (nutritional risk in critically ill) to define their nutritional regiment [30].

The studies employed to develop and validate the previous tools were not created with specifically the septic patient in mind, but there have been several recent studies focused on this population, including linking NRS-2002 to risk stratification [52] and finding an association between sepsis and malnutrition when employing the mNUTRIC score [53]. However, more data are needed to find a definitive tool to employ specifically in the septic patient.

CONCLUSIONS

The safe prescription of nutrition in the critical septic patients involves multiple aspects, owing to the complexity of the pathophysiology, as well as the multiple factors that can intervene in providing adequate nutrition. A clinician that wants to start either enteral or parenteral nutrition should always be aware of: total and specific macronutrient requirements, with a focus on protein (1.2−2 g/kg/day), the requirements of nitrogen, the relationship between noncaloric protein with the total nitrogen, the percentage and total quantity of carbohydrates (no more than 3−4 gr/kg/day) and lipids (no more than 1.5 gr/kg/day), alongside covering water and electrolyte requirements.

The importance of providing optimal nutrition in both your protein and caloric intake cannot be overstated. The nutritional status and the risk involved in the form of nutrition we choose to administer should be evaluated. The studies on which most of the evidence is based to issue recommendations were conducted in general critical patients, with limited exceptions. It is necessary to continue the investigation in the septic patient to be able to know more in depth the applicability of the different recommendations issued.

REFERENCES

[1] Evans L, Rhodes A, Alhazzani W, Antonelli M, Coopersmith C, French C, et al. Surviving sepsis campaign: international guidelines for management of sepsis and septic shock 2021. Crit Care Med 2021; 49(11):e1063−143.

[2] van der Poll T, van de Veerdonk F, Scicluna B, Netea M. The immunopathology of sepsis and potential therapeutic targets. Nat Rev Immunol 2017;17(7):407−20.

[3] De Waele E, Malbrain M, Spapen H. Nutrition in sepsis: a bench-to-bedside review. Nutrients 2020;12(2):395.

[4] Compher C, Bingham A, McCall M, Patel J, Rice T, Braunschweig C, et al. Guidelines for the provision of nutrition support therapy in the adult critically ill patient: the American Society for Parenteral and Enteral Nutrition. J Parenter Enteral Nutr 2022;46(1):12−41.

[5] Singer P, Blaser A, Berger M, Alhazzani W, Calder P, Casaer M, et al. ESPEN guideline on clinical nutrition in the intensive care unit. Clin Nutr 2019;38(1):48−79.

[6] Wasyluk W, Zwolak A. Metabolic alterations in sepsis. J Clin Med 2021;10(11):2412.

[7] Cohen J, Vincent J, Adhikari N, Machado F, Angus D, Calandra T, et al. Sepsis: a roadmap for future research. Lancet Infect Dis 2015;15(5):581−614.

[8] Wasyluk W, Wasyluk M, Zwolak A. Sepsis as a pan-endocrine illness—endocrine disorders in septic patients. J Clin Med 2021;10(10):2075.

[9] Honore P, Hoste E, Molnár Z, Jacobs R, Joannes-Boyau O, Malbrain M, et al. Cytokine removal in human septic shock: where are we and where are we going? Ann Intensive Care 2019;9(1).

[10] Englert J, Rogers A. Metabolism, metabolomics, and nutritional support of patients with sepsis. Clin Chest Med 2016;37(2):321−31.

[11] Lewis A, Billiar T, Rosengart M. Biology and metabolism of sepsis: innate immunity, bioenergetics, and autophagy. Surg Infect 2016;17(3):286−93.

[12] Carré J, Singer M. Cellular energetic metabolism in sepsis: the need for a systems approach. Biochim Biophys Acta Bioenerg 2008;1777(7−8):763−71.

[13] Gentile L, Cuenca A, Efron P, Ang D, Bihorac A, McKinley B, et al. Persistent inflammation and immunosuppression. J Trauma Acute Care Surg 2012;72(6):1491−501.

[14] Mira J, Gentile L, Mathias B, Efron P, Brakenridge S, Mohr A, et al. Sepsis pathophysiology, chronic critical illness, and persistent inflammation-immunosuppression and catabolism syndrome. Crit Care Med 2017;45(2):253−62.

[15] van Niekerk G, Meaker C, Engelbrecht A. Nutritional support in sepsis: when less may be more. Crit Care 2020; 24(1).

[16] Pakos-Zebrucka K, Koryga I, Mnich K, Ljujic M, Samali A, Gorman A. The integrated stress response. EMBO Rep 2016;17(10):1374−95.

[17] Gidalevitz T, Prahlad V, Morimoto R. The stress of protein misfolding: from single cells to multicellular organisms. Cold Spring Harbor Perspect Biol 2011;3(6). a009704-a009704.

[18] Mathew R, Khor S, Hackett S, Rabinowitz J, Perlman D, White E. Functional role of autophagy-mediated proteome remodeling in cell survival signaling and innate immunity. Mol Cell 2014;55(6):916−30.

[19] Zukiene R, Nauciene Z, Ciapaite J, Mildažienė V. Acute temperature resistance threshold in heart mitochondria: febrile temperature activates function but exceeding it collapses the membrane barrier. Int J Hyperther 2010; 26(1):56−66.

[20] Tey S, Khanna R. Autophagy mediates transporter associated with antigen processing-independent presentation of viral epitopes through MHC class I pathway. Blood 2012;120(5):994−1004.

[21] De Waele E, Opsomer T, Honoré PM, Diltoer M, Mattens S, Huyghens L, Spapen H. Measured versus calculated resting energy expenditure in critically ill adult patients. Do mathematics match the gold standard? Minerva Anestesiol 2015;81:272−82.

[22] Zusman O, Kagan I, Bendavid I, Theilla M, Cohen J, Singer P. Predictive equations versus measured energy expenditure by indirect calorimetry: a retrospective validation. Clin Nutr 2019;38(3):1206−10.

[23] Oshima T, Berger M, De Waele E, Guttormsen A, Heidegger C, Hiesmayr M, et al. Indirect calorimetry in nutritional therapy. A position paper by the ICALIC study group. Clin Nutr 2017;36(3):651−62.

[24] Uehara M, Plank L, Hill G. Components of energy expenditure in patients with severe sepsis and major trauma. Crit Care Med 1999;27(7):1295−302.

[25] Hung K, Chen Y, Wang C, Wang Y, Lin C, Chang Y, et al. Insufficient nutrition and mortality risk in septic patients admitted to ICU with a focus on immune dysfunction. Nutrients 2019;11(2):367.

[26] Chapman M, Peake SL, Bellomo R, Davies A, Deane A, Horowitz M, Hurford S, Lange K, Little L, Mackle D, O'Connor S. Energy-dense versus routine enteral nutrition in the critically ill. N Engl J Med 2018;379(19): 1823−34.

[27] Wischmeyer P. Nutrition therapy in sepsis. Crit Care Clin 2018;34(1):107−25.

[28] Preiser J, van Zanten A, Berger M, Biolo G, Casaer M, Doig G, et al. Metabolic and nutritional support of critically ill patients: consensus and controversies. Crit Care 2015;19(1).

[29] Preiser J. High protein intake during the early phase of critical illness: yes or no? Crit Care 2018;22(1).

[30] McClave S, Taylor B, Martindale R, Warren M, Johnson D, Braunschweig C, et al. Guidelines for the provision and assessment of nutrition support therapy in the adult critically ill patient. J Parenter Enteral Nutr 2016;40(2): 159−211.

[31] Koekkoek W, van Setten C, Olthof L, Kars J, van Zanten A. Timing of PROTein INtake and clinical outcomes of adult critically ill patients on prolonged mechanical VENTilation: the PROTINVENT retrospective study. Clin Nutr 2019;38(2):883−90.

[32] Bendavid I, Zusman O, Kagan I, Theilla M, Cohen J, Singer P. Early administration of protein in critically ill patients: a retrospective cohort study. Nutrients 2019; 11(1):106.

[33] Patel J, Rice T, Compher C, Heyland D. Do we have clinical equipoise (or uncertainty) about how much protein to provide to critically ill patients? Nutr Clin Pract 2019;35(3):499−505.

[34] Ardawi M, Newsholme E. Maximum activities of some enzymes of glycolysis, the tricarboxylic acid cycle and

ketone-body and glutamine utilization pathways in lymphocytes of the rat. Biochem J 1982;208(3):743−8.

[35] Grimble R. Basics in clinical nutrition: immunonutrition − Nutrients which influence immunity: effect and mechanism of action. e-SPEN, the European e-Journal of Clinical Nutrition and Metabolism 2009;4(1):e10−3.

[36] Cruzat V, Macedo Rogero M, Noel Keane K, Curi R, Newsholme P. Glutamine: metabolism and immune function, supplementation and clinical translation. Nutrients 2018;10(11):1564.

[37] Newsholme P. Why is L-glutamine metabolism important to cells of the immune system in health, postinjury, surgery or infection? J Nutr 2001;131(9):2515S−22S.

[38] Oudemans-van Straaten H, Bosman R, Treskes M, van der Spoel H, Zandstra D. Plasma glutamine depletion and patient outcome in acute ICU admissions. Intensive Care Med 2000;27(1):84−90.

[39] Lenders C, Liu S, Wilmore D, Sampson L, Dougherty L, Spiegelman D, et al. Evaluation of a novel food composition database that includes glutamine and other amino acids derived from gene sequencing data. Eur J Clin Nutr 2009;63(12):1433−9.

[40] Heyland D, Elke G, Cook D, Berger M, Wischmeyer P, Albert M, et al. Glutamine and antioxidants in the critically ill patient. J Parenter Enteral Nutr 2014;39(4):401−9.

[41] Calder P. Polyunsaturated fatty acids, inflammation, and immunity. Lipids 2001;36(9):1007−24.

[42] Carr A, Rosengrave P, Bayer S, Chambers S, Mehrtens J, Shaw G. Hypovitaminosis C and vitamin C deficiency in critically ill patients despite recommended enteral and parenteral intakes. Crit Care 2017;21(1).

[43] May J, Harrison F. Role of vitamin C in the function of the vascular endothelium. Antioxidants Redox Signal 2013;19(17):2068−83.

[44] Fowler A, Syed A, Knowlson S, Sculthorpe R, Farthing D, DeWilde C, et al. Phase I safety trial of intravenous ascorbic acid in patients with severe sepsis. J Transl Med 2014;12(1).

[45] Marik P, Khangoora V, Rivera R, Hooper M, Catravas J. Hydrocortisone, vitamin C, and thiamine for the treatment of severe sepsis and septic shock. Chest 2017;151(6):1229−38.

[46] Fujii T, Luethi N, Young P, Frei D, Eastwood G, French C, et al. Effect of vitamin C, hydrocortisone, and thiamine vs hydrocortisone alone on time alive and free of vasopressor support among patients with septic shock. JAMA 2020;323(5):423.

[47] Sevransky J, Rothman R, Hager D, Bernard G, Brown S, Buchman T, et al. Effect of vitamin C, thiamine, and hydrocortisone on ventilator- and vasopressor-free days in patients with sepsis. JAMA 2021;325(8):742.

[48] Sanchez Nava V. ICU Manag 2010;10:12−4.

[49] Harvey S, Parrott F, Harrison D, Bear D, Segaran E, Beale R, et al. Trial of the route of early nutritional support in critically ill adults. N Engl J Med 2014;371(18):1673−84.

[50] Reignier J, Boisramé-Helms J, Brisard L, Lascarrou J, Ait Hssain A, Anguel N, et al. Enteral versus parenteral early nutrition in ventilated adults with shock: a randomised, controlled, multicentre, open-label, parallel-group study (NUTRIREA-2). Lancet 2018;391(10116):133−43.

[51] Mancl E, Muzevich K. Tolerability and safety of enteral nutrition in critically ill patients receiving intravenous vasopressor therapy. J Parenter Enteral Nutr 2012;37(5):641−51.

[52] Gao Q, Cheng Y, Li Z, Tang Q, Qiu R, Cai S, et al. Association between nutritional risk screening score and prognosis of patients with sepsis. Infect Drug Resist 2021;14:3817−25.

[53] Larrondo MHM, León PDO, Ginarte RLM, et al. Assessment of nutritional status in critical ill patients by means of two Nutritional Risk Indexes. Rev Habanera Ciencias Méd 2020;19(4):1−14.

CHAPTER 25

Fever in Intensive Care Units

KAZUAKI ATAGI

INTRODUCTION

Fever is a physiological manifestation of the host immune response to infectious or noninfectious agents. It is a host defense mechanism following exposure to external agents, and the resultant increase in body temperature facilitates the host immune response by promoting the synthesis of antibodies, cytokines, activated T cells, polymorphs, and macrophages. However, increased body temperature may be harmful in patients with acute brain injury and cardiac arrest. Therefore, fever should be treated in inpatients who complain of discomfort due to high body temperature.

The presence of fever often leads to a detailed clinical evaluation by an intensivist, prompting diagnostic and therapeutic decision-making. In the event that critically ill patients in the intensive care unit (ICU) develop a fever, they need to be closely monitored and treated. Therefore, a systematic and comprehensive diagnostic approach for ICU patients with fever is required. This article reviews the common infectious and noninfectious causes of fever and its pathogenesis in ICU patients and outlines a rational approach to case management.

DEFINITIONS FOR FEVER

Generally, the average normal body temperature is approximately 37°C (98.6°F), ranging from 36.0 to 37.5°C (96.8–99.5°F) [1,2]; however, the normal body temperature can vary with the time and method of measurement. In healthy individuals, this temperature variation ranges from 0.5 to 1.0°C (0.9–1.8°F) according to the circadian rhythm and menstrual cycle [3]. During exercise, body temperature can rise by 2.0–3.0°C (3.6–5.3°F) [4]. The definition of fever is arbitrary and depends on the purpose for which it is defined. For example, some studies define fever as a core temperature above 38.0°C (100.4°F), whereas other studies define fever as two consecutive elevations above 38.3°C

(101.0°F) [1]. In neutropenic patients, fever is defined as a single oral temperature of ≥38.3°C (≥101.0°F) in the absence of a prominent environmental cause, or an oral temperature elevation of ≥38.0°C (≥100.4°F) for 1 h [1]. A variety of definitions for fever are acceptable, depending on the desired sensitivity associated with using thermal abnormality as an indicator; this decision is often left to the individual ICU practitioner.

While many physiological changes alter body temperature, various environmental and interventional factors in the ICU alter body temperature, including the use of special mattresses, air conditioning, cardiopulmonary bypass, peritoneal lavage, dialysis, and continuous hemofiltration. It is common that the thermoregulatory mechanisms can be affected by drugs as well as disturbances in the central or autonomic nervous systems. Therefore, it is difficult to determine whether the cause of fever is due to physiological changes, drugs, or environmental factors. Although the cause of fever often remains unclear, a joint task force of the Infectious Diseases Society of America and the American College of Critical Care Medicine established in 2008 defined fever as a body temperature of 38.3°C or higher, regardless of its cause [5].

MEASUREMENT OF FEVER

Body temperature can be measured at peripheral or core sites in ICU patients. Core body temperature measurements are considered to be more accurate than peripheral body temperature measurements, with a sensitivity of 64% and a specificity of 96%. Core measurement methods include intravascular (e.g., use of a pulmonary artery catheter), intravesicular, and rectal measurements [6].

Table 25.1 shows the accuracy of the different methods used to measure body temperature. Body temperature is most accurately measured by an intravascular, esophageal, or bladder thermistor, followed by rectal, oral, and tympanic membrane measurements

The Sepsis Codex. https://doi.org/10.1016/B978-0-323-88271-2.00018-3

229

TABLE 25.1
Accuracy of Methods Used for Measuring Temperature (6, 12–16) [5].

Most accurate
  Pulmonary artery thermistor
  Urinary bladder catheter thermistor
  Esophageal probe
  Rectal probe
Other acceptable methods in order of accuracy
  Oral probe
  Infrared ear thermometry
Other methods less desirable
  Temporal artery thermometer
  Axillary thermometer
  Chemical dot

[5]. The intravascular thermistor is the gold standard for body temperature measurement; however, it is not used in most ICU patients [3]. Instead, peripheral temperature measurement is commonly used in many ICU patients. The guidelines state that axillary measurements, temporal artery estimation, and chemical dot thermometers should not be used in ICU patients, and rectal thermometers should not be used in neutropenic patients [5]. Additionally, body temperature measurements are used to follow the patient's progress while in the ICU. For consistency across measurements, the same measurement method and location should be used.

PATHOGENESIS OF FEVER

Body heat is generated by intracellular chemical reactions that release heat during nutrient catabolism. The human body has a basal metabolic rate that is necessary to maintain cellular functions as well as basal heat production, and the circulatory system distributes this metabolically generated heat throughout the body. Body temperature is finely controlled by the hypothalamus, limbic system, lower brainstem, reticular formation, spinal cord, and sympathetic ganglia. This temperature-sensitive region of the preoptic area regulates body temperature in response to signals from the peripheral and trunk sensors in the skin.

Fever is a result of dysregulated body temperature homeostasis. In humans, it is thought to be a protective adaptive response secondary to the release of cytokines in the circulation. Cytokines such as interleukin-1 (IL-1), interleukin-6 (IL-6), and tumor necrosis factor-α (TNF-α) play a central role in the development of fever. The interaction of these cytokines is complex, and each cytokine can regulate its own expression as well as that of other cytokines [7].

In the central nervous system, these cytokines bind to specific receptors located near the preoptic area of the anterior hypothalamus. These stimulated cytokine receptors then activate phospholipase A2, resulting in the release of arachidonic acid from the cell membrane, which acts as a substrate for the cyclooxygenase pathway [8]. Some cytokines appear to increase cyclooxygenase expression, which subsequently results in the direct release of prostaglandin E2 [9]. Additionally, cytokines are able to diffuse across the blood–brain barrier and act directly on the hypothalamus. Cytokine signaling in the hypothalamus can directly affect body temperature homeostasis, leading to decreased heat loss and increased heat production, causing fever [8].

SIGNIFICANCE OF FEVER

Fever complicates up to 70% of all ICU admissions and is often the result of an infection or other severe conditions [9]. In addition, fever in ICU patients is associated with worse prognosis, especially in cases of head trauma and subarachnoid hemorrhage. In an observational study of 24,204 adult ICU admissions, fever ≥39.5°C (103°F) was associated with an increase in mortality (20% vs. 12%), compared with a fever below 39.5°C (103°F) [10]. Based on the origin, the etiology of fever in the ICU can be classified as infectious or noninfectious. Many intensivists believe that it is impossible to differentiate between infectious and noninfectious causes in cases of fever between 38.3°C (100.9°F) and 38.8°C (101.8°F). However, fevers between 38.9°C (102.0°F) and 41°C (105.8°F) are considered to be infectious. On the other hand, patients with a very high fever of 41.1°C (106.0°F) or higher are more likely to have noninfectious causes such as drug-induced fever or hyperthermia. One study reported that patients with high peak temperatures between 39°C (102.2°F) and 39.4°C (102.9°F) had significantly lower hospital mortality than those who had peak temperatures between 36.5°C (97.7°F) and 36.9°C (98.4°F) (odds ratio 0.56, 95% confidence interval [CI] 0.48−0.66) [11]; in contrast, mortality increased with rising temperature in noninfectious cases of fever (odds ratio 2.07, 95% CI 1.68−2.55). A subsequent study (FACE) published in 2012 reported that higher 28-day mortality observed with body temperature >39.5°C (103.1°F) occurred in patients without sepsis but not in patients with sepsis. Certain studies have also shown an inverse relationship between fever and mortality in ICU and emergency patients [12].

FEVER PATTERNS

Usually, the pattern of fever is unlikely to be helpful in its diagnosis. However, some patterns of fever are typically associated with specific etiologies [13]. For example,

sustained fever is often caused by gram-negative bacterial infections or central nervous system injuries [13]. In addition, fever that occurs 48 h after initiation of mechanical ventilation suggests ventilator-assisted pneumonia (VAP). Fever that occurs 10−14 days after antibiotic therapy administered for an intraabdominal abscess may be due to a fungal infection.

CAUSES OF FEVER IN THE ICU

Any disease process that releases the proinflammatory cytokines IL-1, IL-6, and TNF-α results in fever; this includes both infectious and noninfectious causes of fever [14,15] (Table 25.2). The most common causes of infectious fever in the ICU are VAP, central line-associated bloodstream infection (CLABSI), catheter-related urinary tract infections (UTIs), surgical site infections, and bacteremia [15].

Although infections are the most common cause of fever in ICU patients, many other inflammatory diseases

TABLE 25.2
Infectious and Noninfectious Causes of Fever [15].

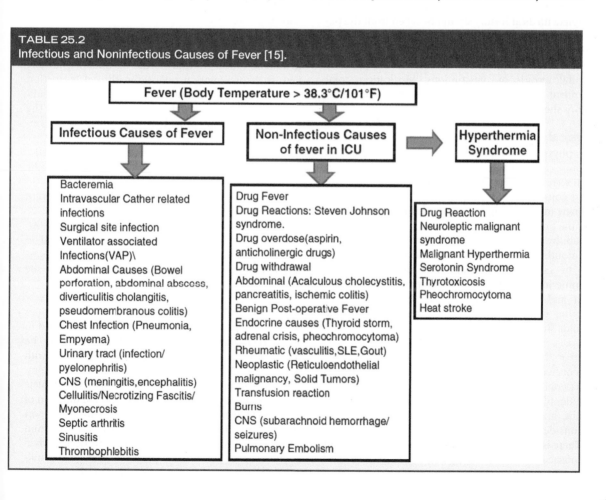

Fever (Body Temperature > 38.3°C/101°F)		
Infectious Causes of Fever	**Non-Infectious Causes of fever in ICU**	**Hyperthermia Syndrome**
Bacteremia Intravascular Cather related infections Surgical site infection Ventilator associated Infections(VAP)\ Abdominal Causes (Bowel perforation, abdominal abscess, diverticulitis cholangitis, pseudomembranous colitis) Chest Infection (Pneumonia, Empyema) Urinary tract (infection/pyelonephritis) CNS (meningitis,encephalitis) Cellulitis/Necrotizing Fascitis/Myonecrosis Septic arthritis Sinusitis Thrombophlebitis	Drug Fever Drug Reactions: Steven Johnson syndrome. Drug overdose(aspirin, anticholinergic drugs) Drug withdrawal Abdominal (Acalculous cholecystitis, pancreatitis, ischemic colitis) Benign Post-operative Fever Endocrine causes (Thyroid storm, adrenal crisis, pheochromocytoma) Rheumatic (vasculitis,SLE,Gout) Neoplastic (Reticuloendothelial malignancy, Solid Tumors) Transfusion reaction Burns CNS (subarachnoid hemorrhage/seizures) Pulmonary Embolism	Drug Reaction Neuroleptic malignant syndrome Malignant Hyperthermia Serotonin Syndrome Thyrotoxicosis Pheochromocytoma Heat stroke

can result in fevers of noninfectious origin. The most common noninfectious fever in the ICU is postoperative fever, caused by drugs, transfusion reactions, and venous thromboembolism. Additionally, infection is not always associated with fever. For example, approximately 10% of septic patients are hypothermic and 35% are normothermic. Patients with sepsis who do not develop fever have a significantly higher mortality rate than septic patients with fever [15,16]. It is unclear why some patients with infections do not develop febrile responses.

A TREATMENT APPROACH FOR CRITICALLY ILL FEBRILE PATIENTS

A systematic approach for treating patients with severe fever in the ICU is to integrate the following points:

Review of History and Records

A thorough review of the patient's medical chart, followed by a complete physical examination, is important for identifying the cause of fever in the ICU. A complete medical history should be taken from the patient or attendant, depending on the circumstances. In addition, medical records of recent treatment or medication should be noted and confirmed with previous hospital records or prescriptions. Medication, total parenteral nutrition, transfusion, and microbiological history should also be assessed.

Physical Examination

On physical examination, the physician should examine chest sounds, quality of sputum and endotracheal secretions, tenderness, or rigidity in the abdomen. Heart sounds should also be carefully monitored for any new murmurs suggestive of endocarditis. Additionally, the presence of diarrhea should be checked for the possibility of *Clostridium difficile* infection. Furthermore, the mouth, skin, joints, and lower extremities should also be examined in detail. It is also necessary to examine intravascular catheters, urinary catheters, and chest and abdominal drains. Finally, any dressings covering the wounds should be removed, and the wounds should be examined.

Interpretation of Survey Data

Patients with fever in the ICU undergo a variety of tests to ascertain the cause of the fever. Laboratory tests include blood cultures, urine cultures, chest radiographs, and other tests. The following points should be considered when interpreting laboratory data:

1. There is an overlap of bacteria between normal and infected tissues in the gastrointestinal tract and genital system.

2. For blood cultures, the number of samples drawn with positive growth and organism growth should be compared.
3. If UTI is suspected, urinalysis should show >10 white blood cells/high-power field and colony-forming unit >105/mL to confirm the diagnosis.

Magnitude of Fever

In cases of fever between 38.3°C (100.9°F) and 38.8°C (101.8°F), it is challenging to differentiate between infectious and noninfectious etiologies. Fever between 38.9°C (102.2°F) and 41°C (105.8°F) is usually the result of infection. Fever above 41.1°C (106.6°F) usually has a noninfectious etiology (e.g., drug-induced fever, transfusion reaction, adrenal insufficiency, thyroid storm, heatstroke, and malignant hyperthermia). Fever patterns are fraught with uncertainty and are unlikely to be useful for diagnosis.

INITIAL INVESTIGATIONS

Blood Cultures

Since the information provided by a positive blood culture can significantly impact patient prognosis and treatment, blood cultures should be obtained for any new fever presentation unless the clinical evaluation strongly suggests a noninfectious cause. Table 25.3 indicates the different methods used for blood cultures. The following guidelines provide 10 recommendations concerning blood culture collection and analysis [5]:

(a) Three to four blood cultures should be obtained within the first 24 h of the onset of fever for the detection of microbial growth.
(b) Single blood cultures are not recommended, except in neonates.
(c) Different sites should be used for each sample. At least 10−20 mL of blood should be collected in blood culture bottles.
(d) If an intravascular device is in place, a separate site should be used for blood collection.

Serum Procalcitonin

The Surviving Sepsis Campaign guidelines published in 2021 state that serum procalcitonin (PCT) can be assessed in adults with sepsis or septic shock with adequate source control [17]. These guidelines recommend that serum PCT is assessed in addition to complete clinical evaluation to determine the optimal duration of therapy. However, there is limited evidence to support this practice. Therefore, we suggest the use of serum PCT in addition to clinical evaluation to decide when to initiate antimicrobials. In previous studies using antimicrobial therapy and clinical evaluation, there was no

TABLE 25.3
Blood Culture Systems [5].

Method	Aerobes	Anaerobes	Yeast	Fungi	Mycobacteria	Comments
Conventional broth-in-bottle	+ +	+ +	+/+ +	+	+	Slower than automated systems
Broth-in-bottle with continuous monitoring	+++	+ +/+++	+ +/+++	+	$+^a$, + + +^{b}	Speeds time to detection compared with intermittent monitoring
Lysis-centrifugation (isolator^c)	+ +/+++	+	+++	+++	+++	Volume cultured is 10 Ml
Antibiotic removal systems (resin bottles)	+ +	+/+ +	+ +	+	+	Greatest yield on staphylococci and yeast compared with conventional systems

+, not recommended; ++, acceptable; +++, best available method.
^{a} Using standard blood culture bottles.
^{b} using special mycobacterial bottles.
^{c} Isolator (Inverness Medical Innovations, Waltham, MA).

difference in short-term mortality or other factors when PCT was assessed. There have been no studies of long-term mortality or other factors related to PCT assessment.

Polymerase Chain Reaction—Based Screening

Rapid molecular diagnostic platforms based on multiplex polymerase chain reaction assays have been developed to quickly screen for a wide variety of pathogens. However, high cost has been a significant factor in preventing the widespread use of such platforms.

Respiratory Tract Sampling and Urine Cultures

Gram staining and culture of the endotracheal aspirate and sputum of febrile patients should be performed if sampling is available.

For patients with a Foley catheter, urine should be collected from the catheter port and transported for culture immediately, or at least within 2 h of collection, for optimal results.

Radiologic Investigations
Chest radiograph

The most commonly indicated radiographic examinations provide information about the appearance of new or worsening lung lesions. However, portable chest radiographs are not sensitive, and new findings may not be easily detected, especially in the presence of preexisting radiographic abnormalities.

Computed tomography scan

Computed tomography (CT) should not be routinely performed in all patients. However, CT scans provide essential information when chest radiographs are difficult to diagnose. They can also help distinguish whether a new or worsening lung lesion has developed. In addition, abdominal CT scans are much more sensitive in detecting hepatobiliary infection/inflammation, psoas hematoma/abscess, pancreatic necrosis, adenopathy, and retroperitoneal collection than ultrasound.

Microbiologic Cultures from Suspected Sites of Infection

Many patients in the ICU have several potential sites of infection, including wounds, catheters, fluid collections, joints, stool (e.g., *C. difficile*), and sinuses. It is prudent to collect samples from such potential sites and culture them, if necessary.

If the patient develops fever during transfusion and the transfusion is stopped, the transfusion bag and its contents should also be sent for culture.

DIAGNOSTIC EVALUATION

It is essential to obtain blood cultures and other appropriate cultures before initiating antibiotic therapy. Many studies have demonstrated that both prior and current antibiotic therapies can reduce the predictive accuracy of invasive diagnostic tests.

INFECTIOUS CAUSES OF FEVER

Common infectious causes of fever in the ICU include VAP, CLABSI, catheter-associated UTI, surgical site infection, and sinusitis.

Ventilator-Assisted Pneumonia

VAP is pneumonia that develops after more than 48 h of ventilator use. VAP is defined by (1) new or increased lung infiltrates on chest radiographs, (2) increased bronchial secretions or abscesses, and (3) increased white blood cells [18].

Central Line-Associated Bloodstream Infection

Intravascular catheter-related infections are generally recognized as fever without localized symptoms. However, other symptoms such as cellulitis at the insertion site, purulent drainage from the insertion site, incidentally detected sepsis or septic shock, pyogenic thrombophlebitis, and endocarditis may also occur. Diagnosis can be confirmed by excluding other possible causes and identifying the typical causative microorganism, such as staphylococcal or streptococcal species.

Catheter-Related UTIs

Catheter-related UTIs may present with symptoms of cystitis, such as suprapubic pain, hematuria, pyuria, or pyelonephritis. However, it often presents with fever without localized symptoms or signs. In such cases, confirmation of bacteriuria facilitates the diagnosis.

Surgical Site Infection

Postoperative patients with fever or shock should be considered for surgical site infections. Abdominal signs may be masked by analgesia or sedation, but it is essential to observe surgical drains for bleeding and discharge of purulent material. Most surgical site infections develop one to four weeks after surgery.

Sinusitis

A common cause of sinusitis is poor drainage of nasal secretions from the sinuses. Therefore, a deviated nasal septum, nasogastric tube, facial trauma, skull base fracture, and nasopharyngeal hematomas cause sinusitis.

Sinusitis is suspected to be caused by purulent nasal discharge, fever, headache, and malodorous breath. A CT scan and sinus fluid collection for examination will increase the accuracy of the diagnosis. *Pseudomonas* accounts for 60% of all infections, while *Staphylococcus aureus* and *Streptococcus* are implicated in 33% of cases.

Postoperative Fever

Fever is common during the first 48 h after surgery. Early postoperative fever is usually noninfectious. However, fever occurring 96 h postoperatively is more likely to be infectious. Therefore, postoperative noninfectious causes, including deep vein thrombosis, pulmonary embolism, drug-induced fever, anesthesia-induced malignant hyperthermia, and acute allograft rejection should be considered.

NONINFECTIOUS CAUSES OF FEVER IN THE ICU

Hyperthermia

Hyperthermia is defined when the body temperature is >41.0°C (105.8°F) and does not respond to pharmacological treatment. In hyperthermia, there is an uncontrolled rise in body temperature associated with a breakdown in the homeostasis of body temperature regulation. Malignant hyperthermia, neuroleptic malignant syndrome, serotonin syndrome secondary to antipsychotics, heatstroke, and endocrine causes (thyrotoxicosis, pheochromocytoma, adrenal crisis, etc.) are common causes of hyperthermia.

Drug-Induced Fever

Drug-induced fever caused by allergies or other causes is difficult to diagnose (Table 25.4) [15]. One can also experience high fever (e.g., 38.9°C [102°F]) without other signs. Such fever does not invariably occur immediately after drug administration. In some cases, the fever occurs days after drug administration and abates after many days. Therefore, drug-induced fever is a diagnosis of exclusion, unless other rash-like signs are observed.

TABLE 25.4
Medicines Associated With Drug Fever [15].

Most common	Barbiturates, phenytoin, antihistaminic, methyldopa, penicillin, salicylates, sulfonamides, amphotericin-B, procainamide, bleomycin
Less common	Isoniazid, para-aminosalicylic acid, streptomycin, rifampicin, propylthiouracil, streptokinase, vancomycin, nitrofurantoin, allopurinol, cephalosporin, hydralazine, azathioprine
Least common	Insulins, tetracycline, digitalis, chloramphenicol

Acute Transfusion Reaction

Fever is the most common side effect of transfusion reactions. Fevers caused due to acute transfusion reactions usually occur within 1–6 h after the start of red blood cell or platelet transfusion and may be accompanied by chills and mild dyspnea (e.g., transfusion-related acute lung injury). These reactions are benign and have no sequelae. Diagnosis is made by clinically ruling out other causes of fever in patients receiving blood transfusions.

TREATMENT OF FEVER IN THE ICU

In patients with sepsis or septic shock, the necessary infection source control measures should be implemented as soon as possible. Moreover, in the case of CLABSI or UTI, the catheter should be removed as soon as possible. Simultaneously, it is essential to perform blood cultures and administer empiric antimicrobial therapy.

Antipyretics and external cooling may be used only if the fever itself is considered harmful, such as when intracranial pressure is elevated or if the body temperature is above 41°C (105.8°F). However, these measures should not be routinely performed in cases of sepsis or septic shock.

REFERENCES

[1] Hughes WT, Armstrong D, Bodey GP, et al. 2002 guidelines for the use of antimicrobial agents in neutropenic patients with cancer. Clin Infect Dis 2002;34:730–51.

[2] Mackowiak PA, Wasserman SS, Levine MM. A critical appraisal of 98.6 degrees F, the upper limit of the normal body temperature, and other legacies of Carl Reinhold August Wunderlich. JAMA 1992;268:1578–80.

[3] Dinarello CA, Cannon JG, Wolff SM. New concepts on the pathogenesis of fever. Rev Infect Dis 1988;10:168–89.

[4] Waterhouse J, Edwards B, Bedford P, et al. Thermoregulation during mild exercise at different circadian times. Chronobiol Int 2004;21:253–75.

[5] O'Grady NP, Barie PS, Bartlett JG, Bleck T, Carroll K, Kalil AC, et al., American College of Critical Care Medicine, Infectious Diseases Society of America. Guidelines for evaluation of new fever in critically ill adult patients: 2008 update from the American College of Critical Care Medicine and the Infectious Diseases Society of America. Crit Care Med 2008;36(4):1330–49.

[6] Niven DJ, Gaudet JE, Laupland KB, Mrklas KJ, Roberts DJ, Stelfox HT. Accuracy of peripheral thermometers for estimating temperature: a systematic review and meta-analysis. Ann Intern Med November 17, 2015;163(10):768–77.

[7] Marik PE. Fever in the ICU. Chest March 2000;117(3):855–69.

[8] Mackowiak PA. Concepts of fever. Arch Intern Med September 28, 1998;158(17):1870–81.

[9] Circiumaru B, Baldock G, Cohen J. A prospective study of fever in the intensive care unit. Intensive Care Med 1999;25:668.

[10] Laupland KB, Shahpori R, Kirkpatrick AW, et al. Occurrence and outcome of fever in critically ill adults. Crit Care Med 2008;36:1531.

[11] Young PJ, Saxena M, Beasley R, et al. Early peak temperature and mortality in critically ill patients with or without infection. Intensive Care Med 2012;38:437–44.

[12] Lee BH, Inui D, Suh GY, Kim JY, Kwon JY, Park J, et al. Association of body temperature and antipyretic treatments with mortality of critically ill patients with and without sepsis: multi-centered prospective observational study. Crti Care February 28, 2012;16(1):R33.

[13] Musher DM, Fainstein V, Young EJ, et al. Fever patterns: their lack of clinical significance. Arch Intern Med 1979;139:1225–8.

[14] Scholz H. Fever. Am J Physiol Regul Integr Comp Physiol April 2003;284(4):R913–5.

[15] G.S. Pangtey and R. Prasad. Fever in intensive care unit. Infectious diseases in the intensive care unit pp 1-13.

[16] Rumbus Z, Matics R, Hegyi P, et al. Fever is associated with reduced, hypothermia with increased mortality in septic patients: a meta-analysis of clinical trials. PLoS One January 12, 2017;12(1):e0170152.

[17] Evans L, Rhodes A, Alhazzani W, et al. Surviving sepsis campaign: international guidelines for management of sepsis and septic shock 2021. Crit Care Med November 2021;49(11):e1063–143.

[18] National Healthcare Safety Network. Pneumonia (Ventilator-associated [VAP] and non-ventilator-associated pneumonia [PNEU]) event. November 27, 2021. https://www.cdc.gov/nhsn/pdfs/pscmanual/6pscvapcurrent.pdf.

CHAPTER 26

Sepsis—In the Era of Antimicrobial Resistance

RAJESH CHANDRA MISHRA • SHARMILI SINHA • REENA SHAH • AHSAN AHMED • AHSINA JAHAN LOPA

INTRODUCTION

Sepsis is one of the leading causes of morbidity and mortality across the globe with an estimate of around 20% of all global deaths with the highest burden in sub-Saharan Africa, Oceania, South Asia, East Asia, and southeast Asia [1]. Bacteria have been found to be the major causative agents for these life-threatening sepsis, with two-thirds of these patients had gram-negative organisms isolated and one-half had gram-positive organisms isolated [2]. An alarming pattern of multi- and pandrug-resistant (PDR) gram-negative bacteria are currently emerging with Enterobacteriaceae, Pseudomonas, and Acinetobacter are the major concerns worldwide. The incidence of PDR organisms has also been reported in healthcare setting in patients with prolonged intensive care unit (ICU) and hospital stay with high mortality rates by Sinha et al. [3]. They are not only found in the patients with healthcare-associated infection but also seen in patients coming from community [4]. This antimicrobial resistance (AMR) poses a global challenge with its impact not only limited to clinical morbidity and mortality but also huge economical impact in terms of loss of life, reduction in GDP, and costing world up to $100 trillion [5].

While AMR is a natural phenomenon which may occur as microbes evolve and mutate, inappropriate use of antibiotics, poor prevention and control of infections, lack of awareness, and numerous other factors are accelerating the pace at which microorganisms emerge and spread such resistance.

Infections caused by antibiotic-resistance germs are difficult to treat and sometimes untreatable. Sepsis due to AMR organisms has emerged as the biggest threat of public health crisis of international concern of the 21st century. Considering the paucity of currently available antimicrobial agents to cover this emerging threat,

the key immediate solution would be their prevention through various protocols such as strict hand hygiene maintenance, implementing VAP bundles as well as through antibiotic stewardship programs.

While the treating physicians rely on clinical expertise and published guidelines to treat with empirical therapy for system-based infectious syndromes, more rapid diagnostic testing for identifying AMR organism early along with the possible modification of guidelines for treatment of community-acquired AMR sepsis according to local microbiological susceptibility data are necessary to reduce mortality and prevent the spread.

Although the best effective strategy to reduce AMR sepsis is still unknown, a multifaceted approach aimed at appropriate initial antibiotic therapy, early identification of AMR and isolate to prevent spread, strengthening surveillance, improving patient and clinician education and awareness regarding the appropriate use of antibiotics with strict policies is most likely to be successful.

EPIDEMIOLOGY OF AMR SEPSIS

AMR organisms-induced sepsis emerged now as a new global public health threat. It has substantially increased morbidity, mortality, and healthcare-associated expenses. By 2050, death attributable to AMR sepsis alone is predicted to be more than 10 million per year which will exceed mortality caused by cancer, diabetes, or road traffic accident [6].

The prevalence of AMR organism varies in different parts of the world. One study found an average of around 50% AMR rate of all nosocomial blood stream infection, including 20.5% and 0.5% of isolated microorganisms with extensively drug-resistant and PDR patterns [7]. Among such bacteria, extended-spectrum beta-lactamase (ESBL) producer *Enterobacteriaceae* seems to be the most prevalent mainly ESBL-producing *Escherichia coli* and *Klebsiella pneumoniae* [4].

Carbapenem-resistant *Acinetobacter baumannii* and carbapenem-resistant or third-generation cephalosporin-resistant *Enterobacteriaceae* have been listed as critical pathogens while vancomycin-resistant *Enterococcus* (VRE) as high priority on the World Health Organization priority list of antibiotic-resistant bacteria [8].

ANTIBIOTIC RESISTANCE—GENETICS

The bacterial chromosome is a circular molecule of DNA that functions as a self-replicating genetic element. Gene expression usually involves transcription of DNA into messenger RNA and translation of mRNA into protein. Extrachromosomal genetic elements such as plasmids and bacteriophages are nonessential replicons which often determine resistance to antimicrobial agents, production of virulence factors, or other functions. The chromosome replicates semiconservatively; each DNA strand serves as template for synthesis of its complementary strand [9].

Any antibiotic use can lead to antibiotic resistance. Antibiotics kill germs like bacteria and fungi, but the resistant survivors remain. Resistance traits can be inherited generation to generation. They can also pass directly from germ to germ by way of mobile genetic elements [9—14]. These are as follows:

1. Plasmids are circles of DNA that can move between cells. Plasmids, supercoiled, circular, double-stranded DNA molecules are replicons that are maintained as discrete, extrachromosomal genetic elements in bacteria. Plasmids usually encode traits that are not essential for bacterial viability and replicate independently of the chromosome. Many plasmids control medically important properties of pathogenic bacteria, including resistance to one or several antibiotics, production of toxins, and synthesis of cell surface structures required for adherence or colonization. Plasmids that determine resistance to antibiotics are often called R plasmids (or R factors). Representative toxins encoded by plasmids include heat-labile and heat-stable enterotoxins of *E. coli*, exfoliative toxin of *Staphylococcus aureus*, and tetanus toxin of *Clostridium tetani*.

2. Transposons are small pieces of DNA that can go into and change the overall DNA of a cell. These can move from chromosomes (which carry all the genes essential for germ survival) to plasmids and back.

3. Phages are viruses that attack bacteria and can carry DNA from germ to germ. Bacteriophages are infectious agents mainly viruses that replicate as obligate intracellular parasites in bacteria. Extracellular phage particles are metabolically inert and consist principally of proteins plus nucleic acid (DNA or RNA, but not both).

To survive the effects of antibiotics, bacteria are constantly finding new defense strategies, called "resistance mechanisms." Bacterial DNA informs how to make specific proteins, which determine the germ's resistance mechanisms which keep changing over time. Once new resistance develops, exposure to antibiotics wipes out susceptible germs and allows the resistant germ to survive and multiply. The surviving germs have resistance traits in their DNA. This genetic information can pass from generation to generation in germs and can also move between germs via mobile genetic elements and other processes. This creates more resistant germs, which continue to spread. These resistance genes can be shared with other bacteria that have not been exposed to antibiotics. Genetic exchanges among bacteria occur by several mechanisms (Fig. 26.1). In transformation, the recipient bacterium takes up extracellular donor DNA. In transduction, donor DNA packaged in a bacteriophage infects the recipient bacterium. In conjugation, the donor bacterium transfers DNA to the recipient by mating. Recombination is the rearrangement of donor and recipient genomes to form new, hybrid genomes. Transposons are mobile DNA segments that move from place to place within or between genomes (Fig. 26.1).

Bacteria those are difficult to eradicate have the right combination of resistance genes; all antibiotics become ineffective, resulting in multidrug-resistant (MDR) sepsis. For example, since beginning of the antibiotic era, the beta (β)-lactam class include the earliest-developed and narrow-spectrum penicillins, broader-spectrum cephalosporins, and the most recently introduced and broadest-spectrum carbapenems. Beta-lactam antibiotics kill bacteria by binding to proteins to stop the bacteria from creating a cell wall or prevent the cell wall from properly forming which is essential for survival. Enterobacteriaceae are a large family of bacteria that are a common cause of infections in hospitals and in the community. Some Enterobacteriaceae can produce enzymes called ESBLs, which break down and destroy beta-lactam antibiotics. Carbapenems are one of the few remaining antibiotics that can treat ESBL-producing bacteria, but resistance enzymes are on the rise and destroying the antibiotics. Some Enterobacteriaceae can produce an enzyme called a carbapenemase that makes carbapenems, penicillins, and cephalosporins ineffective. Bacteria from the

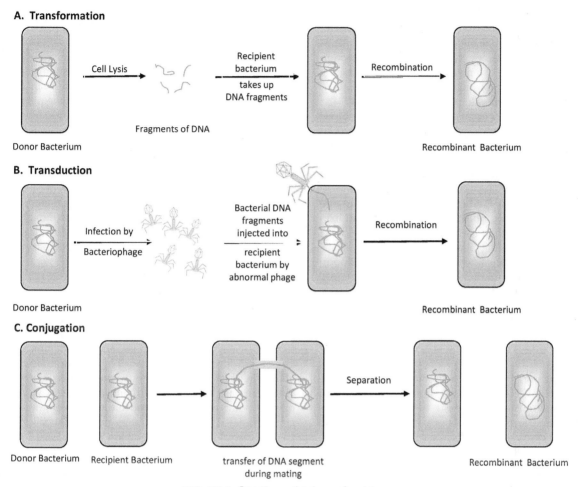

FIG. 26.1 Genetic mechanisms of resistance.

Enterobacteriaceae family, including *Klebsiella pneumoniae K. pneumoniae* and *Escherichia coli*, can produce a carbapenemase and become carbapenemase-resistant Enterobacteriaceae (CRE) [11,12].

Enzymes that CRE produce include *K. pneumoniae* carbapenemase (KPC), Oxacillinase-48 (OXA-48), New Delhi metallo-beta-lactamase (NDM), and Verona integron-encoded metallo-beta-lactamase (VIM).

Another mechanism by which bacteria exert AMR is through their ability to form biofilms. Biofilms are surface-attached bacteria encased in a self-produced extracellular polymeric matrix. This increases resistance to a wide range of stressors including the immune system, disinfectants, and antibiotics. It is usually not one single mechanism that provides the resistance, but rather a combination of several of these mechanisms that manifests the extremely high resistance observed within biofilm cells [11].

Toxin—antitoxin (TA) systems are ubiquitous among bacteria and play an important role in the dissemination and evolution of antibiotic resistance, for example, by maintaining MDR plasmids, by inducing persistence formation and by playing a role in biofilm formation. TA systems are often associated with antimicrobial genes present on the same plasmid as the TA itself, and how that coincidence can act to maintain the

AMR genes even in the absence of the drug. The mutagenic a global response to DNA damage (SOS) system, which is induced by many commonly used antimicrobial drugs, including long-lived drugs such as fluoroquinolones, activates some TA systems, placing a continuing selective pressure on certain TA systems to be mobilized throughout bacterial populations [13].

A common misconception is to think of antibiotic resistance as being exclusively a function of particular resistance mutations or acquired foreign resistance genes. What is less appreciated is that both the environment and the overall genotype of the target bacteria can significantly modulate the phenotypic expression of antibiotic resistance. Knowing the identity of resistance mutations and genes is often insufficient information to accurately predict the resistance phenotype in the clinic. In an age of increasing reliance on DNA sequence data, this dissociation of genotype and phenotype has important consequences for the ability of clinical bacteriology to guide optimal therapy. They also estimate the degree to which there is a genetic "dark matter" of currently unknown (or underappreciated) genes and mutations contributing to resistance in clinical isolates [15].

Clinical and Laboratory Diagnosis of MDR

Early diagnosis and administration of most appropriate antibiotics are essential for best outcome in sepsis and septic shock. Surviving Sepsis Campaign guidelines recommend to give antibiotics with 1 h time period [16]. However, when sepsis is suspected to have been caused by MDR bacteria, it mandates the use of high-grade antimicrobials and multiple agents at the outset so as to cover all possible multidrug-resistant organisms (MDROs). The therapy usually proves costly. Hence, it needs to be based on a combined decision guided by clinical assessment and laboratory diagnosis.

Clinical diagnosis of MDR sepsis
The risk factors for the development of sepsis by MDROs are:
* Prior and prolonged use of antibiotics
* Prolonged stay in hospital and healthcare set ups
* Multiple comorbidities
* High prevalence of MDR bacteria in the hospital

Laboratory diagnosis
It is one of the most important challenges to establish microbiologic diagnosis for MDR organisms from various samples such as blood, urine, tracheal, and other body fluids. The identification of the bacteria

and specific species is essential before antimicrobial susceptibility test (AST) can be performed. The AST remains key to choosing appropriate antimicrobial agents judiciously in these cases as most of these causative agents require combination therapies. It is imperative to understand the presence of inherent resistance genes (if any) so as to target the bacteria with the right antibiotics. With the advent of rapid diagnostic tests which includes the syndromic tests, the turnaround time (TAT) for the identification of the bacterium and resistance genes has become short and thus proven very useful. This helps to target the infections with most specific antibiotics. However, the conventional microbiologic culture sensitivity methods continue to play role in the isolation of microorganisms though the TAT remains long. Following are few rapid diagnostic tests either available in market or in the stage of development.

Matrix-assisted laser desorption ionization time-of-flight mass spectrometry. In this method, bacteria are made to pass through an ionization chamber and pulsed laser are applied. The proteinaceous architecture of each bacterium is unique, and thus identification of each species is accomplished by migration speed of protein which is unique for that particular bacterium. The results are then compared with a reference database. For such process, isolated bacterial colonies or growth isolated from blood cultures or bacterial pellets (purified isolates from positive blood culture) can be utilized. Identification results of MALDI-TOF have around 95% match with the conventional microbiological methods. Hence, it is already in use in many laboratories across the globe.

There is evidence to support that this method of MALDI-TOF plus AMS may help by reducing time to instituting appropriate antibiotic therapy in MDR cases [17,18]. There are also prospects that MALDI-TOF can be useful in detecting resistant bacteria by the identification of drug modification or spectra in relation to the presence of specific resistant mechanisms, e.g., ESBL or KPC. Further research and development is required to explore their impact on therapeutic choices.

Fluorescent in situ hybridization. Specific binding of fluorescent probes of nucleic acids to complementary sequences of the bacterial 16S rRNA is observed. A fluorescent microscope is used to observe binding. Specific probes are chosen according to Gram stain. Gram-negative bacilli (GNB) probes could identify *E. coli*,

Pseudomonas aeruginosa, and *Klebsiella pneumoniae* in 0.3–3 h s with >95% sensitivity and 90% specificity [19,20]. It is claimed to have faster identification of GNB. Studies conducted on this mostly have been directed at gram-positive bacteria [21,22].

Light scattering technology. The technology is based on detecting turbidity from growth of bacteria in liquid media. Few studies indicate around 91% similarity with conventional lab method like broth microdilution [23]. Time to AST is 5 h compared to 48 h of standard microdilution method [24].

Fish combined with time-lapse microscopy. Both identification and AST are designed to be fully automated. Time to identification and AST results after culture positivity may be as short as 1.5 h to 7 h, respectively [25]. There is substantial reduction in time to detection. At least eight GNB species and 15 antibiotics can be studies in this method. This has good agreement with traditional culture methods.

Molecular detection based on NAATs and microarrays. This method is based on the amplification of particular genetic targets. Next by hybridization, a microarray of oligonucleotides probe is used for the identification of targets. Few of these are:

- Verigene BC-GN—This can identify up to four GNB genus and five species and time to isolation is around 2 h after culture sensitivity [26–28].
- Film array BCID—The FilmArray BCID (BioFire Diagnostics, Salt Lake City, UT, USA) consists of a fully automated nested multiplex polymerase chain reaction (PCR) that can identify *P. aeruginosa*, *A. baumannii*, *K. pneumoniae*, *E. coli*, and other members of the Enterobacterales (i.e., Enterobacteriaceae, Proteus, *Enterobacter cloacae* complex, *Klebsiella oxytoca*, *Serratia marcescens*) [29]. It also allows for rapid identification of three resistance markers, but of them only KPC-encoding genes relate to MDR GNB infections. The TAT of the test from positive culture is around 1 h, with high sensitivity and specificity.
- Unyvero System—The Unyvero System (Curetis GmbH, Holzgerlingen, Germany) is a molecular diagnostic platform for the detection of bacteria and fungi, as well as antibiotic resistance genes. This system is able to detect, among others, nonfermenters (*A. baumannii*, *P. aeruginosa*, and *Stenotrophomonas maltophilia*), Proteus spp., nine other members of Enterobacterales at species level (e.g.

K. pneumoniae, *E. coli*) and various antibiotic resistance gene markers [30].

Lateral flow immunoassay for rapid detection of resistance enzymes. These are antibody-based methods which use colloidal gold nanoparticles bound to a nitrocellulose membrane within a lateral flow device. These work on the principle of immunological capture of epitopes specific to resistance enzymes. Various panels for the identification of resistance enzyme exist. The five most widespread carbapenemases found in Enterobacterales (NDM-, KPC-, IMP-, and VIM-type and OXA-48-like), the OXA-23 carbapenemase, the ESBLs of CTX-M-type, and the MCR-1 enzyme (colistin resistance) can be detected by this technique. The yield time is less than 30 min. They are easy to perform, inexpensive, and has high level of sensitivity and specificity when used with bacterial colonies and high sensitivity and positivity [31–33].

Rapid tests on whole blood

- Nucleic acid amplification test-based methods when molecular techniques are applied directly on whole blood, the potential diagnostic advantages are intuitive (i.e., results for both identification and AST are available just a few hours after the blood draw), and several nucleic acid amplification tests (NAATs) have thus been developed over the years for this purpose. However, they have generally shown variable diagnostic performances and possible suboptimal sensitivity (e.g., for the presence of PCR inhibitors in whole blood) or suboptimal specificity [34,35]. Light Cycler SeptiFast, Septi Test, and VYOO assays are few examples [36–38].

  The T2 magnetic resonance nanodiagnostic system (T2 Biosystems, Lexington, MA, USA) can identify Candida (T2Candida panel) and bacteria (T2Bacteria panel) directly on whole blood through a fully automated method [39].

  The conventional culture sensitivity methods continue to remain the standard way for the isolation of bacteria and identification of species with ASTs. Long TAT remains the major limitation of these conventional methods.

Therapeutic implications. It is evident that rapid diagnostic methods will be helpful for rapid identification of causative bacteria and gives information about resistance genes as well. Therefore, these will certainly facilitate the initiation of appropriate antimicrobial agents with more accuracy. However, limitations are lack of availability of such tests at all centers, and TAT may be actually prolonged in certain cases. However, these tests do not cover all bacteria, and few newly emerging resistance mechanisms may be missing in these technology-based tests. Therefore, the diagnosis of MDR sepsis should be equitably based on both clinical assessment and laboratory tests.

TREATMENT
Multidrug-Resistant Gram-Positive Bacteria
Ever since the introduction of penicillin in 1940s, the fight against infections by gram-positive bacteria has been varied. Gram-positive infections can result in a wide variety of diseases, including skin and soft tissue infections, surgical and trauma wound infections, urinary tract infections, gastrointestinal tract infections, pneumonia, osteomyelitis, endocarditis, thrombophlebitis, mastitis, meningitis, toxic shock syndrome, septicemia, and infections of indwelling medical devices [40]. Today, among various pathogenic gram-positive bacteria, *Staphylococcus aureus*, *Streptococcus pneumoniae*, and enterococci stand out as being responsible for global resistance challenges, significant public health burden, and cost to healthcare [41]. Multidrug resistance among gram-positive bacteria, especially methicillin-resistant *S. aureus*, has been a major healthcare concern worldwide [42].

Multidrug-Resistant Gram-Negative Bacteria
The treatment of multidrug-resistant gram-negative bacteria (MDR-GNB) infections in critically ill patients presents many challenges. Effective treatment should be administered as soon as possible, patient's medical history and local microbiological patterns remain essential for guiding empirical treatment choices (Fig. 26.2), to avoid both overtreatment and undertreatment allowing good antimicrobial stewardship principles. Carbapenem-resistant Enterobacteriaceae, *Pseudomonas aeruginosa*, and *A. baumannii* are being reported with increasing frequencies worldwide, although with important variability across regions, hospitals and even single wards and hence needing good infection control practices in these areas.

In the past few years, new treatment options, such as ceftazidime/avibactam, meropenem/vaborbactam, ceftolozane/tazobactam, plazomicin, and eravacycline have become available, and others will become soon, which have provided some much-awaited resources for effectively counteracting severe infections due to these organisms. However, judicious use is imperative for delaying the emergence of resistance to novel agents. Despite important progresses, pharmacokinetic/pharmacodynamic optimization of dosages and treatment duration in critically ill patients has still some areas of uncertainty.

Conclusion: Sepsis caused by MDR organisms is gradually becoming a global threat and emerging as a

Organism	Recommended drugs
MSSA	Cefazolin, Cloxacillin
MRSA	Vancomycin, Daptomycin, Teicoplanin, Linezolid, Ceftaroline, Tigecycline
VISA, hVISA, VRSA	Combination of high-dose daptomycin with another antibiotic including gentamicin, rifampicin, linezolid, trimethoprim-sulfamethoxazole (TMP-SMX), or a β-lactam
VRE	Linezolid, High-dose ampicillin, daptomycin; nitrofurantoin, Fosfomycin (UTI); doxycycline, chloramphenicol, gentamicin, streptomycin (combination therapy)
DRSP	Respiratory fluoroquinolones (moxifloxacin, Gemifloxacin, or levofloxacin), or a beta-lactam alone or in combination with a beta-lactamase inhibitor (high dose amoxicillin or amoxicillin-clavulanate) along with doxycycline

FIG. 26.2 Gram positive organisms and recommended antimicrobial agents [43]. (Kulkarni AP, Nagvekar VC, Veeraraghavan B, Warrier AR, Deepak TS, Ahdal J, Jain R. Current perspectives on treatment of gram-positive infections in India: what is the way forward? Interdiscip Perspect Infect Dis 2019;2019:8. Article ID 7601847. https://doi.org/10.1155/2019/7601847)

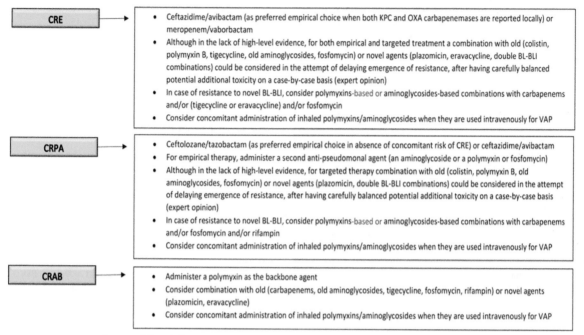

FIG. 26.3 Current Clinical Reasoning for the Treatment of Serious MDR-GNB Infections in Critically Ill Patients. *MDR-GNB*, multidrug-resistant gram-negative bacteria; *CRE*, carbapenem-resistant Enterobacterales; *CRPA*, carbapenem-resistant *Pseudomonas aeruginosa*; *CRAB*, carbapenem-resistant *Acinetobacter baumannii*; *BL-BLI*, β-lactam/β-lactamase inhibitors; *VAP*, ventilator-associated pneumonia [44].

pandemic. Rapid diagnostic tests using PCR-based technology are the way forward for rapid identification of such resistant microorganisms along with resistant genes. Early and timely intervention with appropriate antimicrobial agents remain the cornerstone. Multiresistant bacteria in critically ill patients should be preferably targeted with combination therapy. Emergence of resistant pathogens can be prevented by strict implementation of antimicrobial stewardship programs.

KEY POINTS

1. Sepsis caused by MDR bacteria is a global threat and emerging pandemic.
2. Rapid diagnostic tests like PCR-based panels are useful for fast identification of MDR organisms and the resistant genes.
3. Early and timely treatment with appropriate antibiotics is best recommended.
4. MDR bacteria in ICU should be treated with combination therapy.
5. Prevention is key and solely possible by antibiotic stewardship programs.

REFERENCES

[1] Rudd KE, Johnson SC, Agesa KM, et al. Global, regional, and national sepsis incidence and mortality, 1990–2017: analysis for the Global Burden of Disease Study. Lancet 2020;395:200–11. https://doi.org/10.1016/S0140-6736(19)32989-7. Published online Jan 16.

[2] Sakr Y, Jaschinski U, Wittebole X, Szakmany T, Lipman J, Ñamendys-Silva SA, Martin-Loeches I, Leone M, Lupu MN, Vincent JL. ICON investigators. Sepsis in intensive care unit patients: worldwide data from the intensive care over nations audit. Open Forum Infect Dis November 19, 2018;5(12):ofy313. https://doi.org/10.1093/ofid/ofy313. PMID: 30555852; PMCID: PMC6289022.

[3] Sinha S, Sahu S, Pati J, Ray B, Pattnaik S. Retrospective analysis of colistin-resistant bacteria in a tertiary centre in India. Indian J Med Res March 2019;149:418–22.

[4] Capsoni N, Bellone P, Aliberti S, et al. Prevalence, risk factors and outcomes of patients coming from the community with sepsis due to multidrug resistant bacteria. Multidiscip Respir Med 2019;14:23. https://doi.org/10.1186/s40248-019-0185-4.

[5] https://www.who.int/medicines/technical_briefing/tbs/TBS2016_AMR.

[6] The review on antimicrobial resistance team chaired by O'Neil J. Antimicrobial resistance: tackling a crisis for

the health and wealth of nations. Review on antimicrobial resistance. 2014. Available at: https://www.amr-review.org/sites/default/files/AMR%20Review%20%20P aper%20-%20Tackling%20a%20crisis%20for%20the%2 0health%20and%20wealth%20of%20nations_1.pdf.

[7] Tabah A, Koulenti D, Laupland K, et al. Characteristics and determinants of outcome of hospital-acquired bloodstream infections in intensive care units: the EURO-BACT International Cohort Study. Intensive Care Med 2012;38:1930—45.

[8] Tacconelli E, Carrara E, Savoldi A, et al. WHO Pathogens Priority List Working Group. Discovery, research, and development of new antibiotics: the WHO priority list of antibiotic-resistant bacteria and tuberculosis. Lancet Infect Dis 2018;18(3):318—27. https://doi.org/10.1016/S1473-3099(17)30753-3.

[9] Nikaido H. Multidrug resistance in bacteria. Annu Rev Biochem 2009;78:119—46. https://doi.org/10.1146/annurev.biochem.78.082907.145923.

[10] CDC. Antibiotic resistance threats in the United States. 2019 [Atlanta, GA].

[11] Hall CW, Mah T-F. Molecular mechanisms of biofilm-based antibiotic resistance and tolerance in pathogenic bacteria. FEMS Microbiol Rev 2017. https://doi.org/10.1093/femsre/fux010.

[12] Editorial: bacterial pathogens, antibiotics and antibiotic resistance. fux016 FEMS (Fed Eur Microbiol Soc) Microbiol Rev 2017;41:450—2. https://doi.org/10.1093/femsre/fux016 [Advance Access].

[13] Yang QE, Walsh TR. Toxin-antitoxin systems and their role in disseminating and maintaining antimicrobial resistance. FEMS Microbiol Rev 2017. https://doi.org/10.1093/femsre/fux006.

[14] Baron S. Chapter 5, genetics: medical microbiology. 4th ed. Galveston (TX): University of Texas Medical Branch at Galveston; 1996 [Not mentioned anywhere].

[15] Hughes D, Andersson DI. Environmental and genetic modulation of the phenotypic expression of antibiotic resistance. FEMS Microbiol Rev 2017. https://doi.org/10.1093/femsre/fux004.

[16] Rhodes A, Evans LE, Alhazzani W, Levy M, Antonelli M, Ferrer R, Kumar, et al. Surviving sepsis Campaign: international guidelines for management of sepsis and septic shock: 2016. Crit Care Med March 2017;45(3): 486—552. https://doi.org/10.1097/CCM.000000000000 225.

[17] Wenzler E, Goff DA, Mangino JE, Reed EE, Wehr A, Bauer KA. Impact of rapid identification of Acinetobacter Baumannii via matrix-assisted laser desorption ionization time-of-flight mass spectrometry combined with antimicrobial stewardship in patients with pneumonia and/or bacteremia. Diagn Microbiol Infect Dis 2016;84: 63e8.

[18] Huang AM, Newton D, Kunapuli A, Gandhi TN, Washer LL, Isip J, et al. Impact of rapid organism identification via matrix-assisted laser desorption/ionization time-of-flight combined with antimicrobial stewardship team intervention in adult patients with bacteremia and candidemia. Clin Infect Dis 2013;57:1237e45.

[19] Opota O, Croxatto A, Prod'hom G, Greub G. Blood culture-based diagnosis of bacteraemia: state of the art. Clin Microbiol Infect 2015;21:313e22.

[20] Morgan M, Marlowe E, Della-Latta P, Salimnia H, Novak-Weekley S, Wu F, et al. Multicenter evaluation of a new shortened peptide nucleic acid fluorescence in situ hybridization procedure for species identification of select Gram-negative bacilli from blood cultures. J Clin Microbiol 2010;48:2268e70.

[21] Harris DM, Hata DJ. Rapid identification of bacteria and Candida using PNAFISHz from blood and peritoneal fluid cultures: a retrospective clinical study. Ann Clin Microbiol Antimicrob 2013;12:2.

[22] Ly T, Gulia J, Pyrgos V, Waga M, Shoham S. Impact upon clinical outcomes of translation of PNA FISH-generated laboratory data from the clinical microbiology bench to bedside in real time. Therapeut Clin Risk Manag 2008; 4:637e40.

[23] Pliakos EE, Andreatos N, Shehadeh F, Ziakas PD, Mylonakis E. The costeffectiveness of rapid diagnostic testing for the diagnosis of bloodstream infections with or without antimicrobial stewardship. Clin Microbiol Rev 2018;31.

[24] Barnini S, Brucculeri V, Morici P, Ghelardi E, Florio W, Lupetti A. A new rapid method for direct antimicrobial susceptibility testing of bacteria from positive blood cultures. BMC Microbiol 2016;16:185.

[25] Charnot-Katsikas A, Tesic V, Love N, Hill B, Bethel C, Boonlayangoor S, et al. Use of the accelerate Pheno system for identification and antimicrobial susceptibility testing of pathogens in positive blood cultures and impact on time to results and workflow. J Clin Microbiol 2018;56.

[26] Bork JT, Leekha S, Heil EL, Zhao L, Badamas R, Johnson JK. Rapid testing using the Verigene Gram-negative blood culture nucleic acid test in combination with antimicrobial stewardship intervention against Gram-negative bacteremia. Antimicrob Agents Chemother 2015;59:1588e95.

[27] Claeys KC, Heil EL, Pogue JM, Lephart PR, Johnson JK. The Verigene dilemma:gram-negative polymicrobial bloodstream infections and clinical decision making. Diagn Microbiol Infect Dis 2018;91:144e6.

[28] Walker T, Dumadag S, Lee CJ, Lee SH, Bender JM, Cupo Abbott J, et al. Clinical impact of laboratory implementation of Verigene BC-GN microarray-based assay for detection of gram-negative bacteria in positive blood cultures. J Clin Microbiol 2016;54:1789e96.

[29] Altun O, Almuhayawi M, Ullberg M, Ozenci V. Clinical evaluation of the FilmArray blood culture identification panel in identification of bacteria and yeasts from positive blood culture bottles. J Clin Microbiol 2013;51: 4130e6.

[30] Burrack-Lange SC, Personne Y, Huber M, Winkler E, Weile J, Knabbe C, et al. Multicenter assessment of the

rapid Unyvero Blood Culture molecular assay. J Med Microbiol 2018;67:1294e301.

[31] Hamprecht A, Vehreschild JJ, Seifert H, Saleh A. Rapid detection of NDM, KPC and OXA-48 carbapenemases directly from positive blood cultures using a new multiplex immunochromatographic assay. PLoS One 2018; 13:e0204157.

[32] Riccobono E, Antonelli A, Pecile P, Bogaerts P, D'Andrea MM, Rossolini GM. Evaluation of the KPC K-SeT(R) immunochromatographic assay for the rapid detection of KPC carbapenemase producers from positive blood cultures. J Antimicrob Chemother 2018;73: 539e40.

[33] Takissian J, Bonnin RA, Naas T, Dortet L. NG-test carba 5 for rapid detection of carbapenemase-producing Enterobacterales from positive blood cultures. Antimicrob Agents Chemother 2019;63.

[34] Al-Soud WA, Radstrom P. Purification and characterization of PCR-inhibitory components in blood cells. J Clin Microbiol 2001;39:485e93.

[35] Dubourg G, Raoult D, Fenollar F. Emerging methodologies for pathogen identification in bloodstream infections: an update. Expert Rev Mol Diagn 2019:1e13.

[36] Dark P, Blackwood B, Gates S, McAuley D, Perkins GD, McMullan R, et al. Accuracy of LightCycler((R)) SeptiFast for the detection and identification of pathogens in the blood of patients with suspected sepsis: a systematic review and meta-analysis. Intensive Care Med 2015;41:21e33.

[37] Carrara L, Navarro F, Turbau M, Seres M, Moran I, Quintana I, et al. Molecular diagnosis of bloodstream infections with a new dual-priming oligonucleotidebased multiplex PCR assay. J Med Microbiol 2013;62:1673e9.

[38] Ljungstrom L, Enroth H, Claesson BE, Ovemyr I, Karlsson J, Fr€oberg B, et al. Clinical evaluation of commercial nucleic acid amplification tests in patients with suspected sepsis. BMC Infect Dis 2015;15:199.

[39] Clancy CJ, Nguyen MH. T2 magnetic resonance for the diagnosis of bloodstream infections: charting a path forward. J Antimicrob Chemother 2018;73(Suppl. l):iv2e5.

[40] Nair N, Biswas R, Götz F, Biswas L. Impact of *Staphylococcus aureus* on pathogenesis in polymicrobial infections. Infect Immun 2014;82(6):2162−9 [View at: Publisher Site|Google Scholar].

[41] Woodford N, Livermore DM. Infections caused by Gram-positive bacteria: a review of the global challenge. Infection 2009;59(Suppl. 1):S4−16 [View at: Publisher Site|Google Scholar].

[42] Cornaglia G. Fighting infections due to multidrug-resistant Gram-positive pathogens. Clin Microbiol Infect 2009;15(3):209−11.

[43] Kulkarni AP, Nagvekar VC, Veeraraghavan B, Warrier AR, Deepak TS, Ahdal J, Jain R. Current perspectives on treatment of gram-positive infections in India: what is the way forward? Interdiscip Perspect Infect Dis 2019. https://doi.org/10.1155/2019/7601847. Article ID 7601847, 8 pages, 2019.

[44] Bassetti M, Peghin M, Vena A, Giacobbe DR. Treatment of infections due to MDR gram-negative bacteria. Front Med April 2019;6. Article 74, www.frontiersin.org.

CHAPTER 27

Factors Underlying Racial and Gender Disparities in Sepsis Management

RYOUNG-EUN KO • GEE YOUNG SUH

INTRODUCTION

Despite the standardization of sepsis management, sepsis mortality rates vary widely. This indicates the presence of healthcare disparities, which are defined as "differences in the quality of healthcare that are not due to access-related factors or clinical needs, preferences, and appropriateness of intervention" [1]. Disparities based on demographic factors such as age, race, gender, and socioeconomic status (SES) are observed across the entire healthcare field. For example, National Healthcare Quality and Disparities Report [2], which is a comprehensive overview of healthcare received by the general population in the United Sates, report various disparities in many aspects of healthcare, depending on race and SES. This chapter provides an overview of the current state of the literature on the possible factors that underly racial and gender disparities in sepsis, where such disparities can influence the course of sepsis, and the potential targets for interventions.

RACIAL DISPARITIES

Various patient-based, hospital-based, and community-based factors may be responsible for racial disparities in sepsis, and these factors will be looked at in more detail.

Definition of Race

For better understanding of racial disparities, it is important to understand the definition of race that is frequently used in epidemiological studies. In 1994, in response to the overwhelming demand to reflect the increasing diversity of the United States population, the Office of Management and Budget (OMB) began a comprehensive review of the current racial and ethnic categories in collaboration with the Interagency Committee for the Review of the Racial and Ethnic Standards

[3]. In 1997, the OMB accepted the recommendations of the Interagency Committee and released standards for federal data on race. According to the 1997 revision, "Black" is defined as a person having their origins in any of the Black racial groups of Africa. "White" is defined as a person having their origins in any of the original peoples of Europe, the Middle East, or North Africa. "Asian" is defined as a person having their origins in any of the original peoples of the Far East, Southeast Asia, or the Indian subcontinent. "Hispanic" is defined as a person of Cuban, Mexican, Puerto Rican, or Central American, or other Spanish culture or origin, regardless of race. Several examples in literature defined "minority" races as referring to any race that is nonwhite.

Sepsis-Related Outcomes According to Race

According to studies on the effects of race on sepsis-related mortality, race alone cannot fully explain sepsis-related mortality [4]. However, race-specific patient-based, hospital-based, and community-based factors can influence the differences in sepsis-related outcomes. Several epidemiological studies on sepsis have shown those results. A study conducted by Barnato AE et al. using hospital discharge and US Census data in 68 hospital referral regions in six states showed that there were racial differences in the incidence and outcomes of sepsis. The study reported that Blacks had the highest rate of sepsis (6.08 per 1000) followed by Hispanics (4.06 per 1000) and Whites (3.58 per 1000). In addition, Blacks had the highest age- and gender-standardized hospital mortality rates compared to Hispanics (26.1% vs. 24.6% and 24.2%, $P < .001$) [5]. Prest J et al. analyzed the Multiple Cause of Death (MCOD) database from 2005 to 2018 and showed that Blacks experienced a higher sepsis-related mortality rate than Whites, and Asians had the lowest rates [6].

The Sepsis Codex. https://doi.org/10.1016/B978-0-323-88271-2.00035-3

Patient-Based Factors
Genetic Susceptibility
The latest definition of sepsis is organ dysfunction due to dysregulated host immune response to infection [7], and thus it is understandable why the genetic makeup of a patient may contribute to the host's immunological response, thereby increasing the risk of acquiring infection and/or increasing the risk of developing sepsis secondary to infection. Studies on genetic variants, particularly single-nucleotide polymorphisms (SNPs) are providing evidence that genetic makeup of patients is a determining factor in both inflammatory response and clinical outcomes in patients with sepsis [8–12]. Numerous SNPs linked to an increased predilection to sepsis are located in genes associated with vital inflammatory response pathways. The most studied SNPs are associated with genes related to Toll-like receptors and tumor necrosis factor α pathways [11–14]. A recent metaanalysis conducted to evaluate the effect of host genetic variants on the risk of sepsis showed that 29 variants of 23 genes were significantly associated with risk of sepsis, including eight variants of pattern recognition receptors, 14 variants of cytokines, one variant of an immune-related gene, and six variants of other genes [15]. These findings might be useful in providing insight to the molecular mechanisms in the pathogenesis of sepsis and provide crucial information on individual responses to sepsis.

Multiple genes and gene–environment interactions are required for sepsis development and variations in clinical presentation. However, published genetic epidemiological studies to date have been limited by including mainly Whites, having small sample sizes, and difficulties of genetically defining race [13,16–18]. Furthermore, many of the polymorphisms that have been identified by various gene studies have not been consistently reproduced [15]. Although personalized treatment for sepsis in accordance to an individual's genetic profile may not be available any time soon, this area of research will continue to expand and more individualized approaches to management to sepsis may become feasible in the future.

Chronic Comorbid Conditions
Racial differences in comorbid conditions such as diabetes [19], obesity [20], renal failure [21], chronic obstructive pulmonary disease [22], and human immunodeficiency virus (HIV) [23] infection may increase the susceptibility to infection and sepsis. Racial disparities identified in many of these comorbid conditions show that Blacks experience both an increased prevalence of these conditions and a reduction in life expectancy when compared to Whites [24]. Blacks are also more likely to have chronic comorbid conditions that alter immune function such as diabetes, chronic renal failure, and obesity, which is linked with a high risk of acute organ dysfunction and a relatively poor clinical outcomes [25]. In addition, Blacks more often have inflammatory diseases such as systemic lupus erythematosus and inflammatory bowel disease, which increases their risk of developing sepsis [26–28]. HIV infection is also known to be more frequent in Blacks [23], and significantly higher proportion of Blacks with sepsis have HIV infections compared with Whites [29]. These differences may partially account for the higher sepsis-related hospitalization rates found in Blacks. Better management of these comorbid conditions may bring about reduction in racial disparities seen in sepsis.

Few studies have compared Asians to Whites when it comes to the epidemiology of sepsis. According to the published results based on the National Center for Health Statistics' MCOD dataset, Asians were less likely to experience sepsis-related death (risk ratio [RR] = 0.78, 95% confidence interval [CI] = 0.77–0.78), while Blacks (RR = 2.24, 95% CI = 2.23–2.24) and American Indians (RR = 1.24, 95% CI = 12.4–1.25) were more likely than Whites to experience sepsis-related death [30]. These differences may be related to the characteristics of comorbidities found in Asians, but more studies looking into this question are needed.

Hospital-Based Factors
Some previous studies report there are racial disparities in hospital care of patients with sepsis. Some of these studies suggest that bundle compliance is lower for Blacks when compared to Whites. Mayr FB et al. conducted a prospective observational study of patients with community-acquired pneumonia in 28 hospitals in the United States and compared management differences in Blacks and Whites [31]. This study reported that Blacks were less likely to receive antibiotics within 4 h (odds ratio [OR] = 0.55; 95% CI = 0.43–0.70; $P < .001$) and less likely to receive guideline-adherent antibiotics (OR = 0.72; 95% CI = 0.57–0.91, $P = .006$). Higher intensity of care in Blacks was observed, but these differences were explained by different case-mix and variations in sepsis management across hospitals. However, recent studies did not show racial disparities in initial sepsis management [32,33]. For instance, an observational cohort study investigating timely antibiotic therapy for sepsis by Taylor SP et al. reported that there was no difference among races in the rate of antibiotic administration

within the one-hour of triage in the emergency department for suspected septic shock [32].

Recently, a study reported differences in rates of interhospital transfer of patients with sepsis among Blacks and Whites. A cross-sectional analysis of a 2016 National Inpatient Sample data reported that Blacks had lower odds of interhospital transfer, which suggest that Blacks may not be given access to necessary specialized care [34]. However, this phenomenon could be explained primarily by Whites having a higher likelihood of being admitted to urban teaching hospitals. Several studies have suggested that differences in characteristics of hospitals contribute to racial disparities in sepsis management [30]. These interhospital differences could be potentially modifiable, thus requiring increased efforts for standardized sepsis management. In addition, Blacks are more likely than Whites to be discharged to home instead of receiving being discharged to a long-term acute care hospital for further management, which may reflect insurance status [35]. Minority populations in whom medical care put them under higher financial burden may not be able to manage preexisting comorbidities or functional limitations properly after hospitalizations for sepsis which may lead to worse long-term outcome, such as readmissions.

Community-Based Factors

Community-based factors including employment status, SES, and education level have been linked with variations in susceptibility to numerous diseases including sepsis [36–38]. Moor et al. investigated the characteristics of three regions in the southern United States that had significantly higher age-adjusted sepsis mortality rates from 2003 to 2012 relative to the rest of the United States [39]. These areas were characterized by lower education level, lower income, lower insurance coverage, and higher unemployment rates compared to the rest of the country. A higher level of education has been linked to better health outcomes, such as life expectancy [40,41], but few studies have focused on a correlation between educational status and sepsis mortality. Education may reflect certain nonsocioeconomic characteristics that affect health outcomes, such as problem-solving skills or health literacy, which may be able to partially offset the adversities posed by other socioeconomic variables, including lack of insurance.

Sepsis incidence or prevalence is found to vary depending on many socioeconomic factors [42–45]. Furthermore, SES is purported to be an extremely powerful predictor of sepsis-related deaths [44,46]. Various studies define SES differently, so it is sometimes very difficult to compare the results of one study to another. Goodwin et al. found that people living in medically underserved areas had much higher odds of being admitted for sepsis and were more likely to have sepsis-related deaths [46]. In this study, medically underserved area was defined as a composite index that included the ratio of primary care physicians per 1,000 people, infant mortality rate, the proportion of the population with an income below the poverty rate, and the percentage of the elderly population. Interestingly, in this study, ZIP code–based surrogates of SES, including income and education level had minimal influence on sepsis mortality. Another approach has been to use aggregate SES scores to reflect various aspects of the SES that influence individual's overall ability to access the healthcare system [44,47,48]. A study using the prospectively collected Reasons for Geographic and Racial Differences in Stroke (REGARDS) study database showed that residents in districts with lower aggregate neighborhood SES (nSES) score had increased incidence of sepsis [44]. The nSES score used in this study included factors such as median household income, median home value, percentage of households receiving interest, dividend, or rental fees, percentage of adults completing high school or college, and percentage of working individuals in managerial, executive, or professional occupations.

Preventive health is at the front line of health promotion initiatives, as many diseases can be avoided by access to primary care services and lifestyle modification. However, even after adjustment for demographics and insurance status, centers with higher proportions of Blacks were more likely to have lower visit to primary care [49]. Furthermore, vaccination coverage was remarkably lower among Blacks and Asians when compared to Whites [50]. This result remained after adjusting for age, gender, health insurance, education, usual place of care, the number of physician visits in the past 12 months, and health insurance. Additional efforts are strongly suggested to aid in the improvement of the preventive health of people, for all races.

GENDER DISPARITIES
Effect of Gender on Prevalence and Mortality of Sepsis

Epidemiological studies consistently report a higher prevalence of sepsis and septic shock in men, relative to women with prevalence of 53.7%–64.6% [51–55]. Annane D et al., reported on prospective epidemiology study of more than 8,251 septic shock patients among more than 100,000 intensive care unit (ICU) patients collected from 22 French hospitals over an eight-year period [51]. The study reported that approximately 63.7% of patients with septic shock were men compared to 58.0% for nonseptic shock patients which was statistically significant different. A national prospective cross-sectional survey study in China showed that among 2,322 sepsis patients admitted to participating ICU, 64.6% of patients were men [55]. Some studies report lower prevalence of sepsis in men, such as a study which analyzed Spanish National hospital discharge database for public and private hospitals over a period of 10 years, where 53% of sepsis patients were men [54]. A prospective cohort of sepsis and septic shock patients in South Korea also report about 60% prevalence of men [53,56].

But studies report inconsistent results in mortality outcomes based on gender difference (Table 27.1). As with prevalence, some studies report higher rate of morality in men compared to women. The OutcomeRea study, which was conducted in 12 French ICUs and consisted of data collected over an eight-year period,

reported significant lower hospital mortality in sepsis patients in women which was due to decreased mortality in women who were over 50 years of age [57]. In this study, there was no difference in mortality in patients under 50 years of age. A relatively small prospective study involving 97 patients from Pakistan by Nasir N et al. reported that men with sepsis have a 70% greater mortality rate, and this increased mortality is associated with a higher interleukin-6 plasma level [63]. A retrospective analysis of MCOD recorded in China reported that being a man was independently associated with an increased sepsis-related mortality (RR = 1.582, 95% CI = 1.570–1.595) [61]. A retrospective population-based study in the United States also showed similar results [6]. From 2005 to 2018, the overall sepsis-related mortality rates were found to be higher in men (57 deaths per 100,000) when compared to women (45.1 deaths per 100,000). In a retrospective analysis of MIMIC-III database, Xu et al. reported higher 90-day and one-year mortality and hospital and ICU length of stay in men compared to women [59].

TABLE 27.1
Selected Studies on Gender Disparities in Sepsis

Study	Dates	Country	Number of patients	Designs	Prevalence of men	Mortality outcomes	Accordance to gender (for women compared to men)
Adrie et al. [57]	1997–2005	France	1692	Prospective	63.0%	Hospital	aOR 0.75 (CI 95%, 0.57–0.97)
Nachtigall et al. [58]	2006–2007	Germany	709	Prospective	56.4%	ICU	aOR 1.96 (95% CI, 1.04–3.71)
Xu et al. [59]	2001–12	United States	6134	Retrospective population based (MIMIC-III)	56.4%	One-year	RR 0.930 (CI 95%, 0.857 −0.993)
Van Vught et al. [60]	2011–2014	Netherlands	1533	Prospective (selected critically ill)	61.0%	90-day	aOR 0.94 (CI 95%, 0.74–1.20)
Weng et al. [61]	2015	China	245,105	Retrospective population-based	57.5%	Sepsis-related	RR 0.631 (CI 95%, 0.628 −0.636)
Sunden-Cullberg et al. [62]	2008–15	Sweden	2720	Retrospective	55.5%	30-day	aOR 1.28 (CI 95%, 1.00–1.64)
Prest et al. [6]	2005–18	United States	2,427,907	Retrospective population-based	Not available	Sepsis-related	RR 0.79 (CI 95%, 0.77–0.82)

aOR, adjusted odds ratio; *CI*, confidence interval; *ICU*, intensive care unit; *MIMIC*, Medical Information Mart for Intensive Care; *RR*, risk ratio.

But other studies found no difference in mortality among two genders [60,64]. A prospective observational study performed in two ICUs in the Netherlands reported no difference in mortality between the two genders [60]. Also, a retrospective analysis of APACHE IV database show adjusted OR of mortality in subgroup of sepsis was 1.07 (0.99—1.16, 95% CI, $P = .08$) for women compared to men. There are even reports of increased mortality in women. A prospective, observational study in Germany noted that the mortality of women with sepsis is higher than that of men [58]. A recent systematic review and metaanalysis found uncertain prognostic effect of gender on all-cause ICU and hospital mortality in patients with sepsis admitted to ICUs [65].

Patient-Based Factors

One of the most frequently cited potential factor causing gender difference is levels of different hormones observed in respective gender. Animal studies have shown that estrogens, in particular estradiol, can inhibit the inflammatory response and regulate the immune system to reach a balance of inflammatory and antiinflammatory reactions as well as promote the repair of damaged tissues [66,67]. Septic female proestrus mice have been shown to maintain splenic immune function and, therefore, experience lower mortality rates than in comparable male mice [68]. Estrogen administration has been shown to protect the liver and intestines in male septic rats by reducing oxidative stress, increasing macrophage activity, and reducing mortality [69]. In addition, administration of estrogen receptor agonists (ER-α and ER-β) to septic male or ovariectomized female rats has been shown to significantly reduce sepsis-induced leukocyte-functional capillary interaction and improve intestinal microcirculation [70]. In contrast, testosterone might weaken the immune response against major systemic infections. Testosterone has been shown to have significant immunosuppressive effects on both the innate and adaptive immune systems, by reducing production of immunoglobulins, decreasing cytokine production, and limiting lymphocyte proliferation [71,72].

There may also be nonhormonal-based factors that can influence the differential immune responses. Gender-based disparities in the incidence of sepsis are already observed in neonatal and pediatric sepsis population [73,74] when the difference in level of hormones will be subtle at best [74]. Differences that exist between males and females in their innate immune responses, including differences in cell number, activity, and cytokine production might account for these differences

[75,76]. One such factor might be the X-chromosome. Many genes on the X-chromosome regulate immune function and are important in modulating sex differences in immune response. An X-chromosome mosaicism, which occurs naturally in women, may affect sex-related differences in immune responses [77,78]. Experimental studies show that female X-chromosome mosaicism serve to diversify leukocyte responses during endotoxemia in mice and may result to the dimorphic character of the inflammatory reaction [79,80].

Hospital-Based Factors

It has been reported that the proportion of women receiving optimal care is lower as compared to men in various patient populations, including out-of-hospital cardiac arrest [81], acute coronary syndromes [82], cancer [83,84], stroke [85,86], trauma [87], and posttraumatic intensive care [88]. In the ICU, men are more likely to undergo invasive procedures such as mechanical ventilation and catheterization compared to women [89]. Results of recent Swiss ICU-Registry demonstrate that women are less likely to receive ICU treatment regardless of disease severity [90]. In regard to sepsis, some studies found that men receive recommended sepsis management more frequently than women [62,64]. A retrospective observational study in an urban academic emergency department which included data of 711 sepsis patients reported there was significant delay in antibiotic administration in women with mean time to first antibiotics of 184 min (95% CI, 171—197 min) compared to 153 min (95% CI, 143—163 min) for men ($P < .001$) [64]. A nationwide cohort study of sepsis or septic shock admitted to ICUs within 24 h of presentation to emergency department in Sweden also revealed a marked difference in sepsis management between men and women [62]. The study showed that men had 41.5% completion rate of Hour-1 bundle compared to only 30.0% for women ($P < .001$). Men also had a shorter time to the initiation of antibiotics at 65 min (95% CI, 30—136 min) compared to 87 min (95% CI, 39—172 min) for women ($P < .001$). How these disparities in hospital management process in sepsis according to gender affect mortality and morbidity in sepsis remain to be seen.

Interaction Effects of Gender and SES

There are reports of gender-specific association between SES and medical conditions. For example, a cross-sectional analysis of the CONSTANCES cohort reported higher prevalence of hypertension in men compared to women [91]. Interestingly, SES was strongly associated with hypertension prevalence in women compared to men. Tang et al. analyzed the National Population Health Survey in Canada and showed that after adjustment prevalence of diabetes increased with decreasing SES in women but not in men [92]. These results suggest that a gender-specific approach related to SES intervention may be needed to reduce gender disparities in these patient populations. Up to now, gender differences in the association between SES and sepsis have not been clearly investigated. Future studies are needed to see if such gender-specific interaction with SES exists in sepsis and/or septic shock.

POTENTIAL TARGET FOR INTERVENTIONS TO REDUCE DISPARITIES

Although racial and gender disparities are widely described, studies on interventions to reduce racial and gender disparities remain sparse. There are several studies that report on interventions as part of quality improvement programs [93–95], but no study specifically addresses racial and gender disparities in sepsis management. It is recommended that further research be undertaken to find the appropriate interventions that will hopefully reduce racial and gender disparities.

The presence of an association between susceptibility to sepsis and clinical outcomes to host genomic variations might explain some of the race and gender disparities observed in sepsis. For example, a recent study showed how individual transcriptomic signatures can explain the host response in sepsis, and this type of approach will help in establishing a precision medicine-based approach for management of sepsis and may enable the development of novel targeted therapies [96]. Future research should be focused on discovering ways to reduce individual disparities by uncovering genomic insights and social determinants of health.

Hospital-based interventions should focus on decreasing interhospitals and intrahospital variations in sepsis management regardless of patient race and gender. In a systematic review, Fitzgerald and Hurst report that healthcare professionals exhibit implicit biases that lead to a negative evaluation of a person on the basis of irrelevant characteristics such as race or gender [97]. Interventions to improve adherence to standardized treatment protocols such as the sepsis bundle proposed eased by Surviving Sepsis Campaign might be a way to remove this kind of biases which might lead to disparities in sepsis management [98,99].

The community needs to focus on individuals with low SES. Patients who are in the lower SESs have more comorbidities and hurdles to access to healthcare, for example, lack of service availability and the financial burden of care. As a result, the risk of death from sepsis

may increase in such individuals. Many reports in the literature recommended interventions aimed at preventing sepsis by optimization of comorbidities and provision of vaccinations for lower SESs [100,101]. Achieving this requires a multidisciplinary, multifaceted team approach. Approaches targeting social networks or support and self-care for individuals with low SES have been shown to affect health outcomes [102]. Social networks are important for both preventive care and the transition from hospital to postsepsis care.

CONCLUSION

Sepsis is a common life-threatening condition that is associated with high mortality and long-term morbidity in survivors. The relationship between race, gender, and sepsis is complex, and there are data suggesting existence of racial and gender disparities in management and outcome of sepsis. By understanding these complex interactions, effective interventions aimed at addressing these disparities can be instituted.

REFERENCES

[1] Institute of Medicine Committee on, U., R. Eliminating, and C. Ethnic Disparities in Health. In: Unequal treatment: confronting racial and ethnic disparities in health care, Smedley BD, Stith AY, Nelson AR, editors. National Academies Press (US) Copyright 2002 by the National Academy of Sciences; 2003. All rights reserved: Washington (DC).

[2] 2019 National Healthcare Quality and Disparities Reports. https://www.ahrq.gov/research/findings/nhqrdr/index.html.

[3] Office of Management and Budget. https://obamawhitehouse.archives.gov/omb/fedreg_1997standards.

[4] Galiatsatos P, et al. Health disparities and sepsis: a systematic review and meta-analysis on the influence of race on sepsis-related mortality. J Racial Ethn Health Disparities 2019;6(5):900–8.

[5] Barnato AE, et al. Racial variation in the incidence, care, and outcomes of severe sepsis: analysis of population, patient, and hospital characteristics. Am J Respir Crit Care Med 2008;177(3):279–84.

[6] Prest J, Sathananthan M, Jeganathan N. Current trends in sepsis-related mortality in the United States. Crit Care Med 2021;49(8):1276–84.

[7] Singer M, et al. The third international consensus definitions for sepsis and septic shock (Sepsis-3). JAMA 2016; 315(8):801–10.

[8] Gao JW, et al. Association between the TLR2 Arg753Gln polymorphism and the risk of sepsis: a meta-analysis. Crit Care 2015;19:416.

[9] Teuffel O, et al. Association between tumor necrosis factor-alpha promoter -308 A/G polymorphism and susceptibility to sepsis and sepsis mortality: a systematic review and meta-analysis. Crit Care Med 2010;38(1): 276–82.

[10] Thair SA, et al. A single nucleotide polymorphism in NF-κB inducing kinase is associated with mortality in septic shock. J Immunol 2011;186(4):2321−8.

[11] Georgescu AM, et al. Evaluation of TNF-α genetic polymorphisms as predictors for sepsis susceptibility and progression. BMC Infect Dis 2020;20(1):221.

[12] Feng B, et al. Association of tumor necrosis factor α -308G/A and interleukin-6 -174G/C gene polymorphism with pneumonia-induced sepsis. J Crit Care 2015;30(5):920−3.

[13] Bronkhorst MW, et al. Single-nucleotide polymorphisms in the Toll-like receptor pathway increase susceptibility to infections in severely injured trauma patients. J Trauma Acute Care Surg 2013;74(3):862−70.

[14] Kothari N, et al. Tumor necrosis factor gene polymorphism results in high TNF level in sepsis and septic shock. Cytokine 2013;61(2):676−81.

[15] Lu H, et al. Host genetic variants in sepsis risk: a field synopsis and meta-analysis. Crit Care 2019;23(1):26.

[16] Hahn EC, et al. Association of HLA-G 3′UTR polymorphisms and haplotypes with severe sepsis in a Brazilian population. Hum Immunol 2017;78(11−12):718−23.

[17] Grube M, et al. Donor nucleotide-binding oligomerization-containing protein 2 (NOD2) single nucleotide polymorphism 13 is associated with septic shock after allogeneic stem cell transplantation. Biol Blood Marrow Transplant 2015;21(8):1399−404.

[18] Redfern RL, Reins RY, McDermott AM. Toll-like receptor activation modulates antimicrobial peptide expression by ocular surface cells. Exp Eye Res 2011;92(3):209−20.

[19] Harris MI. Noninsulin-dependent diabetes mellitus in black and white Americans. Diabetes Metab Rev 1990; 6(2):71−90.

[20] Ogden CL, et al. Trends in obesity prevalence by race and hispanic origin-1999−2000 to 2017−2018. JAMA 2020; 324(12):1208−10.

[21] Muntner P, et al. End-stage renal disease in young black males in a black-white population: longitudinal analysis of the Bogalusa Heart Study. BMC Nephrol 2009;10:40.

[22] Fuller-Thomson E, Chisholm RS, Brennenstuhl S. COPD in a population-based sample of never-smokers: interactions among sex, gender, and race. Int J Chronic Dis 2016;2016:5862026.

[23] Williams LD, et al. Trajectories of and disparities in HIV prevalence among Black, white, and Hispanic/Latino men who have sex with men in 86 large U.S. metropolitan statistical areas, 1992−2013. Ann Epidemiol 2021; 54:52−63.

[24] Esper AM, et al. The role of infection and comorbidity: factors that influence disparities in sepsis. Crit Care Med 2006;34(10):2576−82.

[25] Ellis KR, et al. Chronic disease among African American families: a systematic scoping review. Prev Chronic Dis 2020;17:E167.

[26] Feldman CH, et al. Epidemiology and sociodemographics of systemic lupus erythematosus and lupus nephritis among US adults with Medicaid coverage, 2000−2004. Arthritis Rheum 2013;65(3):753−63.

[27] Afzali A, Cross RK. Racial and ethnic minorities with inflammatory bowel disease in the United States: a systematic review of disease characteristics and differences. Inflamm Bowel Dis 2016;22(8):2023−40.

[28] Stojan G, Petri M. Epidemiology of systemic lupus erythematosus: an update. Curr Opin Rheumatol 2018; 30(2):144−50.

[29] Dombrovskiy VY, et al. Occurrence and outcomes of sepsis: influence of race. Crit Care Med 2007;35(3): 763−8.

[30] Jones JM, et al. Racial disparities in sepsis-related in-hospital mortality: using a broad case capture method and multivariate controls for clinical and hospital variables, 2004−2013. Crit Care Med 2017;45(12): e1209−17.

[31] Mayr FB, et al. Do hospitals provide lower quality of care to black patients for pneumonia? Crit Care Med 2010; 38(3):759−65.

[32] Taylor SP, et al. Hospital differences drive antibiotic delays for black patients compared with white patients with suspected septic shock. Crit Care Med 2018; 46(2):e126−31.

[33] Madsen TE, Napoli AM. Analysis of race and time to antibiotics among patients with severe sepsis or septic shock. J Racial Ethn Health Disparities 2017;4(4): 680−6.

[34] Shannon EM, Schnipper JL, Mueller SK. Identifying racial/ethnic disparities in interhospital transfer: an observational study. J Gen Intern Med 2020;35(10): 2939−46.

[35] Lane-Fall MB, et al. Insurance and racial differences in long-term acute care utilization after critical illness. Crit Care Med 2012;40(4):1143−9.

[36] Pathirana TI, Jackson CA. Socioeconomic status and multimorbidity: a systematic review and meta-analysis. Aust N Z J Publ Health 2018;42(2):186−94.

[37] Soto GJ, Martin GS, Gong MN. Healthcare disparities in critical illness. Crit Care Med 2013;41(12):2784−93.

[38] Assari S. Life expectancy gain due to employment status depends on race, gender, education, and their intersections. J Racial Ethn Health Disparities 2018; 5(2):375−86.

[39] Moore JX, et al. Black-white racial disparities in sepsis: a prospective analysis of the REasons for Geographic and Racial Differences in Stroke (REGARDS) cohort. Crit Care 2015;19(1):279.

[40] Cantu PA, et al. Increasing education-based disparities in healthy life expectancy among U.S. Non-hispanic whites, 2000−2010. J Gerontol B Psychol Sci Soc Sci 2021;76(2):319−29.

[41] Shkolnikov VM, et al. The changing relation between education and life expectancy in central and eastern Europe in the 1990s. J Epidemiol Community Health 2006;60(10):875−81.

[42] O'Brien Jr JM, et al. Insurance type and sepsis-associated hospitalizations and sepsis-associated mortality among US adults: a retrospective cohort study. Crit Care 2011; 15(3):R130.

[43] Rush B, et al. Association of household income level and in-hospital mortality in patients with sepsis: a nationwide retrospective cohort analysis. J Intensive Care Med 2018;33(10):551−6.

[44] Donnelly JP, et al. Association of neighborhood socioeconomic status with risk of infection and sepsis. Clin Infect Dis 2018;66(12):1940−7.

[45] Wang HE, et al. Chronic medical conditions and risk of sepsis. PLoS One 2012;7(10):e48307.

[46] Goodwin AJ, et al. Where you live matters: the impact of place of residence on severe sepsis incidence and mortality. Chest 2016;150(4):829−36.

[47] Storm L, et al. Socioeconomic status and risk of intensive care unit admission with sepsis. Acta Anaesthesiol Scand 2018;62(7):983−92.

[48] Galiatsatos P, et al. The association between neighborhood socioeconomic disadvantage and readmissions for patients hospitalized with sepsis. Crit Care Med 2020;48(6):808−14.

[49] Brown EJ, et al. Racial disparities in geographic access to primary care in Philadelphia. Health Aff 2016;35(8): 1374−81.

[50] Lu PJ, et al. Racial and ethnic disparities in vaccination coverage among adult populations in the U.S. Vaccine 2015;33(Suppl. 4):D83−91.

[51] Annane D, et al. Current epidemiology of septic shock: the CUB-Réa Network. Am J Respir Crit Care Med 2003;168(2):165−72.

[52] Sands KE, et al. Epidemiology of sepsis syndrome in 8 academic medical centers. JAMA 1997;278(3):234−40.

[53] Jeon K, et al. Characteristics, management and clinical outcomes of patients with sepsis: a multicenter cohort study in Korea. Acute Crit Care 2019;34(3):179−91.

[54] Darbà J, Marsà A. Epidemiology, management and costs of sepsis in Spain (2008−2017): a retrospective multicentre study. Curr Med Res Opin 2020;36(7):1089−95.

[55] Xie J, et al. The epidemiology of sepsis in Chinese ICUs: a national cross-sectional survey. Crit Care Med 2020; 48(3):e209−18.

[56] Park S, et al. Normothermia in patients with sepsis who present to emergency departments is associated with low compliance with sepsis bundles and increased in-hospital mortality rate. Crit Care Med 2020;48(10): 1462−70.

[57] Adrie C, et al. Influence of gender on the outcome of severe sepsis: a reappraisal. Chest 2007;132(6):1786−93.

[58] Nachtigall I, et al. Gender-related outcome difference is related to course of sepsis on mixed ICUs: a prospective, observational clinical study. Crit Care 2011;15(3):R151.

[59] Xu J, et al. Association of sex with clinical outcome in critically ill sepsis patients: a retrospective analysis of the large clinical database MIMIC-III. Shock 2019; 52(2):146−51.

[60] van Vught LA, et al. Association of gender with outcome and host response in critically ill sepsis patients. Crit Care Med 2017;45(11):1854−62.

[61] Weng L, et al. Sepsis-related mortality in China: a descriptive analysis. Intensive Care Med 2018;44(7): 1071−80.

[62] Sunden-Cullberg J, Nilsson A, Inghammar M. Sex-based differences in ED management of critically ill patients with sepsis: a nationwide cohort study. Intensive Care Med 2020;46(4):727−36.

[63] Nasir N, et al. Mortality in sepsis and its relationship with gender. Pakistan J Med Sci 2015;31(5):1201−6.

[64] Mahmood K, Eldeirawi K, Wahidi MM. Association of gender with outcomes in critically ill patients. Crit Care 2012;16(3):R92.

[65] Antequera A, et al. Sex as a prognostic factor for mortality in critically ill adults with sepsis: a systematic review and meta-analysis. BMJ Open 2021;11(9):e048982.

[66] Harnish DC. Estrogen receptor ligands in the control of pathogenic inflammation. Curr Opin Invest Drugs 2006; 7(11):997−1001.

[67] Straub RH. The complex role of estrogens in inflammation. Endocr Rev 2007;28(5):521−74.

[68] Zellweger R, et al. Females in proestrus state maintain splenic immune functions and tolerate sepsis better than males. Crit Care Med 1997;25(1):106−10.

[69] Sener G, et al. Estrogen protects the liver and intestines against sepsis-induced injury in rats. J Surg Res 2005; 128(1):70−8.

[70] Sharawy N, et al. Estradiol receptors agonists induced effects in rat intestinal microcirculation during sepsis. Microvasc Res 2013;85:118−27.

[71] Angele MK, et al. Gender differences in sepsis: cardiovascular and immunological aspects. Virulence 2014;5(1): 12−9.

[72] Gubbels Bupp MR, Jorgensen TN. Androgen-induced immunosuppression. Front Immunol 2018;9:794.

[73] Bindl L, et al. Gender-based differences in children with sepsis and ARDS: the ESPNIC ARDS Database Group. Intensive Care Med 2003;29(10):1770−3.

[74] Watson RS, et al. The epidemiology of severe sepsis in children in the United States. Am J Respir Crit Care Med 2003;167(5):695−701.

[75] Klein SL, Flanagan KL. Sex differences in immune responses. Nat Rev Immunol 2016;16(10):626−38.

[76] Jaillon S, Berthenet K, Garlanda C. Sexual dimorphism in innate immunity. Clin Rev Allergy Immunol 2019; 56(3):308−21.

[77] Spolarics Z, et al. Inherent X-linked genetic variability and cellular mosaicism unique to females contribute to sex-related differences in the innate immune response. Front Immunol 2017;8:1455.

[78] Libert C, Dejager L, Pinheiro I. The X chromosome in immune functions: when a chromosome makes the difference. Nat Rev Immunol 2010;10(8):594−604.

[79] Chandra R, et al. Female X-chromosome mosaicism for gp91phox expression diversifies leukocyte responses

during endotoxemia. Crit Care Med 2010;38(10): 2003—10.

[80] Chandra R, et al. Female X-chromosome mosaicism for NOX2 deficiency presents unique inflammatory phenotype and improves outcome in polymicrobial sepsis. J Immunol 2011;186(11):6465—73.

[81] Jeong JS, et al. Gender disparities in percutaneous coronary intervention in out-of-hospital cardiac arrest. Am J Emerg Med 2019;37(4):632—8.

[82] Blomkalns AL, et al. Gender disparities in the diagnosis and treatment of non-ST-segment elevation acute coronary syndromes: large-scale observations from the CRUSADE (can rapid risk stratification of unstable angina patients suppress adverse outcomes with early implementation of the American College of Cardiology/American Heart Association guidelines) national quality improvement initiative. J Am Coll Cardiol 2005;45(6):832—7.

[83] Tabaac AR, et al. Gender identity disparities in cancer screening behaviors. Am J Prev Med 2018;54(3):385—93.

[84] Kim SE, et al. Sex- and gender-specific disparities in colorectal cancer risk. World J Gastroenterol 2015;21(17): 5167—75.

[85] Reeves MJ, et al. Sex differences in stroke: epidemiology, clinical presentation, medical care, and outcomes. Lancet Neurol 2008;7(10):915—26.

[86] Doelfel SR, et al. Gender disparities in stroke code activation in patients with intracerebral hemorrhage. J Stroke Cerebrovasc Dis 2021;30(12):106119.

[87] Marcolini EG, et al. Gender disparities in trauma care: how sex determines treatment, behavior, and outcome. Anesthesiol Clin 2019;37(1):107—17.

[88] Larsson E, et al. Impact of gender on post- traumatic intensive care and outcomes. Scand J Trauma Resuscitation Emerg Med 2019;27(1):115.

[89] Samuelsson C, et al. Gender differences in outcome and use of resources do exist in Swedish intensive care, but to no advantage for women of premenopausal age. Crit Care 2015;19(1):129.

[90] Todorov A, et al. Gender differences in the provision of intensive care: a Bayesian approach. Intensive Care Med 2021;47(5):577—87.

[91] Neufcourt L, et al. Gender differences in the association between socioeconomic status and hypertension in France: a cross-sectional analysis of the CONSTANCES cohort. PLoS One 2020;15(4):e0231878.

[92] Tang M, Chen Y, Krewski D. Gender-related differences in the association between socioeconomic status and self-reported diabetes. Int J Epidemiol 2003;32(3): 381—5.

[93] Gatewood MO, et al. A quality improvement project to improve early sepsis care in the emergency department. BMJ Qual Saf 2015;24(12):787—95.

[94] Nguyen HB, et al. Implementation of a bundle of quality indicators for the early management of severe sepsis and septic shock is associated with decreased mortality. Crit Care Med 2007;35(4):1105—12.

[95] Pepper DJ, et al. Evidence underpinning the centers for medicare & medicaid services' severe sepsis and septic shock management bundle (SEP-1): a systematic review. Ann Intern Med 2018;168(8):558—68.

[96] Davenport EE, et al. Genomic landscape of the individual host response and outcomes in sepsis: a prospective cohort study. Lancet Respir Med 2016;4(4):259—71.

[97] FitzGerald C, Hurst S. Implicit bias in healthcare professionals: a systematic review. BMC Med Ethics 2017; 18(1):19.

[98] Evans L, et al. Surviving sepsis campaign: international guidelines for management of sepsis and septic shock 2021. Intensive Care Med 2021;47(11):1181—247.

[99] Evans L, et al. Surviving sepsis Campaign: international guidelines for management of sepsis and septic shock 2021. Crit Care Med 2021;49(11):e1063—143.

[100] Rhee C, et al. Prevalence, underlying causes, and preventability of sepsis-associated mortality in US acute care hospitals. JAMA Netw Open 2019;2(2):e187571.

[101] Richardson A, Morris DE, Clarke SC. Vaccination in Southeast Asia—reducing meningitis, sepsis and pneumonia with new and existing vaccines. Vaccine 2014; 32(33):4119—23.

[102] Galobardes B, et al. Indicators of socioeconomic position (part 1). J Epidemiol Community Health 2006; 60(1):7—12.

CHAPTER 28

Sepsis in Special Populations

MARIE BALDISSERI • LAURA S. JOHNSON • MICHAEL MAZZEI • MARY JANE REED

SEPSIS AND OBESITY

Obesity has risen to the level of a national and a global epidemic. According to the most recent WHO Global Health Observatory data, nearly two billion adults worldwide are overweight, and 650 million of these individuals are obese [1]. The global prevalence of obesity has nearly tripled between 1975 and 2016. In the United States, nearly 70% of adults in the United States are overweight, and 35% are defined as obese. As a result, over 25% of patients admitted to intensive care units (ICUs) are overweight and obese [2]. Historically, sepsis represents the most common cause for admission to the ICU and the most common cause of death in the ICU, with global in-hospital mortality of 15%—25% [3,4]. As a result, the comanagement of obesity and sepsis in critically ill patients occurs with increasing regularity and unique challenges.

The "Obesity Paradox" of Sepsis

The "obesity paradox" is a well-described phenomenon in which obese patients have lower-than-expected mortality outcomes than similar patients without obesity. A recent metaanalysis demonstrated that in studies of adults admitted to the intensive care unit (ICU) with sepsis, adjusting for other baseline variables, patients who are overweight or obese have reductions in short-term mortality compared to those with normal body mass indices (BMIs) [5]. A recent retrospective review of over 55,000 patients with sepsis across 139 US hospitals demonstrated similar findings of 30-day mortality inversely proportional to BMI, with significantly lower mortality in patients with higher BMI compared with those with normal BMI [6]. In a prospective analysis of over 1400 patients with severe sepsis by Prescott et al., higher BMI was also associated with statistically significant improved one-year mortality [7].

Several physiologic rationales have been proposed for these mortality reductions. Increased adipose tissue and lipoprotein in patients with obesity may more effectively bind and inactivate lipopolysaccharide and other toxic bacterial products released during sepsis [8]. Increased adiposity is also correlated with several endocrinological and immune responses, which may confer a survival benefit. For example, obesity is associated with increased renin—angiotensin system activity; while this promotes chronic hypertension, it may exert a protective hemodynamic effect during sepsis [9]. In general, patients who are overweight have been found to receive less fluid and pressors per kilogram during the first four days of treatment, which has been demonstrated as conferring a survival benefit [10]. Additionally, excess adipose tissue may provide a greater reserve of energy during the catabolic septic state.

The degree of inflammatory response is also highlighted as an explanation for the differential outcomes of sepsis between patients with and without obesity, although data are somewhat conflicting in this regard [11]. For example, increased adiposity has been associated with greater tumor necrosis factor (TNF) production, which may augment host defenses and soluble TNF receptors, which might subsequently bind excess TNF and ameliorate its secondary harmful effects [12]. The magnitude of the inflammatory interleukin-6 (IL-6) response has also been shown to be somewhat muted in obese patients [10]. Conversely, several animal models of obesity in sepsis have highlighted an augmented inflammatory response. For example, Vachharajani et al. have demonstrated increased endovascular dysfunction and a more pronounced cerebral microvascular inflammatory response in septic mice [13]. In another animal study by Singer et al., mice with obesity secondary to leptin receptor mutations demonstrate a potentiated thrombogenic and inflammatory response to sepsis [14].

The role of adiponectin in sepsis is also an area of study. Adiponectin is an antiinflammatory cytokine that is synthesized in adipose cells and stored in adipose tissue. However, adiponectin levels demonstrate a paradoxical deficiency in obesity and a subsequent increase in serum levels with weight loss [15,16]. The exact role of adiponectin is unclear in sepsis; levels are depressed in sepsis as well as morbid obesity, and this, in turn, has been associated with insulin resistance, increased microvascular dysfunction, and a potentiated inflammatory response [17,18]. However, outcome studies have demonstrated improved outcomes among critically ill individuals with low adiponectin levels and worse mortality outcomes among critically ill patients with high serum adiponectin levels [19,20]. Leptin is another immunomodulatory cytokine that is elevated among patients with obesity; its exact role in sepsis is unclear, but it is thought to play a regulatory role in cytokine production and cell-mediated immunity, and leptin levels are markedly increased in sepsis [21].

Overall, significant uncertainty exists regarding the direction and extent of obesity's effect on mortality in adults with sepsis. Individual studies continue to show conflicting results and a variety of effect sizes. In a recent review of the literature, for example, Trivedi et al. identified a total of seven high-quality studies designed to delineate the relationship between obesity and sepsis mortality. Of these studies, three demonstrated no significant association between obesity and mortality, one observed increased mortality among obese patients, and three studies found lower mortality among obese patients [22]. It is also not clear that the "obesity paradox" demonstrates beneficial effects beyond the short term. For example, in a recent retrospective analysis by Robinson et al., a protective effect of obesity was demonstrated at one month after a sepsis diagnosis; yet, the converse was seen at the 180-day and one-year postsepsis mark, with significantly increased odds of death seen among patients with obesity [23]. This significant variance in findings suggests that the effect of obesity on sepsis outcomes remain poorly understood and may be partially explained by differences in study design or inclusion criteria.

Challenges in the Management of Septic Patients with Obesity

Fluid resuscitation: Despite the weight-based Surviving Sepsis Campaign recommendations for standardized initial fluid resuscitation of 30 mL/kg, it has been demonstrated in several studies that obese patients receive relatively lower fluid volumes than nonobese patients [10,24,25]. The optimal resuscitative strategy for obese patients is unknown. Weight-based fluid administration recommendations do not specify whether actual, ideal, or adjusted body weight (ABW) should be used to calculate resuscitative volumes. Research that has been directed toward optimal volume dosing strategies in obesity has been met with mixed or

conflicting results; for example, after adjusting for condition- and treatment-related variables, Taylor et al. found that volume dosing based on ABW was associated with improved mortality compared to total body weight (TBW); conversely, Kiracofe-Hoyte et al. found that septic patients who were dosed with 30 mL/kg doses based on TBW had a shorter time to hemodynamic instability and a lower risk of death in the hospital compared to patients with lower volume dosing strategies [26,27]. Other studies have shown that obese patients have lower vasopressor dosing by weight; it is unclear whether vasopressors should be dosed based on weight or not. Future research should be directed toward clarifying adequate fluid resuscitation in obesity and more clearly establishing tools to assess volume status and requirements in these patients accurately.

Mechanical ventilation: There are several deleterious effects that obesity has on the patient in need of respiratory support in the setting of sepsis. Vital capacity, functional residual capacity, and total lung capacity are decreased in obesity, and the chest wall and lung tissue compliance may be affected. As a result, the risk of developing atelectasis is increased. Other adverse sequelae of obesity include increases in upper and lower airway resistance and impairment of oxygen and carbon dioxide exchange [28]. Ventilatory management of the septic patient with obesity represents a significant challenge to the intensive care physician; strategies to improve pulmonary mechanics include reverse Trendelenburg positioning and early use of adjuncts such as prone positioning or inhaled nitrous oxide in the setting of severe hypoxemia. Low tidal volume lung ventilation, a mainstay of acute respiratory distress syndrome management, should be provided based on ideal body weight [29].

Nursing care: There are challenges to caring for patients with obesity related to their habitus and nursing requirements. Patients with obesity require more resources to reposition and transfer in and out of bed adequately; this has direct consequences related to the development of hospital-acquired sequelae of critical illness. Indeed, in a retrospective review of critically injured trauma patients, obesity was associated with several complications, including pneumonias, urinary tract infections, deep venous thrombosis, and decubitus ulcers [30]. There is evidence to suggest that the odds of these adverse events occurring scale directly with increasing BMI [31]. Patients with obesity in the ICU are more likely to require the use of extra or specialty resources such as special bed or mattresses, specialty commodes, and overbed trapezes; patients with obesity are more likely to require multiple personnel resources for position and transfer and are significantly less likely to transition to out-of-bed activity [32]. With nursing shortages being so prevalent, the allocation of additional hospital resources to septic patients with obesity should be anticipated.

Antibiotic dosing: While the early initiation of broad-spectrum antibiotics has been a mainstay of early goal-directed therapy for sepsis, obesity is a known risk factor for inadequate serum antibiotic concentrations and failure of antibiotic treatment [33]. Antibiotics are classified as either lipophilic (fat-soluble such as macrolides, quinolones, and tigecycline) or hydrophilic (water-soluble such as β-lactams and aminoglycosides); lipophilic agents achieve a higher volume of distribution due to binding to adipose tissue, and as a result, are more greatly affected by obesity [34]. As a result, lipophilic drugs are more likely to be dosed, according to TBW. Conversely, the volume of distribution may be overestimated in patients with obesity if dosing is based on TBW; if the drug is hydrophilic, ABW may be more appropriate for dosing in this instance [35]. In addition to the volume of distribution, obesity has additional effects on the glomerular filtration rate of the kidneys, which can in turn further alter antibiotic clearance [36].

An example of an antibiotic that is susceptible to underdosing in obesity is vancomycin. This antibiotic is commonly used in sepsis and is likely the most well-researched from the standpoint of the effects of obesity. It has been demonstrated that patients with obesity are more likely to receive inadequate doses of vancomycin, resulting in subtherapeutic levels and the potential persistence of bacterial infection [37]. A recent retrospective study demonstrated that vancomycin is frequently underdosed in sepsis, with 28.3% of overweight patients receiving an appropriate first dose compared to 51.1% of nonoverweight people [38]. Furthermore, the frequency and proportion of underdosing are shown to correlate linearly with increasing BMI directly. Overweight patients spend a smaller fraction of their course within the therapeutic range for vancomycin and have longer hospital lengths of stay, more treatment failures, and higher mortality [38]. A retrospective study of beta-lactam and fluoroquinolone in the emergency department to obese patients demonstrated appropriate initial dosing rates of between 1% and 8% [39].

In general, dosing of antibiotics in sepsis and obesity is grossly underresearched. However, attempts have been made to compile limited data and provide preliminary protocols for the dosing of antibiotics in obesity. For example, Meng et al. has provided a systematic review of dosing guidelines and provided recommendations for antimicrobial dosing in obesity, shown in Table 28.1 [40].

As the population with obesity continues to climb, obesity in sepsis will exert increasing influence on the healthcare system. Despite the suggestion of improved outcomes in sepsis for this population, obesity brings several unique issues that can significantly impact the quality of care if not recognized. These include differences in the initial resuscitation, nursing requirements, ventilator management, and antibiotic administration. Despite the significant impact of obesity on sepsis treatment, the current body of evidence for the management of these patients remains sparse. Further research should be directed to developing a more individualized approach to the patient with obesity and sepsis, more clearly defining the physiologic consequences of obesity, and targeting interventions that will improve the care of this challenging group.

SEPSIS AND CANCER
Introduction

Cancer occurs in approximately 16.8% of all sepsis patients [40]. Although death rates from cancer have decreased over time partly due to improved patient selection for ICU admission as well as improvements in treatments, cancer still remains one of the leading causes of death worldwide. Severe sepsis is associated with 8.5% of all cancer deaths [41]. In-hospital mortality rates for cancer patients with sepsis are 43%−55% higher than for those without underlying cancer [40−45]. Although deaths from sepsis are higher in adult and pediatric cancer patents compared to the general population, it appears that mortality rates for cancer patients with sepsis are improving. A study by Cooper et al. in 2019 showed that mortality rates in cancer patients with sepsis have decreased to 26% in 2014 compared to 31% in 2003 [46].

Cancer has been reported to be the most common comorbid medical condition in sepsis [40]. Incidence rates of severe sepsis in cancer patients are four times higher than in patients without cancer. Cancer patients are estimated to be 10 times more susceptible to sepsis and infections [40,42,47]. It is estimated that up to 20% of cancer patients develop sepsis [40,48]. Cancer patients with neutropenia, acute leukemia, advanced disease, or delay in admission to the ICU have a higher rate of bacteremia of 10%−30%, and sepsis and septic shock with higher mortality rates [49,50]. A higher mortality rate of up to 15% has been seen in young adult cancer patients with sepsis compared to similarly aged patients without cancer [48]. However, this difference in mortality rate appeared to decrease with increasing age when comparing cancer patients with sepsis and

TABLE 28.1
Recommended Antimicrobial Dosing in Obesity

Amoxicillin**	Consider upper limit of normal dosing in Severe Infections (e.g., up to 1 g PO q8h)
Ampicillin*	Consider upper limit of normal dosing in severe infections (e.g., up to 2 g q4h)
Amikacin	Use ABW for initial dose; adjust by TDM
Aztreonam*	Consider upper end of normal dosing in severe infections (e.g., 2 g q6–8h)
Cefazolin*	Consider upper limit of normal dosing in severe infections (e.g., up to 2 g q8h continuous or 1.5–2 g q6h intermittent dosing)
Ceftaroline	No change, consider q8h dosing
Ceftazidime	Up to 2 g q8h prolonged infusion
Ceftazidime/avibactam	No change
Ceftolozane/tazobactam	No change
Cefepime	Up to 2 g q8h prolonged infusion
Cephalexin**	Consider upper end of normal dosing in severe infections (e.g., 500–1000 mg q6h)
Ciprofloxacin*	Consider upper end of normal dosing in severe infections (e.g., up to 400 mg IV q8h or 750 mg PO q12h)
Clindamycin	600 mg q6h or 900 mg q8h IV; 450–600 mg q6h or 600–900 mg q8h PO; consider max dose 2.7 g/day in severe infections; 4.800 g/day in life-threatening infections
Colistin	Use IBW, consider maximum dose of 360 mg/day
Dalbavancin	No change
Daptomycin	Consider using ABW
Doripenem	No change; consider extended infusion in severe infections
Ertapenem	No change
Gentamicin	Use ABW for initial dose; adjust by TDM
Levofloxacin	750 g q24h for most infections; consider 1000 g q24h for gram negative organisms
Linezolid	No change
Meropenem	No change, consider extended infusion in severe infections
Moxifloxacin	No change
Nafcillin*	Consider upper end of normal dosing in severe infections (e.g., up to 2 g q4h)
Oritavancin	No change
Piperacillin-tazobactam	Up to 4.5g q8h (prolonged infused over 4 h) or 4.5g q6h (30-min infusion); prolonged infusions preferred for critically ill obese patients
Polymyxin B*	Consider ABW toward higher doses, consider maximum dose 200 mg or 2 million u/day
Tedizolid	No change
Telavancin*	No change; consider a maximum of 1000 mg/dose
Tigecycline	No change
Trimethoprim/Sulfamethoxazole*	Up to 320 mg PO q12h or 8–10 mg/kg of ABW per day in divided doses
Tobramycin	Use ABW for initial dose; adjust by TDM
Vancomycin	Considering load 20–25 mg/kg by TBW (consider a maximum of 2.5 g) followed by 10–15 mg/kg by TBW q12h (consider a maximum of 2 g/dose), then adjust by level; consider initial maximum daily dose of 4.5 g (including load)

* = insufficient data; ** = no data; ABW = adjusted body weight [IBW + 0.4 × (TBW-IBW)]; TBW = total body weight, IBW = ideal body weight [Male: 50.0 + 2.3 × (number of inches over 5 ft); Female: 45.5 + 2.3 × (number of inches over 5 ft)].
(Adapted from Meng L, Mui E, Holubar MK, et al. Comprehensive guidance for antibiotic dosing in obese adults. J Pharm Pharmacol 2017; 37: 1415–1431).

those cancer patients without sepsis [44]. Increasing age does not appear to be a factor in cancer-related sepsis compared to the general population [41]. In neutropenic cancer patients, 10%−20% of patients will develop bacteremia after cytotoxic chemotherapy and up to 60% of patients after stem cell transplantation with mortality rates as high as 40% [50,51]. Neutropenic sepsis is a leading cause of deaths from sepsis as a complication of cancer therapies [52]. Neutropenic patients who are afebrile or hypothermic have a higher incidence of severe sepsis and septic shock and increased in-hospital morbidity [52]. The longer the duration of neutropenia and the more severe can lead to higher rates of neutropenic sepsis [53]. Neutropenic patients appear to have a higher risk of acute kidney injury and increased levels of IL-6 and interleukin-8 in response to fighting infection [54]. Cancer patients with COVID-19 appear to have a higher rate of adverse events. It is now estimated that COVID-19 patients with known malignancies are 30% more likely to develop sepsis and to develop thromboembolism [55,56].

Hospital admission rates, length of stay, and hospital costs are increased threefold in cancer patients with severe sepsis. Length of stay and hospital costs are nearly three times higher in cancer patients with severe sepsis than those patients without severe sepsis [41]. Readmission rates 30 days after the initial hospital stay are higher at 23.2% compared to 20.1% for noncancer-related sepsis admissions [44]. It is estimated that more than one in five hospitalizations from sepsis are cancer-related [5]. Compared to those without a prior history of cancer, cancer survivors have more than double the risk of developing sepsis. In a study of hospital discharge data, it was found that there were 16.4 cases of sepsis per 1000 patients who had cancer [41]. The incidence of cancer was four times higher in these cancer survivors [41]. Other studies have shown that cancer survivors had a higher incidence of sepsis (12.66% vs. 3.81%) believed to be secondary to chronic altered immunity and additional morbidities [57,58]. Cancer patients with underlying psychiatric illnesses such as anxiety, depression, and substance abuse have also been found to have a higher risk for sepsis [59].

The type of cancer influences the incidence of severe sepsis in cancer patients, with hematologic tumors being nine times more likely than those with solid tumors, to experience an episode of severe sepsis although the mortality rates for severe sepsis were similar [41]. Taccone also found in European ICUs that patients with hematological tumors had much rates of sepsis-related death up to 58% [43].

Pathogenesis

Death from cancer results either from direct invasion of the malignant cells of solid organs or into the circulation or the lymphatic system. Patients with malignancies are susceptible to infections primarily because of their depressed immunologic state with defenses that are significantly compromised by ongoing therapies with chemotherapeutic agents. However, in addition, other factors increase the susceptibility rate of cancer patients to sepsis that include frequent hospitalizations, more frequent operative procedures, and procedures with in-dwelling catheters and devices, malnutrition, and concurrent illnesses. Cancer patients are more susceptible to opportunistic infections as a result of their underlying immunosuppression from both their malignancy and from the chemotherapy as well [50].

Diagnosis

It can be difficult to diagnose sepsis in neutropenic cancer patients who often have presenting signs and symptoms that are nonspecific. Lack of fever and an elevated white blood cell count are standard criteria that clinicians use for most patients with sepsis but are often absent in the neutropenic cancer patient with sepsis. It is important that the clinician has a high index of suspicion for sepsis in cancer patients who present with evidence of end-organ dysfunction such as altered mental status, decreased blood pressures especially with a wide pulse pressure, and other signs of end-organ dysfunction such as decreased urine output, and increased liver enzymes.

Serum lactate levels can be helpful in the diagnosis of sepsis reflecting significant tissue hypoperfusion. Unfortunately, in some cancer patients, serum lactate levels can be elevated from the patient's underlying oncologic disease. In a single-center retrospective analysis, hyperlactatemia was more frequently observed in cancer patients with sepsis as compared to noncancer patients (65% vs. 49.1%) and associated with lower survival rates (65.4% vs. 85.7%) [60]. Although in general, lactate levels may be elevated in cancer patients and these elevated levels remain a means of risk stratification for sepsis in cancer patients.

Are the present diagnostic tools and scoring systems appropriate for cancer patients with suspected sepsis? Systemic inflammatory response syndrome (SIRS) criteria are commonly utilized in septic patients. However, as previously reported, the SIRS criteria tend to be sensitive but not very specific [61,62]. These criteria have not been demonstrated to be ideal criteria for cancer patients with sepsis and have not been validated in trials looking at specific criteria such as qSOFA and MEWS in cancer patients [63]. A single-center study by Mato et al. in 2009 examined the utility of SIRS criteria in predicting the onset of septic shock in hospitalized patients with hematologic malignancies who were mostly nonneutropenic [64]. The predictive values in this study were fever, tachypnea, and tachycardia. Certainly, additional multicenter studies would contribute further to these limited although compelling results. Biomarkers have also been used as methods of utilization in identifying cancer patients who are at risk for sepsis. Numerous biomarkers have been studied, but only a few are in clinical use [61,65]. Biomarker panels and gene expression tests are now being evaluated in studies, although no biomarker has qualified as an ideal biomarker as of yet [61,66].

Early diagnosis and identification of sepsis can be complicated in immunocompromised patients. Although methods for improved and faster identification of organisms have been identified from blood cultures, they are not readily available yet [67]. A high index of suspicion of sepsis still remains the main predictor of diagnosis and outcome. Although it is well established that early administration of antibiotics in sepsis decreases hospital mortality, the question remains as to whether we should take a different approach to patients in cancer patients with sepsis considering their higher risk of sepsis from prior episodes of sepsis and frequent administration of antibiotic regimens. Admittedly these patients are more complex due to several facts such as periods of neutropenia, use of prophylactic antibiotics, use of granulocyte colony-stimulating factor (G-CSF), use of indwelling central venous catheters, as well as ongoing chemotherapy [68]. Complicating the diagnosis of sepsis and further confounding the diagnosis of sepsis in cancer patients is that certain cancers such as anaplastic large cell lymphomas and relapsing T-cell lymphomas can mimic sepsis with symptoms such as fever and elevated white blood cell counts [69,70]. In addition, cancer treatments such as interleukin-2 and chimeric antigen receptor T-cell therapies can also cause sepsis-like symptoms such as SIRS, shock, vascular endothelial leak syndrome, and multiple organ dysfunction [71].

Prevention and Treatment of Sepsis

The most effective strategies to decrease and prevent sepsis include hand hygiene. Additional prophylactic methods include vaccination, judicious use of antibiotics, avoiding indiscriminate use of antibiotics, and finally, sepsis awareness among patients, as well as in the community. Specific strategies to decrease sepsis include appropriate antibiotic prophylaxis and treatment and prevention of neutropenia, with the ancillary use of G-CSF and granulocyte-macrophage stimulating factor [G(M)-CSF].

SEPSIS AND SOLID ORGAN TRANSPLANT RECIPIENTS

Introduction

Solid organ transplants have increased yearly through 2019 [72]. As immunosuppressive regimens have improved, infection and sepsis have surpassed graft rejection as a significant cause of morbidity and mortality in solid organ transplant recipients (SOTRs) [73]. An accurate incidence of sepsis in SOTR is not known. Estimates of sepsis in SOTR range from 20% to 60%, with resultant mortality of 5%–40% [74]. Conventional wisdom is that SOTRs have higher mortality from sepsis. However, some studies suggest that SOTR may have lower mortality depending on organ transplanted; lung recipients have higher overall sepsis mortality [75,76]. Immunosuppression does not appear to increase mortality in SOTR with COVID-19 infection [77].

Diagnosis

Sepsis, as defined by surviving sepsis campaign international guidelines, is "life-threatening organ dysfunction resulting from dysregulated host response to infection" [78]. The immunosuppressives used in SOTR may blunt this response, making the diagnosis of sepsis more difficult. SOTRs tend to have diminished symptoms and attenuated clinical and radiologic findings. These patients often present with minor fever, minor leukocytosis, more thrombocytopenia, and increased end-organ failure [74]. Detailed history, thorough physical examination, and a high index of suspicion are crucial in diagnosing sepsis in the SOTR. Exposure history to sick contacts, medication compliance, environmental exposure, and travel history often overlooked in the immunocompetent patient are essential questions in the SOTR [79]. Inflammatory markers such as procalcitonin (PCT) are valuable in identifying systemic but not localized bacterial infections or viral infections. The cutoff value of PCT in SOTR systemic bacterial infection has not been fully identified. Also, the PCT can be elevated after surgery and administration of some immunosuppressives such as antithymocyte globulin. The PCT should be used as a supportive tool but not the sole test in diagnosing infection in the SOTR [79,80].

SOTRs are more susceptible to both common infections as well as opportunistic infections. This is multifactorial based on pretransplant medical conditions of the recipient, infectious status of the donor, and type of organ transplanted. Intraoperative factors such as longer length of operation, blood transfusions, prolonged ischemia time of organ, and other complications can increase the risk of infection. Posttransplant, the level of immunosuppression, antimicrobial prophylaxis use, cytomegalovirus infection, and nontransplant complications contribute to the risk of infection in the SOTR [81]. Knowledge of the timeline from initial transplantation and beyond is essential to help identify the possible etiology of infection in these patients, where on the timeline often reflects the net immunosuppressive state of the patient and exposure to infectious sources [81,82] (See Fig. 28.1).

The net immunosuppressive state of the SOTR contributes to the susceptibility to infection and possible pathogens. Immunosuppressive regimens often include induction dosing, T-cell–depleting regimens, B-cell depression agents, and high-dose corticosteroids. The peritransplant medical condition of the SOTR is also contributory, including malnutrition, diabetes mellitus control, critical illness, and mechanical pulmonary or circulatory support. The initial four weeks after transplant, patients are at risk for healthcare-associated infections. Surgical site infections, catheter and device-related infections, ventilator-associated pneumonia, Clostridioides difficile, and anastomotic complications are possible causes of sepsis during this period. As SOTRs are often exposed to multidrug-resistant organisms (MDROs), empiric treatment must include this coverage [81].

The subsequent period, generally up to six months, reflects the peak time of immunosuppression. Infections during this time often reflect the sum effect of drug immunosuppression, antiinfectious prophylaxis, and host defenses. Opportunistic infections, especially in patients without prophylaxis, can occur. Latent or recurrent infections also occur more often during this timeframe. Community-acquired and MDRO infections are persistently possible throughout the posttransplant period [81].

After six months, if the graft is functioning, drug-induced immunosuppression can usually be decreased, leading to chronic immunosuppression. Any increase in immunosuppression for rejection can return the SOTR to a greater immunosuppressive state, increasing the chance of additional opportunistic infections [82].

Specific organ transplants have more common site infections. Kidney transplant patients' most common infection requiring hospitalization is urinary tract infection. Liver transplant patients with biliary stenosis, hepatic artery thrombosis, or bilioenteric anastomosis have a higher risk of cholangitis and hepatic abscess. Lung transplant recipients have posttransplant lung denervation with decreased cough reflex, loss of lymphatics, and impaired mucociliary clearance, which contributes to a higher risk of pneumonia [83].

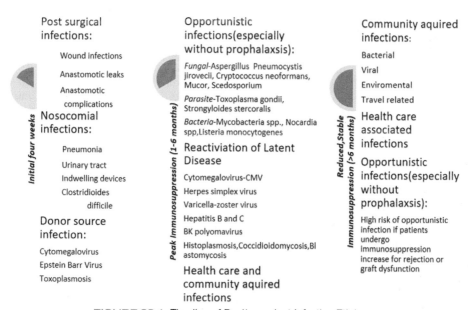

FIGURE 28.1 Timeline of Posttransplant Infection Etiology.

Treatment

The therapeutic approach to the septic SOTR does not differ from the nontransplant septic patient such as resuscitation, end-organ perfusion, expedient administration of broad antiinfectives based on possible etiologies, and source control if necessary. The level of immunosuppression during active infection is usually decreased; however, this should be done in consultation with the transplant care team as the risk of rejection needs to be considered. Adrenal insufficiency should be considered in those patients who have been on chronic steroids [84].

Significant drug interactions can occur with antimicrobials and immunosuppressives. Drug levels, if available, should be monitored closely. Common medications often used in septic patients also can have significant interactions with immunosuppressive drugs. Changes in renal or hepatic function can add additional pharmacodynamics to immunosuppressives. Careful daily review of medications is essential, and pharmacist consultation is prudent [85].

In summary, the septic SOTR requires a high index of suspicion for infection with detailed history and physical examination. The broad differential for infectious pathogens can be narrowed with knowledge of net immunosuppressive state based on the timeline from transplant, history of previous infections, type of graft, and active prophylaxis.

BURNS AND SEPSIS

Introduction

Over two million people sustain a thermal or chemical trauma yearly, with nearly 200,000 resulting in deaths. While death rates have been decreasing in high-income countries, the rates in middle- and low-income countries remain significant. For those who do not die, disability-adjusted life years are significantly impacted, and healthcare systems worldwide spend many millions of US$ per year caring for these patients [86,87]. Burn injury has a profound impact on patient life, with functional recovery often impeded by significant variables, including the rapidity at which patients can achieve wound closure [88].

As with many patients in the ICU, if a patient with a large burn survives their initial insult, the primary cause of death is multiple organ dysfunction syndrome (MODS) directly related to sepsis. While a lot of attention has been paid to the diagnosis and treatment of sepsis over the decades, all sepsis trials have excluded burn patients for two key reasons [89,90]. The first is that burn patients have lost the primary barrier to infection in sustaining their injury. While the skin serves a wide variety of homeostatic, immune-modulatory, and cosmetic functions, it primarily acts as a barrier to infection. Until wounds are closed, the risk for sepsis persists, leaving the patient and surgical team in a race to complete wound excision and definitive closure before MODS can occur. Secondly, burn patients develop a profound hypermetabolic response to injury that persists for months after the initial insult [91,92]. The ongoing exposure to inflammatory mediators results in baseline changes to many variables that comprise standard sepsis criteria: heart rate, respiratory rate, temperature, and white blood cell count.

Diagnosis

Therefore, the standard diagnostic components of sepsis in the general population are of limited value in a patient population whose injury complex results in changes that can last for months after even wound closure [93]. Recognizing this problem, the American Burn Association held a Consensus Conference in 2007 to, among other topics, identify criteria for sepsis in adult and pediatric burn patients that would be more discriminating than those used for the general population (Table 28.2) [94]. Since then, several groups have attempted to improve upon these criteria's diagnostic sensitivity and specificity, primarily focusing on the adult population. Mann-Salinas and colleagues were the first to attempt to optimize the approach, identifying six criteria for identifying burn sepsis with bacteremia [93]. While more sensitive for this population than the ABA consensus criteria, the potential for patients to have sepsis in the absence of positive blood cultures is not addressed by these criteria. More recent studies have attempted to address this and other limitations with variable results; while bacteremia is one potential source of sepsis in the burn-injured population, other infectious organisms and other locations can also make patients profoundly ill [95–101]. Timing is also a critical difference when assessing sepsis in the burn patient. Throughout what is often an extended hospital stay, burn patients may continue to develop sepsis episodically until all wound beds are closed [102,103]. Additionally, extended use of indwelling devices for venous access, ventilation, and bladder drainage can increase the risks for device-related infections and subsequent sepsis; ultimately, burn patients are not free from the risk of sepsis until well after they are discharged [104].

Treatment

Initiation of antimicrobial coverage for burn patients with sepsis requires an understanding of the common

TABLE 28.2
ABA Criteria 2007

SEPSIS		
Three or more of the following:		
Temperature >39°C or <36.5°C		
Progressive tachycardia	Adults >110	
	Children >2 standard deviations above age-specific norms (85% age-adjusted max heart rate)	
Progressive tachypnea	Adults not intubated >25 bpm Adults intubated MV > 12 L/min	
	Children >2 standard deviations above age-specific norms (85% age-adjusted max respiratory rate)	
Thrombocytopenia (does not apply until >3d after injury)	Adults <100,000	
	Children <2 standard deviations below age-specific norms	
Hyperglycemia (in the absence of preexisting diabetes mellitus)	Untreated plasma glucose >200 mg/dL or equivalent mM/L	
	Insulin resistance	Adults: Intravenous insulin >7U/h IV
		Adults/Children: >25% increase in insulin requirements over 24 h
Inability to continue enteral feeding >24 h	Abdominal distention	
	Enteral feeding intolerance	Adults: Residual > 2x feeding rate
		Children: Residual >150 mL/hr.
	Uncontrollable diarrhea	Adults: >2500 mL/day
		Children: >400 mL/day
Required that documented infection be identified one of the following:		
Culture positive infection		
Pathologic tissue source identified		
Clinical response to antimicrobials		
Septic shock		
Above + shock like hemodynamic parameters defined in the 2004 Surviving Sepsis Campaign		

organisms found in the burn unit. Of the gram-positive organisms, *Staphylococcus aureus* remains among the leading causes of burn wound infection, with variable methicillin resistance rates; less commonly seen are streptococci and enterococci [105,106]. Early infections (within 3—7d of injury) are most likely to be gram-positive, while later infections are more likely to be gram-negative organisms. *Pseudomonas* remains the most common organism, gram-positive or negative,

associated with mortality, typically manifesting after the first-week postinjury [107]. Additional gram-negative organisms seen in burn wounds include *Acinetobacter* and *Enterobacteriaceae*. Nonbacterial causes of burn wound infection include fungal species, most commonly Candida spp. and Aspergillus spp, and viruses primarily of the herpesvirus group [105,106]. While neither fungal nor viral infection is particularly associated with sepsis, the persistence of open wounds due to local infection by fungus or virus can perpetuate the risk for systemic infection by bacteria.

Prevention of burn sepsis is at the forefront of burn treatment strategies. Regular interval exchanges of indwelling devices, use of ventilator liberation strategies, and attention to appropriate nutritional support all have their role in preventing infection, along with strict adherence to infection control practices [104]. Short courses of targeted antimicrobial agents based on local patterns of wound colonization can be coupled with physical isolation of patients, appropriate use of personal protective equipment, and handwashing to reduce the development and potential outbreak of resistant strains [106].

Early excision of the burn-injured tissue is the best definitive treatment for the prevention of sepsis. Multiple studies have demonstrated a decrease in bacterial cell count in quantitative tissue cultures and subsequent rate of sepsis diagnoses with early excision versus late (within 72 h of time of injury or at the extreme 10 or more days from the time of injury) [108–110]. Until surgery can be performed; however, topical antimicrobial agents including silver sulfadiazine, cerium nitrate-silver sulfadiazine, mafenide acetate, or bacitracin can be used based on the region of the body injured and the depth of injury at that location. Systemic antimicrobial dosing in the burn unit is complicated by changes in the volume of distribution, renal function, and the hypermetabolic state of injury, increasing the metabolism of antimicrobial drugs. A multidisciplinary approach to management is often critical to maintaining an appropriate safety profile. Fungal infection needs to be treated with wide local excision and systemic antifungal agents, while viral infections can be controlled with oral and topical antiviral agents [106].

Ultimately, more work is necessary to optimize the care of burn patients to prevent or manage sepsis. A better understanding of the inflammatory response to injury coupled with the incorporation of enhanced pathogen detection practices and the development of novel skin substitutes will allow for more complete management of this patient population to minimize the impact of sepsis on morbidity and mortality.

REFERENCES

[1] WHO Global Health Observatory. Obesity and overweight. June 9, 2021. Retrieved from, https://www.who.int/news-room/fact-sheets/detail/obesity-and-overweight.

[2] Ogden CL, Carroll MD, Kit BK, et al. Prevalence of childhood and adult obesity in the United States, 2011-2012. JAMA 2014;311:806–14.

[3] Angus DC, Linde-Zwirble WT, Lidicker J, et al. Epidemiology of severe sepsis in the United States: analysis of incidence, outcome, and associated costs of care. Crit Care Med 2001;29:1303–10.

[4] Fleischmann C, Scherag A, Adhikari N, et al. Assessment of global incidence and mortality of hospital-treated sepsis. Current estimates and limitations. Am J Respir Crit Care 2016;193:259–72.

[5] Pepper DJ, Sun J, Welsh J, et al. Increased body mass index and adjusted mortality in ICU patients with sepsis or septic shock: a systematic review and meta-analysis. Crit Care 2016;20:1–10.

[6] Pepper DJ, Demirkale CY, Sun J, et al. Does obesity protect against death in sepsis? A retrospective cohort study of 55,038 adult patients. Crit Care Med 2019;47:643.

[7] Prescott HC, Chang VW, O'Brien Jr, et al. Obesity and one-year outcomes in older Americans with severe sepsis. Crit Care Med 2014;42:1766.

[8] Ulevitch RJ, Johnston AR, Weinstein DB. New function for high density lipoproteins. Their participation in intravascular reactions of bacterial lipopolysaccharides. J Clin Invest 1979;64:1516–24.

[9] Galic S, Oakhill JS, Steinberg GR. Adipose tissue as an endocrine organ. Mol Cell Endocrinol 2010;316:129–39.

[10] Wacharasint P, Boyd JH, Russell JA, et al. One size does not fit all in severe infection: obesity alters outcome, susceptibility, treatment, and inflammatory response. Crit Care 2013;17:1–10.

[11] Kolyva AS, Zolota V, Mpatsoulis D, et al. The role of obesity in the immune response during sepsis. Nutr Diabetes 2014;4. e137–e137.

[12] Winkler G, Kiss S, Keszthelyi L, et al. Expression of tumor necrosis factor (TNF)-a protein in the subcutaneous and visceral adipose tissue in correlation with adipocyte cell volume, serum TNF-a, soluble serum TNF-receptor-2 concentrations and C-peptide level. Eur J Endocrinol 2003;149:129–35.

[13] Vachharajani V, Russell JM, Scott KL, et al. Obesity exacerbates sepsis-induced inflammation and microvascular dysfunction in mouse brain. Microcirculation 2005;12:183–94.

[14] Singer G, Stoke KY, Terao S, et al. Sepsis-induced intestinal microvascular and inflammatory responses in obese mice. Shock 2009;31:275–9.

[15] Arita Y, Kihara S, Ouchi N, et al. Paradoxical decrease of an adipose-specific protein, adiponectin, in obesity. Biochem Biophys Res Commun 1999;257:79–83.

[16] Yang WS, Lee WJ, Funahashi T, et al. Weight reduction increases plasma levels of an adipose-derived anti-inflammatory protein, adiponectin. J Clin Endocrinol Metab 2001;86:3815–9.

[17] Venkatesh B, Hickman I, Nisbet J, et al. Changes in serum adiponectin concentrations in critical illness: a preliminary investigation. Crit Care 2009;13:1–5.

[18] Teoh H, Quan A, Bang KA, et al. Adiponectin deficiency promotes endothelial activation and profoundly

exacerbates sepsis-related mortality. Amer J Physiol Endocrinol Metab 2008;295:E658−64.

[19] Koch A, Sanson E, Voigt S, et al. Serum adiponectin upon admission to the intensive care unit may predict mortality in critically ill patients. J Crit Care 2011;26:166−74.

[20] Walkey AJ, Rice TW, Konter J, et al. Plasma adiponectin and mortality in critically ill subjects with acute respiratory failure. Crit Care Med 2010;38:2329.

[21] Behnes M, Brueckmann M, Lang S, et al. Alterations of leptin in the course of inflammation and severe sepsis. BMC Infect Dis 2012;12:1−11.

[22] Trivedi V, Bavishi C, Jean R. Impact of obesity on sepsis mortality: a systematic review. J Crit Care 2015;30:518−24.

[23] Robinson JD. Examining body mass index and sepsis mortality at one year after sepsis. VCU; 2020. p. 1−140.

[24] Rhodes A, Evans LE, Alhazzani W, et al. Surviving sepsis campaign: international guidelines for management of sepsis and septic shock. Intensive Care Med 2017;43:304−77.

[25] Arabi YM, Dara SI, Tamim HM, et al. Clinical characteristics, sepsis interventions and outcomes in the obese patients with septic shock: an international multicenter cohort study. Crit Care 2013;17:1−13.

[26] Taylor SP, Karvetski CH, Templin MA, et al. Initial fluid resuscitation following adjusted body weight dosing is associated with improved mortality in obese patients with suspected septic shock. J Crit Care 2018;43:7−12.

[27] Kiracofe-Hoyte BR, Doepker BA, Riha HM, et al. Assessment of fluid resuscitation on time to hemodynamic stability in obese patients with septic shock. J Crit Care 2021;63:96−201.

[28] Bahammam AS, Al-Jawder SE. Managing acute respiratory decompensation in the morbidly obese. Respirology 2012;17:759−71.

[29] Hibbert K, Rice M, Malhotra A. Obesity and ARDS. Chest 2012;142:785−90.

[30] Yaegashi M, Jean R, Zuriqat M, et al. Outcome of morbid obesity in the intensive care unit. J Intensive Care Med 2005;20:147−54.

[31] Newell MA, Bard MR, Goettler CE, et al. Body mass index and outcomes in critically injured blunt trauma patients: weighing the impact. J Am Coll Surg 2007;204:1056−61.

[32] Winkelman C, Maloney B. Obese ICU patients: resource utilization and outcomes. Clin Nurs Res 2005;14:303−23.

[33] Longo C, Bartlett G, MacGibbon B, et al. The effect of obesity on antibiotic treatment failure: a historical cohort study. Pharmacoepidemiol Drug Saf 2013;22:970−6.

[34] Leykin Y, Miotto L, Pellis T. Pharmacokinetic considerations in the obese. Best Pract Res Clin Anaesthesiol 2011;25:27−36.

[35] Meng L, Mui E, Holubar MK, et al. Comprehensive guidance for antibiotic dosing in obese adults. J Pharm Pharmacol 2017;37:1415−31.

[36] Pai MP. Estimating the glomerular filtration rate in obese adult patients for drug dosing. Adv Chron Kidney Dis 2010;17:e53−62.

[37] Hall R, Payne K, Rahman AP. Multicenter evaluation of vancomycin dosing: emphasis on obesity. Am J Med 2008;121:515−8.

[38] Koyanagi M, Anning R, Loewenthal M, et al. Vancomycin: audit of American guideline-based intermittent dose administration with focus on overweight patients. Br J Clin Pharmacol 2020;86:958−65.

[39] Roe JL, Fuentes JM, Mullins ME. Underdosing of common antibiotics for obese patients in the ED. Am J Emerg Med 2012;30:1212−4.

[40] Martin GS, Mannino DM, Eaton S, et al. The epidemiology of sepsis in the U.S. from 1979 through 2000. N Engl J Med 2003;348:1546−54.

[41] Williams MD, Braun LA, Cooper LM, et al. Crit Care 2004;8:R291−8.

[42] Danai PA, Moss M, Mannino DM, et al. The epidemiology of sepsis in patients with malignancy. Chest 2006;129:1432−40.

[43] Taccone FS, Artigas AA, Sprung CL, et al. Crit Care 2009;13:R15.

[44] Hensley MK, Donnelly JP, Carlton EF, et al. Epidemiology and outcomes of cancer-related versus non-cancer-related sepsis hospitalizations. Crit Care Med 2019;47:1310−6.

[45] Basu SK, Fernandez ID, Fisher SG, et al. Length of stay and mortality associated with febrile neutropenia among children with cancer. J Clin Oncol 2005;23:7958−66.

[46] Cooper AJ, Keller SP, Chan C, et al. Improvements in sepsis associated mortality in hospitalized patients with cancer versus those without cancer: a 12-year analysis using clinical data. Ann Am Thorac Soc 2020;17:466−73.

[47] Moore JX, Akinyemiju T, Bartolucci A, et al. A prospective study of cancer survivors and risk of sepsis within the REGARDS cohort. Cancer Epidemiol 2018;55:30−8.

[48] Rhee C, Dantes R, Epstein L, et al. Incidence and trends of sepsis in US hospitals using clinical vs claims data. JAMA 2017;318:1241−9.

[49] Kochanek M, Schalk E, von Bergwelt-Baildon M, et al. Management of sepsis in neutropenic cancer patients: 2018 guidelines from the infectious diseases working party (AGIHO) and intensive care working party (iCHOP) of the German society of hematology and medical oncology (DGHO). Ann Hematol 2019;98:1051−69.

[50] Kern WV, Roth JA, Bertz H, et al. Contribution of specific pathogens to bloodstream infection mortality in neutropenic patients with hematologic malignancies: results from a multicentric surveillance cohort study. Transpl Infect Dis 2019;21:e13186.

[51] Gustinetti G, Mikulska M. Bloodstream infections in neutropenic cancer patients: a practical update. Virulence 2016;7:280−97.

[52] Tavakoli A, Carannante A. Nursing care of oncology patients with sepsis. Semin Oncol Nurs 2021;21:151130.

[53] Strojnik K, Mahkovic-Hergouth K, Novakovic BJ, et al. Outcome of severe infections in afebrile neutropenic cancer patients. Radiol Oncol 2016;50:442−8.

[54] Reilly JP, Anderson BJ, Hudock KM, et al. Neutropenic sepsis is associated with distinct clinical and biological characteristics: a cohort study of severe sepsis. Crit Care 2016;20:222.

[55] Alpert N, Rapp JL, Marcellino B, et al. Clinical course of cancer patients with COVID-19: a retrospective cohort study. JNCI Cancer Spectr 2021;5. pkaa085.

[56] Alpert N, Taioli E. Clinical characteristics and outcomes of COVID-19-infected cancer patients: a systematic review and meta-analysis. J Natl Cancer Inst 2021;113: 501−2.

[57] Moore JX, Akinyemiju T, Bartolucci A, et al. A prospective study of community mediators on the risk of sepsis after cancer. J Intensive Care Med 2020; 35:1546−55.

[58] Moore JX, Akinyemiju T, Bartolucci A, et al. Mediating effects of frailty indicators on the risk of sepsis after sepsis. J Intensive Care Med 2020;35:708−19.

[59] Liu Q, Song H, Andersson TM, et al. Psychiatric disorders are associated with increased risk of sepsis following a cancer diagnosis. Cancer Res 2020;80:3436−42.

[60] Lopez R, Rodrigo P-A, Baus F, et al. Outcomes of sepsis and septic shock in cancer patients; focus on lactate. Front Med 2021;8:603275.

[61] Vincent JL, Opal SM, Marshall JC, et al. Sepsis definitions: time for change. Lancet 2013;381:774−5.

[62] Sprung CL, Sakr Y, Vincent JL, et al. An evaluation of systemic inflammatory response syndrome signs in the Sepsis Occurrence in Acutely Ill Patients (SOAP) study. Intensive Care Med 2006;32:421−7.

[63] Alberti C, Brun-Buisson C, Goodman SV, et al. Influence of systemic inflammatory response syndrome and sepsis on outcome of the critically ill infected patients. Am J Respir Crit Care Med 2003;168:77−84.

[64] Mato A, Fuchs BD, Heitjan DF, et al. Utility of the systemic inflammatory response syndrome (SIRS) criteria in predicting the onset of septic shock in hospitalized patients with hematologic malignancies. Cancer Biol Ther 2009;8:1095−100.

[65] Reinhart K, Bauer M, Riedemann NC, et al. New approaches to sepsis: molecular diagnostics and biomarkers. Clin Microbiol Rev 2012;25:609−34.

[66] Sutherland A, Thomas M, Brandon RA, et al. Development and validation of a novel molecular biomarker diagnostic test for the early detection of sepsis. Crit Care 2011;15:R149.

[67] Leisenfeld O, Lehman L, Hunfeld K-P, et al. Molecular diagnosis of sepsis: new aspects asnd recent developments. Eur J Microb Immunol (Bp) 2014;4: 1−25.

[68] Freifeld AG, Bow EJ, Sepkowitz KA, et al. Clinical practice guideline for the use of antimicrobial agents in neutropenic patients with cancer: 2010 update by the Infectious Disease Society of America. Clin Infect Dis 2011;52:e56−93.

[69] Mosunjac MB, Sundstrom JB, Mosunjac MI. Unusual presentation of anaplastic large cell lymphoma with clinical course mimicking fever of unknown origin and sepsis: autopsy study of five cases. Croat Med J 2008; 49:660−8.

[70] Boland C, Layios N, Ferrant A, et al. Relapsing T-cell lymphoma mimicking adult respiratory distress syndrome and sepsis. Leuk Lymphoma 2006;47:1989−90.

[71] Caorsi C, Quintana E, Valdés S, et al. Continuous cardiac output and hemodynamic monitoring: high temporal correlation between plasma TNF-alpha and hemodynamic changes during a sepsis-like state in cancer immunotherapy. J Endotoxin Res 2003;9:91−5.

[72] Aubert O, et al. COVID-19 pandemic and worldwide OrganTransplantation: a population-based study. Lancet Public Health 2021;6(10):e709−19 [MEDLINE—Academic. Web].

[73] Riella LV. Understanding the causes of mortality post-transplantation—there is more than meets the eye. Brazilian Journal of Nephrology 2018;40(2):102−4. Web. Oct 7, 2021.

[74] Kalil AC, Sandkovsky U, Florescu DF. Severe infections in critically ill solid organ transplant recipients. Clin Microbiol Infect 2018;24(12):1257−63 [Web].

[75] Donnelly JP, et al. Inpatient mortality among solid organ transplant recipients hospitalized for sepsis and severe sepsis. Clin Infect Dis 2016;63(2):186−94. Web. 9/26/2021.

[76] Kalil AC, et al. Is bacteremic sepsis associated with higher mortality in transplant recipients than in non-transplant patients? A matched case-control propensity-adjusted study. Clin Infect Dis 2014;60(2): 216−22. Web. 9/26/2021.

[77] Heldman MR, Kates OS. COVID-19 in solid organ transplant recipients: a review of the current literature [published online ahead of print, 2021 Jun 29]. Curr Treat Options Infect Dis 2021:1−16. https://doi.org/10.1007/s40506-021-00249-6.

[78] Evans L, Rhodes A, Alhazzani W, Antonelli M, Coopersmith CM, French C, Machado FR, Mcintyre L, Ostermann M, Prescott HC, Schorr C, Simpson S, Wiersinga WJ, Alshamsi F, Angus DC, Arabi Y, Azevedo L, Beale R, Beilman G, Belley-Cote E, Burry L, Cecconi M, Centofanti J, Coz Yataco A, De Waele J, Dellinger RP, Doi K, Du B, Estenssoro E, Ferrer R, Gomersall C, Hodgson C, Hylander Møller M, Iwashyna T, Jacob S, Kleinpell R, Klompas M, Koh Y, Kumar A, Kwizera A, Lobo S, Masur H, McGloughlin S, Mehta S, Mehta Y, Mer M, Nunnally M, Oczkowski S, Osborn T, Papathanassoglou E, Perner A, Puskarich M, Roberts J, Schweickert W, Seckel M, Sevransky J, Sprung CL, Welte T, Zimmerman J, Levy M. Surviving sepsis campaign: international guidelines for management of sepsis and septic shock 2021. Crit Care Med 2021;49(11):e1063−143. https://doi.org/10.1097/CCM.0000000000005337. Web. Oct 7, 2021.

[79] Florescu DF, Kalil AC. Survival outcome of sepsis in recipients of solid organ transplant. Seminars in respiratory and critical care medicine 42 2021;5:717–25 [Web].

[80] Coppock D, et al. Role of procalcitonin in management of infection in solid organ transplantation recipients: review. OBM Transplantation 2019;3(1):1. Web. Oct 13, 2021.

[81] Timsit J-F, et al. Diagnostic and therapeutic approach to infectious diseases in solid organ transplant recipients, 45. Springer Science and Business Media LLC; 2019 [Web].

[82] Guenette A, Husain S. Infectious complications following solid organ transplantation. Critical Care Clinics 35 2019;1:151–68. Web. Oct 7, 2021.

[83] McCreery RJ, Florescu DF, Kalil AC. Sepsis in immunocompromised patients without human immunodeficiency virus. J Infect Dis 2020;222(Suppl. ment_2): S156–65. Web. 9/26/2021.

[84] Bafi AT, Tomotani DY, de Freitas FG. Sepsis in solid-organ transplant patients. Shock 2017;47(1S Suppl. 1): 12–6.

[85] Sparkes T, Lemonovich TL. Interactions between anti-infective agents and immunosuppressants—guidelines from the American society of transplantation infectious diseases community of practice. Clin Transplant 2019; 33:e13510.

[86] WHO WHO. Burns. 2018 [Internet] [cited 2021 Sep 9]. Available from: https://www.who.int/news-room/fact-sheets/detail/burns.

[87] ABA ABA. Burn incidence fact sheet. 2016 [Internet]. 2016 [cited 2021 Sep 9]. Available from: https:// ameriburn.org/who-we-are/media/burn-incidence-fact-sheet/%3E.

[88] Haug VF, Tapking C, Panayi AC, Thiele P, Wang AT, Obed D, Hirche C, Most P, Kneser U, Hundeshagen G. Long-term sequelae of critical illness in sepsis, trauma and burns: A systematic review and meta-analysis. J Trauma Acute Care Surg 2021;91(4):736–747. https://doi.org/ 10.1097/TA.0000000000003349. PMID: 34252062.

[89] Seymour CW, Liu VX, Iwashyna TJ, Brunkhorst FM, Rea TD, Scherag A, et al. Assessment of clinical criteria for sepsis for the third international consensus definitions for sepsis and septic shock (sepsis-3). JAMA, J Am Med Assoc February 23, 2016;315(8):762–74.

[90] Shankar-Hari M, Phillips GS, Levy ML, Seymour CW, Liu VX, Deutschman CS, et al. Developing a new definition and assessing new clinical criteria for septic shock for the third international consensus definitions for sepsis and septic shock (Sepsis-3) original investigation | caring for the critically ill patient. JAMA 2016;315(8):775–87.

[91] Williams FN, Herndon DN, Jeschke MG. The hypermetabolic response to burn injury and interventions to modify this response. Clin Plast Surg. 2009;36(4): 583–96. https://doi.org/10.1016/j.cps.2009.05.001. PMID: 19793553; PMCID: PMC3776603.

[92] Jeschke MG, Gauglitz GG, Kulp GA, Finnerty CC, Williams FN, Kraft R, et al. Long-term persistance of the pathophysiologic response to severe burn injury.

[93] Mann-Salinas EA, Baun MM, Meininger JC, Murray CK, Aden JK, Wolf SE, et al. Novel predictors of sepsis outperform the American burn association sepsis criteria in the burn intensive care unit patient. J Burn Care Res January 1, 2013;34(1):31–43.

[94] Greenhalgh DG, Saffle JR, Holmes JH, Gamelli RL, Palmieri TL, Horton JW, et al. American burn association consensus conference to define sepsis and infection in burns. J Burn Care Res 2007;28(6):776–90.

[95] Yoon J, Kym D, Hur J, Kim Y, Yang HT, Yim H, et al. Comparative usefulness of sepsis-3, burn sepsis, and conventional sepsis criteria in patients with major burns. Crit Care Med 2018;46(7):e656–62.

[96] Yan J, Hill WF, Rehou S, Pinto R, Shahrokhi S, Jeschke MG. Sepsis criteria versus clinical diagnosis of sepsis in burn patients: a validation of current sepsis scores. Surgery December 1, 2018;164(6):1241–5.

[97] Walker SAN, Cooper A, Peragine C, Elligsen M, Jeschke MG. Development and validation of a screening tool for early identification of bloodstream infection in acute burn injury patients. Surgery 2021;170(2): 525–31.

[98] Schultz L, Walker SAN, Elligsen M, Walker SE, Simor A, Mubareka S, et al. Identification of predictors of early infection in acute burn patients. Burns 2013;39(7): 1355–66.

[99] Rech MA, Mosier MJ, Zelisko S, Netzer G, Kovacs EJ, Afshar M. Comparison of automated methods versus the American burn association sepsis definition to identify sepsis and sepsis with organ dysfunction/septic shock in burn-injured adults. J Burn Care Res 2017; 38(5):312–8.

[100] Keen A, Knoblock L, Edelman L, Saffle J. Effective limitation of blood culture use in the burn unit. J Burn Care Rehabil 2002;23(3):183–9.

[101] Hill DM, Percy MD, Velamuri SR, Lanfranco J, Romero Legro I, Sinclair SE, et al. Predictors for identifying burn sepsis and performance vs existing criteria. J Burn Care Res 2018;39(6):982–8.

[102] Johnson LS, Shupp JW, Pavlovich AR, Pezzullo JC, Jeng JC, Jordan MH. Hospital length of stay—does 1% TBSA really equal 1 day? J Burn Care Res 2011;32(1).

[103] Taylor SL, Sen S, Greenhalgh DG, Lawless MB, Curri T, Palmieri TL. Not all patients meet the 1 day per percent burn rule: a simple method for predicting hospital length of stay in patients with burn. Burns March 1, 2017;43(2):282–9.

[104] Greenhalgh DG. Sepsis in the burn patient: a different problem than sepsis in the general population. Burn Trauma 2017;5(1):1–10.

[105] Norbury W, Herndon DN, Tanksley J, Jeschke MG, Finnerty CC. Infection in burns. Surg Infect 2016; 17(2):250–5.

[106] Church D, Elsayed S, Reid O, Winston B, Lindsay R. Burn wound infections. Clin Microbiol Rev 2006; 19(2):403—34.

[107] Altoparlak U, Erol S, Akcay MN, Celebi F, Kadanali A. The time-related changes of antimicrobial resistance patterns and predominant bacterial profiles of burn wounds and body flora of burned patients. Burns 2004;30(7):660—4.

[108] Barret JP, Herndon. Effects of burn wound excision on bacterial colonization and invasion. Plast Reconstr Surg February 2003;111(2):744—50.

[109] Hart DW, Wolf SE, Chinkes DL, Beauford RB, Mlcak RP, Heggers JP, et al. Effects of early excision and aggressive enteral feeding on hypermetabolism, catabolism, and sepsis after severe burn. J Trauma 2003;54(4):755—64.

[110] Hart DW, Wolf SE, Chinkes DL, Gore DC, Mlcak RP, Beauford RB, et al. Determinants of skeletal muscle catabolism after severe burn. Ann Surg 2000;232(4): 455—65.

CHAPTER 29

Comprehensive Management of Sepsis in Pediatrics

ELISABETH ESTEBAN • JUAN CARLOS DE CARLOS • JUAN IGNACIO SÁNCHEZ •
JAVIER GIL ANTON

EPIDEMIOLOGY

Sepsis remains the main cause of morbidity and mortality in the pediatric population worldwide. The incidence and prevalence of sepsis have undergone radical changes in recent years. Thanks to medical advances, community-acquired sepsis has been reduced in healthy patients, as it was traditionally caused by microorganisms now covered by international immunization schedules. On the other hand, both the incidence and prevalence have increased in patients with underlying disorders and those with compromised immune systems. In the pediatric population, this higher incidence has been particularly apparent in children under five years of age and is related to gastrointestinal and respiratory infections and infections taking hold during the neonatal period. Its mortality is higher in patients under five, reflected especially in data coming from developing countries. Thus, a prevalence of 6%−8% has been estimated for developed countries, while the rate in countries located in sub-Saharan Africa can reach as high as 23%. Among pediatric patients, a mortality rate of up to 25% in cases of severe sepsis and septic shock has been observed [1−3].

DEFINITION

Pediatric definitions of sepsis are not currently as clearly standardized as those for adults. The latter were updated in 2016 following the Third International Consensus, also known as Sepsis-3 [4].

Prior consensus definitions were based on systemic inflammatory response syndrome (SIRS). In 2005, the Consensus Conference in Barcelona, composed of pediatric experts, unveiled the pediatric definitions, which were adapted to the philosophy of the definitions for adults and were also based on SIRS criteria [5] (Tables 29.1 and 29.2). These definitions are complex, and in some studies, discrepancies with the clinical criteria have been detected.

To date, these have been the most common criteria used to define and classify pediatric patients with sepsis.

In the Surviving Sepsis Campaign that was part of the 2016 Consensus [6], the concept of severe sepsis was eliminated. Sepsis is life-threatening organ dysfunction caused by a dysregulated immune response to an infection. To define this organ dysfunction that sepsis produces, the use of the SOFA score is suggested. As the same time, the use of a simplified score, quick-SOFA, is proposed as the means for the initial clinical detection [4]. However, there are no pediatric recommendations. In the consensus on practical clinical parameters for hemodynamic support in children and newborns with septic shock, published in 2017 [7], septic shock is considered to be when an infection is suspected and there are one or more signs of inadequate tissue perfusion or arterial hypotension.

Lastly, the pediatric Consensus of the Surviving Sepsis Campaign, published in 2020 [8], recognizes that the revision of the pediatric definitions is something that is currently pending. Its recommendations include identifying the condition as sepsis when associated with organ dysfunction and septic shock when associated with cardiovascular dysfunction, following the definitions from 2005. As for the criteria for organ dysfunction, it does not specify what these should be. Among others, the Goldstein (2005) criteria or the SOFA score adapted to pediatrics [9,10], in line with the Sepsis-3 definitions, may be used.

The Sepsis Codex. https://doi.org/10.1016/B978-0-323-88271-2.00019-5

TABLE 29.1

Pediatric Definitions of Sepsis. International Consensus Conference on Pediatric Sepsis (2005) [5]

SEPSIS:

Suspected or confirmed infection and two out of four criteria, of which at least one must be temperature or leukocyte count:

- Central T > 38.5°C or < 36°C.
- Tachycardia >2 SD for the age (Table 29.2).

Not due to other causes (external stimuli, drugs, or pain) or unexplained and persistent >30 min or Bradycardia <10% tile in children <1 year (Table 29.2) not due to other causes (vagal stimulation, beta blockers, congenital cardiopathy) or that is unexplained and persistent >30 min.

- Tachypnea >2 SD (Table 29.2) or need for mechanical ventilation due to an acute process not attributable to other causes like underlying neuromuscular disease or anesthesia.
- Leukocytosis or leukopenia for the age (Table 29.2) (not attributable to other causes like chemotherapy) or >10% immature forms.

SEVERE SEPSIS:

Sepsis with organ dysfunction: Cardiovascular dysfunction or acute respiratory distress syndrome or two or more dysfunctions in the other organs.

Cardiovascular dysfunction:

Despite correct volume expansion with isotonic fluids ($\geq$40 mL/kg in 1 h):
Blood pressure <5% tile for the age or SAP <2 SD below the norm for the age (Table 29.2)
or
Need for vasoactive drugs to maintain BP within a normal range (dopamine >5 µg/kg/min or any dose of adrenaline, noradrenaline, or dobutamine).
or
Two of the following signs or symptoms of tissue hypoperfusion:
− Unexplained metabolic acidosis: base deficit < −5 mEq/L.
− Elevated arterial lactate: >2 times above normal.
− Oliguria: <0.5 mL/kg/h.
− Prolonged capillary refill time: >5 s.
− Central-peripheral temperature difference: >3°C.

Respiratory dysfunction:

PaO_2/FiO_2 <300, without prior cyanotic heart disease or pulmonary disease.
If PaO_2/FiO_2 $\leq$200, with bilateral infiltration, acute onset, and no evidence of heart failure, it would be ARDS.
or
$PaCO_2$ > 65 (or > 20 mmHg over the basal $PaCO_2$)
or
Proven need for O_2 or requirements of >50% of FiO_2 for SpO_2 $\geq$ 92%
or
Need for nonelective invasive or noninvasive mechanical ventilation (if the patient is within the postoperative period, a suspected infection that impedes extubation is required).

Neurological dysfunction:

Glasgow coma scale score $\leq$11 or sudden change with a decrease of $\geq$3 points with respect to a normal basal score.

Hematologic dysfunction:

Platelet count <80,000/mm^3 or 50% decrease from the previous value in past three days (in chronic hematology/oncology patients)
or
International normalized ratio (INR) > 2.

Renal dysfunction:

Serum creatinine $\geq$2 times higher than the limit for the age or double the basal value.

Hepatic dysfunction:

Total bilirubin $\geq$4 mg/dL (not in neonates) or ALT two times higher than the normal limit for their age.

SEPTIC SHOCK:

Sepsis with cardiovascular dysfunction.

TABLE 29.2

Parameters to Define Tachycardia, Bradycardia, Tachypnea, Leukocytosis, and Arterial Hypotension, From the International Consensus Conference on Pediatric Sepsis (2005) [5]

Age	Tachycardia HR >95% tile for Beats per min	Bradycardia HR <5% tile for Beats per min	Tachypnea RR >95% tile for Breaths per min	Leukocytes/mm3 >95%tile or <5% tile	SAP mmHg
<7 days	>180	<100	>50	34,000	<59
7d–1 month	>180	<100	>40	>19,500 or <5000	<69 (79)
1m–1 year	>180	<90	>34	>17,500 or < 5000	<75
2–5 years	>140		>22	>15,500 or <6000	<74
6–12 years	>130		>18	>13,500 or < 4500	<83
13–17 years	<110		>14	>11,000 or < 4500	<90

IDENTIFYING SEPSIS, CLINICAL PRESENTATION, AND COMPLEMENTARY DIAGNOSTIC TESTS

Various tools and systematized screening or early detection packages have been described, which can help detect this condition quickly and with less variability. Although none have proven to be superior, they can be useful to alert physicians and detect sepsis early, so that it may be confirmed based on clinical judgment. A myriad of warning systems based on computerized medical records can also help make this early diagnosis. It is recommended that each center have a rapid detection system in place, in the form of a code or electronic alarm (Table 29.3).

INITIAL CLINICAL ASSESSMENT

The immediate clinical evaluation based on priorities should be initiated by applying the Pediatric Assessment Triangle as a primary survey (appearance, work of breathing, and circulation to the skin). Circulation is fundamentally affected in sepsis, presenting as either compensated shock or decompensated shock (affecting the patient's state of consciousness).

As far as their *appearance*, septic children usually present as exhausted, fussy, hypotonic, confused, irritable, and/or anxious. These changes in appearance can be indicators of reduced cerebral perfusion or a neurological source of infection.

As for *respiration*, tachypnea may be observed; this is the body's way of compensating for metabolic acidosis. Signs of more serious respiratory difficulty may point to a pulmonary source of infection such as pneumonia. In more extreme cases, a reduced level of consciousness can leave the child unable to maintain an open airway.

As regards the *circulation*, we may observe a change in the perfusion, manifesting as paleness, acrocyanosis, or mottled skin. The extremities are usually cold to the touch (except in "warm shock"), and the pulse can be accelerated, bounding, or even weak. Capillary refill time is another consideration and should be measured at the nail bed, placing the extremity at the level of the heart. A measurement under two seconds is considered normal.

This quick initial assessment will allow us to establish priorities for our actions. This should be followed by a systematic evaluation using the ABCDE approach, a more thorough physical examination, and complementary diagnostic tests.

When performing the physical examination, remember that blood pressure in initial phases of shock in children can be normal, thanks to compensatory mechanisms such as tachycardia and increased peripheral resistance. Only in the more advanced phases of shock, arterial hypotension appears. Thus, diagnosing sepsis should be done without waiting for arterial hypotension to appear, basing judgment on the other clinical manifestations. In children and especially in infants, maintaining cardiac output in the initial phases of shock is done by increasing cardiac frequency. Thus, tachycardia is the earliest sign and beats per minute can reach remarkably high readings. By contrast, bradycardia is an especially alarming late sign, as it can indicate impending cardiovascular arrest.

There can be a series of manifestations on the skin as a consequence of hemodynamic stress and

TABLE 29.3

Flowchart for the Clinical Detection of Sepsis in Children. https://secip.com/images/uploads/2020/07/Sepsis.pdf [15]

Suspicion of infection:
Does the patient have a history suggestive of infection?
Clinical presentation typical of source of infection?
Abnormal temperature (>38.5°C or <36°C)?
Do they have risk factors for serious infection?[a]

NO → **RE-EVALUATE**

↓ **YES**

Do they have any other signs that cannot be explained by another cause?
- Persistent tachycardia or bradycardia for their age
- Persistent tachypnea for their age, need for oxygen or assisted ventilation
- Altered state of consciousness: irritability, drowsiness, lethargy, hypotonia
- Presents arterial hypotension[b]
- Presents signs of tissue hypoperfusion: abnormal pulse, capillary refill time, or coloration
- Petechiae or purpura
- Appearance or sensation (of patient, family, or healthcare personnel) of severity

NO → **RE-EVALUATE**

↓ **YES**

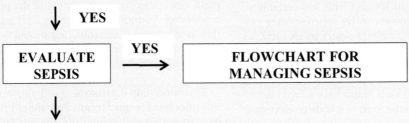

EVALUATE SEPSIS — **YES** → **FLOWCHART FOR MANAGING SEPSIS**

↓

Does the patient show any signs of hypoperfusion or organ dysfunction?
- Arterial hypotension (blood pressure <95%tile for the age) or need for vasoactive drugs to maintain correct pressure[b]
- Signs of tissue hypoperfusion
- Signs of organ dysfunction

↓

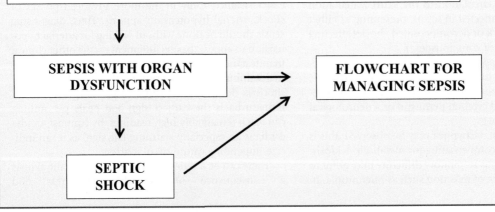

SEPSIS WITH ORGAN DYSFUNCTION → **FLOWCHART FOR MANAGING SEPSIS**

↓

SEPTIC SHOCK

[a]Immunodeficiency, immunosuppression, neoplastic disease, asplenia, organ transplant, invasive device.
[b]Criteria from the International Consensus Conference on Pediatric Sepsis (2005) [5].

compensatory vasoconstriction. This is an early indicator of low cardiac output even when blood pressure is normal.

Other times, during so-called "warm shock," cutaneous vasodilation predominates initially, and we observe hot, vasodilated skin with a flash capillary refill and a bounding pulse.

Another common sign is oliguria, which is secondary to reduced renal perfusion.

The manifestations of septic shock on a neurological level are related to compromised cerebral perfusion. The patient can present initially as anxious, agitated, and/or irritable and later become confused, apathetic, exhausted, and/or fussy. A progressive change in consciousness may appear as confusion and even potentially coma. These can also be manifestations of a neurological source of infection, which should be suspected if the neurological involvement is disproportional to the hemodynamic stress and/or there are meningeal signs, focality, and/or convulsions.

Fever is a sign that is almost always present, although it may not appear in newborns, very young infants, or immunocompromised patients. In stages where shock is established, the presence of thermal instability is common, characterized by a spiking fever and hypothermia.

Manifestations of the causal microorganisms themselves can also be observed. Of these, cutaneous manifestations can be particularly significant. Petechiae and ecchymosis may be observed, and these lesions are highly suggestive of sepsis secondary to *Neisseria meningitidis*. The presence of ecthyma gangrenosum insinuates an infection by *Pseudomonas aeruginosa*, and varicella-like lesions, erythroderma, and/or exanthema can be a sign of streptococcal toxic shock syndrome.

Taking the *personal medical history* should include aspects related to the current clinical status, vaccination, relevant medical background, allergies, previous antibiotic therapy, and colonizations.

ADDITIONAL DIAGNOSTIC TESTS FOR SEPSIS

In a patient with suspected sepsis, we should carry out additional diagnostic tests to help confirm the diagnosis, establish its severity, pinpoint the source of infection, and determine the causal agent. Initially, we should perform (Table 29.4):
- Blood test + blood culture
  - Blood count, C-reactive protein, procalcitonin, acid–base balance, lactate, electrolytes and

TABLE 29.4 Useful Complementary Diagnostic Tests in Children With Sepsis	
Objective	**Diagnostic Tests**
Support the clinical diagnosis of sepsis	Blood count[a] C-reactive protein[a], procalcitonin[a] Other markers of bacterial infection
Evaluate the systemic repercussions, severity, and prognosis	Blood gases[a] Lactate[a] Coagulation[a] Glucose[a] Electrolytes, Ca^{2+a} Urea, creatinine[a] Transaminase, bilirubin[a] Troponin, NT-ProBNP Ultrasound and echocardiogram[a]
Determine the original source of infection[c]	Urine exam[a] CSF exam[b] Imaging studies targeting the (potential) source of infection (e.g., chest X-ray or ultrasound)[a]
Ascertain the etiological agent (microbiological diagnosis)	Blood culture[a] Urine culture[b] CSF culture[b] Other cultures in accordance with the suspected diagnosis[b] Rapid diagnostic techniques (PCR)[b]

[a] Recommended in the initial treatment approach for sepsis.
[b] Based on clinical suspicion.
[c] Useful both when sepsis is suspected and in order to administer a more targeted empirical antibiotic treatment and take specific interventional measures to control the source of infection.

ionized calcium, glucose, blood coagulation test, bilirubin, urea, creatinine, and transaminase.
  - Polymerase chain reaction (PCR) for *N. meningitidis* and *Streptococcus pneumoniae*.
  - In patients who are fitted with a central venous access device, collect both a central and peripheral blood sample. If this is not possible, collect at least two consecutive samples from the catheter. If it is a device with multiple lumens, a sample should be collected from each of them. The minimum total volume should not be less than 1–2 mL in infants and 4–5 mL in children (in accordance with the instructions on the blood culture bottle).
- Lumbar puncture (depending on age and clinical presentation)
  - Determine the best moment to perform this based on the stability of the patient.

- Basic exam, Gram stain, culture, PCR for *N. meningitidis* and *S. pneumoniae*.
- Urinalysis
  - Basic exam, Gram stain, urine culture.
  - Catheterization should be employed in infants and incontinent patients.
- Imaging tests
  - These should be based on the suspected source of infection and the clinical stability of the patient.

Here are some considerations to bear in mind when performing additional diagnostic tests on children:

- In newborns and infants, besides leukocytosis, the presence of leukopenia is also frequently observed. The presence of leukopenia and neutropenia can be signs of a poor prognosis in septic patients.
- Lactate: Elevated lactate level is one of the signs of tissue hypoperfusion and can increase (>2 mmol/L) in severe sepsis. However, lactate is not always high in children with sepsis-induced tissue hypoperfusion.
- Lumbar puncture is contraindicated if the patient is unstable, there are signs of intracranial hypertension, or there is a serious coagulopathy with platelets under $50,000/mm^3$ or a control prothrombin time under 50%.

ETIOLOGY AND TREATMENT WITH ANTIMICROBIALS

The etiology of sepsis/septic shock in pediatrics has changed in recent decades fundamentally due to two factors:

- The immunization of the population against the typical causal agents of community-acquired sepsis, such as *Neisseria meningitidis*, *S. pneumoniae*, and *Haemophilus influenzae* type B, has greatly reduced the prevalence of these pathogens.
- Today, many children with sepsis have at least one chronic disease (complex or noncomplex), have been exposed to healthcare settings, are immunocompromised, or have had or currently have invasive devices. These patients are at considerable risk of colonization and infection by antibiotic-resistant microorganisms, including methicillin-resistant *Staphylococcus aureus*, *Clostridium difficile*, *Pseudomonas* sp., and fungal infections.

Before prescribing an empirical antibiotic treatment, we should understand the prevalence of the different microorganisms in our environment and their antibiotic resistance profile.

Correct treatment with broad-spectrum antibiotics is a fundamental part of effectively treating sepsis and is associated with a lower mortality when coupled with early, quick support with fluids [11]. By contrast, the incorrect use of antibiotics is associated with a greater mortality in adult patients with septic shock [12].

There is currently scarce data to guide the administration of empirical antimicrobial treatment in pediatric sepsis, particularly for previously healthy patients or those with specific chronic diseases. However, the implementation of a protocol based on the risk profile of the chronic illness has been shown to improve empirical antibiotic treatment in children with sepsis [8,13]. We propose a wide-spectrum empirical antibiotic therapy, which will vary in accordance with the age, source of infection, context (community-acquired infection or healthcare-related/nosocomial infection), and the presence of any known immunodeficiency. The first dose should be administered in the first hour after septic shock is detected, ideally after drawing a sample for a blood culture, as long as this does not delay the administration of antibiotics beyond the recommended time frames. In the case of sepsis, the administration of the antibiotic within the first three hours can be considered [8,14]. The empirical treatment should be reevaluated 48 hours after it is initiated. If no pathogen is identified and a bacterial/fungal infection is considered improbable, the empirical antibiotic treatment should be suspended to reduce unnecessary exposure to antibiotics or antifungal agents. However, in many children with a clinical diagnosis of septic shock, no pathogen is isolated. Patients with microbiology results for that are negative for bacteria can have negative blood cultures due to pretreatment with antibiotics, the absence of bacteremia (for example, bacterial pneumonia despite a true bacterial infection), low culture yields, or sepsis related to viral infections. Therefore, the decision to continue, reduce, or suspend antimicrobial therapy should often be taken based on medical judgment and indirect clinical information. This should take into account the clinical presentation, site and type of infection, host risk factors, and clinical improvement and should always be made in accordance with an antibiotic use optimization program. Each center should have an empirical antibiotic therapy guide based on their antibiotic policies and resistance profile (Table 29.5).

CONTROLLING THE SOURCE OF INFECTION

All patients with sepsis/septic shock should be evaluated for the presence of a source of infection that can be eradicated via control methods [14].

An anatomical source of infection should be established as early as possible and quickly diagnosed or excluded, within the first six hours of the onset of this

TABLE 29.5
Proposal for Empirical Antibiotic Therapy Based on Suspicion of Infection

	Community-Acquired Infection	Nosocomial Infection
AGE <1 MONTH		
No shock or meningitis	AMPICILLIN + GENTAMICIN	VANCOMYCIN + AMIKACIN/PIPERACILLIN-TAZOBACTAM
Shock and/or meningitis	AMPICILLIN + CEFOTAXIME	**Meningitis:** CEFTAZIDIME + VANCOMYCIN **Suspicion of GNB:** MEROPENEM + VANCOMYCIN ± AMIKACIN
AGE >1 MONTH		
No shock or meningitis	CEFTRIAXONE	PIPERACILLIN-TAZOBACTAM
Shock and/or meningitis	• CEFOTAXIME + VANCOMYCIN (if meningitis, respiratory/osteoarticular source of infection, or toxic shock syndrome) + CLINDAMYCIN/LINEZOLID (if toxic shock syndrome, necrotizing fasciitis, suspicion of anaerobic causal agent in ORL or respiratory source) • **Abdominal source of infection:** PIPERACILLIN-TAZOBACTAM/MEROPENEM	• **meningitis:** CEFTAZIDIME ± VANCOMYCIN (if central line catheter/CSF device/postoperative period). • **Shock:** MEROPENEM + VANCOMYCIN ± AMIKACIN

disease pattern whenever possible [14], especially in cases of diffuse peritonitis, necrotizing fasciitis, pyomyositis, intestinal ischemia, etc. Once the source has been pinpointed, treatment efforts should be initiated to eradicate the causal pathogen and bring the clinical symptoms under control.

HEMODYNAMIC THERAPY

For hemodynamic therapy, we refer to the protocol for diagnosing and treating septic shock and sepsis associated with organ dysfunction issued by the Spanish Society of Pediatric Intensive Care, published in 2020 [15]. See the quick guide in Table 29.6. This update is based on guidelines from the American College of Critical Care Medicine, published in 2017, which include a series of recommendations that are quite different from previous protocols [7]: (a) initial use of adrenaline administered via peripheral IV or intraosseous access, definitively relegating dopamine, (b) usefulness of intraosseous access using an intraosseous infusion (IO) drill, which also provides a safer way of using vasopressor agents in comparison to a central line, (c) need to establish adequate perfusion pressure with the aim of maintaining organ perfusion,

and (d) monitoring the central venous oxygen saturation (ScvO$_2$) with the aim to keep it above 70%. However, an extremely high ScvO$_2$ can be a sign of mitochondrial dysfunction or the sepsis pattern characterized by vasodilation and high cardiac output. For the remaining treatments, this protocol is based on the recent 2020 Surviving Sepsis guide [8], which we've adapted to the realities of the healthcare setting in the pediatric intensive care unit.

INITIAL RESUSCITATION AND FLUID-REFRACTORY SHOCK (SEE TABLE 29.6)

- Upon clinical suspicion of sepsis, treatment should be initiated without waiting for the results of complementary diagnostic tests or transfer. This initial phase should be completed in 60 minutes.
- Administer high-flow oxygen therapy via reservoir mask, and if needed and available, high-flow nasal oxygen therapy or even continuous positive airway pressure.
- Engage in the ABC sequence for resuscitation: if necessary, initiate cardiopulmonary resuscitation or provide respiratory support by opening the airway, intubating, and ventilating.

TABLE 29.6

Quick Guide: Flowchart for the Hemodynamic Management of Sepsis in Children

Recognize change in the perfusion / state of consciousness
High-flow O2 (reservoir mask, nasal cannulation)
Peripheral IV/Intraosseous (IO) access

If no data suggestive of fluid overload (rales, crepitant crackles, hepatomegaly), administer volume expansion 10-20 mL/kg (max. 60 mL/kg) until perfusion is improved. Discontinue if signs of fluid overload appear
Correct hypoglycemia o hypocalcemia
Administer antibiotic therapy

Fluid-refractory shock

IV/IO adrenaline 0.05-0.3 µg/kg/min
IV/IO/IM atropine/ketamine for central line and intubation, if necessary
If the objective monitoring data indicate warm shock, administer noradrenaline > 0.05 µg/kg/min

Catecholamine-resistant shock

Consider intubation
Normal MAP-CVP for the age, SvO2 >70%
Advanced monitoring: cardiac index (CI) and systemic vascular resistance index (SVRI)
OBJECTIVE : CI= 3.5–5.5 L/min/m^2 SVRI = 80 × (MAP–CVP)/CI= 800–1600 dyne-s/cm^5/m^2

Cold shock with normal BP
ScvO2 < 70% / Hb > 10 g/dL
despite adrenaline

1. Add milrinone

2. If CO < 3.3 / increased systemic resistance: add nitroprusside

3. If no response, consider levosimendan

Cold shock with low BP
ScvO2 < 70% / Hb > 10 g/dL
despite adrenaline

1. Add noradrenaline to normalize diastolic BP

2. If CO < 3.3: add dobutamine, enoximone, levosimendan, or milrinone

Warm shock with low BP
ScvO2 > 70% despite having administered noradrenaline
and optimized blood volume

1. Add vasopressin, terlipressin, or angiotensin

2. If CO < 3.3: add adrenaline, dobutamine, enoximone, or levosimendan

Persistent catecholamine-resistant shock

Rule out and treat pericardial effusion, pneumothorax, and intrabdominal pressure >12 mmHg
Control source of infection

Refractory shock

ECMO

- Monitor the heart rate (HR), respiratory rate (RR), continuous electrocardiogram, pulse oximetry, and blood pressure (BP) (noninvasive).
- In 5–10 min, obtain a peripheral intravenous (IV) access, or intraosseous access using an IO drill (sedation and/or analgesia may be needed) in lieu of this, until a central line can be placed.
- Take a blood sample for analysis: blood culture, blood count, arterial blood gases, electrolytes, ionized calcium, urea, creatinine, transaminase, lactate, and coagulation.
- Volume resuscitation in health systems in which there are pediatric critical care units available: 10–20 mL/kg every 5–10 min, up to 60 mL/kg in the first hour, administered repeatedly while monitoring response until target values are achieved. Consider interrupting the administration of volume if signs of volume overload appear (crepitant crackles, hepatomegaly, etc.). Administering volume should not compete with antibiotic therapy that requires IV access points to be established.
- Volume resuscitation in health systems in which there are no pediatric critical care units available: If the patient does not present with hypotension, administering a bolus infusion is not recommended, as fluid overload may be more harmful than beneficial. If the patient does present with hypotension, being more restrictive when administering volume is advisable. A bolus of 10–20 mL/kg up to 40 mL/kg is recommended, interrupting administration if fluid overload is detected.
- Correct hypocalcemia (10% calcium gluconate, 0.5 mL/kg, max. 10 mL) and hypoglycemia (10% dextrose, 2.5 mL/kg).
- Periodically evaluate the need to intubate based on the state of consciousness, cardiorespiratory situation, and response to treatment. Correct prior hemodynamic resuscitation will reduce the risk of instability during intubation. Before intubating, it is recommended to have initiated volume expansion and the inotropic or vasoactive agent. For intubation, ketamine, atropine and rocuronium may be used.
- Initiate antibiotic therapy as soon as possible after samples are drawn, always within the first hour of clinical suspicion in the case of septic shock and within three hours if there is organ dysfunction without shock. Taking samples should not result in a delay in starting treatment.
- During the initial resuscitation, the achievement of objectives is assessed via basic monitoring parameters: HR, RR, SpO$_2$, BP, and clinical parameters, palpable pulse without a difference between central

and peripheral sites, warm extremities without temperature gradients, and a normal level of consciousness.
- If instability continues despite fluid administration, this is considered fluid-refractory shock and treatment with inotropic agents and/or vasopressors is the recommended course of action. Adrenaline (0.05–0.3 µg/kg/min) would be the initial inotropic agent of choice, this being especially useful in cases of cardiac dysfunction. If shock is accompanied by a pattern of low systemic resistance, it would be better to use noradrenaline (>0.05 µg/kg/min). As merely clinical estimations are unreliable, the use of objective parameters such as analyzing pulse wave, echocardiography, and SvO2 is recommended to establish the pathophysiology of the shock. The use of both vasoactive agents in diluted perfusion via peripheral IV is admissible while waiting for a central line to be placed. However, in our opinion, establishing an intraosseous access would be a better choice.

CATECHOLAMINE-RESISTANT SHOCK

If the aforementioned treatment does not yield the desired results, intensifying monitoring is recommended, adding the following tools to the clinical objectives: SvcO2 >70% and cardiac index (CI) = 3.5–5.5 L/min/m^2. It must be taken into consideration that central venous pressure (CVP) values will be influenced by the possible coexistence of mechanical ventilation and changes in the ventricular compliance; therefore, it is not useful in estimating preload. Blood volume will be assessed using other means (global end-diastolic volume, ultrasound), titrating the effect of fluids and pharmaceuticals on the cardiac output. Systemic vascular resistance index is calculated using blood pressure parameters and cardiac output: SVRI = 80 × (MAP-CVP)/CI. The normal reference range is 800–1600 dyne-s/cm^5/m^2.

Depending on the pattern of systemic resistance and cardiac output, children with septic shock can present with three possible scenarios:
- Pattern 1: Normal BP/low CO/high SVR:
  The inovasodilator of choice to be added to adrenaline is milrinone. Nitroprusside is the second-line treatment, followed by levosimendan if this fails.
- Pattern 2: Low BP/low CO/low SVR:
  Add noradrenaline to the adrenaline. Once blood pressure has been recovered, dobutamine, enoximone, levosimendan, or milrinone may be started in order to raise the CO.
- Pattern 3: Low BP/high CO/low SVR:

If increasing the dose of noradrenaline fails to yield the desired target values, vasopressin, angiotensin, or terlipressin must be used to try and decrease the noradrenaline. The effect of these pharmaceuticals can reduce the CO and make it necessary to introduce inovasodilators: adrenaline, dobutamine, or levosimendan.

Indeed, in this complex situation, the apparently paradoxical combination of vasodilators and vasoconstrictive inotropic pharmaceuticals may be necessary, given the need to simultaneously manage the blood volume, cardiac contractility, and systemic vascular resistance. For this, we need objective monitoring parameters in addition to the clinical evaluation such as ultrasound/transpulmonary thermodilution/NIRS/$ScvO_2$, with the aim of maintaining cardiac output.

PERSISTENT CATECHOLAMINE-RESISTANT SHOCK AND REFRACTORY SHOCK

If despite the above the shock has not been reverted, the presence of complications such as cardiac tamponade, pneumothorax, and abdominal compartment syndrome should be investigated.

Lastly, the use of venoarterial extracorporeal membrane oxygenation (ECMO) should be considered in the case of refractory shock or sepsis-associated respiratory failure that does not respond to other therapies. ECMO can be venovenous in acute respiratory distress syndrome (ARDS) and refractory hypoxemia.

OTHER THERAPEUTIC MEASURES

Corticosteroids: Hydrocortisone is reserved for patients who have not responded to fluids and vasoactive agents. Doses of 100 mg/m^2/day (max. 200 mg/day in adults) may be sufficient.

Glucose: Blood sugar should be monitored in order to avoid hypoglycemia. Limits of 180 mg/dL to initiate insulin perfusion and 140 mg/dL to discontinue it seem reasonable.

Sedation: IV ketamine (1−2 mg/kg), in combination with IV atropine (0.2 mg/kg, max. 1 mg), is recommended for intubation, even in patients with tachycardia. Fentanyl and benzodiazepines in low doses are possible alternatives. Etomidate, propofol, and barbiturates are not recommended. The use of rocuronium facilitates intubation. Midazolam-fentanyl perfusions can be well-suited for maintenance under mechanical ventilation.

Thyroid hormone: The routine use of levothyroxine is not recommended.

Calcium: In patients who require vasoactive support, ionized calcium levels should be maintained.

Antipyretics: Their use to increase patient comfort and reduce metabolic demand is rational.

Hemoderivatives: For stable patients, maintaining Hb > 7 mg/dL is recommended. "Stable" is understood as the patient having a sustained MAP without having increased vasoactive support in two hours. If the patient is unstable, an objective is not established, but we suggest evaluating the contribution of the Hb level to oxygen transport = $CI \times Hb \times 1.39 \times SpO2$, which is especially important in situations such as hypoxemia, myocardial ischemia, or acute hemorrhage.

Prophylactic transfusions of platelets or plasma should not be administered in children who are not bleeding, despite abnormal blood analysis values.

There are no established ranges for performing invasive procedures, but a lower limit of 50,000 platelets seems prudent (guide for adults). In addition, ultrasound-guided catheterization is recommended due to its significantly lower rate of complications.

Mechanical ventilation: Bear in mind the repercussions that positive intrathoracic pressure can have on venous return and CVP. The patient's hemodynamic situation can be affected by intubation, and thus this maneuver should be preceded by volume expansion unless there are data suggestive of right-sided heart failure. As a whole, ventilation will facilitate left heart function and will compromise that of the right.

ARDS: Noninvasive ventilation may be initiated in patients with ARDS who are responding to the initial resuscitation and do not require intubation for other reasons. However, in severe sepsis/shock, noninvasive ventilation should not delay intubation, and the recommended strategies for pediatric ARDS (PALICC) should be used: protective ventilation with low tidal volumes (4−8 mL/kg), optimal positive end-expiratory pressure to obtain correct recruitment, plateau pressure ≤30 cm H_2O, driving pressure <15 cm H_2O, permissive hypercapnia, use of prone position, and neuromuscular blockade if necessary. Nitric oxide is reserved for situations of refractory hypoxemia.

Hemofiltration: Consider early use when there is a positive fluid balance after initial resuscitation that is uncontrolled with restriction and diuretics. High-volume hemofiltration is not recommended.

Nutrition: Early initiation (48 h) of progressive enteral nutrition is the method of choice for patients in whom escalating vasoactive support is not required. Ordering parenteral nutrition should be delayed until the seventh day. Nasogastric tube feeding is prioritized over transpyloric tube feeding if there are no specific indications to do otherwise. Prophylaxis for stress ulcers is not recommended, except in high-risk patients.

Prophylaxis for deep vein thrombosis: Not recommended as a routine practice.

Immunoglobulin: We discourage its routine use and recommend this exclusively for toxic shock syndrome, especially streptococcal toxic shock syndrome, and for patients with a known humoral immunodeficiency or immune-compromised patients with low immunoglobulin levels.

REFERENCES

[1] Rudd KE, Johnson SC, Agesa KM, Shackelford KA, Tsoi D, Kievlan DR, et al. Global , regional , and national sepsis incidence and mortality, 1990–2017: analysis for the global burden of disease study. Lancet 2020;395: 200–11. https://doi.org/10.1016/S0140-6736(19)32989-7. Available from:.

[2] Yébenes JC, Ruiz-Rodriguez JC, Ferrer R, Clèries M, Bosch A. Epidemiology of sepsis in Catalonia: analysis of incidence and outcomes in a European setting. Ann Intensive Care 2017;7(19):1–10.

[3] Weiss SL, Fitzgerald JC, Pappachan J, Wheeler D, Jaramillo-bustamante JC, Salloo A, et al. Global epidemiology of pediatric severe sepsis: the sepsis prevalence , outcomes , and therapies study. Am J Respir Crit Care Med 2015;191(10):1147–57.

[4] Singer M, Deutschman CS, Seymour CW, et al. The third international consensus definitions for sepsis and septic shock (Sepsis-3). JAMA 2016;315:801–10.

[5] Goldstein B, Giroir B, Randolph A, International Consensus Conference on Pediatric Sepsis. International pediatric sepsis consensus conference: definitions for sepsis and organ dysfunction in pediatrics. Pediatr Crit Care Med 2005;6:2–8.

[6] Rhodes A, Evans LE, Alhazzani W, et al. Surviving sepsis campaign: international guidelines for management of sepsis and septic shock: 2016. Intensive Care Med 2017; 43:304–77.

[7] Davis AL, Carcillo JA, Aneja RK, et al. The American College of critical care medicine clinical practice parameters for hemodynamic support of pediatric and neonatal septic shock: executive summary. Pediatr Crit Care Med 2017 2017;18:884–90.

[8] Weiss SL, Peters MJ, Alhazzani W, et al. Surviving sepsis campaign international guidelines for the management of septic shock and sepsis-associated organ dysfunction in children. Pediatr Crit Care Med 2020; 21:e52–106.

[9] Matics TJ, Sanchez-Pinto LN. Adaptation and validation of a pediatric sequential organ failure assessment score and evaluation of the sepsis-3 definitions in critically ill children. JAMA Pediatr 2017;171(10):e172352.

[10] Schlapbach LJ, Straney L, Bellomo R, et al. Prognostic accuracy of age-adapted SOFA, SIRS, PELOD-2, and qSOFA for in-hospital mortality among children with suspected infection admitted to the intensive care unit. Intensive Care Med 2018;44:179–88.

[11] Evans IVR, Phillips GS, Alpern ER, et al. Association between the New York sepsis care mandate and in-hospital mortality for pediatric sepsis. JAMA 2018;320: 358–367 3.

[12] Kumar A, Ellis P, Arabi Y, et al. Cooperative antimicrobial therapy of septic shock database research group: initiation of inappropriate antimicrobial therapy results in a fivefold reduction of survival in human septic shock. Chest 2009;136:1237–48.

[13] Karsies TJ, Sargel CL, Marquardt DJ, et al. An empiric antibiotic protocol using risk stratification improves antibiotic selection and timing in critically ill children. Ann Am Thorac Soc 2014;11:1569–75.

[14] Evans L, Rhodes A, Alhazzani W, Antonelli M, Coopersmith CM, French C. Surviving sepsis campaign: international guidelines for management of sepsis and septic shock. Intensive Care Med 2021. https://doi.org/ 10.1007/s00134-021-06506-y.

[15] Sánchez JI, de Carlos JC, Gil AJ. Protocolo de diagnóstico y tratamiento del shock séptico y de la sepsis asociada a disfunción orgánica [Protocol for the diagnosis and treatment of septic shock and sepsis associated with organ dysfunction]. Sociedad y Fundación Española de Cuidados Intensivos Pediátricos. https://secip.com/images/uploads/2020/07/Sepsis.pdf.

CHAPTER 30

Maternal Sepsis

LUIS ANTONIO GORORDO-DELSOL • GRACIELA MERINOS-SÁNCHEZ •
LUCILA NIEVES-TORRES • JEANETTE ZÚÑIGA ESCORZA

INTRODUCTION

It seems that the conceptual definition of Sepsis-3 [1–3] can be applied almost indistinctly to the obstetric population, so it can be specified that maternal sepsis is a life-threatening condition defined as one or more organ dysfunctions resulting from an infection during pregnancy, childbirth, postabortion, or the postpartum period up to 42 days [4–6]; however, the risk factors, detection routes, and treatment have some peculiarities in this population.

Sepsis is the cause of one out of every five deaths in the world [7]; the World Health Organization estimates 5.2 million annual cases of maternal sepsis worldwide, that is, 11 out of every 1000 live births, which sepsis is the third leading cause of maternal death on the planet [6]; in high-income countries (HICs), it occurs in 0.6 per 1000 live births, while in low-middle income countries (LMICs), it represents 12–15 per 1000 live births; this gap of 20 times more cases of maternal sepsis in LMICs than in HICs suggests that it is a priority issue that can be mitigated with simple and low-cost measures, education for patients and families, health personnel, and access to a reduced list of essential resources, but that discussion is beyond the scope of this chapter [4–6].

PHYSIOLOGICAL CHANGES DURING PREGNANCY AND RISK FACTORS

Maternal sepsis can be the result of obstetric and non-obstetric factors present during pregnancy and/or its care, for example, the performance of diagnostic or therapeutic procedures that facilitate the entry of pathogens, the indication of unnecessary caesarean sections, indiscriminate use of antimicrobials, preexisting pathologies, and/or manifested during pregnancy, which can be exacerbated due to causes of their own or unrelated to pregnancy [8]. The adaptive physiological changes that occur during pregnancy are of particular interest when understanding the predisposition of pregnant women to acquire serious infections and develop sepsis.

Some immunological changes may render the body's defenses incapable of initiating, maintaining, and regulating the inflammatory response to infection [9], which may trigger organ damage to systems already overworked to adaptively compensate for uterine demand.

Cardiopulmonary changes are of particular interest, such as an increase in plasma volume of up to 50% and tachycardia of 10–20 beats per minute over baseline, which generates an increase in normal cardiac output of up to 40%, or changes such as decreased venous return due to the weight of the gravid uterus, decreased systemic vascular resistance, and even changes in coagulation that favor thrombosis. Respiratory changes include tachypnea, increased oxygen consumption of 20%, decreased functional residual capacity up to 25%, and therefore decreased $PaCO_2$, thus decreasing the buffering capacity of the respiratory system [10–12].

DIAGNOSIS

The most common signs and symptoms of maternal sepsis are like those of any infection: fever, chills, asthenia, adynamia, myalgia, arthralgia, tachycardia, tachypnea, etc. [8]; however, these are often underestimated by the patient and her caregivers, since many may have these "general symptoms" such as discomforts, "typical of pregnancy", which generates delays in treating infections and therefore of sepsis. Some other obstetric data that may be related to sepsis are abdominal pain, uterine activity outside the expected period, anemia, uterine atony, obstetric hemorrhage, and vaginal discharge, among others [13].

As in other cases of sepsis, the clinical diagnosis depends, first, on the integration of an infectious syndrome and, second, on its support with laboratory or cabinet studies; however, it must be understood that

The Sepsis Codex. https://doi.org/10.1016/B978-0-323-88271-2.00030-4

TABLE 30.1
Stages of Pregnancy and Reference Values in Range and Average [14]

Stage	Temperature (°C)	Leukocytes (10⁹/L)	Breathing rate (rpm)	PaCO₂ (kPa)	Pulse (Lpm)
First trimester	36.6 a 37.6 (37.1)	3.5 a 12.0 (8.0)	7.5 a 16.5 (12)	27 a 34 (31)	55 a 92.5 (75)
Second trimester	36.6 a 37.3 (36.9)	3.5 a 13.5 (8.5)	10 a 21 (15)	26 a 37 (32)	55 a 95 (75)
Third trimester	35.2 a 38.1 (36.6)	3.5 a 14.0 (9.0)	8 a 24 (16.5)	23 a 36 (30)	60 a 105 (82)
Peripartum	35.8 a 37.5 (36.6)	3.5 a 17.5 (10.5)	8 a 25 (17)	18 a 34 (27)	54 a 107 (80)
Postpartum (48 h)	–	6.5 a 23.0 (14.5)	9.5 a 21.5 (15.5)	24 a 34 (29)	65 a 90 (78)
Postpartum (4 a 12 weeks)	35.9 a 36.8 (36.4)	4.0 a 9.5 (6.5)	7 a 19 (12.5)	31 a 42.5 (36.6)	51 a 85 (68)

pregnant women may have some changes that may even appear differently at each stage (Table 30.1) [14].

Some scales can help identify patients at risk, for example, the Sepsis in Obstetric Score (Table 30.2) greater than six points has an AUC-ROC of 0.92−0.97 to predict admission to the intensive care unit, need for telemetry, positive cultures, and fetal tachycardia, making it a very useful tool even in environments with limited resources [15]. Another widely accepted scale is the modified SOFA for obstetrics (omSOFA) [16], which proposes some simple adjustments to an already known scale, where some "standardized" values are taken into account for the obstetric patient during the third trimester of pregnancy (Table 30.3).

TREATMENT

Fortunately, other chapters of this book have already masterfully addressed the pillars of sepsis treatment, which are applicable, in their foundation and particularities, to maternal sepsis: antimicrobials directed at the site of infection and supported by local epidemiology, microbiological approach efficient, evaluation of the response to volume and fluid therapy, early initiation of vasopressors and inotropes when warranted, surgical resolution of the site of infection, etc. On the other hand, there is not enough evidence to recommend the opposite, since it seems that there are no (nor will there be) controlled clinical trials in pregnant women where these treatments are put on

TABLE 30.2
Sepsis in Obstetric Score [15]

Item	Abnormally high rate				Normal	Abnormally low rate			
Points	+4	+3	+2	+1	0	+1	+2	+3	+4
Temperature (oC)	>40.9	39−40.9		38.5−38.9	36−38.4	34−35.9	32−33.9	30−31.9	<30
Systolic blood pressure (mmHg)					>90		70−90		<70
Hearth rate	>179	150−179	130−149	120−129	<119				
Breathing frequency	>49	35−49		25−35	12−24	10−11	6−9		<5
Leukocytes (mm³)	>39.9		25−39.9	17−24.9	5.7−16.9	3−5.6	1−2.9		<1
Immature cells (%)			>10%		<10%				
Lactate (mmol/L)			>4		<4				

TABLE 30.3
Obstetric Modified SOFA [16]

Item	0	1	2
PaO_2/FiO_2	≥400	300–400	<300
Platelets (mm³)	≥150,000	100,000–150,000	<100,000
Bilirubin (mg/dL)	≤1.17	1.17–1.87	>1.87
Mean arterial pressure (mmHg)	≥70	<70	Need for any vasopressor
State of alert	Alert	Wake up to verbal encouragement	Wake up to nociceptive stimulus
Creatinine (mg/dL)	<1.0	1.0–1.36	>1.36

trial, so we are left with indirect evidence and few observational studies. The controversy will continue to seek the midpoint between a resolution of the pregnancy, the treatment of the infection, and the control of sepsis, in some very obvious cases, in others where a consensus will have to be reached between Obstetrics, Critical Medicine, Neonatology, and more for the greatest benefit of the patient and the product of pregnancy.

PERSPECTIVES

In short, maternal sepsis is a challenge for the multidisciplinary healthcare team, the evolution of its physiological changes during pregnancy, preexisting and acquired diseases can make detection, stratification, and treatment even more complex, so increasing public knowledge and toward health personnel is of great impact for primary prevention and timely care.

REFERENCES

[1] Singer M, Deutschman CS, Seymour CW, Shankar-Hari M, Annane D, Bauer M, et al. The third international consensus definitions for sepsis and septic shock (Sepsis-3). JAMA 2016;315(8):801–10. https://doi.org/10.1001/jama.2016.0287.

[2] Seymour CW, Liu VX, Iwashyma TJ, Brunkhorst FM, Rea TD, Scherag A, et al. Assessment of clinical criteria for sepsis for the third international consensus definition for sepsis and septic shock (Sepsis-3). JAMA 2016;315(8):762–74. https://doi.org/10.1001/jama.2016.0288.

[3] Shankar-Hari M, Phillips GS, Levy M, Seymour CW, Liu VX, Deutschman CS, et al. Developing a new definition an assessing new clinical criteria for septic shock. JAMA 2016;315(8):775–86. https://doi.org/10.1001/jama.2016.0289.

[4] World Health Organization. Statement on maternal sepsis (Internet). Geneva: WHO; 2017 (citado el 1 de marzo de 2022) Disponible en: https://www.paho.org/en/documents/who-statement-maternal-sepsis-2017.

[5] World Health Organization. Global report on the epidemiology and burden of sepsis: current evidence, identifying gaps and future directions (Internet). 1a edición. Geneva: WHO; 2020 (citado el 1 de marzo de 2022) Disponible en:. https://www.who.int/publications/i/item/9789240010789.

[6] de Salud S. Prevención, diagnóstico y tratamiento de la sepsis materna (Internet). Edición; 2018. Ciudad de México: CENETEC; 2018 (consulta: 1 de marzo de 2022) Disponible en, https://cenetec-difusion.com/gpc-sns/.

[7] Rudd KE, Johnson SC, Agesa KM, Shackelford KA, Tsoi B, Rhodes-Kievlan D, et al. Global, regional, and national sepsis incidence and mortality, 1990-2017: analysis for the Global Burden of Disease Study. Lancet 2020; 395(10219):200–11. https://doi.org/10.1016/S0140-6736(19)32989-7.

[8] Nares-Torices MA, Monares-Zepeda E, Hernández-Pacheco JA. Capítulo 24. Sepsis en obstetricia. En Gorordo-Delsol LA. Sepsis: fisiopatología, diagnóstico y tratamiento. 1a edición. Ciudad de México: Intersistemas SA de CV; 2016. p. 319–35.

[9] Abu-Raya B, Michalski C, Sadarangani M, Lavoie PM. Maternal immunological adaptation during normal pregnancy. Front Immunol 2020;11:575197. https://doi.org/10.3389/fimmu.2020.575197.

[10] Chu J, Johnston TA, Geoghegan J. The royal college of obstetricians and gynaecologists. BJOG 2019;127(5): e14–52. https://doi.org/10.1111/1471-0528.15995.

[11] Queensland Clinical Guidelines. Trauma in pregnancy (Internet). Queensland: QCG; 2019 (citado el 1 de marzo de 2022) Disponible en: https://www.health.qld.gov.au/__data/assets/pdf_file/0013/140611/g-trauma.pdf.

[12] Cusick SS, Tibbles CD. Trauma in pregnancy. Emerg Med Clin 2007;25(3):861–72. https://doi.org/10.1016/j.emc.2007.06.010.

[13] Barton JR, Sibai BM. Severe sepsis and septic shock in pregnancy. Obstet Gynecol 2012;120(3):689–706. https://doi.org/10.1097/AOG.0b013e318263a52d.

[14] Bauer MS, Bauer S, Rajala B, MacEachern MP, Polley LS, Childers D, et al. Maternal physiologic parameters in relationship to systemic inflammatory response syndrome criteria: a systematic review and meta-analysis. Obstet Gynecol 2014;124:535—41. https://doi.org/10.1097/AOG.0000000000000423.

[15] Albright CM, Ali TN, Lopes V, Rouse DJ, Anderson BL. The Sepsis in Obstrtric Score: a model to identify risk of morbidity from sepsis in pregnancy. Am J Obstet Gynecol 2014;211(1):39.e1—8. https://doi.org/10.1016/j.ajog.2014.03.010.

[16] Bowyer L, Robinson HL, Barrett H, Crozier TM, Giles M, Idel I, et al. SOMANZ guidelines for the investigation and management sepsis in pregnancy. Aust N Z J Obstet Gynaecol 2017;57(5):540—51. https://doi.org/10.1111/ajo.12646.

CHAPTER 31

Role of Preventive Measures in Sepsis

JORGE E. SINCLAIR AVILA • JORGE E. SINCLAIR DE FRÍAS • LORENZO J. OLIVERO

INTRODUCTION

Sepsis is a clinical syndrome defined as a life-threatening organ dysfunction caused by a dysregulated host response to infection [1] and is a common final pathway of many infectious diseases worldwide. It can lead to tissue damage, organ failure, and death.

Although information on the global epidemiology of sepsis is difficult to find, in 2017, the Global Burden of Disease Study reported an incidence estimated of 48.9 million cases of sepsis worldwide and 11 million sepsis-related deaths, representing 19.7% of all global deaths [2]. This study also report that more than half of all sepsis cases worldwide occurred among children, many of them neonates. Globally, an estimated 84% of neonatal deaths due to infections are preventable [3].

The World Health Organization's (WHO's) first global report on sepsis in 2020 reveals that sepsis frequently results from infections acquired in health-care settings. Almost half (49%) of patients with sepsis in intensive care units (ICUs) acquired the infection in the hospital and an estimate of 27% and 42% of hospitalized and ICU patients, respectively, will die from sepsis [3]. In the same way, mortality rates increase linearly according to sepsis' severity, being $\geq 10\%$ in sepsis and $\geq 40\%$ in septic shock [1,4].

As mentioned, sepsis has a negative impact, increasing the rate of short-term complications and in-hospital mortality; however, it also increases the rate of the long-term complications and general mortality. Over one-third of sepsis survivors die within the first year, 40% are rehospitalized within 90 days of discharge, and one-sixth experience significant morbidity [3].

In 2018, Paoli et al. conducted a six-year retrospective observational database study in which records of more than 65.9 million patients (20% of US population) between various academic and private hospitals were reviewed. They found over 2.5 million of sepsis cases, and the costs obtained from billing records were analyzed. They reported a mean hospital length of stay of 7.7, 10, and 12.6 days, a mean ICU length of stay of 5.1, 6.2, and 7.2 days, and a cost of 16,324, 24,638, and 38,298 USD for sepsis without organ dysfunction, severe sepsis, and septic shock (according to previous definition of sepsis), respectively. Moreover, sepsis represents an estimated total annual cost of $16.7 billion nationally [5].

CHALLENGES

Although public health organizations have been doing enormous efforts to create strategies to recognize and treat infections in their earlier stages, those measures represent a continuous challenge for health organizations.

First, because more than 50%–80% of sepsis cases are from unknown origin, this means that there is not a recognized source of infection [2]. This is important because if there is not an identifiable pathogen, it will be difficult to create specific preventable measures (e.g., vaccine development, improvement of diagnostic test, disease surveillance, etc.)

In addition, the diagnosis of sepsis is challenging for many reasons. Sepsis is a syndrome with no classical findings, sometimes mimicking other conditions. Moreover, there is no definitive diagnostic test; therefore, its diagnosis is based on the latest expert's consensus guidelines and criteria.

Finally, disparities in sepsis incidence and mortality exist among low- and middle-income countries, particularly in sub-Saharan Africa and South-East Asia. The highest sepsis burden is found in locations with scarce resources and limited capacity to prevent, identify, or treat sepsis, accounting for 85% of sepsis cases and sepsis-related deaths worldwide [2].

The Sepsis Codex. https://doi.org/10.1016/B978-0-323-88271-2.00012-2

ETIOLOGY AND RISK FACTORS

The majority of the known etiology of sepsis account for diarrheal illness, lower respiratory tract infections, health-care–related infections, and maternal-fetal diseases including the neonatal period [2]. Antimicrobial resistance is another challenging factor in sepsis outcome as it complicates the ability to treat infections, especially in health-care–associated infections (HCAIs) [2]. Also, the use of implanted devices such a urinary catheter, port-a-cath, central venous catheter, and endotracheal tube is an important cause of sepsis and infections, in general, among hospitalized patients [1].

Others, but not less important are abdominal, skin and soft tissue and genitourinary tract infections [1].

For a better development of preventive strategies, we first need to expose the main risk factors for sepsis. As mentioned, an important factor is ICU admission, as almost 50% of ICU patients have a nosocomial infection [6], therefore, increasing their risk of sepsis. Other important risk factors include extreme ages (<1 year or >75 years) [7], malignancy [8,9], primary comorbidities (diabetes mellitus, cirrhosis, community acquired pneumonia, bacteremia, alcoholism), immunosuppression (neutropenia, corticosteroid treatment), recent antibiotic treatment, and invasive medical devices (e.g., endotracheal tubes, intravenous lines, urinary catheters) [1,10]. Thereby, public policies have various edges to address preventable sepsis and improve the quality of care.

Nonetheless, mortality of sepsis has decreased overall [4,11–14]. In a six-year study from 2004 to 2010, there was a 59% in-hospital mortality reduction, from 21.2% in 2004 to 8.7% in 2010 [15]. Similar results were obtained in a 12-year study of 101,064 ICU patients with sepsis and septic shock in which 50% risk reduction was observed from 35% to 18%. This important reduction was stratified by multiple variables such as comorbidities, underlying disease, severity, age, and the rise in incidence of sepsis over time, suggesting that the mortality reduction may be due to improved management strategies for sepsis.

PREVENTIVE MEASURES

WHO focuses these preventive measures in two main steps:
1. Prevention of microbial transmission and infection
2. Prevention of an infection evolving into sepsis.

Prevention of Microbial Transmission and Infection

Measures that address infection prevention are relatively simple and well known to most health workers; however, the high disparity of socioeconomic status between different nations makes these measures difficult to fulfill in certain contexts. These include hand hygiene, global access to vaccination, outbreak response, food safety, prevention of HCAIs, using personal protective equipment (PPE), management of chronic conditions, and education for patients and families [16].

Standard precautions

We group in this section a set of basic measures used for the care for all patients. These include the practice of hand hygiene, safe injection practices, respiratory hygiene, and the use of appropriate PPE (e.g., gloves, gowns, surgical masks, etc.), especially when there is a risk of exposure to body fluids or other potentially infective material.

Hand hygiene. Health care-acquired infection is one of the most important preventable causes of death and morbidity between hospitalized patients, being hand hygiene the most important measure to prevent it. In all settings, emphasis on handwashing as a primary infection control measure has not been misplaced and should continue. However, despite its simplicity, hand hygiene is still poorly practiced in health-care settings.

WHO shows up some interesting key facts [17]:
- One in four health-care facilities do not have basic water services, resulting in more than 1.8 billion people currently lacking basic water services at their health-care facility, while 712 million have no running water at their health-care facility.
- One in three facilities lack hand hygiene facilities at the point of care.
- Compliance with hand hygiene best practices is only around 9% during care of critically ill patients in low-income countries.
- Levels of hand hygiene compliance for high-income countries rarely exceed 70%, calling for additional efforts to improve practices all over the world.

In health-care facilities, it is recommended to maintain an infection prevention and occupational health program and assure that one individual with training in infection prevention is employed by or regularly available to manage the facility's infection prevention program. In addition, assuring the availability of sufficient and proper supplies to address those programs must be guaranteed.

The Centers for Disease Control and Prevention (CDC) recommends main situations where hand hygiene should be performed:
1. Before and after contact with a patient or objects in their immediate vicinity.
2. Before performing an aseptic task.
3. After contact with blood, body fluids, or contaminated surfaces.

Nevertheless, due to the increasing rate of irritant contact dermatitis resulting from hand hygiene measures [18], situations mentioned above can be done with wither soaps with water or alcohol-based hand rubs, except in situations where hands are visibly dirty in which hand washing with either nonantimicrobial soap or antimicrobial soap with water is necessary. Therefore, the two general options are [19]:

- Antiseptic hand rub: for unsoiled hands (preferred and the most effective method).
- Soap and water: for soiled hands.

Barriers to hand hygiene compliance also exist, for example, work overload and time constraints, poor situational awareness of the instances when hand hygiene should be performed, intolerance or aversion to certain disinfectant formulations, and lack of a safety culture at the workplace [20].

Certain measures have been proposed to improve health-care workers hand hygiene adherence, for example, periodically monitoring the hand hygiene episodes and opportunities within the ward, in which designated hand hygiene observers or electronic hand hygiene systems monitor compliance and provide immediate feedback (e.g., real-time data visualization of each hospital floor's hand hygiene process measures, verbal feedback on improper technique, etc.). In addition, repeating training sessions on hand hygiene frequently increases situational awareness [21].

Other proposed strategies are increasing the number of hand hygiene stations and visual reminders (e.g., posters) and provide them at easily accessible locations, and monitor the volume and quantity of alcohol-based hand rubs [22].

Appropriate hand hygiene prevents up to 50% of avoidable infections acquired during health-care delivery, including those affecting the health work force. The WHO hand hygiene strategy has proved to be highly effective, leading to a significant improvement in key hand hygiene indicators, a reduction in HCAIs and antimicrobial resistance, and substantially helping to stop outbreaks.

Similarly, regular and frequent hand washing at home and public places should be a common and mandatory practice, reducing contagiousness of diseases. This measure itself has been shown to reduce the transmission of many viral diseases [23]. It is important to apply this measure at all times including home, public spaces (e.g., mall, restaurants, etc.), and health-care settings: outpatient/inpatient environment, operation rooms, and ICUs.

Blood-borne infections and safe injection practices. Another common group of preventable infections are caused by blood-borne pathogens that are infectious microorganism in human blood, including but not limited to, hepatitis B virus (HBV), hepatitis C

virus (HCV), and human immunodeficiency virus (HIV). Particularly, these infections can become chronic and decrease the body's ability to respond to others pathogens, for example, immunocompromised state of cirrhosis caused by HBV/HCV caused by HIV itself. This group of disease can occur in a variety of settings, from the use of recreational drugs and unprotected sexual practices to occupational workers exposed to needlesticks or other sharp-related injuries.

Specific measures need to be assured to decrease blood-borne infections outside health-care facility. Creation of public programs enhancing protective factors and reversing or reducing risk factors addressing all forms of drug abuse including legal and illegal drugs in local communities targeting specific population based of demography risk to improve program effectiveness is a reasonable measure to target recreational drug use. These programs must be designed to enhance family bonding, parental monitoring, good social behaviors, and self-control [24]. And in the case of sexual transmitted infections: abstinence, vaccination, reducing the number of sexual partners, mutual monogamy, and use of condoms are the main measures [25].

In health-care setting, planning safe handling and disposal before any procedure is one the measures to reduce the risk of needle accident within health-care workers. Use of gloves and aseptic techniques, single-use disposable syringe, needle alternatives when available, devices with safety features, immediately discard on a sharp container, proper handling containers, and rapid-acting response if an accident occur are the most important strategies to decrease the risk of acquiring an infection from needle accident [26].

Respiratory hygiene. Practices used to control the transmission of respiratory infections (e.g., influenza, COVID-19) include placing a mask on coughing patients, covering the mouth and maintain a distance of 3—6 feet from others when coughing or sneezing, proper dispose of tissues after use, and performing hand hygiene after coughing or sneezing or coming into contact with respiratory secretions [27].

Personal protective equipment. PPE is a group of physical barriers that protects against microorganism, chemicals, and radiation hazards. PPE includes gloves, face shields, respirators, gowns, mask, and others. Evidence has shown that its' use decreases the risk of in-hospital infections. Table 31.1 summarizes some of the main components of PPE.

Health-care—associated infections

HCAIs and nosocomial infection are infections acquired in a hospital or other health-care facility that were not present or incubating at the time of admission. Clinical signs and symptoms typically manifest 48 h or more after admission.

There are certain factors that have been shown to increase the risk of getting a health-care infection [28]:

A. Underlying health status: advanced age, malnutrition, alcoholism, heavy smoking, chronic lung disease, and diabetes.

B. Acute disease process: surgery, trauma, and burns.

C. Invasive procedures: endotracheal or nasal intubation, central venous catheterization, extracorporeal renal support, surgical drains, nasogastric tube, tracheostomy, and urinary catheter.

D. Treatment: blood transfusion, recent antimicrobial therapy, immunosuppressive treatments, stress ulcer prophylaxis, recumbent position, parenteral nutrition, and length of stay.

In 2002, there were 1.7 million HAIs, and 5.8% of those died [29]. The direct economic burden of HAIs in the United States is estimated to be between $28 and $34 billion annually, of which $25 to $32 billion could have been prevented [30].

The most common types of HAIs include central line–associated bloodstream infection (CLABSI), catheter-related urinary tract infection (CAUTI), ventilator-associated pneumonia (VAP), and surgical site infection (SSI). Moreover, an increasing number of HAIs are caused by multidrug-resistant organisms [31].

Intravascular catheter-related infection. Intravascular catheter-related blood stream infection (CRBSI) is a primary bloodstream infection in a patient with an intravascular catheter accessed >48 h prior or within 48 h of catheter removal that can be attributed to the presence of an intravascular catheter.

The most common cause is attributed to CLABSI [19]. Nonetheless, its incidence is decreasing in some areas, possibly as a result of prevention efforts [32,33]. For example, 25,000 fewer CLABSIs occurred in the ICUs of the United States between 2009 and 2001 (59% reduction). It is also estimated that 6000 lives were saved during this period with an estimated financial saving of $414 million USD in potential excess health-care costs [32].

Some recommendations have been proved to decrease CRBSIs. Choosing a catheter with the fewest lumens, with antiseptic or antimicrobial properties, avoiding femoral lines in adults if possible, and performing strict aseptic technique with ultrasound guidance have been shown to decrease rates of CRBSIs [31]. In addition, considering peripherally inserted central catheter has shown to lower the rates of infections compared to CVCs [34], but this measure is still controversial.

Catheter-related urinary tract infection. CAUTI is a symptomatic urinary tract infection occurring in a patient with an indwelling urinary catheter or within 48 h after removal of a urinary catheter. One of the main factors related to CAUTI/bacteriuria is the duration of catheterization. CAUTIs account for up to 40%

Item of PPE	Indications
TABLE 31.1 Personal Protective Equipment [27].	
Gloves	• Contact with blood, body fluids, secretions, excretions, contaminated items, mucous membranes, and nonintact skin.
Gown	• During procedures and patient care activities when contact of clothing/exposed skin with blood/body fluids, secretions, and excretions is anticipated.
Mask, eye protection (goggles), face shield	• When procedures and patient care activities are likely to generate splashes or sprays of blood, body fluids, secretions (e.g., suctioning and endotracheal intubation). • During aerosol-generating procedures on patients with suspected or proven infections transmitted by respiratory aerosols (e.g., severe acute respiratory syndrome), wear a fit-tested N95 or higher respirator in addition to gloves, gown, and face/eye protection.

Note: Adapted from Seigel et al. Am J Infect Control 2007 Dec; 35(10 Suppl 2): S65-164. https://doi.org/10.1016/j.ajic.2007.10.007.

of nosocomial infections, resulting in bacteremia in up to 4% of cases, which has a mortality rate of around 13% [28,34,35].

Some important strategies for addressing CAUTIs are classified in procedural and postprocedural strategies. Procedural strategies include considering whether routine catheterization is necessary or if alternative options could be used instead, clean intermittent catheterization, use of condom catheters, selecting the smallest catheter necessary to provide adequate drainage, and use of sterile technique during insertion.

Postprocedural strategies focus primarily on daily care of the catheter assuring proper function and a clean environment. These include cleaning the genital area with soap and water, ensuring urine flow, and maintaining a sterile closed system. Use of prophylactic antibiotics used to be a common practice around acute-care settings; however, it is not recommended as it has not shown good efficacy and their use can lead to antibiotic resistance [35].

Ventilator-associated pneumonia. VAP is a type of hospital-acquired pneumonia that develops ≥ 48 h after endotracheal intubation. VAP is associated with prolonged length of mechanical ventilation and days of hospitalization [36,37]; the cost associated with VAP has been estimated at up to USD $40,000 per patient [38].

Common risk factors for VAP are older age, malnutrition, chronic renal failure, anemia, and chronic lung disease, among others [39,40]. Reintubation or prolonged intubation, mechanical ventilation for acute respiratory distress syndrome, frequent ventilator circuit changes, use of muscle relaxants, and the presence of an intracranial pressure monitor are other important factors related to VAP [41–43].

Strategies to prevent VAP include the use of alternative options such as noninvasive positive-pressure ventilation and oral rather than nasal intubation, which prevents contamination with sinus pathogens. In addition, using the lower sedation possible, considering also daily breaks of sedation, early mobilization, minimizing secretion pooling, maintain ventilation circuits, and oral care with sterile water are also important strategies while taking care of intubated patients [31,44].

Surgical site infection. SSI is defined as an infection arising within 30 days of a surgical procedure at the site of the surgical incision. It represents around 20% of all HCAI [45]. Its incidence is around 5% of all surgical wounds. The annual cost of SSI is extremely high

in the United States, estimated from $3.5 to $10 billion annually [45]. As other HAIs, SSIs are related not only with an increased length of stay but also to emergency department visits and readmissions [45].

Several number of risk factors are involved in the development of SSI, from modifiable (underlying health state, lifestyle behaviors, glycemic control, etc.) and nonmodifiable (sex, age) to procedural and postprocedural-related factors, such surgical attire, hand scrubbing, wound classification, the duration and complexity of the surgical procedure, and the surgical technique (e.g., open vs. laparoscopic) as the most important. In addition, the WHO reports that antimicrobial resistance is also a significant factor in the development of an SSI [46].

Strategies involved in SSI prevention prior the surgery are use of alcohol-based surgical skin preparation, treating all infections, advising patients to bath or shower the night before surgery, promote smoking cessation, and the use of prophylactic antibiotics when indicated. During the procedure, it is recommended to maintain normothermia, blood glucose levels <200 mg/dL, and for patients with normal pulmonary function undergoing general anesthesia with endotracheal intubation, it is recommended to administer increased FIO_2 during surgery and after extubation in the immediate postoperative period [47]. Inspect dressings regularly and change when needed, avoid the use of antimicrobial agents to the incision, and minimize blood loss to avoid the need for transfusion are the most important measures after surgery [45,47].

Vaccination

Vaccination is one of the public health measures that has the greatest impact on reduction of the burden from infectious diseases and associated mortality, especially in children.

Childhood vaccination coverage is generally high; there are around 15 different preventable diseases and essentially determine the first pediatrician visits early in life. Human papillomavirus and meningococcal vaccinations are recommended for adolescents. Adulthood immunizations include diphtheria, pertussis, and tetanus boosters, and vaccines to prevent influenza, pneumococcal pneumonia, and hepatitis A and B. There are also special schedules for immunocompromised patients as well as for travelers. COVID-19 vaccination is the newest vaccine and is recommended for children, adolescents, and adults.

Comprehensive vaccination programs were developed and became the cornerstone of good public health intervention, improving primary care strategies in developing countries, decreasing mortality in childhood, and improving quality of life.

It is estimated that vaccines prevent up to three million deaths each year worldwide [48]. Since its development, the primary focus of vaccination programs has been childhood vaccination; however, recently there have been promising developments in adult vaccination, with a growing emphasis on pregnant women and the elderly.

Vaccines have important health, social, and economic benefits, helping economic growth everywhere by lowering morbidity and mortality. The annual return on investment in vaccination has been calculated to be between 12% and 18% [49].

Food safety and water sanitization

Infectious diarrheal disease is the leading cause of sepsis and the second cause of sepsis-related deaths since 1990 [2]. Infectious diarrhea is caused by bacteria, virus, and parasites. According to the CDC, an estimated one in every six people in the United States is affected by a foodborne illness annually. Risk factors include the cross-contamination of food and improper handling and storage. CDC recommends four steps for food safety:

1. Clean: Washing your hands and work surfaces before, during, and after preparing food.
2. Separate: Separating raw meat, poultry, seafood, and eggs from ready-to-eat foods to prevent cross-contamination.
3. Cook: Cooking food to the right internal temperature to kill harmful bacteria.
4. Chill: Store food at a proper temperature to prevent bacteria multiplication.

Prevention of the evolution of sepsis

As mentioned, certain population of patients are particularly at high risk of developing sepsis. Patients with age corresponding to early childhood and elderly adults are the most affected. In 2017, the WHO global sepsis report found that 41.5% (20.3 million) of incident sepsis cases and 26.4% (2.9 million) deaths related to sepsis worldwide were among children younger than five years. Among elderly patients, the incidence of sepsis increases disproportionately for patients with age >65 years; actually, age has proven to be an independent predictor of mortality in sepsis [1]. Obesity, diabetes, cancer, and other immunosuppressed patients are also population at risk [9,50].

CONCLUSIONS

Prevention of sepsis has an enormous implication in public health policies and government expenditure, as well as improving health-care quality and standard of care. We have seen how incidence of sepsis has been decreasing in the last decade with the implementation, improvement, and constant updating of the prevention measures carried out by multiple health entities worldwide. We need to continue in this same pathway by adapting new strategies to reduce the burden of sepsis, especially in underdeveloped countries.

REFERENCES

[1] Singer M, Deutschman CS, Seymour CW, Shankar-Hari M, Annane D, Bauer M, et al. The third international consensus definitions for sepsis and septic shock (Sepsis-3). JAMA [Internet] February 23, 2016;315(8):801–10. Available from, https://pubmed.ncbi.nlm.nih.gov/26903338.

[2] Rudd KE, Johnson SC, Agesa KM, Shackelford KA, Tsoi D, Kievlan DR, et al. Global, regional, and national sepsis incidence and mortality, 1990–2017: analysis for the Global Burden of Disease Study. Lancet [Internet]. January 18, 2020 [cited 2022 Apr 14];395(10219):200–211. Available from: https://www.thelancet.com/journals/lancet/article/PIIS0140-6736(19)32989-7/fulltext#.Ylh2TxAAn-U.mendeley.

[3] WHO. Global report on the epidemiology and burden of sepsis [Internet]. 2020 [cited 2022 Apr 20]. Available from https://apps.who.int/iris/bitstream/handle/10665/334216/9789240010789-eng.pdf.

[4] Kaukonen K-M, Bailey M, Pilcher D, Cooper DJ, Bellomo R. Systemic inflammatory response syndrome criteria in defining severe sepsis. N Engl J Med [Internet] March 17, 2015;372(17):1629–38. https://doi.org/10.1056/NEJMoa1415326. Available from.

[5] Angus DC, Linde-Zwirble WT, Lidicker J, Clermont G, Carcillo J, Pinsky MR. Epidemiology of severe sepsis in the United States: analysis of incidence, outcome, and associated costs of care. Crit Care Med [Internet] 2001;29(7). Available from, https://journals.lww.com/ccmjournal/Fulltext/2001/07000/Epidemiology_of_severe_sepsis_in_the_United.2.aspx.

[6] Zaragoza R, Ramírez P, López-Pueyo MJ. Infección nosocomial en las unidades de cuidados intensivos. Enferm Infecc Microbiol Clín [Internet] 2014;32(5):320–7. Available from, https://www.sciencedirect.com/science/article/pii/S0213005X14000597.

[7] Martin GS, Mannino DM, Moss M. The effect of age on the development and outcome of adult sepsis*. Crit Care Med [Internet] 2006;34(1). Available from, https://journals.lww.com/ccmjournal/Fulltext/2006/010

00/The_effect_of_age_on_the_development_and_outco me.3.aspx.

[8] Torres VB, Azevedo LC, Silva UV, Caruso P, Torelly AP, Silva E, et al. Sepsis-associated outcomes in critically ill patients with malignancies. Ann Am Thorac Soc [Internet] June 18, 2015 [cited 2022 Apr 20];150618124156002. Available from, http://www.atsjournals.org/doi/10. 1513/AnnalsATS.201501-046OC.

[9] Williams MD, Braun LA, Cooper LM, Johnston J, Weiss RV, Qualy RL, et al. Hospitalized cancer patients with severe sepsis: analysis of incidence, mortality, and associated costs of care. Crit Care [Internet] 2004;8(5): R291. https://doi.org/10.1186/cc2893. Available from.

[10] Gauer RL. Early recognition and management of sepsis in adults: the first six hours. Am Fam Physician 2013;1(88): 44–53.

[11] Meyer N, Harhay MO, Small DS, Prescott HC, Bowles KH, Gaieski DF, et al. Temporal trends in incidence, sepsis-related mortality, and hospital-based acute care after sepsis. Crit Care Med [Internet] 2018;46(3). Available from, https://journals.lww.com/ccmjournal/Fulltext/201 8/03000/Temporal_Trends_in_Incidence,_Sepsis_Relat ed.2.aspx.

[12] Lagu T, Rothberg MB, Shieh M-S, Pekow PS, Steingrub JS, Lindenauer PK. Hospitalizations, costs, and outcomes of severe sepsis in the United States 2003 to 2007. Crit Care Med [Internet] 2012;40(3). Available from, https:// journals.lww.com/ccmjournal/Fulltext/2012/03000/Hos pitalizations,_costs,_and_outcomes_of_severe.7.aspx.

[13] Dombrovskiy VY, Martin AA, Sunderram J, Paz HL. Rapid increase in hospitalization and mortality rates for severe sepsis in the United States: a trend analysis from 1993 to 2003*. Crit Care Med [Internet] 2007;35(5). Available from, https://journals.lww.com/ccmjournal/Fulltext/20 07/05000/Rapid_increase_in_hospitalization_and_mor tality.4.aspx.

[14] Martin GS, Mannino DM, Eaton S, Moss M. The epidemiology of sepsis in the United States from 1979 through 2000. N Engl J Med [Internet] April 17, 2003;348(16): 1546–54. https://doi.org/10.1056/NEJMoa022139. Available from.

[15] Miller RR, Dong L, Nelson NC, Brown SM, Kuttler KG, Probst DR, et al. Multicenter implementation of a severe sepsis and septic shock treatment bundle. Am J Respir Crit Care Med [Internet]. July 1, 2013 [cited 2022 Apr 20]; 188(1):77–82. Available from: http://www.atsjournals. org/doi/abs/10.1164/rccm.201212-2199OC.

[16] WHO. Sepsis [Internet]. 2020 [cited 2022 Apr 20]. Available from https://www.who.int/news-room/fact-sheets/ detail/sepsis.

[17] WHO. World hand hygiene day [Internet]. Key facts and figures. 2021 [cited 2022 Apr 20]. Available from https://www.who.int/campaigns/world-hand-hygiene-day/2021/key-facts-and-figures.

[18] Larson E, Girard R, Pessoa-Silva CL, Boyce J, Donaldson L, Pittet D. Skin reactions related to hand hygiene and

selection of hand hygiene products. Am J Infect Control [Internet] December 1, 2006;34(10):627–35. https:// doi.org/10.1016/j.ajic.2006.05.289. Available from.

[19] Mermel LA, Allon M, Bouza E, Craven DE, Flynn P, O'Grady NP, et al. Clinical practice guidelines for the diagnosis and management of intravascular catheter-related infection: 2009 update by the Infectious Diseases Society of America. Clin Infect Dis [Internet] July 1, 2009; 49(1):1–45. https://doi.org/10.1086/599376. Available from.

[20] Pittet D, Hugonnet S, Harbarth S, Mourouga P, Sauvan V, Touveneau S, et al. Effectiveness of a hospital-wide programme to improve compliance with hand hygiene. Lancet [Internet] October 14, 2000;356(9238):1307–12. https://doi.org/10.1016/S0140-6736(00)02814-2. Available from.

[21] Alexandre R. Marra, MD and Michael B. Edmond, MD, MPH M. Innovations in promoting hand hygiene compliance [Internet]. The PSNet Collection. 2014 [cited 2022 Apr 22]. Available from: https://psnet.ahrq.gov/ perspective/innovations-promoting-hand-hygiene-comp liance.

[22] Larson E. A causal link between handwashing and risk of infection? Examination of the evidence. Infect Control January 1988;9(1):28–36.

[23] Wong VWY, Cowling BJ, Aiello AE. Hand hygiene and risk of influenza virus infections in the community: a systematic review and meta-analysis. Epidemiol Infect [Internet]. May 23, 2014 [cited 2022 Apr 15];142(5):922–932. Available from: https://www.cambridge.org/core/ product/identifier/S095026881400003X/type/journal_ article.

[24] National Institute on Drug Abuse. NIDA. Prevention principles. [Internet]. 2020 [cited 2022 Apr 20]. Available from https://nida.nih.gov/publications/preventing-drug-use-among-children-adolescents/prevention-principles.

[25] CDC. The centers for disease control and prevention. Sexually transmitted diseases (STDs): prevention [Internet]. [cited April 20, 2022]. Available from: https://www.cdc.gov/std/prevention.

[26] Occupational Safety and Health Administration (OSHA). United States Department of Labor. Bloodborne pathogens and needlestick prevention [Internet]. [cited April 20, 2022]. Available from https://www.osha.gov/ bloodborne-pathogens.

[27] Siegel JD, Rhinehart E, Jackson M, Chiarello L, Committee HCICPA. 2007 guideline for isolation precautions: preventing transmission of infectious agents in health care settings. Am J Infect Control [Internet] December 2007;35(10 Suppl. 2):S65–164. Available from, https:// pubmed.ncbi.nlm.nih.gov/18068815.

[28] Inweregbu K, Dave J, Pittard A. Nosocomial infections. Cont Educ Anaesth Crit Care Pain [Internet] February 1, 2005;5(1):14–7. https://doi.org/10.1093/bjaceaccp/mki 006. Available from.

[29] Klevens RM, Edwards JR, Richards CLJ, Horan TC, Gaynes RP, Pollock DA, et al. Estimating health care-associated infections and deaths in U.S. hospitals, 2002. Public Health Rep 2007;122(2):160−6.

[30] Scott RD. The direct medical costs of healthcare-associated infections in U.S. hospitals and the benefits of prevention. In: Division of Healthcare Quality Promotion National Center for Preparedness, Detection, and Control of Infectious Diseases Coordinat [Internet]. [cited April 20, 2022]. Available from https://www.cdc.gov/HAI/pdfs/hai/scott_costpaper.pdf.

[31] Yokoe DS, Anderson DJ, Berenholtz SM, Calfee DP, Dubberke ER, Ellingson KD, et al. A compendium of strategies to prevent healthcare-associated infections in acute care hospitals: 2014 updates. Infect Control Hosp Epidemiol [Internet] August 2014;35(8):967−77. Available from, https://pubmed.ncbi.nlm.nih.gov/25026611.

[32] Centers for Disease Control and Prevention (CDC). Central line-associated blood stream infections−United States 2001, 2008, and 2009. Vital Signs [Internet] 2011;60(8):243. Available from, https://www.cdc.gov/mmwr/preview/mmwrhtml/mm6008a4.htm.

[33] Centers for Disease Control and Prevention (CDC). Bloodstream infection event (central line-associated bloodstream infection and non-central line associated bloodstream infection) [Internet]. National Healthcare Safety Network. 2022 [cited 2022 Apr 20]. p. 48. Available from https://www.cdc.gov/nhsn/pdfs/pscmanual/4psc_clabscurrent.pdf.

[34] Maki DG, Kluger DM, Crnich CJ. The risk of bloodstream infection in adults with different intravascular devices: a systematic review of 200 Published Prospective Studies. Mayo Clin Proc [Internet] September 1, 2006;81(9):1159−71. https://doi.org/10.4065/81.9.1159. Available from.

[35] Hooton TM, Bradley SF, Cardenas DD, Colgan R, Geerlings SE, Rice JC, et al. Diagnosis, prevention, and treatment of catheter-associated urinary tract infection in adults: 2009 international clinical practice guidelines from the Infectious Diseases Society of America. Clin Infect Dis [Internet] March 1, 2010;50(5):625−63. https://doi.org/10.1086/650482. Available from.

[36] Kalil AC, Metersky ML, Klompas M, Muscedere J, Sweeney DA, Palmer LB, et al. Management of adults with hospital-acquired and ventilator-associated pneumonia: 2016 clinical practice guidelines by the Infectious Diseases Society of America and the American Thoracic Society. Clin Infect Dis [Internet] September 1, 2016; 63(5):e61−111. https://doi.org/10.1093/cid/ciw353. Available from.

[37] Muscedere JG, Day A. Heyland1 DK. Mortality, attributable mortality, and clinical events as end points for clinical trials of ventilator-associated pneumonia and hospital-acquired pneumonia. Clin Infect Dis [Internet] August 1, 2010;51(Supplement_1):S120−5. https://doi.org/10.1086/653060. Available from.

[38] Kollef MH, Hamilton CW, Ernst FR. Economic impact of ventilator-associated pneumonia in a large matched cohort. Infect Control Hosp Epidemiol [Internet] 2012; 33(3):250−6. Available from, https://www.cambridge.org/core/article/economic-impact-of-ventilatorassociated-pneumonia-in-a-large-matched-cohort/96D7E72FB75A086924708F1807270BB7.

[39] Tejerina E, Frutos-Vivar F, Restrepo MI, Anzueto A, Abroug F, Palizas F, et al. Incidence, risk factors, and outcome of ventilator-associated pneumonia. J Crit Care [Internet] 2006;21(1):56−65. Available from, https://www.sciencedirect.com/science/article/pii/S0883944105001942.

[40] Sopena N, Heras E, Casas I, Bechini J, Guasch I, Pedro-Botet ML, et al. Risk factors for hospital-acquired pneumonia outside the intensive care unit: a case-control study. Am J Infect Control [Internet] January 1, 2014; 42(1):38−42. https://doi.org/10.1016/j.ajic.2013.06.021. Available from.

[41] Torres A, Gatell JM, Aznar E, el-Ebiary M, Puig de la Bellacasa J, González J, et al. Re-intubation increases the risk of nosocomial pneumonia in patients needing mechanical ventilation. Am J Respir Crit Care Med [Internet]. July 20, 1995 [cited 2022 Apr 29];152(1):137−141. Available from http://www.ncbi.nlm.nih.gov/pubmed/7599812.

[42] Ranjan N, Chaudhary U, Chaudhry D, Ranjan KP. Ventilator-associated pneumonia in a tertiary care intensive care unit: analysis of incidence, risk factors and mortality. Indian J Crit Care Med [Internet] April 2014; 18(4):200−4. Available from, https://pubmed.ncbi.nlm.nih.gov/24872648.

[43] Kollef MH, Shapiro SD, Von Harz B, Prentice D, John St R, Silver P, et al. Patient transport from intensive care increases the risk of developing ventilator-associated pneumonia. Chest [Internet] September 1, 1997;112(3):765−73. https://doi.org/10.1378/chest.112.3.765. Available from.

[44] Centers for Disease Control and Prevention (CDC). Patient safety component manual [Internet]. National Healthcare Safety Network (NHSN). 2022 [cited 2022 Apr 20]. Available from: https://www.cdc.gov/nhsn/pdfs/pscmanual/pcsmanual_current.pdf.

[45] Anderson DJ, Podgorny K, Berríos-Torres SI, Bratzler DW, Dellinger EP, Greene L, et al. Strategies to prevent surgical site infections in acute care hospitals: 2014 update. Infect Control Hosp Epidemiol [Internet] 2014;35(6):605−27. Available from, https://www.cambridge.org/core/article/strategies-to-prevent-surgical-site-infections-in-acute-care-hospitals-2014-update/B2BF77B215DED9C1C2B87BAAC7817ECF.

[46] World Health Organization. WHO. Important issues in the approach to surgical site infection prevention. Global guidelines for the prevention of surgical site infection; 2016.

[47] Berríos-Torres SI, Umscheid CA, Bratzler DW, Leas B, Stone EC, Kelz RR, et al. Centers for disease control and prevention guideline for the prevention of surgical site

infection. JAMA Surg [Internet] August 1, 2017;152(8): 784–91. https://doi.org/10.1001/jamasurg.2017.0904. Available from.

[48] Rémy V, Zöllner Y, Heckmann U. Vaccination: the cornerstone of an efficient healthcare system. J Mark Access Heal policy [Internet] August 12, 2015;3. https://doi.org/10.3402/jmahp.v3.27041. Available from, https://pubmed.ncbi.nlm.nih.gov/27123189.

[49] Andre FE, Booy R, Bock HL, Clemens J, Datta SK, John TJ, et al. Vaccination greatly reduces disease, disability, death and inequity worldwide. Bull World Health Organ [Internet] February 2008;86(2):140–6. Available from, https://pubmed.ncbi.nlm.nih.gov/18297169.

[50] Falagas ME, Kompoti M. Obesity and infection. Lancet Infect Dis [Internet] July 1, 2006;6(7):438–46. https://doi.org/10.1016/S1473-3099(06)70523-0. Available from.

CHAPTER 32

Value of the Protocolization and Sepsis Performance Improvement Program in Early Identification

CARLOS SANCHEZ

INTRODUCTION

We often hear that the best medicine is the one that prevents; however, sometimes prevention gets out of hand and the next level that we have to work on is the early identification of diseases, mainly in those conditions where timely intervention makes the difference between life and death, where "time is money", such is the case of sepsis. This principle of early identification deserves a coordination that involves several factors, such as community awareness and education, hospital environment and culture, interdisciplinary and multiprofessional management, evidence-based management structure, development, and implementation of protocols, data collection, verification of indicators. quality, feedback from the patient, family, and health personnel, among many other factors [1].

The spotlight on quality and safety in health care is well recognized. Through decreasing clinical variation in patient management, increasing adherence to evidence-based guidelines, monitoring processes, and measuring outcomes, clinicians can improve the quality of care in the intensive care unit (ICU) [2]. Process improvement has been defined as the actual improvement of a process by focusing on efficiency as well as effectiveness.

The basic components include assessing performance, providing feedback, conducting evaluations, and making process improvement changes. The work of Donabedian [3–5] introduced a model for assessing the quality of medical practice, including structure, process, and outcome parameters. Juran [6], who originally coined the term total quality management, and Deming (see https://www.deming.org/), who outlined concepts of continuous quality improvement, have contributed to the emphasis on quality improvement within performance improvement activities.

It is important to bear in mind that in order to improve the results in patients with sepsis in our hospitals and community, the first thing we must do is characterize the problem. A study must be carried out that allows us to know how sepsis is affecting us and to verify each step of the process that goes from the attention in the triage to the follow-up of the patient to the discharge.

The identification of patients with possible sepsis is critically important because real-time recognition and evidence-based interventions substantially improve survival. No point-of-care tests are currently available to accurately predict patients with, or those likely to imminently develop, sepsis; currently, however, nurses at the bedside must rely on clinical judgment, potentially augmented by patient matrix, in order to target sepsis among their patients with infection.

UNIFORMITY AND PROTOCOLIZATION

One of the most important problems we face worldwide in the diagnosis of sepsis is the lack of uniformity of criteria, although it is true that in 2016, the third international consensus for the diagnosis of sepsis was published [7]; not all health personnel know these criteria. On the other hand, there are those who use outdated, nonspecific, and even not validated criteria; of course, this leads to problems in the triage of patients, to diagnostic difficulties in the emergency department, ICU, and regular hospitalization rooms. This variability in the criteria used leads not only to diagnostic errors but also makes data collection less reliable.

Understanding that sepsis is a dysregulated response of the host to an infection and that it leads to failure of organs with compromise for life [7], our alert systems must be focused on determining these failures as soon

The Sepsis Codex. https://doi.org/10.1016/B978-0-323-88271-2.00017-1

as possible, including identifying patients that could develop organic failures before they occur; this can be worked from the clinical diagnosis, laboratory and artificial intelligence. In this context, it is very important to use protocols for the diagnosis of sepsis, and it is necessary that we all "speak the same language"," thus reducing the possibility of making mistakes. Hospitals continue to link reimbursement to sepsis quality matrix, and many healthcare organizations have leveraged clinicians to address methods that may improve outcomes. To improve compliance with the use of the sepsis bundles, many interventions have been suggested to aid clinicians and providers. However, currently there is no one intervention that has been identified to improve overall bundle compliance [8].

The preparation and protocolization is not something that should be established only for the first moments in the care of patients with suspected sepsis, but rather, the creation and activation of strategies aimed at facilitating the diagnosis of sepsis, as well as its identification of focus, germ, and initiation of the correct timely treatment are necessary to optimize results. The establishment of the sepsis code allows us to facilitate and work in a more organized way in the diagnosis of the patient with sepsis, and this leads us to the need to have rapid response teams in the identification and management of these critically ill patients; of course, this team directly and actively involves the nursing staff.

EARLY WARNING DIGITAL SYSTEMS AND ARTIFICIAL INTELLIGENCE

Early warning digital systems and artificial intelligence are tools that are used more and more by hospitals every day; this type of software provides us with many advantages in the early diagnosis of sepsis, since it can not only predict sepsis in a large part of patients but also allows us a more accurate diagnosis in those patients who have unusual or atypical symptoms and signs. With the publication in 2019 on the phenotypes of sepsis [9], artificial intelligence has helped us to identify patterns of organic failures that make us "buy time" by getting ahead in hours and sometimes even days before the failure of the organs. Electronic reminders may promote positive social change because earlier recognition of sepsis by nurses may lead to a reduction of healthcare costs through improved management of sepsis patients in acute care settings [10].

A systematic review of the 16 articles reviewed (see Appendix A) highlights that electronic sepsis screening tools and alerts are used in various ways, some that trigger the bedside nurse to contact a physician for further instruction and others that trigger notification

of a specialty trained team. In a study by [11], the electronic sepsis alert and provider notification preceded ICU transfer by a median of four hours. In a randomized controlled trial where the charge nurse was notified via a paging system and subsequently expected to contact the provider for orders, 70% of patients in the intervention group had received greater than one intervention, or bundle element, compared to the control group ($P = 0.018$) [12].

In two studies, a sepsis team was activated based on a positive sepsis screen. In one study, the physician was expected to validate the sepsis alert before activating a sepsis team [13] compared to automated overhead activation based on electronic screening [14]. Sepsis bundle compliance was significantly higher ($P < 0.01$) in the postintervention group in each of the three studies where a specially trained team was activated based on an automated sepsis alert [13–15]. There was also a notable decline in discharge to hospice, with an increase in survival at discharge and discharge to home [13–15]. One study showed a sevenfold reduction in mortality postimplementation of a code sepsis team [14].

Two studies assessed nurse-initiated protocols (NIPs) in early identification and treatment of sepsis. Bruce et al. [16] found that upon a positive sepsis screen, the bedside nurse was to contact the provider for validation to use NIPs. Bruce et al. [16] found no significant differences in morality, fluid administration, or hospital length of stay.

Comparatively, a study by Gatewood et al. [17] demonstrated that allowing the nurse to automatically initiate sepsis specific order sets that included diagnostic studies, as well as to administer the first liter of fluid resuscitation prior to contacting the physician resulted in a 154% improvement in sepsis bundle compliance and a prepost intervention mortality reduction from 13.3% to 11.1%.

Standardized order sets are interventions that have been studied for use in guiding early identification and management of sepsis. In three of four studies, if the provider acknowledged that sepsis was present, the electronic health record (EHR) opened a sepsis management tool offering evidence-based orders (Hooper et al. Semlar et al., Kurczewski et al.). In a study by Hooper et al. [18], sepsis assessments were performed by providers after an automated text alert was triggered by the EHR in 185 of 220 of cases. Hooper et al. [18] found that the sepsis management tool was opened in less than 60% of cases in the study by Semlar et al. [12] and orders placed via the tool less than 30% of the time.

The results of this systematic review suggest that evidence-based sepsis care implemented within the recommended timeline based on early identification through electronic triggers will improve patient outcomes, and that a specially trained team should be considered to improve sepsis bundle compliance. Results also support that bundled care driven only by physician orders often include missed components. Findings support the use of multiple tools and a collaborative approach to bundled sepsis care [8].

HIGH-FIDELITY SIMULATION

High-fidelity simulation is another strategy to implement and improve the diagnosis of sepsis; to date, medical simulation has been popular, especially in anesthesiology, medical emergency, and critical care fields [19,20]. There are many courses using simulation such as in patient safety [21] and practice of skills in emergency conditions [22,23]. It has many benefits for students that include meeting a real experience, no harm to patients, and it is a student-centered learning style [19]. Teaching hospitals are exposed to additional risks of patients' experience of adverse events while providing resident training. Within the ICU environment, where the costs of adverse events are high, teaching trainees in a manner that minimizes medical errors is now a paramount issue. In addition, critical care training in ICUs is further hindered by the difficulties in (1) ensuring exposure of learners to a broad range of clinical situations with a risk-free method and (2) assessing learner performance under standardized conditions [24].

A study showed that a medical simulation course helps students understand better compared with a case-based discussion in the management of shock [10]. Students gained more knowledge and skill in emergency situations than in problem-based learning [19]. A recent randomized study suggested that high-fidelity simulation improves students' knowledge and communication about advanced life support [20]. Moreover, in septic shock resuscitation, students had better knowledge and skills in resuscitation compared with a precourse assessment.

REFERENCES

[1] Kleinpell. Targeting sepsis as a performance improvement metric AACN. Advanced Critical Care 2014;25(2): 179–86.

[2] Chelluri LP. Quality and performance improvement in critical care. Indian J Crit Care Med 2008;12:67–76.

[3] Donabedian A. Evaluating the quality of medical care. Milbank Q 1966;4:166–206.

[4] Donabedian Q. The quality of care: how can it be assessed? JAMA 1988;260:1743–8.

[5] Donabedian A. Explorations in quality assessment and monitoring: the definition of quality and approaches to its assessment. Ann Arbor, MI: Health Administration Press; 1980.

[6] Juran JM. Made in the U.S.A.: a renaissance in quality. Harv Bus Rev 1993;71:42–7.

[7] Singer M. The Third International Consensus Definitions for Sepsis and Septic Shock (Sepsis-3). JAMA 2016; 315(8):801–10.

[8] Delawder JM. An interdisciplinary code sepsis team to improve sepsis bundle compliance in the emergency department. In: Doctor of nursing practice (DNP) final clinical projects; 2018. p. 20.

[9] Christopher W. Seymour derivation, validation, and potential treatment implications of novel clinical phenotypes for sepsis. JAMA 2019;321(20):2003–17.

[10] Maria M, Lindo. Evaluation of automated reminders to reduce sepsis mortality rates. Walden Dissertations and Doctoral Studies Collection 2017.

[11] Alsolamy S, Al Salamah M, Al Thagafi M, Al-Dorzi HM, Marini AM, Aljerian N, et al. Diagnostic accuracy of a screening electronic alert tool for severe sepsis and septic shock in the emergency department. BMC Med Inform Decis Mak 2014;14:105. https://doi.org/10.1186/s12911-014-0105-7. PMID: 25476738; PMCID: PMC4261595.

[12] Semler M., Weavind L., Hooper M., Rice T., Gowda S., Nádas A., et al. An electronic tool for the evaluation and treatment of sepsis in the ICU: a randomized controlled trial. Crit Care Med. Submitted for publication. https://doi.org/10.1097/CCM.0000000000001020.

[13] Hayden GE, Tuuri RE, Scott R, Losek JD, Blackshaw AM, Schoenling AJ, Nietert PJ, Hall GA. Triage sepsis alert and sepsis protocol lower times to fluids and antibiotics in the ED. Am J Emerg Med 2016;34(1):1–9. https://doi.org/10.1016/j.ajem.2015.08.039. Epub 2015 Aug 28. PMID: 26386734; PMCID: PMC4905767.

[14] La Rosa PS, Brooks JP, Deych E, Boone EL, Edwards DJ, Wang Q, et al. Hypothesis testing and power calculations for taxonomic-based human microbiome data. PLoS ONE 2012;7(12):e52078. https://doi.org/10.1371/journal.pone.0052078.

[15] Umscheid CA, Betesh J, VanZandbergen C, Hanish A, Tait G, Mikkelsen ME, French B, Fuchs BD. Development, implementation, and impact of an automated early warning and response system for sepsis. J Hosp Med 2015; 10(1):26–31. https://doi.org/10.1002/jhm.2259. Epub 2014 Sep 26. PMID: 25263548; PMCID: PMC4410778.

[16] Bruce HR, Maiden J, Fedullo PF, Kim SC. Impact of nurse-initiated ED sepsis protocol on compliance with sepsis bundles, time to initial antibiotic administration, and in-hospital mortality. J Emerg Nurs 2015 Mar;41(2): 130–7. https://doi.org/10.1016/j.jen.2014.12.007. Epub 2015 Jan 19. PMID: 25612516.

[17] Gatewood MO, Wemple M, Greco S, Kritek PA, Durvasula R. A quality improvement project to improve early sepsis care in the emergency department. BMJ Qual Saf 2015 Dec;24(12):787–95. https://doi.org/

10.1136/bmjqs-2014-003552. Epub 2015 Aug 6. PMID: 26251506.

[18] Hooper MH, Weavind L, Wheeler AP, Martin JB, Gowda SS, Semler MW, Hayes RM, Albert DW, Deane NB, Nian H, Mathe JL, Nadas A, Sztipanovits J, Miller A, Bernard GR, Rice TW. Randomized trial of automated, electronic monitoring to facilitate early detection of sepsis in the intensive care unit. Crit Care Med 2012 Jul;40(7):2096–101. https://doi.org/10.1097/CCM.0b013e318250a887. PMID: 22584763; PMCID: PMC4451061.

[19] Scalese RJ, Obeso VT, Issenberg SB. Simulation technology for skills training and competency assessment in medical education. J Gen Intern Med 2008;23(Suppl. 1):46–9.

[20] McGaghie WC, Issenberg SB, Petrusa ER, Scalese RJ. A critical review of simulation-based medical education research: 2003–2009. Med Educ 2010;44(1):50–63.

[21] Nishisaki A, Keren R, Nadkarni V. Does simulation improve patient safety? Self-efficacy, competence, operational performance, and patient safety. Anesthesiol Clin 2007;25(2):225–36.

[22] Bond WF, Lammers RL, Spillane LL, et al. The use of simulation in emergency medicine: a research agenda. Acad Emerg Med 2007;14(4):353–63.

[23] Bond W, Kuhn G, Binstadt E, et al. The use of simulation in the development of individual cognitive expertise in emergency medicine. Acad Emerg Med 2008;15(11):1037–45.

[24] Pamplin JC. Prolonged, high-fidelity simulation for study of patient care in resource-limited medical contexts and for technology comparative effectiveness testing. Crit Care Explor July 2021;3(7).

CHAPTER 33

Long-Term Sequelae of Sepsis

AHMED REDA TAHA

INTRODUCTION

Having survived a septic episode does not count as a happy ending for our patients. Until recently, no one understood that saving someone's life and surviving sepsis could cause them harm and suffering for months or years afterward. Focusing on mortality outcomes following critical illness, we would have never been prepared for the reality of the postsepsis sequelae, such as physical and neuropsychological dysfunction, costly ongoing health care, and leads to financial and mental devastation for families [1].

With technological advances, many critically ill septic patients now survive previously fatal illnesses, generating an enlarging population of intensive care unit (ICU) survivors. While some critical condition is an acute event with minimal long-term effects, we are now aware that a substantial number of patients are left in a chronic state with increased risks of mortality and morbidity. Understanding how critical illness may affect mortality after hospital discharge is essential to measuring the actual value of intensive care and targeting therapeutic and palliative interventions that will improve survival and quality of life following critical illness. Intensive care physicians should utilize a further understanding of the epidemiology and control of medical vulnerabilities after sepsis to help sepsis survivorship [2].

Multiple studies have shown that sepsis survivors are at increased risk for death, which will persist for at least two years after sepsis hospitalization. Although that is related mainly to the lasting consequences of sepsis, both the epidemiology and biology of sepsis are crucial to understand (Fig. 33.1).

LONG-TERM DERANGEMENTS IN SEPSIS SURVIVORS

Postsepsis Immunopathy

In sepsis survivors, the observed health deterioration that leads to frequent rehospitalizations is primarily the effect of long-term immune derangement. Although there is no substantial evidence to support this assumption, a lot of the new studies carry good insights [3].

The long-term immune dysfunction in sepsis is dependent on epigenetic and metabolic cellular reprogramming. Roquilly et al. [4] found that alveolar macrophages and circulating monocytes showed evidence of reprogramming six months after the inflammation was resolved in humans with systemic inflammation. A signal is generated to prevent phagocytosis when this molecule binds to the universal cell receptor CD47.

Upon bacterial reinfection, reprogrammed alveolar macrophages are hampered in their phagocytic capacity. According to the research group's earlier paper, they also demonstrated that primary infection could alter the local environment in the tissue, thereby altering antigen-presenting cells that are impaired in terms of T-cell activation, resulting in immune suppression and increased susceptibility to long-term secondary infections [5].

As the reduced response to secondary infectious insults (i.e., postsepsis immunopathy) is thought to be a common sequela of sepsis, a murine study using cecal ligation and puncture model of sepsis reported trained (boosted) immunity at the cellular level, with an altered gene expression profile of naive bone marrow monocytes.

Monitoring circulating inflammatory markers or cell-based immune-suppressive markers, such as human leukocyte antigen D-related on monocytes (mHLA-DR), could help identify individuals at risk for secondary infections and/or worsening of chronic medical conditions [6,7].

At long-term follow-up, both circulating interleukin-7 and programmed cell death protein-1 (PD-1) levels remained elevated, suggesting chronic inflammation and immunosuppression [8].

Yende et al. found that most sepsis survivors develop persistent inflammation and immunosuppression, leading to a greater risk of hospital readmission and

The Sepsis Codex. https://doi.org/10.1016/B978-0-323-88271-2.00007-9

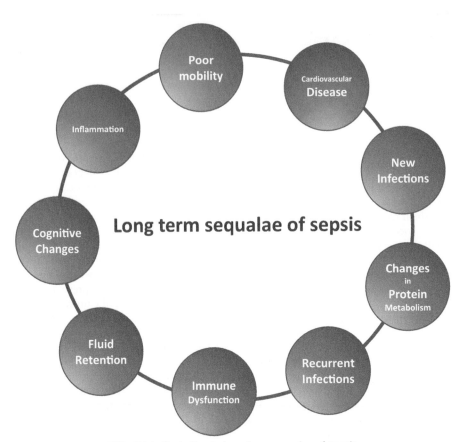

FIG. 33.1 Illustration to long-term sequalae of sepsis.

mortality within one year. Two phenotypes of sepsis survivors were identified based on the biomarkers of inflammation (C-reactive protein) and immunosuppression (PD-1) [9].

The "hyperinflammation and immunosuppression" phenotype observed in 70% of the cohort was significantly higher than the "normal" phenotype (odds ratio 1.4–8.3, P0.01), rehospitalizations, and rehospitalization and/or death specific to cardiovascular disease or cancer. The phenotypes had similar presepsis health status, and the associations were significant even after adjusting for demographics, comorbidities, and acute sepsis severity. Persistent inflammation and immunosuppression are common among sepsis survivors and are associated with poor long-term outcomes. Sepsis survivors suffer long-term immune derangements, as found in these findings [9].

Cardiovascular Disease After Sepsis

Infection is a significant trigger of acute coronary syndromes. It produces high levels of ischemia, endothelial dysfunction, procoagulant states, and inflammatory cellular infiltration (e.g., T-cells, macrophages, and neutrophils) within atherosclerotic plaques. These infectious sequelae can increase the short-term risk of cardiovascular events, including stroke, myocardial infarction, and fatal coronary artery disease [10,11]. The recruitment of inflammatory cells contributes to acute coronary syndromes by producing cytokines, proteases, coagulation factors, free radicals, and vasoactive intermediates that increase endothelial damage, disrupt the fibrous cap, and start the formation of thrombi. In addition, the residual inflammatory and procoagulant state can extend for years after the infection resolves and raise a survivor's risk of cardiovascular diseases

[12,13]; hospitalization for severe pneumonia carried a fourfold increase in developing cardiovascular disease in the first 30 days postinfection and remained elevated for 10 years [14].

Both atherosclerosis and sepsis are inflammatory states associated with increased short- and long-term risk of cardiovascular disease. Ref. [15] found that survivors of severe sepsis had a 13-fold increased risk of developing cardiovascular events compared with unmatched controls and a 1.9-fold increased risk compared with matched population controls [15]. This 1.9-fold increase in risk is similar to the risk of developing cardiovascular events in cigarette smokers and patients with diabetes and hypercholesterolemia. Contrary to the other organ systems, the cardiovascular system exhibits a unique feature: 45% of patients who survived sepsis had no preexisting cardiovascular disease; yet, 25.9% of these patients developed subsequent cardiovascular events [15]. These findings suggest that survivors of postsepsis syndrome may be predisposed to developing chronic illnesses where none previously existed.

Estimating the Magnitude of the Problem

In long-term studies of ICU populations, death rates are either reported for all critically ill septic patients or subgroups that share clinical or therapeutic characteristics. Critical illness definitions often use the admission to an ICU as a proxy [16,17]. In defining a group this way, some septic patients who are cared for elsewhere may be missed or include patients who do not have exceptionally severe illnesses. Alternatively, we can focus on one or more subgroups of septic patients, such as those with severe sepsis, additional acute respiratory distress syndrome (ARDS), prolonged mechanical ventilation, or the elderly [18]. Despite studies of subgroups of septic patients providing vital information about that specific population, the results may not apply to other critically ill septic patients. The majority of studies calculate the long-term mortality starting from the time of ICU admission and include deaths in the hospital. Recent population-based studies have estimated long-term mortality among patients who survive sepsis based on the date of discharge from the hospital. Considering the high hospital mortality rate associated with most critically ill septic populations, the latter approach allows for a more accurate assessment of posthospitalization mortality [17,18]. It is, therefore, crucial to use caution when comparing mortality across studies, since including or excluding hospital deaths can significantly change mortality estimates [19–21] (Fig. 33.2).

Mechanistic Hypotheses of Injury and Repair

Fundamental insights into the biology of conditions such as sepsis have been gained from basic and translational research, leading to the development of significant new therapeutic paradigms [22]. Most patients who suffer from these life-threatening diseases lack access to safe and effective therapies that target specific cellular and molecular processes. Many challenges face researchers who wish to translate experimentally generated mechanistic hypotheses into clinically effective interventions. In well-established animal models of severe illness, assumptions of generalizability may not be valid, according to recent analyses. Experimental paradigms and disease models must be thoroughly revised to close this translational gap. The discovery of how tissues and organs undergo repair and remodeling during disease and after serious injury will likely lead to many novel insights into postcritical illness recovery [23,24]. Comorbid conditions such as genetic susceptibility and cognitive or physiological reserve are influential in the pathophysiologic continuum that extends from acute illness to recovery. A growing body of recent research has demonstrated that tissue regeneration and reorganization mechanisms that accompany ARDS, acute kidney injury, myocardial ischemia, and muscle wasting in critical illness are highly dynamic. Together, these findings have opened a new window on the processes of tissue regeneration that, together with a burgeoning understanding of regenerative biology and medicine, will likely impact the way we approach critically ill patients. Many long-term complications of critical illness can be attributed to neurologic or muscular injuries sustained during acute infection [25,26]. A major focus of critical illness research is unraveling the mechanisms that lead to sepsis-associated encephalopathy, cerebral infarction, and structural muscle changes.

The Recovery from Critical Illness in Randomized Clinical Trials

The Improving Mortality during Post-Acute Care Transitions for Sepsis (NCT03865602) is a pragmatic randomized controlled trial (RCT) that evaluates the impact of a STAR (Sepsis Transition and Recovery) program on mortality rates. Three hospitals are randomized 1:1 to the STAR program versus usual care for 708 sepsis survivors. A centrally located nurse navigator will provide telephone counseling and eHealth support to facilitate best practices for postsepsis care (medication optimization, screening for new impairments/symptoms, monitoring existing comorbidities, and

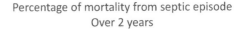

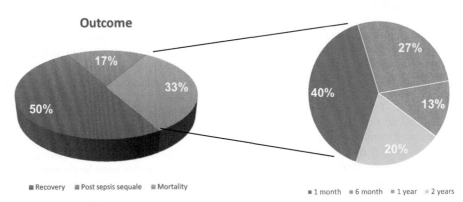

FIG. 33.2 **Patient Outcomes Following Sepsis** Approximately half of patients who survived a hospitalization for sepsis achieved a complete or near complete recovery at two years after discharge; one-third of total patients died during this period; and one-sixth of these patients remained with one or more of the serious, lasting complications of postsepsis sequalae. (Data presented from Refs. [2,3,6,13,33].)

palliative care referral when needed). 30-day readmission rates or mortality are the primary outcomes [27].

Former ICU patients participated in a randomized controlled study to determine the impact of a web-based educational resource that includes short videos about common life support and its sequelae (NCT04317144). A total of 330 ICU survivors will be assigned to access the web-based resource. Their primary outcome is self-reported posttraumatic stress disorder (PTSD) symptoms 2, 6, and 12 months after the ICU stay [27].

An RCT assessing the impact of the Prevnar vaccine after an ICU stay for sepsis considers the benefit of the pneumococcal vaccine to accelerate immune recovery (NCT03565159). The Prevnar vaccine will be compared to a placebo in 214 ICU survivors. The primary outcome is time to infection-related rehospitalization or death. A secondary outcome was the evaluation of immune recovery patterns [27].

Implications for Quality of Life, Return to Work, Finances, and Social Relationships

The quality of life for sepsis survivors is often severely diminished, and they are frequently unable to return to work or resume their prior roles [28,29]. An analysis of 51 studies examining the return employment of 7267 patients and 858 family caregivers was conducted [30].

Based on pooled estimates (among those previously employed), the return to employment rate at 3, 6, and 12 months was 33%, 55%, and 56%, respectively [30]. Improvement in psychosocial health was associated with being able to return to work [30]. Studies have found that caregivers have fewer work hours and lower wages [30,31]. An observational study of 46 ARDS survivors participating in the Reevaluation of Systemic Early Neuromuscular Blockade (ROSE) trial examined how the financial burden of their hospitalization was perceived [31]. Two-thirds of patients reported financial burden owing to out-of-pocket medical expenses and lost income. Many patients reported additional costs as well. Financial toxicity can lead to impaired mental/physical health, increased dependence on others, and specific material hardships [31]. Clinical outcomes following the downstream consequences of financial toxicity include impaired mental/physical health, increased dependency, and material hardships. Most sepsis survivors are satisfied with their outcome, despite the extensive morbidity they encounter. A cohort study of 1453 Dutch patients who survived for one year following an ICU stay found that only 67 (5%) considered their outcome unacceptable [32]. A cohort study of 1453 Dutch patients who survived for one year following an ICU stay found that only 67 (5%) considered their outcome unacceptable [32]. As part of the survey, patients were asked whether they considered themselves in an acceptable condition following their ICU treatment (agree/disagree/neutral) [32]. It was associated with lower quality of life, lower cognitive and physical functioning, and greater anxiety and depressive symptoms when individuals disagreed with this statement. However, a significant finding was that no line could be drawn between an unacceptable outcome and a level of quality-of-life impairment [32].

A Review of Critical Care Management

The complex clinical management of patients with post-sepsis remains challenging due to a variety of clinical sequelae, a variety of interventions, and a limited body of evidence. An earlier review on enhancing recovery from sepsis recorded several effective practices for preventing rehospitalization and promoting recovery, including medication optimization, screening for impairments, monitoring for common and preventable causes of medical deterioration, and referral to palliative care for selected patients [33]. Taylor et al. [33] examined their association with risk-adjusted outcomes in a cohort of sepsis survivors from 10 USA hospitals. Sixty-two percent of 189 sepsis survivors had their medications optimized, 65% had functional or mental health impairments screened, 46% were monitored for common causes of health deterioration, and 58% had care alignment processes documented (e.g., goals of care discussion, palliative care referral). Patients who received these practices had lower odds of rehospitalization or death; however, only 20% of them received all four within 90 days of sepsis hospitalization—indicating that better strategies are needed to implement these recommendations [34].

The importance of medication optimization has been underscored by a study using data from the US Department of Veterans Affairs health-care system [35]. The discontinuation rate of statins in ICU and sepsis survivors ranged from 10% to 15% across hospitals [35]. Despite this, rates of new antipsychotic initiation ranged from 2% to 4% across hospitals (in the absence of new or prior mental health diagnoses) [35]. While the appropriateness of these medication changes cannot be determined, this and prior studies suggest a high rate of inappropriate discontinuation of chronic medications and accidental continuation of medications initiated for temporary symptoms control during critical illness [36,37]. Moreover, prior multicenter RCTs have shown that complex medication optimization interventions can reduce rehospitalizations, underscoring the necessity of this practice. Finally,

specialized follow-up programs have been suggested to meet the complex and multifaceted needs of survivors of sepsis and other critical illnesses [38].

In a Cochrane review on follow-up services for improving long-term outcomes in ICU survivors, only five studies (four randomized, one observational) with 1707 participants were included in the review [39]. Analyses of the four randomized interventions found no difference in health-related quality of life or mortality at 12 months post-ICU discharge [39]. There was insufficient evidence to draw conclusions about depression/anxiety, physical function, or cognitive function. According to the study, there is insufficient evidence to determine whether post-ICU follow-up services improve health outcomes.

Even though randomized clinical trials do not support ICU follow-up services, they remain a critical arena for learning about survivorship and testing novel approaches to supporting recovery. ICU follow-up services are organized and structured differently across centers [40]. Based on a qualitative study of 66 ICU survivors on three continents—52 who attended follow-up programs and 14 who did not—researchers identified five key components of successful ICU recovery programs: continuity of care, symptom management, normalization and expectations management, internal and external validation of the process, and reducing feelings of guilt and hopelessness [40]. In addition, a qualitative study of 15 sepsis survivors identified 11 domains of health-related quality of life as critically important to survivors: psychological impairment, control over one's life, walking ability, return to everyday living, cognitive impairment, family support, daily living, access to health care, fatigue, physical impairment (including pain), and self-perception [41]. Moreover, many of these domains considered important to survivors are not captured in existing quality of life measures (e.g., SF-36, 5Q5D) [40,41]—which may explain the apparent disconnect between the high reported satisfaction with ICU follow-up programs and the apparent lack of benefit in trials using existing outcome instruments.

The concept of peer support is also evolving to support ICU survivors and their families. Evidence for peer support in critically ill patients is limited, just as for follow-up programs in ICUs [42]. An analysis of eight studies involving 92 patients and 192 family members found that peer support reduced psychological morbidity and increased social support [42]. Due to the limited evidence supporting ICU follow-up and peer support programs, it may be difficult to obtain the resources needed to develop and maintain such programs [43]. Recently, a large-scale qualitative assessment of two learning collaboratives (of ICU follow-up and peer support programs) identified barriers to the implementation of peer support and ICU follow-up programs [43]. The human experience of survivorship was identified as a key enabler for recruiting physicians to work in ICU follow-up programs and obtaining interest and funding from hospital administrators [43]. In a systematic review of nonpharmacologic interventions to prevent or mitigate adverse long-term outcomes among ICU survivors, six categories of interventions were identified: exercise and rehabilitation programs; ICU follow-up programs; psychosocial support programs; diaries, information, and education [44]. A total of 36 studies with a total of 5165 patients were included. Most were single-center studies. In addition to diaries and exercise programs, there was inconclusive evidence that other types of interventions had a positive impact on mental outcomes [44]. A large, recent, claims-based study from Germany suggests that inpatient rehabilitation may significantly improve five-year survival rates from sepsis [39]. This study examined 83,974 hospital patients with septic shock, sepsis, or severe infections.

Compared to noninfectious hospitalized controls matched by age, sex, comorbidity, and dependency, these survivors had an increased risk of death at least five years postsepsis [45]. Most sepsis survivors were treated in inpatient rehabilitation centers (14.5% of septic shock patients, 6.3% of sepsis patients, and 3.3% of severe infection patients). In contrast, patients receiving inpatient rehabilitation had a reduced five-year mortality rate (adjusted hazards ratio 1/4 0.81, $P < .001$) [45]. They conclude that specialized rehabilitation programs may improve long-term survival after sepsis.

Deb et al. analyzed the data of Medicare beneficiaries who survived sepsis hospitalization and were referred to home health-care services; Deb et al. assessed whether earlier follow-up was associated with reduced 30-day readmission rates. In particular, the study examined the effects of initiating home care services within two days of discharge from the hospital and having the first physician follow-up within seven days of discharge. A study of 170,000 patients found that 28% had early home health care and physician follow-up, 45% had early home health care, 11% had early physician follow-up, and 16% had neither [46]. A combination of home health care and physician follow-up lowered 30-day readmissions by 7%, despite neither of them affecting readmission in isolation [46].

Physiologic Reserve and Loss of Biologic Complexity

As an increasingly recognized prognostic determinant of survival and functional outcome for critically ill patients, "physiologic reserve" is defined as the critical threshold of physiological adaptation that an individual can mount in response to acute illness and/or trauma before suffering decompensation and death. Unfortunately, this concept can be difficult to apply to the bedside, since there is no discrete diagnostic test or measure for physiologic reserve. A surrogate clinical marker such as the presence and severity of the frail phenotype can provide insight into the "physiologic reserve." Clinically, frailty can be defined as the accumulation of deficits that, while individually insignificant, collectively contribute to increased risk of chronic diseases, vulnerability to adverse events, and diminished physiologic reserves. Despite the lack of specific studies evaluating the value of frailty assessment in critically ill patients, research has shown that frailty is associated with the increased complexity of supportive care, prolonged hospitalization, increased mortality, and long-term institutionalization for the elderly and those undergoing major cardiovascular surgery. A routine assessment of frailty in all critically ill patients may provide additional prognostic information that can be incorporated into discussions with patients and/or family members regarding ICU admission and support and the withdrawal of such support after time-limited trials of advanced life support in the ICU. In addition, frailty assessment could identify patients who need intensive rehabilitative support during and after critical care to optimize their outcomes [47].

In addition to its ability to withstand and adapt to a variety of external environmental stressors, the human body is a complex biologic system. As a system, the response to such stressors is typically highly elaborate, although its apparent randomness has an overall structure and stability. The application of nonlinear dynamics (chaos theory) to biological systems has better understood the processes underlying their function during the past two decades. System complexity (the number of ways the system can detect a change in its baseline state, process that change, and generate a distinct response) determines its ability to adapt to baseline changes and its resiliency to catastrophic failures. In response to a stimulus, the biologic system mounts a multimodal adaptive response that temporarily reduces the variability apparent within the system [48].

The baseline complexity of a system and its ability to reduce complexity in response to a stimulus seem to determine its ability to adapt to a stimulus without experiencing catastrophic failure. Conceptually, senescence, disease, or injury affects a system's ability to detect changes in the baseline state or adapt to those changes. The result is that the system's output is simplified, less complex, or less "random." Therefore, quantifying changes in the complexity of a biological system can provide valuable insight into its homeostatic functioning.

Data from human studies confirm this supposition, showing that loss of output variability in the dynamics of healthy organ system function is an early sign of dysfunction. Furthermore, in various organ systems, physiologic aging and disease can lead to a loss of complexity (see Table 33.1).

A number of these changes have also been associated with adverse outcomes of patients, such as cardiovascular events, falls, fractures, and mortality. A reduction in complexity is associated with a reduction in the repertoire of possible physiologic responses to stressors, a diminished ability to adapt to perturbations, and a diminished threshold for decompensation (e.g., with less significant episodes of acute illness or injury). Once a critical threshold is exceeded, the aggregate

system may no longer be able to maintain a steady-state, and an accelerated and catastrophic dysregulation occurs. This theoretical, critical threshold can be interpreted as a "physiologic reserve" [49].

Clinical syndromes of frailty are phenotypic expressions of this process. Initially described in the geriatric population, frailty is a syndrome in which minor deficiencies accumulate, which may not be significant, but collectively may contribute to an impossible burden of disease and vulnerability to adverse events. The prevalence and severity of frailty vary greatly across age groups despite being closely related to aging and aging. Nonlinear dynamics best describe the phenomenon since the number of deficits appears to be more significant than the specific deficits themselves [50]. When the repertoire of physiologic responses to environmental stressors decreases, the ability to adapt and respond is reduced, resulting in greater vulnerability to adverse clinical events and outcomes. The concept of "punished inefficiency" also plays a part in which many physiological impairments lead to physiologic inefficiency [51]. In addition to reduced complexity of physiologic responses, frail patients consume more than their already diminished energy [50].

As a result of its syndromic nature, frailty can be difficult to define and characterize. The operational definition proposed by Fried and colleagues [50] is one of the most widely accepted methods for measuring frailty. However, there are limitations to this definition, including the lack of cognitive and psychological domains, the stratification of frail, prefrail, or nonfrail categories, and the lack of validation of each of the five criteria [50–53].

A prospective study evaluating the five Fried criteria and cognitive impairment and depression in a cohort of 754 independent elderly patients, followed for up to 7.5 years, emphasizes these limitations. In this study, slow gait speed was the strongest predictor of adverse outcomes (OR 3.8, 5.9, 2.5, and 2.7 for chronic disability, long-term nursing home stay, injurious fall, and death). Low physical activity was the second strongest factor [54]. Cognitive impairment (defined as a score on the Folstein Mini-Mental Status Examination <24) [55] showed a greater prognostic value when compared to the other three criteria. Many different scoring systems have been developed to recognize better and treat frailty, all of which have advantages and disadvantages. Compared to the other three criteria, it showed a greater predictive value. Each domain was represented differently in the published scoring systems [56]. A comprehensive tool to measure frailty was identified in this review as the Frailty Index (FI), which

TABLE 33.1

Overview of Changes in Complexity That can Occur to Various Organ Systems in Response to Aging or Disease

Complexity change	Example condition(s)
Loss of heart rate variability	Aging, critical illness, trauma, ischemic heart disease, congestive heart failure (CHF), prior to the onset of atrial fibrillation, and ventricular fibrillation
Loss of temperature curve complexity	Critical illness
Respiratory rate complexity	Aging, CHF
Alterations in gait dynamics	Aging, Parkinson's disease
Pulsatile hormone release	Aging, sleep disturbance
Blood pressure variability	Aging, critical illness
Electroencephalographic evoked potentials	Aging, critical illness

utilizes a detailed 70-item inventory of clinical deficits to determine the presence and quantify the severity of frailty [57]. Its comprehensive nature makes it difficult to incorporate into the busy, often chaotic clinical critical care medicine practice, even when used for research purposes.

A Conceptual Framework for Frailty in Critical Care

In addition, critically ill patients may be vulnerable to frailty development, and nonlinear dynamics may explain many of these observed phenomena. Critical illness involves a catastrophic disruption of homeostasis: acute stressors overwhelm physiologic reserves, requiring somatic support to maintain life [58]. Critically ill patients have a heightened vulnerability to adverse outcomes and events, just like frail elderly patients. Short-term risks involve unpredictable clinical deterioration, regardless of age or premorbid functional reserve. It has been suggested that the severity of acute perturbation necessary to cause critical decompensation is variable, and it is affected by: (1) the rapidity with which the stressor induces change within the system, (2) the current level of physiologic instability, and (3) whether somatic support can improve physiology. In concept, life-supportive technology can be viewed as enhancing the output of the biological system, providing time for the system to adapt and heal; however, in most circumstances, it does not directly affect the underlying processes that lead to decompensation [59]. Subacute critical illness presents a more challenging problem. Organ dysfunction results from catastrophic disruption of the system, but the specific organs that fail in a particular patient at a specific time and in a specific way remain unpredictable. However, in critical care, one commonly observed symptom is the rapid onset of severe muscle wasting, motor weakness, and functional impairment over days to weeks. This process would typically take years to develop in an outpatient setting. The neuromuscular dysfunction associated with critical illness occurs in 5%–10% of critically ill patients. It is associated with an increased risk of ICU mortality, prolonged hospitalization and rehabilitation, and reduced quality of life after discharge [60]. There has been some speculation that critical illness may be a manifestation of rapid development of frailty due to its shared features of weakness, muscle wasting, poor functional status, neurocognitive dysfunction, and the psychological effects of depression and caregiver burnout. Additionally, functional dependence after critical illness is associated with two of the most distinctive phenotypic features of frailty: the inability to walk and

weak upper extremity muscles [60]. Muscle loss and weakness are strongly associated with complications in ICU, suggesting that interventions that prevent or minimize muscle wasting may improve outcomes. Nonlinearity implies that treatments affecting only one aspect of a process are more likely to fail, unless that treatment targets a single etiological factor that results in a cascade of decompensation or can affect multiple processes simultaneously.

In terms of predicting short- and long-term functional outcomes and the ability of a patient to heal, there are no well-validated tools that clearly distinguish survivors from nonsurvivors at the time of presentation to ICU with an episode of critical illness [61]. Furthermore, medical practitioners' high degree of confidence regarding the outcome of an individual patient and the effect of specific interventions on that outcome is in stark contrast to their limited accuracy in making these predictions. Therefore, in spite of the fact that critical care practitioners do prognostication every day, this process is fraught with error [62,63].

Unfortunately, many other illness severities scoring systems, such as the APACHE score, are not helpful for the care of individual patients, as these tools were designed to compare patient populations rather than predict patients' survival probability. The results of a systematic review comparing doctors' predictions with those of validated scoring systems found that physicians were twice as accurate in identifying patients who died before ICU discharge, but both were only moderately accurate [64]. In terms of physicians' predictions of the outcome, one caveat relates to perception: the prediction of low chances of survival by physicians is strongly associated with the self-fulfilling prophecy of withdrawal of life-supporting measures and death, independent of the severity of the illness [65]. In terms of outcome in critical illness, frailty and physiologic reserve have yet to be clearly elucidated. The independent prognostic value of premorbid functional status and ICU is controversial

Results support the hypothesis that physiologic reserve plays an important role, and when it is exhausted, recovery from critical illness may be significantly prolonged or impossible. As a result, investigators are now trying to identify biomarkers that, together with clinical prediction rules, can aid in reliably prognosticating more effectively to determine a clinically useful measure of the "physiologic age" of the patient (see Table 28.3). In the noncritical illness literature, detecting the syndrome of frailty in geriatric and perioperative populations has gained popularity as a significant potential "biomarker" of prognosis.

The lack of critical care-specific data, the multiplicity of definitions, and the heterogeneity of patient populations prevent us from drawing firm conclusions about the consequences of frailty. Data are emerging that suggest some measures of frailty may be useful in predicting not only mortality but also intensity of care, adverse events, and functional outcome of elderly patients following hospitalization, including those requiring ICU admission [65].

As a result of the interaction between acute critical illness, comorbid diseases, preillness functional status, and physiologic reserve, long-term mortality after critical illness varies widely.

Even so, for most groups of critically ill patients, the majority of deaths among ICU survivors occur during the first 6–12 months following hospital discharge, suggesting there may be a window of opportunity for future studies and potential interventions. It, therefore, must no longer be an endpoint of success but rather the beginning of an assessment of biochemical, physiologic, and cognitive markers that are necessary to reliably predict long-term mortality and provide the foundation for palliative and therapeutic interventions that will improve care after critical illness.

Cognitive Impairment After Sepsis

Both the lay public and medical professionals consider admission to the ICU a tragic occurrence. Though the ICU experience may be harrowing, we are aware of the life-changing "legacy" of cognitive and behavioral problems that ICU survivors face in the months and years following critical illness. Over the past decade or so, investigators have published data that clearly illustrate a spectrum of acquired or exacerbated "neck-up" disorders that severely compromise the lives of our patients and seriously delay or prevent their recovery. A potentially life-altering, "dementia-like" long-term cognitive impairment affects 60%–80% of ICU survivors and is most frequently characterized by memory and executive dysfunction. It impacts patients' ability to return to work, find their car in a parking lot, go shopping, etc. Although many people can recall the names of people they know well, they have difficulty remembering new events, facts, and their schedules.

Added to these extremely troubling neuropsychological deficits are mood disorders such as major depression and PTSD. Unfortunately, the two diagnoses (depression and PTSD) are often missed, despite their prevalence in 25%–30% and 10%–20% of ICU survivors, respectively. As a profession, we are just beginning to address risk factors for these "newly acquired" or "accelerated from baseline" diseases. As health-care

professionals, how can we incorporate these issues into our work?

It's essential to visualize a patient arriving on a gurney with a life-threatening disease, such as pneumonia or cholecystitis, and then to remind yourself that, during the ensuing days under your care, this person with a "lung or gall bladder problem" will also acquire new neuropathic and neuromuscular conditions. Therefore, our attention should be focused primarily on these two new elements of disease burden during and after our patients' ICU stays.

It is just now that we are beginning to address the risk factors for these "newly acquired" and "accelerated from baseline" diseases. It is also essential to recognize that these two categories of body decay are inextricably linked. We would be wise to identify the following modifiable risk factors during our patients' ICU stay and recovery: total exposure to potent psychoactive medications, duration of delirium, sleep deficits and derangements, and periods of immobilization. It is at a pivotal time of dramatic change in critical care, both within the walls of the ICU and beyond into the world of cognitive and physical rehabilitation after ICU discharge.

In the last decade and a half, cognitive impairment among sepsis survivors has been increasingly studied. Sepsis survivors have been shown to display marked cognitive deficits following critical illness, generating significant knowledge. Nearly 20 studies report that cognitive problems persist for years, often without premorbid cognitive problems, in more than two out of three individuals after hospital discharge. There are, however, many key questions remaining, including the trajectory of change over time, whether ICU survivors continue to experience cognitive decline, and how cognitive impairments relate to the so-called "real-world" outcomes (ecological validity). The trajectory of change over time has been extensively examined in other populations, but it has rarely been studied following intensive care due to the limited duration of follow-up used (usually only looked at one-time point). Therefore, much remains unknown about the long-term natural history and recovery of ICU-acquired cognitive impairments.

Research is needed to better understand whether persistent cognitive decline occurs after or is exacerbated by critical illness, particularly in older populations, and whether differential risk factors lead to specific patterns of outcomes. The increasing rates of Alzheimer's disease may be in part due to the effects of critical illness and its treatment, although this remains to be proven. Many questions remain in terms of the functional or real-world effects of cognitive impairments common in ICU survivors. This has received little attention. These outcomes include driving, managing medications, managing finances (e.g., balancing a checkbook), shopping for groceries, and understanding maps in other cognitively impaired populations. Often, functional outcomes are difficult to measure and require specialized facilities and extensive training.

Furthermore, there are no or limited normative data for tasks of ecological validity, such as managing medications. We should not let these obstacles dim our enthusiasm for determining the impact of cognitive deficits on real-world activities, since these studies will better understand the functional consequences of post-ICU cognitive impairments. ICU survivors continue to experience cognitive impairment. The popular media and clinical settings and research settings have begun paying more attention to this phenomenon in recent years. The current efforts to improve post-ICU morbidities are promising, and rehabilitation studies after intensive care are inspiring. However, there is still much to learn. In addition to addressing the fundamental questions elucidated in this chapter, future efforts should reflect the increasing sophistication and granularity of assessments of cognitive outcomes. With time, these efforts will directly impact the quality of life and well-being of ICU survivors, ultimately enhancing public health.

Intensive Care Follow-up Clinics

In the current state of evidence, following up with patients in an ICU is not beneficial or cost-effective. However, we should not diminish the importance of these long-term outcomes or abandon our patients once they leave the ICU. Qualitative research conducted with patients and their families has found that some aspects of follow-up services are subjectively helpful. The challenge is to develop and implement longitudinal models of care that begin the day a patient enters the ICU and continue after they leave. Aiming to prevent morbidities through early rehabilitation activities | [66] and managing delirium [67], both of which impact long-term outcomes. One intervention that may reduce PTSD symptoms is the use of a diary of ICU events kept by health-care providers and given to patients after discharge [68]. A follow-up model should utilize technology, such as telemedicine and electronic health records, to engage and communicate with primary health-care providers, rehabilitation facilities, and our patients and reach out to patients beyond urban areas where tertiary ICUs are usually located. Future research and design of follow-up models should integrate control groups and well-planned outcome analyses,

including cost-effectiveness. Additionally, researchers should carefully consider the tools they use to assess these outcomes and their validity in ICU survivors, particularly those with cognitive impairments and psychiatric morbidities. Finally, models should be longitudinal, beginning with the ICU stay and continuing throughout acute care. Specialists and primary care physicians should communicate with their patients throughout that period [69].

REFERENCES

[1] Ashbaugh DG, Bigelow DB, Petty TL Levine BE. Acute respiratory distress in adults. Lancet 1967;2:319–23.

[2] Needham DM, Davidson J, Cohen H, et al. Improving long-term outcomes after discharge from intensive care unit: report from a stakeholders' conference. Crit Care Med 2012;40:502–9.

[3] Shankar-Hari M, Harrison DA, Ferrando-Vivas P, et al. Risk factors at index & hospitalization associated with longer-term mortality in adult sepsis survivors. JAMA Netw Open 2019;2:e194900.

[4] Roquilly A, Jacqueline C, Davieau M, et al. Alveolar macrophages are & epigenetically altered after inflammation, leading to long-term lung immuno- paralysis. Nat Immunol 2020;21:636–48.

[5] Roquilly A, McWilliam HEG, Jacqueline C, et al. Local modulation of antigen- presenting cell development after resolution of pneumonia induces long-term susceptibility to secondary infections. Immunity 2017;47. 135–147.e135.

[6] Zorio V, Venet F, Delwarde B, et al. Assessment of sepsis-induced immuno- suppression at ICU discharge and 6 months after ICU discharge. Ann Intensive Care 2017; 7:80.

[7] Rubio I, Osuchowski MF, Shankar-Hari M, et al. Current gaps in sepsis immunology: new opportunities for translational research. Lancet Infect Dis 2019;19:e422–36.

[8] Riche F, Chousterman BG, Valleur P, et al. Protracted immune disorders at one year after ICU discharge in patients with septic shock. Crit Care 2018;22:42.

[9] Yende S, Kellum JA, Talisa VB, et al. Long-term host immune response trajectories among hospitalized patients with sepsis. JAMA Netw Open 2019;2:e198686.

[10] Corrales-Medina VF, Madjid M, Musher DM. Role of acute infection in triggering acute coronary syndromes. Lancet Infect Dis 2010;10(2):83–92.

[11] Corrales-Medina VF, Musher DM, Shachkina S, Chirinos JA. Acute pneumonia and the cardiovascular system. Lancet (London, England) 2013;381(9865): 496–505.

[12] Yende S, D'Angelo G, Kellum JA, et al. Inflammatory markers at hospital discharge predict subsequent mortality after pneumonia and sepsis. Am J Respir Crit Care Med 2008;177(11):1242–7.

[13] Yende S, D'Angelo G, Mayr F, et al. Elevated hemostasis markers after pneumonia increases one-year risk of all-cause and cardiovascular deaths. PLoS One 2011;6(8): e22847.

[14] Corrales-Medina VF, Alvarez KN, Weissfeld LA, et al. Association between hospitalization for pneumonia and subsequent risk of cardiovascular disease. JAMA 2015; 313(3):264−74.

[15] Yende S, Linde-Zwirble W, Mayr F, Weissfeld LA, Reis S, Angus DC. Risk of cardiovascular events in survivors of severe sepsis. Am J Respir Crit Care Med 2014;189(9): 1065−74.

[16] Wunsch H, Angus DC, Harrison DA. Linde-zwirb in the United States and United Kingdom. Am J Respir Crit Care Med 2011;183:1666−73. le WT, Rowan KM. Comparison of medical admissions to intensive care units.

[17] Kahn JM, Benson NM, Appleby D, Carson SS, Iwashyna TJ. Long-term acute care hospital utilization after critical illness. JAMA 2010;303:2253−9.

[18] Keenan SP, Dodek P, Chan K, et al. Intensive care unit admission has minimal impact on long-term mortality. Crit Care Med 2002;30:501−7.

[19] Dragsted L. Outcome from intensive care. A five year study of 1,308 patients. Dan Med Bull 1991;38:365−74.

[20] Wright JC, Plenderleith L, Ridley SA. Long-term survival following intensive care: subgroup analysis and comparison with the general population. Anaesthesia 2003;58: 637−42.

[21] Williams TA, Dobb GJ, Finn JC, et al. Determinants of long-term survival after intensive care. Crit Care Med 2008;36:1523−30.

[22] Dyson A, Singer M. Animal models of sepsis: why does preclinical efficacy fail to translate to the clinical setting? Crit Care Med 2009;37:S30−7.

[23] Seok J, Warren HS, Cuenca AG, et al. Genomic responses in mouse models poorly mimic human inflammatory diseases. Proc Natl Acad Sci USA 2013;110:3507−12.

[24] Perel P, Roberts I, Sena E, et al. Comparison of treatment effects between animal experiments and clinical trials: systematic review. BMJ 2007;334:197.

[25] Fisher M, Feuerstein G, Howells DW, et al. Update of the stroke therapy academic industry roundtable preclinical recommendations. Stroke 2009;40:2244−50.

[26] Iwashyna TJ, Ely EW, Smith DM, Langa KM. Long-term cognitive impairment and functional disability among survivors of severe sepsis. JAMA 2010;304:1787−94.

[27] Kowalkowski M, Chou SH, McWilliams A, et al. Structured, proactive care coordination versus usual care for Improving Morbidity during Post-Acute Care Transitions for Sepsis (IMPACTS): a pragmatic, randomized controlled trial. Trials 2019;20:660.

[28] Wu A, Gao F. Long-term outcomes in survivors from critical illness. Anaesthesia 2004;59:1049−52.

[29] Gill TM, Feinstein AR. A critical appraisal of the quality of quality-of-life measurements. JAMA 1994;272: 619−26.

[30] McPeake J, Mikkelsen ME, Quasim T, et al. Return to employment after critical illness and its association with psychosocial outcomes. a systematic review and meta-analysis. Ann Am Thorac Soc 2019;16:1304−11.

[31] Hauschildt KE, Seigworth C, Kamphuis LA, et al. Financial toxicity after acute & respiratory distress syndrome: a National Qualitative Cohort Study. Crit Care Med 2020;48:1103.

[32] Kerckhoffs MC, Kosasi FFL, Soliman IW, et al. Determinants of self-reported & unacceptable outcome of intensive care treatment 1 year after discharge. Intensive Care Med 2019;45:806−14.

[33] Prescott HC, Angus DC. Enhancing recovery from sepsis. JAMA 2018;319:62−75.

[34] Taylor SP, Chou SH, Sierra MF, et al. Association between adherence to & recommended care and outcomes for adult survivors of sepsis. Ann Am Thorac Soc 2020;17: 89−97.

[35] Coe AB, Vincent BM, Iwashyna TJ. Statin discontinuation and new antipsychotic use after an acute hospital stay vary by hospital. PLoS One 2020;15:e0232707.

[36] Bell CM, Brener SS, Gunraj N, et al. Association of ICU or hospital admission with unintentional discontinuation of medications for chronic diseases. JAMA 2011;306: 840−7.

[37] Scales DC, Fischer HD, Li P, et al. Unintentional continuation of medications intended for acute illness after hospital discharge: a population-based cohort study. J Gen Intern Med 2016;31:196−202.

[38] Ravn-Nielsen LV, Duckert ML, Lund ML, et al. Effect of an in-hospital multifaceted clinical pharmacist intervention on the risk of readmission: a randomized clinical trial. JAMA Intern Med 2018;178:375−82.

[39] Schofield-Robinson OJ, Lewis SR, Smith AF, et al. Follow-up services for improving long-term outcomes in intensive care unit (ICU) survivors. Cochrane Database Syst Rev 2018;11:CD012701.

[40] McPeake J, Boehm LM, Hibbert E, et al. Key components of ICU recovery programs: what did patients report provided benefit? Crit Care Explor 2020;2:e0088.

[41] Konig C, Matt B, Kortgen A, et al. What matters most to sepsis survivors: a & qualitative analysis to identify specific health-related quality of life domains. Qual Life Res 2019;28:637−47.

[42] Haines KJ, Beesley SJ, Hopkins RO, et al. Peer support in critical care: a systematic review. Crit Care Med 2018;46: 1522−31.

[43] Haines KJ, McPeake J, Hibbert E, et al. Enablers and barriers to implementing ICU follow-up clinics and peer support groups following critical illness: the thrive collaboratives. Crit Care Med 2019;47:1194−200.

[44] Geense WW, van den Boogaard M, van der Hoeven JG, et al. Nonpharmacologic interventions to prevent or mitigate adverse long-term outcomes among ICU survivors: a systematic review and meta-analysis. Crit Care Med 2019; 47:1607−18.

[45] Rahmel T, Schmitz S, Nowak H, et al. Long-term mortality and outcome in hospital survivors of septic shock, sepsis, and severe infections: the importance of aftercare. PLoS One 2020;15:e0228952.

[46] Deb P, Murtaugh CM, Bowles KH, et al. Does early follow-up improve the outcomes of sepsis survivors discharged to home healthcare? Med Care 2019;57:633—40.

[47] Varela M, Ruiz-Esteban R, De Juan M. Chaos, fractals, and our concept of disease. Perspect Biology Med 2010;53:584—95.

[48] Lipsitz LA, Goldberger AL. Loss of 'complexity' and aging. Potential applications of fractals and chaos theory to senescence. JAMA 1992;267:1806—9.

[49] Yates FE. Complexity of a human being: changes with age. Neurobiol Aging 2002;23:17—9.

[50] Fried LP, Tangen CM, Walston J, et al. Frailty in older adults: evidence for a phenotype. J Gerontol A Biol Sci Med Sci 2001;56:M146—56.

[51] Weiss CO. Frailty and chronic diseases in older adults. Clin Geriatr Med 2011;27:39—52.

[52] Chaves PH, Varadhan R, Lipsitz LA, et al. Physiological complexity underlying heart rate dynamics and frailty status in community-dwelling older women. J Am Geriatr Soc 2008;56:1698—703.

[53] Kang HG, Costa MD, Priplata AA, et al. Frailty and the degradation of complex balance dynamics during a dual-task protocol. J Gerontol A Biol Sci Med Sci 2009;64:1304—11.

[54] Rothman MD, Leo-Summers L, Gill TM. Prognostic significance of potential frailty criteria. J Am Geriatr Soc 2008;56:2211—6.

[55] Folstein MF, Folstein SE, McHugh PR. 'Mini-mental state'. A practical method for grading the cognitive state of patients for the clinician. J Psychiatr Res 1975;12:189—98.

[56] de Vries NM, Staal JB, van Ravensberg CD, Hobbelen JS, Olde Rikkert MG, Nijhuis-van der Sanden MW. Outcome instruments to measure frailty: a systematic review. Ageing Res Rev 2011;10:104—14.

[57] Rockwood K, Andrew M, Mitnitski A. A comparison of two approaches to measuring frailty in elderly people. J Gerontol A Biol Sci Med Sci 2007;62:738—43.

[58] Seely AJ, Christou NV. Multiple organ dysfunction syndrome: exploring the paradigm of complex nonlinear systems. Crit Care Med 2000;28:2193—200.

[59] McDermid RC, Bagshaw SM. Frailty: a new conceptual framework in critical care medicine. In: Vincent JL, editor. Annual update in intensive care and emergency medicine. Berlin: Springer; 2011. p. 117—9.

[60] Van der Schaaf M, Dettling DS, Beelen A, Lucas C, Dongelmans DA, Nollet F. Poor functional status immediately after discharge from an intensive care unit. Disabil Rehabil 2008;30:1812—8.

[61] Ferreira FL, Bota DP, Bross A, Melot C, Vincent JL. Serial evaluation of the SOFA score to predict outcome in critically ill patients. JAMA 2001;286:1754—8.

[62] Copeland-Fields L, Griffin T, Jenkins T, Buckley M, Wise LC. Comparison of outcome predictions made by physicians, by nurses, and by using the Mortality Prediction Model. Am J Crit Care 2001;10:313—9.

[63] Frick S, Uehlinger DE, Zuercher Zenklusen RM. Medical futility: predicting outcome of intensive care unit patients by nurses and doctors—a prospective comparative study. Crit Care Med 2003;31:456—61.

[64] Sinuff T, Adhikari NK, Cook DJ, et al. Mortality predictions in the intensive care unit: comparing physicians with scoring systems. Crit Care Med 2006;34:878—85.

[65] Rocker G, Cook D, Sjokvist P, et al. Clinician predictions of intensive care unit mortality. Crit Care Med 2004;32:1149—54. 59.

[66] Jones C, Backman C, Capuzzo M, et al. Intensive care diaries reduce new onset post traumatic stress disorder following critical illness: a randomised, controlled trial. Crit Care 2010;14:R168.

[67] Schweickert WD, Pohlman MC, Pohlman AS, et al. Early physical and occupational therapy in mechanically ventilated, critically ill patients: a randomised controlled trial. Lancet 2009;373:1874—82.

[68] Girard TD, Jackson JC, Pandharipande PP, et al. Delirium as a predictor of long-term cognitive impairment in survivors of critical illness. Crit Care Med 2010;38:1513—20.

[69] Azoulay E, Pochard F, Kentish-Barnes N, et al. Risk of post-traumatic stress symptoms in family members of intensive care unit patients. Am J Respir Crit Care Med 2005;171:987—94.

CHAPTER 34

New Diagnostic and Therapeutic Perspectives

JUAN CARLOS RUIZ-RODRÍGUEZ • LUIS CHISCANO-CAMÓN •
ERIKA-PAOLA PLATA MENCHACA • RICARD FERRER

INTRODUCTION

In recent years, new initiatives to improve the diagnosis and treatment of sepsis have been developed. Precision medicine brings a new approach to patient management, allowing specific subgroups of patients to benefit from specific therapeutic strategies that could not be idoneous for the general population of sepsis patients. Among various promising instruments under investigation, which may serve as diagnostic or therapeutic tools, advances in nanotechnology have played a significant role. Herein, new developments for the management of sepsis, the role of precision medicine, and current opportunities for its implementation will be reviewed.

THE ROLE OF TRANSLATIONAL RESEARCH

Translational research facilitates the advent of new diagnostic and therapeutic tools that could be useful in clinical practice. These tools are based on discoveries in basic science and take advantage of a new paradigm for the management of sepsis and its related processes: precision medicine. The scope of the development of translational research initiatives in sepsis is outstanding, needing interdisciplinary work between basic and clinical research teams (Fig. 34.1). Although routine laboratory tests can address several questions that surge at the bedside, the development of new technologies and advances in molecular biology can also impact daily clinical practice.

Translational Research in the Understanding of Sepsis Pathophysiology

Among the mechanisms underlying sepsis-induced cellular dysfunction, various interesting issues are being assessed. Specific abnormalities have been described in the majority of organ systems that are affected by sepsis. The most striking evidence has shown that sepsis causes a major insult that leads to the failure of different cellular forms irrespective of their specialization. However, does a common global defect underlie all forms of sepsis-induced cellular dysfunction? Are there particular mechanisms of failure? Do cells of the same embryologic origin become dysfunctional in a different way from other cell types? Do specialized cells with comparable functions develop unique forms of dysfunction that differ from cells with different differentiation? Since endothelial cells are present in virtually all organ systems, does endothelial cell dysfunction in a particular organ determines endothelial dysfunction in another organ system? Besides, there is cross talk between various structures that modulate organ function.

The mechanisms of sepsis recovery have been scantily studied, creating a field of interest in basic sepsis translational research [1]. What mechanisms and specific intermediaries are pivotal in sepsis recovery? What cellular and subcellular metabolic, energetic, immune, endocrine, intestinal, neuronal, and vascular mechanisms mediate sepsis recovery? Can subcellular, cellular, tissue, or organ-specific dysfunction be improved or mitigated by stimulating the main recovery pathways? Can the degree and duration of sepsis recovery be modulated? [2] The approach to these uncertainties will help solve clinical questions and guide research priorities in sepsis and septic shock.

Sepsis-induced immunosuppression, or immunoparalysis, is triggered and promoted by elevated levels of endotoxin and antiinflammatory cytokines [3,4]. However, there is a lack of knowledge regarding its pathophysiology, prevention, diagnosis, and treatment.

The Sepsis Codex. https://doi.org/10.1016/B978-0-323-88271-2.00015-8

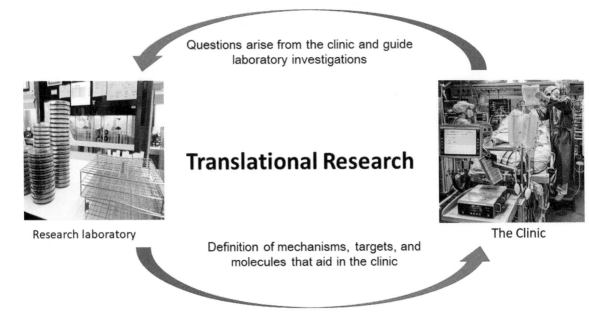

Questions arise from the clinic and guide
laboratory investigations

Translational Research

Research laboratory

The Clinic

Definition of mechanisms, targets, and
molecules that aid in the clinic

FIG. 34.1 Role of translational research. Basic science research engages clinical practice and vice versa.

Several studies have found reactivations of viruses in critically ill patients were not related to a previous immunosuppression state, and its presence has been associated with adverse outcomes [5]. In a study of 560 critically ill sepsis patients, the authors reported that critically ill sepsis patients had high cumulative viral DNA detection rates in the blood (cytomegalovirus [24%], Epstein–Barr virus [53%], herpes simplex virus [14%], human herpes virus-6 [10%], and torque teno virus [78%]) [6] when compared with noncritically ill and age-matched healthy controls. Well-designed studies are necessary to delineate the role and clinical relevance (if any) of pharmacological prophylaxis against viral reactivations in critically ill sepsis patients.

Translational Research and Improvements in Conventional Sepsis Treatment

Administration of intravenous fluids during sepsis resuscitation improves hemodynamics and tissue perfusion; it is considered a cornerstone of treatment and one of the main pillars of sepsis management [7]. However, previous studies have not been designed to demonstrate the importance of intravenous fluids administration during the initial treatment of the different subgroups of patients according to their severity. The best intravenous fluid for early sepsis resuscitation is unknown. Individualized fluid management should be determined when considering the heterogeneity of sepsis patients, as it will improve patient outcomes.

The achievement of pharmacokinetic (PK) and pharmacodynamic (PD) targets is essential for antibiotic stewardship in critically ill patients [8]. Recommendations on dosing and timing of antibiotics were formerly based on studies performed in the general population [9]. This is not adequate for patients with sepsis and septic shock, in whom antimicrobial stewardship should be managed differently. Numerous studies report variations in PK/PD in patients with septic shock; its effect on bacteriological effectiveness and patient outcomes remains to be elucidated. In addition, there is low-quality evidence supporting the use of combined empiric antibiotic treatment, although early antibiotic treatment has been associated with decreased mortality in septic shock [10]. Adequately designed randomized controlled trials should evaluate whether combination therapy is useful to decrease mortality in septic shock. Similar to antimicrobial stewardship, the early diagnosis of sepsis could reduce mortality, shorten the duration of hospitalization, and lower costs [11].

Future directions regarding early diagnosis strategies and most conventional and adjuvant therapies for sepsis are yet to be shaped [12]. Sepsis banks are biomedical research support units that comprise a resource for the development of translational biomedical research on sepsis. In these banks, blood, plasma, and serum samples are obtained from sepsis patients to obtain information on biomarkers. Furthermore, bedside evaluations of the immune system function, the performance of microbiological rapid diagnostic tests may help identify the causing organism and immune system dysregulation. Clinical data should be available for the scientific community to improve knowledge, diagnosis, prevention, and treatment of sepsis [13]. A more comprehensive clinical approach may provide new insights on sepsis management.

NEW MOLECULES FOR ADJUVANT TREATMENT OF SEPSIS

Translational science research has contributed to the study of several molecules in phase II—III clinical trials.

Nangibotide

Human TREM-1 (Triggering Receptor Expressed on Myeloid Cells) is a 30-kDa glycoprotein of the immunoglobulin superfamily. TREM-1 is expressed at late stages of myeloid cell differentiation [14], and it associates with DAP12 for signaling and function [15]. TREM-1 amplifies Toll-like receptor (TLR)-initiated responses against microbial challenges and potentiates the secretion of proinflammatory chemokines and cytokines in response to bacterial and fungal infections. Blockade of TREM-1 reduces inflammation and increases survival in animal models of bacterial sepsis. Nangibotide is a 12 amino acid peptidic fragment derived from TREM-like transcript-1 (TELT-1), a receptor protein of TREM-1 family. Nangibotide can bind to TREM-1 ligand and modulate the amplification of the immune response caused by the activation of TREM-1 in sepsis.

In preclinical animal studies performed in peritonitis with septic shock patients, analogs of nangibotide showed an improvement of inflammatory response and organ function, cardiovascular status, and survival [16,17]. In a recent phase IIa clinical trial that investigated the safety and tolerability of three doses of nangibotide in septic shock, nangibotide-treated patients improved organ function biomarkers. This effect was larger in the subgroup of patients with high circulating soluble TREM-1 (sTREM-1) levels. A phase 2b clinical trial is currently being conducted to evaluate its efficacy, safety, and tolerability in patients with septic shock (efficacy, safety, and tolerability of nangibotide in patients with septic shock) (ASTONISH, ClinicalTrials.gov NCT04055909) [18].

Recombinant Alkaline Phosphatase

Alkaline phosphatase (AP) is an endogenous homodimeric enzyme present in many cells and organs (e.g., intestines, placenta, liver, bone, kidney, and granulocytes) that exerts detoxifying effects through dephosphorylation of endotoxins and other proinflammatory compounds, including extracellular adenosine triphosphate by hydrolysis [19,20]. AP may also attenuate the innate immune response induced by endotoxin release, as dephosphorylation of endotoxin abolishes its biological activity and the dephosphorylated LPS acts as a TLR 4 antagonist [21]. In animal models of sepsis, the AP administration attenuates the inflammatory response and reduces mortality [22].

There are some trials evaluating the effects of AP in sepsis (STOP-AKI). The Safety, Tolerability, Efficacy, and QoL Study of Human recAP in the treatment of patients with sepsis-associated acute kidney injury trial is a double-blind, placebocontrolled, dose-finding adaptive phase 2a/2b trial that enrolled 301 adults with sepsis-associated acute kidney injury [23]. The optimal therapeutic dose of recombinant AP was 1.6 mg/kg. The three-day treatment did not improve kidney function in the first week of treatment, but all-cause mortality at day 28 was lower in recombinant AP group versus placebo (14.4% vs. 26.7%, difference 12.3% [95% CI, 1.9%—22.7%]; $P = .02$). This effect persisted to day 90 (17.1% vs. 29.3%, difference 12.2% [95% CI, 1.3%—23.0%]; $P = .03$) [23]. A clinical phase 3 study, the REVIVAL phase III pivotal trial (ClinicalTrials.gov Identifier: NCT04411472), to investigate the effect of recombinant AP on 28-day mortality in patients with sepsis-associated acute kidney injury is underway.

Adrecizumab

Adrenomedullin (ADM), a 52 amino acid peptide belonging to the calcitonin gene-related peptide family [24], plays an important role in sepsis. ADM has immunomodulation and endothelial barrier-stabilizing properties, maintaining vascular integrity [25]. Its tropism for the vascular endothelium, interstitium, and smooth muscle, and its vasodilatory properties may contribute to sepsis hypotension and increased vascular permeability. At high concentrations, ADM leads to excessive vasodilation, and increased plasma levels of ADM are associated with high vasopressor requirements, multiorgan dysfunction, and mortality [26—28].

Adrecizumab (HAM8101) is a nonneutralizing anti-ADM antibody with epitope specificity for the N-terminal moiety of ADM. By binding to ADM, adrecizumab does not entirely block ADM function, though it reduces its capacity to elicit a second messenger response. Under normal conditions, the concentration of ADM is higher in the interstitium than in the circulating blood. The net effect is an increase of adrecizumab-bound ADM in the blood circulation, pulled from the interstitium, and only partial functional inhibition of ADM. Because of this redistribution, the ADM concentration in the interstitium decreases, and ADM cannot act on smooth muscle cells to exert its vasodilatory activity. Thus, adrecizumab can reduce vasodilation by subtracting excessive levels of interstitially located ADM. The increased net activity of ADM in the blood circulation could promote stabilization of endothelial permeability [29].

Preclinical studies performed in a porcine model of sepsis have shown that the administration of adrecizumab reduced the progression to septic shock, renal granulocyte extravasation, and inflammatory response [30]. The AdrenOSS-2 study, a phase 2a double-blind, randomized, placebocontrolled biomarker-guided trial, addressed the safety and tolerability of adrecizumab in patients with septic shock and elevated plasma concentrations of circulating biologically active ADM (>70 pg/mL) [31]. Adrecizumab was well tolerated and showed a favorable safety profile. Although it was not the primary objective of the study, an improvement in multiorgan dysfunction was observed. A subsequent study, the ENCOURAGE study, is a phase IIb/III clinical trial that will assess adrecizumab (4 mg/kg) in septic shock patients immediately after initiation of vasopressors. Interestingly, this study combines predictive and prognostic enrichment strategies with the primary objective of reducing 28-day mortality and the SOFA score.

Apoptotic Cells

Allocetra-OTS (early apoptotic cells) is a cell-based therapeutic composed of donor apoptotic cells. The product contains allogeneic mononuclear enriched cells in a liquid suspension with at least 40% early apoptotic cells. The apoptotic cells contribute to the maintenance of peripheral immune homeostasis. Allocetra-OTS was shown to have a beneficial effect on cytokine storms with downregulation of both anti- and proinflammatory cytokines. Experimental animal models have demonstrated that the apoptotic cell infusion in mice is associated with a reduction in circulating proinflammatory cytokines, suppression of polymorphonuclear neutrophil infiltration in target organs, decreased serum LPS levels, and decreased mortality [32]. Van Heerden et al. performed a phase Ib clinical trial with Allocetra-OTS in 10 patients with sepsis and SOFA scores ranging from 2 to 6 [33]. All 10 patients survived, while matched historical controls had a mortality rate of 27%. They concluded that infusion of apoptotic cells to patients with mild-to-moderate sepsis was safe and had a significant immunomodulating effect, leading to early resolution of the cytokine storm.

A phase II study evaluating the efficacy, safety, and tolerability of different doses and regimens of Allocetra-OTS to treat organ failure in sepsis patients (NCT04612413) is currently underway.

Seraph 100 Microbind Affinity Blood Filter

A promising new therapeutic strategy is hemoperfusion with Seraph 100 Microbind Affinity Blood Filter (Seraph 100) (ExThera Medical Corporation, Martinez, CA, USA). Seraph 100 is an extracorporeal broad-spectrum adsorbent hemoperfusion device to reduce pathogens (bacteria, viruses, and fungi) and cytokines from the bloodstream. It has a functional core formed by ultra-high molecular weight polyethylene beads, modified to contain end-point attached heparin on the surface, mimicking a naturally mammalian cell surface. The heparin-binding proteins are common in bacteria; therefore, similar binding properties are presupposed within the filter due to charge interactions [34]. Some studies have shown that *Staphylococcus aureus*, including methicillin-resistant *S. aureus* (MRSA), adheres to the heparinized beads [35,36]. In patients with bacteremia, hemoperfusion with Seraph 100 induces a significant reduction of bacterial load with a significant increase in time to positivity in blood cultures (ClinicalTrials.gov Identifier: NCT02914132). A new study (Reduction of Pathogen Load From the Blood in Septic Patients with Suspected, life-threatening bloodstream infection, ClinicalTrials.gov Identifier: NCT04260789) is underway.

CALO2

CALO2, a novel antitoxin agent, is a mixture of liposomes that can capture bacterial toxins responsible for inflammation and organ injury.

Preclinical data show that CALO2 improves survival in mice with severe pneumonia and bacteremia combined with antibiotics. Laterre et al. performed the first-in-human, double-blind, dose-escalation, placebo-controlled, randomized trial in patients with severe community-acquired pneumococcal pneumonia who required intensive care unit (ICU) admission and had been identified as being infected with *Streptococcus pneumoniae* [37]. Patients were assigned to two stages (low-dose CAL02 or placebo and high-dose CAL02 or placebo). CALO2 was safe and well tolerated. A trend to a faster resolution was observed in the high-dose CAL02 group for the clinical cure at the early test of cure, time to cure, change in SOFA score, inflammatory biomarkers, and ICU length of stay. These results suggest a new strategy for the treatment of sepsis and provide a solid basis for a larger clinical study.

NANOTECHNOLOGY

The emergence of nanotechnology and its incorporation into precision medicine have allowed proposing new solutions to improve the diagnosis and treatment of sepsis.

Nanodiagnosis of Sepsis

Nanotechnology can aid in the development of fast, sensitive, and accurate methods for sepsis detection. Several nanoparticles (NPs) have been investigated to improve the diagnosis of sepsis: magnetic (MNPs), gold (AuNPs), fluorescent (silica and quantum dots), and lipid-based NPs.

AuNPs are the most used due to their easy chemical and tunable optical properties. Various technologies have been proposed for the detection of microorganisms. Storhoff et al. developed a colorimetric detection method for identifying nucleic acid sequences based on the distance-dependent optical properties of AuNPs. The authors applied this method to the rapid detection of *mecA* gene in MRSA genomic DNA samples with good results [38]. The qualitative identification of gram-positive microorganisms and genes associated with bacterial infection is possible with silver-enhanced AuNPs (Verigene test, Nanosphere Inc, IL, USA) [39]. Dey et al. detected *Escherichia coli* with a point-of-care device inspired by lens-free interferometric microscopy, encompassing a plasmonic Au nanohole substrate and custom microarrays [40]. Also, it is possible to detect *S. aureus* with diffusometric DNA nanosensors, composed of 200 nm fluorescent polystyrene beads sandwiched with MRSA and 80 nm AuNPs oligonucleotide probes [41].

Nanotechnology also allows the early detection of sepsis biomarkers. Belushkin et al. developed a portable digital AuNPs-enhanced plasmonic imager that enables rapid detection of procalcitonin (PCT) and C-reactive protein [42].

Nanotreatment Technologies for Sepsis

Nanoscale drug delivery platforms have proven to enhance the blood circulation time of antimicrobial agents, overcome the predominant issue of underdosing, and minimize the arising adverse side effects [43,44]. Additionally, alternative antisepsis "nano" therapeutic strategies have been explored using NPs to enable lipopolysaccharide neutralization, blood purification (from inflammatory mediators, pathogens, and endotoxins), TLR inhibition, and immune system modulation (immunomodulatory NPs).

Nanotherapeutics have also developed antimicrobial adjuvants. There is a class of NPs, metal and metal oxide NPs, such as silver (AgNPs), zinc oxide, copper oxide, titanium oxide, and aluminum oxide that possess inherent antimicrobial properties [45]. AgNPs, often called nanoantibiotics [46], serve as antibacterial agents against gram-negative, gram-positive, and drug-resistant pathogens. The mechanisms behind AgNPs bactericidal activity remain unclear. NP-based antimicrobial delivery has also been demonstrated to overcome the predominant issues of biofilms and intracellular microbes. Biofilm-forming bacteria are characterized by a rigid structure that blocks the entrance of antimicrobial agents [47]. For instance, the encapsulation of antibiotics with lipid- and polymer-based NPs acts as a protective shield from enzymes and improves antimicrobial efficacies against biofilm-forming bacteria [48]. AmBisome, Abelcet, and Amphotec, which are different liposomal formulations of the same antifungal agent, amphotericin B, are additional nanotechnology applications to eliminate fungi.

Nanotechnology can improve the PKs of antibiotics through engineered targeted NP-based drug delivery systems. For instance, the surface modification of NPs with molecules that selectively bind to specific receptors onto bacterial walls can enhance the accumulation of a higher dose of antibiotic at the desired spot and minimize toxicity [49].

Another therapeutic strategy is the nanoinhibition of TLR signaling. Nanoantagonists can modulate and suppress TLR signaling [50]. Several cationic lipids have been recognized for their TLR4 modulating activity, including positively charged liposomes formed by cationic amphiphiles. Peptide-AuNP hybrids inhibit TLR4-signaling, acting as antiinflammatory agents [51]. The nanoimmunomodulation can reprogram the immune system to block the uncontrollable secretion of inflammatory cytokines by specifically targeting inflammatory immune cells.

Nanotheranostics Technologies for Sepsis

The recently developed nanoplatforms could be useful for the diagnosis and treatment of sepsis simultaneously. AuNPs present optical and thermal properties with diagnostic and therapeutic applications. Zharov et al. developed an in vitro thermal-based laser method for the simultaneous detection and clearance of *S. aureus* using AuNPs conjugated with antiprotein A antibodies [52]. Carbon nanotubes also have nanotheranostic proprieties. Their high binding affinity to bacteria surfaces and their strong absorbance in near-infrared enable bacteria elimination by efficiently converting laser energy into thermal energy.

FUTURE DIRECTIONS

Sepsis management comprises well-structured and protocolized interventions that undergo continuous revising. The 2021 Surviving Sepsis Campaign (SSC) guidelines summarize the best available evidence for sepsis management. Although the scientific community is aware that implementing the SSC guidelines recommendations is associated with a reduction in mortality [53], sepsis mortality remains unacceptably high [54]. All patients should receive the fundamental pillars of sepsis treatment: infection control, initial resuscitation, and multiorgan support. Still, it is also possible that certain subpopulations of patients may benefit from specific therapies.

There is significant heterogeneity in sepsis, which can be anticipated due to the existing differences in age, causing microorganisms, type of focus, and patient comorbidities. There are two different stages in the inflammatory response at the pathophysiological level: the proinflammatory response and the antiinflammatory response. These may vary among individuals or within the same individual, depending on the continuum of severity ranging that patient is going through.

As a consequence of sepsis heterogeneity, clinical progression in sepsis differs among patients. Low-risk patients may receive conventional management to ensure a good prognosis, though high-risk patients, who may progress to organ dysfunction and death, may require adjuvant-specific therapies based on their pathophysiological characteristics (Fig. 34.2). All this gives rise to the development of precision medicine in sepsis to individualize the management of septic patients and try to identify different endotypes or subgroups of patients based on genetic or biological differences. Precision medicine allows the characterization of homogeneous subgroups of patients who experience similar evolutionary patterns and responses to specific treatments.

Recently, new technologies to detect different evolutionary patterns or in response to several therapies have been developed. The "omic" platforms (e.g., proteomics, metabolomics, transcriptomics, genomics, epigenetics, and bioinformatics) aid in selecting specific endotypes or phenotypes of sepsis patients that are indistinguishable from a clinical point of view. Also, they provide the basis for tailoring therapies to the different endotypes or

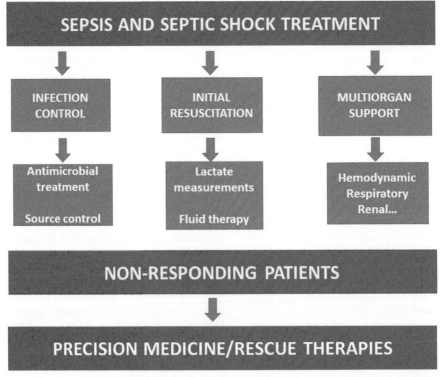

FIG. 34.2 Precision medicine and rescue therapies in sepsis patients nonresponders to conventional therapy.

PRECISION MEDICINE IN SEPSIS

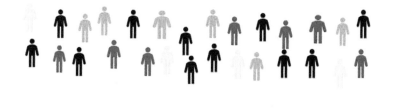

| Procalcitonin | Immunoglobulins | EAA | IL-6 |

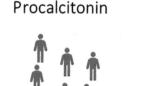 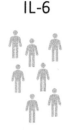

| Vitamin C, hidrocortisone and thiamine combination therapy | Immunoglobulin therapy | Endotoxin Hemoadsorption | Cytokine Hemoadsorption |

FIG. 34.3 Current tools for Precision Medicine in sepsis.   *EAA*, endotoxin activity assay; *IL-6*, interleukin 6.

phenotypes of patients [55−61]. The "omic" profiles are not yet routinely available in clinics.

Biomarkers have been suggested as means of aiding the early diagnosis of sepsis. They are clinical tools to recognize particular subpopulations of patients and to predict their prognosis or response to certain treatments. Plasma levels of PCT, immunoglobulins, and interleukin 6 (IL-6), and the endotoxin activity assay (EAA) (Fig. 34.3) are among the most used biomarkers. PCT, a widely available test, allows the identification of patients with hyperinflammatory profiles who could benefit from high-dose vasopressors, vitamin C, hydrocortisone, and thiamine [62]. Immunoglobulin profile is useful to identify patients with primary or sepsis-induced hypogammaglobulinemia that could be candidates to receive adjuvant treatment with immunoglobulins [63], although it is controversial. IL-6 levels are increased in some patients that could benefit from cytokine hemoadsorption. Hemoadsorption may have a role as rescue therapy in a particular subgroup of patients with refractory septic shock, hyperlactatemia, multiorgan failure, and extreme hypercytokinemia. Patients with refractory septic shock and severe multiorgan dysfunction, with adequate control of the focus and EAA 0.6−0.9, could be candidates for endotoxin hemoadsorption [64].

The early sepsis identification in preclinical stages has become a ubiquitous need that should be further refined in the near future. Technological advances on real-time clinical and physiological monitoring platforms equipped with artificial intelligence have been helpful to detect sepsis early in hospitalized patients by displaying alerts to clinical teams. Identifying early biomarkers by analyzing databases of sepsis banks will also contribute to the predictive enrichment of clinical decision support systems. The implementation of point-of-care devices for the determination of new biomarkers and causing microorganisms and their resistance mechanisms will allow the early initiation of therapeutic measures for sepsis [40,42].

REFERENCES

[1] Perner A, Gordon AC, Angus DC, Lamontagne F, Machado F, Russell JA, Timsit JF, Marshall JC, Myburgh J, Shankar-Hari M, Singer M. The intensive care medicine research agenda on septic shock. Intensive Care Med 2017;43(9):1294−305.

[2] Cohen J, Vincent JL, Adhikari NK, Machado FR, Angus DC, Calandra T, Jaton K, Giulieri S, Delaloye J, Opal S, Tracey K, van der Poll T, Pelfrene E. Sepsis: a roadmap for future research. Lancet Infect Dis 2015;15:581–614.

[3] Boomer JS, To K, Chang KC, et al. Immunosuppression in patients who die of sepsis and multiple organ failure. JAMA 2011;306:2594.

[4] Hotchkiss RS, Coopersmith CM, McDunn JE, Ferguson TA. The sepsis seesaw: tilting toward immunosuppression. Nat Med 2009;15:496–7.

[5] Papazian L, Hraiech S, Lehingue S, et al. Cytomegalovirus reactivation in ICU patients. Intensive Care Med 2016;42: 28–37.

[6] Walton AH, Muenzer JT, Rasche D, et al. Reactivation of multiple viruses in patients with sepsis. PLoS One 2014; 9:e98819.

[7] Cecconi M, De Backer D, Antonelli M, et al. Consensus on circulatory shock and hemodynamic monitoring. Task force of the European Society of Intensive Care Medicine. Intensive Care Med 2014;40:1795–815.

[8] Roberts JA, Abdul-Aziz MH, Davis JS, Dulhunty JM, Cotta MO, Myburgh J, Bellomo R, Lipman J. Continuous versus Intermittent betalactam infusion in severe sepsis. A meta-analysis of individual patient data from randomized trials. Am J Respir Crit Care Med 2016;194:681–91.

[9] Ferrer R, Martin-Loeches I, Phillips G, Osborn TM, Townsend S, Dellinger RP, Artigas A, Schorr C, Levy MM. Empiric antibiotic treatment reduces mortality in severe sepsis and septic shock from the first hour: results from a guideline-based performance improvement program. Crit Care Med 2014;42:1749–55.

[10] Seymour CW, Gesten F, Prescott HC, Friedrich ME, Iwashyna TJ, Phillips GS, Lemeshow S, Osborn T, Terry KM, Levy MM. Time to treatment and mortality during mandated emergency care for sepsis. N Engl J Med 2017;376:2235–44.

[11] Huang AM, Newton D, Kunapuli A, Gandhi TN, Washer LL, Isip J, Collins CD, Nagel JL. Impact of rapid organism identification via matrix-assisted laser desorption/ionization time-of-flight combined with antimicrobial stewardship team intervention in adult patients with bacteremia and candidemia. Clin Infect Dis 2013; 57:1237–45.

[12] Coopersmith C, De Backer D, Deutschman C, Ferrer R, Ishaq L, Machado F, et al. Surviving sepsis campaign: research priorities for sepsis and septic shock. Intensive Care Med 2018;44:1400–26.

[13] Ferrer R, Ruiz-Rodriguez JC, Larrosa N, Llaneras J, Molas E, González-López JJ. Sepsis code implementation at Vall d'Hebron university hospital: rapid diagnostics key to success. ICU Manag Pract 2017;17(4):214–5.

[14] Bouchon A, Dietrich J, Colonna M. Cutting edge: inflammatory responses can be triggered by TREM1, a novel receptor expressed on neutrophils and monocytes. J Immunol 2000;164:4991–5.

[15] Lanier LL, Bakker AB. The ITAM-bearing transmembrane adaptor DAP12 in lymphoid and myeloid cell function. Immunol Today 2000;21:611–4.

[16] Derive M, Boufenzer A, Bouazza Y, Groubatch F, Alauzet C, Barraud D, Lozniewski A, Leroy P, Tran N, Gibot S. Effects of a TREM-like transcript 1-derived peptide during hypodynamic septic shock in pigs. Shock 2013;39:176–82.

[17] Derive M, Bouazza Y, Sennoun N, Marchionni S, Quigley L, Washington V, Massin F, Max JP, Ford J, Alauzet C, Levy B, McVicar DW, Gibot S. Soluble TREM-like transcript-1 regulates leukocyte activation and controls microbial load. J Immunol 2012;188:5585–92.

[18] Francois B, Lambden S, Gibot S, Derive M, Olivier A, Cuvier V, Witte S, Grouin JM, Garaud JJ, Salcedo-Magguilli M, Levy M, Laterre PF. Rationale and protocol for the efficacy, safety and tolerability of nangibotide in patients with septic shock (ASTONISH) phase IIb randomised controlled trial. BMJ Open 2021;11:e042921.

[19] Koyama I, Matsunaga T, Harada T, Hokari S, Komoda T. Alkaline phosphatases reduce toxicity of lipopolysaccharides in vivo and in vitro through dephosphorylation. Clin Biochem 2002;35:455–61.

[20] Bentala H, Verweij WR, Huizinga-Van der Vlag A, van Loenen-Weemaes AM, Meijer DK, Poelstra K. Removal of phosphate from lipid A as a strategy to detoxify lipopolysaccharide. Shock 2002;18:561566.

[21] Wy CA, Goto M, Young RI, Myers TF, Muraskas J. Prophylactic treatment of endotoxic shock with monophosphoryl lipid A in newborn rats. Biol Neonate 2000;77: 191–5.

[22] Su F, Brands R, Wang Z, et al. Beneficial effects of alkaline phosphatase in septic shock. Crit Care Med 2006;34: 2182–7.

[23] Pickkers P, Mehta RL, Murray PT, Joannidis M, Molitoris BA, Kellum JA, Bachler M, Hoste EAJ, Hoiting O, Krell K, Ostermann M, Rozendaal W, Valkonen M, Brealey D, Beishuizen A, Meziani F, Murugan R, de Geus H, Payen D, van den Berg E, Arend J, STOP-AKI Investigators. Effect of human recombinant alkaline phosphatase on 7-day creatinine clearance in patients with sepsis-associated acute kidney injury: a randomized clinical trial. JAMA 2018;320:1998–2009.

[24] Poyner DR, Sexton PM, Marshall I, Smith DM, Quirion R, Born W, et al. International Union of Pharmacology. XXXII. The mammalian calcitonin gene-related peptides, adrenomedullin, amylin, and calcitonin receptors. Pharmacol Rev 2002;54:233–46.

[25] Geven C, Kox M, Pickkers P. Adrenomedullin and adrenomedullin-targeted therapy as treatment strategies relevant for sepsis. Front Immunol 2018;9:292.

[26] Marino R, Struck J, Maisel AS, et al. Plasma adrenomedullin is associated with short-term mortality and vasopressor requirement in patients admitted with sepsis. Crit Care 2014;18:R34.

[27] Caironi P, Latini R, Struck J, Hartmann O, Bergmann A, Maggio G, Cavana M, Tognoni G, Pesenti A, Gattinoni L, Masson S, ALBIOS Study Investigators. Circulating biologically active adrenomedullin (bio-ADM) predicts hemodynamic support requirement and mortality during sepsis. Chest 2017;152:312–20.

[28] Nishio K, Akai Y, Murao Y, et al. Increased plasma concentrations of adrenomedullin correlate with relaxation of vascular tone in patients with septic shock. Crit Care Med 1997;25:953–7.

[29] Geven C, Pickkers P. The mechanism of action of the adrenomedullin-binding antibody adrecizumab. Crit Care 2018;22:159.

[30] Thiele C, Simon TP, Szymanski J, Daniel C, Golias C, Hartmann O, Struck J, Martin L, Marx G, Schuerholz T. Effects of the non-neutralizing humanized monoclonal anti-adrenomedullin antibody adrecizumab on hemodynamic and renal injury in a porcine two-hit model. Shock 2020;54:810–8.

[31] Laterre PF, Pickkers P, Marx G, Wittebole X, Meziani F, Dugernier T, et al. AdrenOSS-2 study participants. Safety and tolerability of nonneutralizing adrenomedullin antibody adrecizumab (HAM8101) in septic shock patients: the AdrenOSS-2 phase 2a biomarker-guided trial. Intensive Care Med November 2021;47(11):1284–94 [Epub ahead of print].

[32] Ren Y, Xie Y, Jiang G, Fan J, Yeung J, Li W, Tam PK, Savill J. Apoptotic cells protect mice against lipopolysaccharide-induced shock. J Immunol 2008;180:4978–85.

[33] van Heerden PV, Abutbul A, Sviri S, Zlotnick E, Nama A, Zimro S, El-Amore R, Shabat Y, Reicher B, Falah B, Mevorach D. Apoptotic cells for therapeutic use in cytokine storm associated with sepsis- a phase Ib clinical trial. Front Immunol 2021;12:718191.

[34] Seffer MT, Eden G, Engelmann S, Kielstein JT. Elimination of Staphylococcus aureus from the bloodstream using a novel biomimetic sorbent haemoperfusion device. BMJ Case Rep 2020;13:e235262.

[35] Mattsby-Baltzer I, Bergstrom T, McCrea K, Ward R, Adolfsson L, Larm O. Affinity apheresis for treatment of bacteremia caused by Staphylococcus aureus and/or methicillin-resistant S. aureus (MRSA). J Microbiol Biotechnol 2011;21:659–64.

[36] Henry BD, Neill DR, Becker KA, et al. Engineered liposomes sequester bacterial exotoxins and protect from severe invasive infections in mice. Nat Biotechnol 2015;33:81–8.

[37] Laterre PF, Colin G, Dequin PF, Dugernier T, Boulain T, Azeredo da Silveira S, Lajaunias F, Perez A, François B. CAL02, a novel antitoxin liposomal agent, in severe pneumococcal pneumonia: a first-inhuman, double-blind, placebo-controlled, randomized trial. Lancet Infect Dis 2019;19:620–30.

[38] Storhoff JJ, Lucas AD, Garimella V, Bao YP, Müller UR. Homogeneous detection of unamplified genomic DNA sequences based on colorimetric scatter of gold nanoparticle probes. Nat Biotechnol 2004;22:883–7.

[39] Scott LJ. Verigene® gram-positive blood culture nucleic acid test. Mol Diagn Ther 2013;17:117–22.

[40] Dey P, Fabri-Faja N, Calvo-Lozano O, Terborg RA, Belushkin A, Yesilkoy F, Fàbrega A, RuizRodriguez JC, Ferrer R, González-López JJ, Estévez MC, Altug H, Pruneri V, Lechuga LM. Label-free bacteria quantification in blood plasma by a bioprinted microarray based interferometric point-of-care device. ACS Sens 2019;4:52–60.

[41] Wang JC, Tung YC, Ichiki K, Sakamoto H, Yang TH, Suye SI, Chuang HS. Culture-free detection of methicillin-resistant Staphylococcus aureus by using self-driving diffusometric DNA nanosensors. Biosens Bioelectron 2020;148:111817.

[42] Belushkin A, Yesilkoy F, González-López JJ, Ruiz-Rodríguez JC, Ferrer R, Fàbrega A, Altug H. Rapid and digital detection of inflammatory biomarkers enabled by a novel portable nanoplasmonic imager. Small 2020;16:e1906108.

[43] Etheridge ML, Campbell SA, Erdman AG, Haynes CL, Wolf SM, McCullough J. Biol Med 2013;9:1.

[44] Cooper DL, Conder CM, Harirforoosh S. Nanoparticles in drug delivery: mechanism of action, formulation and clinical application towards reduction in drug-associated nephrotoxicity. Expert Opin Drug Deliv 2014;11:1661–80.

[45] Li X, Robinson SM, Gupta A, Saha K, Jiang Z, Moyano DF, Sahar A, Riley MA, Rotello VM. Functional gold nanoparticles as potent antimicrobial agents against multi-drug-resistant bacteria. ACS Nano 2014;8:10682–6.

[46] Khan ST, Musarrat J, Al-Khedhairy AA. Countering drug resistance, infectious diseases, and sepsis using metal and metal oxides nanoparticles: current status. Colloids Surf B Biointerfaces 2016;146:7083.

[47] Mohammed YHE, Manukumar HM, Rakesh KP, Karthik CS, Mallu P, Qin HL. Vision for medicine: Staphylococcus aureus biofilm war and unlocking key's for anti-biofilm drug development. Microb Pathog 2018;123:339–47.

[48] Alipour M, Suntres ZE, Lafrenie RM, Omri A. Attenuation of Pseudomonas aeruginosa virulence factors and biofilms by co-encapsulation of bismuth-ethanedithiol with tobramycin in liposomes. J Antimicrob Chemother 2010;65:684–93.

[49] Zhu X, Radovic-Moreno AF, Wu J, Langer R, Shi J. Nanomedicine in the management of microbial infection - overview and perspectives. Nano Today 2014;9:478–98.

[50] Gao W, Xiong Y, Li Q, Yang H. Inhibition of toll-like receptor signaling as a promising therapy for inflammatory diseases: a journey from molecular to nano therapeutics. Front Physiol 2017;8:508.

[51] Wesche-Soldato DE, Swan RZ, Chung CS, Ayala A. The apoptotic pathway as a therapeutic target in sepsis. Curr Drug Targets 2007;8:493–500.

[52] Zharov VP, Mercer KE, Galitovskaya EN, Smeltzer MS. Photothermal nanotherapeutics and nanodiagnostics for selective killing of bacteria targeted with gold nanoparticles. Biophys J 2006;90:619–27.

[53] Levy MM, Rhodes A, Phillips GS, Townsend SR, Schorr CA, Beale R, Osborn T, Lemeshow S, Chiche JD, Artigas A, Dellinger RP. Surviving Sepsis Campaign: association between performance metrics and outcomes in a 7.5-year study. Crit Care Med January 2015;43(1):3–12.

[54] Yébenes JC, Ruiz-Rodriguez JC, Ferrer R, Clèries M, Bosch A, Lorencio C, Rodriguez A, Nuvials X, Martin-Loeches I, Artigas A. SOCMIC (catalonian critical care society) sepsis working group. Epidemiology of sepsis in

catalonia: analysis of incidence and outcomes in a European setting. Ann Intensive Care December 2017;7(1):19.

[55] Maslove DM, Tang BM, McLean AS. Identification of sepsis subtypes in critically ill adults using gene expression profiling. Crit Care October 4, 2012;16(5):R183.

[56] Davenport EE, Burnham KL, Radhakrishnan J, Humburg P, Hutton P, Mills TC, Rautanen A, Gordon AC, Garrard C, Hill AV, Hinds CJ, Knight JC. Genomic landscape of the individual host response and outcomes in sepsis: a prospective cohort study. Lancet Respir Med April 2016;4(4):259−71.

[57] Sweeney TE, Azad TD, Donato M, Haynes WA, Perumal TM, Henao R, Bermejo-Martin JF, Almansa R, Tamayo E, Howrylak JA, Choi A, Parnell GP, Tang B, Nichols M, Woods CW, Ginsburg GS, Kingsmore SF, Omberg L, Mangravite LM, Wong HR, Tsalik EL, Langley RJ, Khatri P. Unsupervised analysis of transcriptomics in bacterial sepsis across multiple datasets reveals three robust clusters. Crit Care Med June 2018;46(6): 915−25.

[58] Bauzá-Martinez J, Aletti F, Pinto BB, Ribas V, Odena MA, Díaz R, Romay E, Ferrer R, Kistler EB, Tedeschi G, Schmid-Schönbein GW, Herpain A, Bendjelid K, de Oliveira E. Proteolysis in septic shock patients: plasma peptidomic patterns are associated with mortality. Br J Anaesth November 2018;121(5):10651074.

[59] Cambiaghi A, Pinto BB, Brunelli L, Falcetta F, Aletti F, Bendjelid K, Pastorelli R, Ferrario M. Characterization of a metabolomic profile associated with responsiveness to therapy in the acute phase of septic shock. Sci Rep August 29, 2017;7(1):9748.

[60] Gårdlund B, Dmitrieva NO, Pieper CF, Finfer S, Marshall JC, Taylor Thompson B. Six subphenotypes in septic shock: latent class analysis of the PROWESS Shock study. J Crit Care October 2018;47:70−9.

[61] Seymour CW, Kennedy JN, Wang S, Chang CH, Elliott CF, Xu Z, Berry S, Clermont G, Cooper G, Gomez H, Huang DT, Kellum JA, Mi Q, Opal SM, Talisa V, van der Poll T, Visweswaran S, Vodovotz Y, Weiss JC, Yealy DM, Yende S, Angus DC. Derivation, validation, and potential treatment implications of novel clinical phenotypes for sepsis. JAMA May 28, 2019;321(20):2003−17.

[62] Marik PE, Khangoora V, Rivera R, Hooper MH, Catravas J. Hydrocortisone, vitamin C, and thiamine for the treatment of severe sepsis and septic shock: a retrospective before-after study. Chest June 2017;151(6):1229−38.

[63] Welte T, Dellinger R, Ebelt H, Ferrer M, Opal S, Singer M. Efficacy and safety of trimodulin, a novel polyclonal antibody preparation, in patients with severe community-acquired pneumonia: a randomized, placebo-controlled, double-blind, multicenter, pase II trial (CIGMA study). Intensive Care Med 2018;44: 438−48.

[64] Ruiz-Rodríguez JC, Chiscano-Camón L, Palmada C, Ruiz-Sanmartin A, Pérez-Carrasco M, Larrosa N, et al. Endotoxin and cytokine sequential hemoadsorption in septic shock and multi-organ failure. Blood Purif 2022;51(7): 630−3.

CHAPTER 35

Artificial Intelligence in Sepsis

MICHIEL SCHINKEL • KETAN PARANJAPE • PRABATH W.B. NANAYAKKARA •
W. JOOST WIERSINGA

INTRODUCTION

Since the dawn of the Information Age in the mid-20th century, the use of data in medicine has become increasingly important [1]. The Information Age was characterized by relatively small datasets organized for a specific purpose and presented in a meaningful context. Clinicians used these data to enhance their understanding of disease processes and improve their decision-making. A major challenge during this time was determining how to use all the available information effectively. This issue became even more apparent with the shift to electronic health record (EHR) systems and monitoring devices in the late 1990s and early 2000s [2]. EHR systems facilitate new ways to store and process patient data such as vital signs, test results, and administered medications [3]. With the exponential growth of patient data stored in healthcare systems worldwide, physicians often feel overwhelmed by its abundance and find it impossible to process the data efficiently. Therefore, there is a need to apply novel technologies such as artificial intelligence (AI) to comb through all these data and generate clinically relevant insights.

AI is the scientific discipline that aims to design and understand systems that mimic human cognition [3]. In the age of AI, intellectual processes such as the ability to reason and make decisions will increasingly be displayed by machines [1]. At the heart of AI's value proposition lies the ability to process and learn from large amounts of data and detect patterns of information [3]. State-of-the-art AI tools are increasingly able to act on those data patterns.

Compared to other industries, the healthcare industry has been relatively slow to adopt AI [4]. Among the medical specialties, radiology and cardiology have been at the forefront in developing and testing AI for medical use [5]. In 2016, the United States Food and Drug Administration (FDA) approved a deep learning model for analyzing cardiovascular magnetic resonance images

as the first AI-based medical device [5]. Another 28 tools, ranging from breast density detection via mammography to triage of time-sensitive conditions in the emergency department (ED), have been approved by the FDA. Over the last decade, the sepsis research field has also shown considerable interest in AI applications. Thus far, results have been mixed [3]. The absence of a gold standard case definition of sepsis is one of the main issues that preclude the optimal use of AI models in this field [6]. However, the intrinsic complexity of the sepsis syndrome, in which multiple and sometimes poorly understood mechanisms play a role, seems to be a perfect area for AI assistance regarding its pathogenesis, diagnosis, treatment, and prognosis [3]. This chapter will introduce the basic concepts of some of the most widely used AI techniques. After that, we will systematically discuss the latest AI developments for sepsis and address the challenges we need to overcome to mainstream AI in sepsis management. An explanation of the terms used throughout this chapter can be found in Table 35.1.

A HIGH-LEVEL OVERVIEW OF ARTIFICIAL INTELLIGENCE TECHNIQUES IN HEALTHCARE

Subfields of Artificial Intelligence

To fully appreciate the latest AI developments for sepsis, we need to understand what AI is. As stated before, we can think of AI as the scientific discipline that aims to design and understand computer systems that mimic human cognition [3]. Within the broader field of AI, many subfields seek to emulate different aspects of human cognition. Examples are computer vision (e.g., image recognition in radiology), robotics (e.g., robot-assisted surgery), and natural language processing (e.g., extracting free-text information from electronic patient records) [7]. However, the most tangible manifestation of AI thus far is machine learning [8]. Machine

TABLE 35.1
An Explanation of Specialized Terms Used Throughout This Chapter

Term	Explanation
Artificial intelligence (AI)	The scientific discipline that aims to design and understand computer systems that mimic human cognition. AI has many subfields such as robotics, computer vision, and machine learning.
Machine learning	Machine learning is the subfield of AI that uses data and algorithms to emulate human learning. Popular techniques within the machine learning domain are supervised learning, unsupervised learning, and reinforcement learning.
Endotypes	Endotypes are subgroups within a condition that are distinguished by pathobiological mechanisms.
Phenotypes	Phenotypes are subgroups within a condition that are distinguished by observable traits.

learning is the AI discipline that uses data and algorithms to emulate human learning and has emerged as the most popular AI discipline in the field of sepsis research [3]. We can further subdivide machine learning broadly into supervised learning, unsupervised learning, and reinforcement learning. In the following paragraphs, we will discuss these machine learning disciplines in more detail and examine sepsis-related cases in which they may be helpful. These concepts are also presented visually in Fig. 35.1.

Supervised Machine Learning

Supervised learning is perhaps the most established area of machine learning. In supervised learning, we train models to learn the associations between inputs and outputs [8]. The inputs can come from any data source, and the outputs can include quantities (regression problems) or class labels (classification problems). When the algorithms have learned the associations between these inputs and outputs, they can predict future outcomes based on new inputs. There is a wide variety of supervised machine learning algorithms with unique characteristics and use cases. Well-known examples include random forests, logistic regression, gradient boosted trees, and deep neural networks.

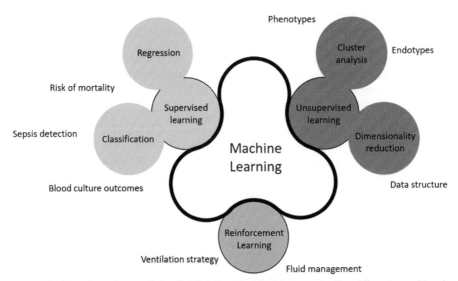

FIG. 35.1 **Machine Learning and its Subfields.** The figure presents the different machine learning subfields (supervised learning, unsupervised learning, and reinforcement learning). Attached to those subfields are the specific techniques within them (e.g., regression and classification within supervised learning). We also show sepsis-specific examples of how those techniques are used. These examples are based on the models we discuss throughout the chapter.

Unsupervised Machine Learning

With unsupervised learning, the data are unlabeled, and the main goal is to learn about the structure of the data rather than specific outcomes [8]. Data inputs are treated as points, and the distances between those points are calculated to find closely related data. Examples of unsupervised learning methods are dimensionality reduction and clustering.

Reinforcement Learning

A third machine learning type, which is recently gaining much interest, is reinforcement learning. Reinforcement learning works in situations with sequential actions, where each step affects the following [8]. The aim is to find a series of actions to optimize a specific outcome, such as survival rates. This type of machine learning does not require labeled data. Instead, the algorithm receives feedback once it has completed the task and will, through trial and error, find the path to the outcome with the most significant (long-term) benefit.

The highly complex clinical management of patients with sepsis is a good use case for reinforcement learning [9]. The treatment is based on several principles and actions, including administering antibiotics, source control, fluid resuscitation, the use of vasopressors, mechanical ventilation, and managing secondary organ failure [10]. Combinations of all these interventions will yield different outcomes. Reinforcement learning can be valuable when finding the optimal sequence of these actions for the individual patient.

MACHINE LEARNING FOR SEPSIS

In the past decade, the number of machine learning papers published in the peer-reviewed literature in the health domain has increased more than 20-fold, with similar numbers in the sepsis field [3,5]. Researchers have developed several hundred machine learning algorithms to aid this syndrome's detection, diagnostic work-up, treatment, and prognostication. We will now discuss some key studies to provide a conceptual framework for the sepsis field's general approaches.

Sepsis Detection

A large part of the literature on machine learning for sepsis focuses on early detection or prediction and primarily uses supervised learning techniques. Predicting the onset of sepsis hours or even days before it happens has much value due to the time-sensitive benefits of the sepsis treatments. Physicians can intensify patient monitoring, optimize diagnostic testing, and initiate therapies early on with these predictions. Investigators have developed at least a dozen such algorithms to predict sepsis onset in the ED, hospital ward, or intensive care unit (ICU) [3,11–18]. The best performing algorithms show reasonably good accuracy using demographics, vital signs, and biomarkers [3]. Up to half of these models are trained on online databases available to researchers worldwide, such as the Medical Information Mart for Intensive Case (MIMIC) and electronic ICU, which significantly expedites the model development and validation phases [3,19,20]. However, few studies have demonstrated the clinical benefits of using such models [3,21].

A well-known sepsis prediction study is the one by Nemati and colleagues [15]. Out of the 27.527 patients admitted to the ICU in their study population, 2.375 developed sepsis according to the sepsis-3 criteria [6]. The model by Nemati et al. predicted sepsis four hours before its onset with an area under the curve (AUC) of the receiver operating characteristics of 0.85. This modified Weibull-Cox proportional hazards model used 65 variables, including high-resolution bedside monitoring data, clinical features, laboratory data, and demographic information. The authors also expanded the prediction window to 12 h before sepsis onset, losing little performance with an AUC of 0.83.

Machine learning has also contributed toward sepsis detection through unsupervised methods, such as cluster analysis. The heterogeneity within the sepsis population has complicated the accurate detection of sepsis and the development of new and effective treatments [22]. In the past few years, clustering techniques have emerged to find subgroups within the sepsis population with similar characteristics. We can then evaluate these subgroups based on their likelihood of responding to specific treatments, otherwise known as population enrichment [23]. Clustering can happen at various levels. Several researchers have derived sepsis subtypes from transcriptomic analyses of circulating immune cells, commonly called endotypes [24,25]. A study by Davenport and colleagues discovered two distinct sepsis response states following ICU admission, which they named SRS1 and SRS2 [24]. SRS1 was associated with signs of immunosuppression such as T-cell exhaustion and endotoxin tolerance. The overall mortality in this group was higher than in the SRS2 type (hazard ratio of 2.4). Other investigators found four distinct sepsis endotypes among ICU patients (Mars1-4) [24]. The Mars1 endotype seemed to provide the most robust classification and was associated with high mortality rates and decreased innate and adaptive immune pathways expression, similar to the SRS1 type by Davenport.

In both these studies, the endotypes were not simply distinguishable by clinical characteristics [24,25]. In contrast, other studies specifically aimed to find such sepsis subgroups based on readily available clinical data and laboratory results instead of complex transcriptome analyses. Seymour and colleagues sought to find clinical phenotypes in a cohort of 20.189 sepsis patients in various wards across 12 community and academic hospitals in the United States [26]. Their study used consensus k-means clustering based on 29 clinical and laboratory variables and derived four distinct sepsis phenotypes. These four phenotypes show considerable overlap with the endotypes we discussed above. For example, the δ phenotype characterized by cardiovascular and liver dysfunction has high mortality rates and resembles the SRS1 and Mars1 clusters [26]. These examples of unsupervised clustering to classify sepsis patients into more homogeneous subgroups show that these methods can detect fairly robust patterns, irrespective of the procedure or variables used. Recognizing these patterns will be one of the keys to the success of any new immune-directed therapy as it may identify patients who can benefit the most from a specific intervention [27]. Using clustering algorithms can even help optimize the use of existing treatment strategies. Researchers have shown that clustering techniques could discover subgroups of sepsis patients likely or unlikely to benefit from early antibiotic treatment [28].

Diagnostic Work-Up

The diagnostic work-up of patients with acute infections and (potential) sepsis can include multiple tests to detect a pathogen and estimate disease severity [29]. Unfortunately, some pathogen detection methods have minimal utility for the initial clinical management since turnaround times for those results can take between hours to days. We can potentially leverage predictive tools based on supervised learning to use routinely available data to innovate pathogen testing and increase its utility in the initial phases of the diagnostic work-up. Most of the work in this field has focused on blood cultures rather than other pathogen tests. This may be because blood cultures present a reasonably good gold standard test compared with different cultures, and physicians liberally use them. Blood culture testing is one of the main diagnostic tests in the sepsis diagnostic work-up. Of the septic patients, 38%−69% have bloodstream infections [30]. While blood cultures can yield significant insights into the optimal antimicrobial strategy, the results will usually take 24−72 h.

In the past decade, researchers have designed multiple machine learning algorithms to predict blood culture results. When these predictions are accurate, we can use them as a proxy for the eventual culture outcome and use them in the early stages of the diagnostic work-up to determine an appropriate treatment strategy. They can be especially helpful in detecting patients at low risk of a bloodstream infection to reduce blood culture draws and unneeded antibiotic therapy. A 2015 review presented 15 such prediction models, with AUCs of up to 0.79 during validation in an ED, hospital ward, or ICU setting [31]. Some of these models, such as one by Shapiro et al. performed similarly well in external validation cohorts, indicating the robustness of those findings [32]. The Shapiro study prospectively included 3730 consecutive ED patients who had a blood culture taken. The robustness of the predictions may be due to the detailed patient characteristics documented as part of the study, such as suspicion of endocarditis, which are usually not included in these types of prediction models when they are based on retrospective data. Though they may have increased performance and robustness, these variables make it harder for such a model to be implemented in the clinic since they will have to be documented every time one uses the tool. Since the 2015 review, advances in machine learning have been apparent through more complicated (deep) neural networks and better performances of AUCs up to 0.99 during internal validations [33,34]. Notably, overfitting to the respective datasets is a genuine concern. Expectedly, external validation of the study by Roimi and colleagues shows a dramatic loss in predictive performance with a drop in AUC from 0.92 to 0.60.

Researchers have also created algorithms to predict a pathogen's susceptibility to certain antibiotics [35]. These algorithms can be highly relevant for sepsis since the results of susceptibility testing in case of a potential bacterial causative agent will only be known 24−72 h after starting the empiric antibiotic therapy. Yelin and colleagues, for instance, showed that antibiotic resistance to empirical treatment for urinary tract infections (UTIs) was highly predictable. Combining patient demographics, past UTI characteristics, and purchase history of antibiotics gave the best predictive performance. The physicians' overall empirical antibiotic mismatch rate was 8.5% (95% CI: 8.03−9.05), while this was just 5.1% (95% CI: 4.69−5.48) for algorithmic drug recommendations.

Sepsis Management

Traditionally, sepsis clinical trials have focused on testing the efficacy of standalone interventions or combinations of interventions at a given time point, such as early treatment with antibiotics, early goal-directed therapy, or the use of immunomodulatory drugs [10,36,37]. These studies rarely consider the sequence of the particular actions that would yield the optimal outcome, while the management of sepsis in practice is a sequential process. With the rapid emergence of reinforcement learning, we now have the technology to evaluate those sequential processes and dynamically optimize the sepsis management strategies.

A pioneering study on reinforcement learning for sepsis created an artificially intelligent clinician to learn optimal vasopressor and fluid usage in the ICU [9]. This study by Komorowski et al. uses a Markov decision process, which provides a mathematical framework to model the patient's state when that state is only partially represented within the data. They analyzed the treatments of actual clinicians and computed the average effect of different therapies on 90-day survival. They then compared these effects to those of strategies generated by their AI model. When the actual clinicians chose treatment policies that overlapped with the actions proposed by the AI clinician, the mortality rates were the lowest. Interestingly, the AI clinician suggested earlier and higher doses of vasopressors, providing new insights into fluid management for sepsis.

To optimize mechanical ventilation strategies in critically ill patients, researchers have also developed a reinforcement learning algorithm called VentAI [38]. Through the sequential decision-making process characteristic of reinforcement learning, the VentAI algorithm changed the specific ventilation strategy more than twice as often as physicians would. On top of that, the VentAI algorithm avoided high FiO_2 (>55%) while preferring FiO_2 levels of 50%–55%. Compared with physician policies, these AI ventilation strategies seemed to decrease the chance of 90-day mortality.

Over the next few years, reinforcement learning will likely be the primary machine learning method used to optimize sepsis management. Although reinforcement learning for sepsis is still very much in its infancy, there lies great promise in the dynamics of these algorithms and their ability to find optimal sequences of steps, which mirrors clinical practice. So far, researchers have only developed reinforcement learning models for specific interventions like fluid management or mechanical ventilation. To create models that include all potential interventions, one needs larger datasets than those currently available [9].

Prognostication of Sepsis Patients

A final area in which machine learning can contribute in the sepsis field is prognostication. Giving physicians a reasonable estimate of the patient's prognosis can help decide which patients need hospital or ICU admission and how long they should stay there. Furthermore, some patients who initially do not seem to have sepsis may still decline rapidly and have a high risk of (sepsis-related) mortality [39]. These patients may benefit significantly from, for instance, the early administration of antibiotics. Researchers have proposed various supervised machine learning models that predict mortality. For example, a model created by Dybowski and colleagues predicts in-hospital mortality for sepsis patients [40]. In this study, the authors used a technique called Classification and Regression Trees to select 11 variables (out of 157) as inputs to an artificial neural network. The neural network reached an AUC of 0.863 and performed significantly better than a logistic regression model (AUC = 0.753) in the same dataset. The neural network in this study slightly outperforms most other published supervised learning prognostication models and the widely used APACHE-II score [3,41].

CHALLENGES WITH AI FOR SEPSIS

The fast-growing interest in AI for sepsis and its ever-increasing possibilities generate new challenges along the way. The main challenge at this point is getting AI models implemented. While researchers have created numerous algorithms for sepsis, few of them have made it into clinical practice [3]. Among 494 studies on machine learning tools for the ICU, of which 37 (7.5%) focused on sepsis exclusively, 476 (96.4%) were retrospective studies, and 378 (80.9%) were classified as having a high risk of bias [3,21]. Only 10 (2.0%) studies were clinical trials to evaluate the real-world benefits of using the machine learning models, and none of the 494 studies reported on model integration in clinical practice [21]. Here we will discuss many of the barriers to AI implementation. Detailed discussions of regulatory issues, ethical dilemmas, and privacy aspects are outside the scope of this chapter.

Machine Learning and the Sepsis Definition

A significant issue with using machine learning for sepsis is that the definition of sepsis does not lend itself to predictive modeling with supervised learning techniques. This is most apparent when we look at the prediction of sepsis onset. With supervised machine learning, one needs labeled data. When we label a patient as having sepsis or not, this represents a broad continuum of disease, inevitably making it harder to predict any one case correctly. Furthermore, the sepsis definition consists mainly of vital parameters and laboratory results. These parameters should not be used in a prediction model since having predictor variables that are part of the outcome definition will lead to overestimated results [3,42]. A solution to the challenges described above is using supervised learning only in settings where we can better define the outcome label, such as predicting mortality or other sepsis-related complications. And, for sepsis detection, unsupervised (unlabeled; data-driven) approaches may be preferred for now.

Clinical Evaluation and Implementation in Different Settings

Another barrier to implementing AI for sepsis is the clinical evaluation of these systems in different settings. The importance of a robust validation, which should include metrics intuitive to clinicians in the emergency room, regular wards, and ICU, was recently illustrated by the validation of the Epic Sepsis Model (ESM) [43,44]. This proprietary algorithm is developed by the EHR vendor Epic and aims to predict the onset of sepsis. The algorithm is integrated into their EHR system and used in hundreds of hospitals worldwide [44]. The ESM is a penalized logistic regression model based on 80 variables, among which are vital signs and laboratory results [44]. When investigators aimed to validate the ESM a few years after its widespread adoption, they showed that the algorithm detected sepsis with an AUC of just 0.63 in their population of 2.552 sepsis patients among 38.455 hospitalizations [44]. Clinicians would have evaluated 109 patients based on an ESM alert to detect one case of sepsis earlier than they would otherwise. On top of that, the model calibration as visualized in calibration plots was inadequate since the model tended to predict extremely high probabilities for sepsis compared to the actual probabilities.

Given that the initially reported performance of the ESM was much better (AUC of 0.76−0.83), this validation clearly illustrates some consistent misconceptions about the development and deployment of predictive models in healthcare [44]. First of all, clinical and operational heterogeneity causes predictive models to perform differently across hospitals and settings [45]. Thus, one cannot deploy a model in a new environment and expect the same results. Furthermore, even the most rigorously validated models will inevitably experience a drop in performance over time. This performance drift usually results from shifts in the patient mix and clinical protocols, which happen quickly in healthcare [46]. To overcome the problems that were illustrated by the ESM validation, we need to take several steps. Model developers should be encouraged to think about how their models should be updated over time and to maintain a stable performance. Researchers have already proposed strategies for this, such as recalibration under case-mix shifts and intercept correction when outcome rates in the data change [46]. External validation is still an essential aspect during model development. It may indicate whether the model finds a valid and somewhat reproducible signal. However, site-specific training will always be required to adapt to a hospital system's intricacies and reach the best performance [43]. Medical journals can be advised to guide peer reviewers to understand the dynamic nature of these algorithms and focus on the proposed (re)training protocols rather than specific external validation performances.

The Trade-off Between Performance and Explainability

Some state-of-the-art AI techniques, such as deep learning networks, offer impressive increases in performance over what we have seen in the past decade. However, these types of models usually have no way of explaining how they make a particular prediction. An example is "Deep Patient," where researchers used deep learning to predict the onset of schizophrenia but did not give any clue how it could do so [47]. This phenomenon is known as the "black box." It may be hard to trust such a prediction for a condition that even an experienced psychiatrist cannot predict. This is why the healthcare industry, particularly the care for critically ill patients with sepsis, provides a great incentive to favor explainable models over those with high performance [43]. Explainability enables the physicians to verify the system in situations with an increased risk of unintended bias and where the consequences of wrong predictions can be fatal. For now, that means that we should only use deep learning models with great caution and that an explainable AI model should be preferred [43].

Artificial Intelligence Training in Medical Education

A final challenge on the road to getting AI for sepsis embedded in routine clinical practice lies in education. Globally, medical training emphasizes memorization-based learning and has not yet transitioned from the age of information to the age of AI [1]. Thus, at the point when state-of-the-art machine learning algorithms for sepsis can be integrated into clinical practice, physicians may not be ready to appreciate the value and pitfalls of these tools entirely nor be able to supervise them [48]. Few studies have explicitly aimed to find the barriers among end-users that could prevent the implementation of machine learning tools in practice. One study showed that about one in five key stakeholders in laboratory medicine does not see any value in AI [49]. There seems to be a disconnect between the views of data scientists and the medical community. Furthermore, the study results raise the concern that specific knowledge on AI in the medical community is still lacking. Additional studies on the barriers and facilitators of AI adoption among end-users are needed. The lack of training on the basics of machine learning during medical education may arguably contribute to the slow maturation of clinical AI implementation. Fortunately, there does seem to be some movement in the right direction. In 2018, the American Medical Association was one of the first to adopt a policy on AI, encouraging research on how to change the medical curriculum to address AI [48]. Consequently, a detailed framework on how to embed education on AI through all stages of medical training has been proposed [48].

CONCLUSIONS

The use of AI for sepsis will bring us ever closer to the idea of precision medicine, where one can tailor the diagnostic work-up and treatment for a particular patient. Unsupervised machine learning helps us detect meaningful subtypes of sepsis patients with similar characteristics, and supervised learning can further help decrease the sepsis population's heterogeneity [26,50]. We still have much to learn about how we can effectively use AI for these purposes. In this chapter, we have discussed some of the foreseen roadblocks on that path. Over the next three to five years, the clinical implementation of AI tools for sepsis will mature, and we will likely see the first of such models' regulatory approval for day-to-day practice. After seeing the first standalone machine learning tools in clinical practice for specific use cases, they will need to be integrated into broader platforms over the coming years. Continuous improvements in the already promising field of reinforcement learning can play a primary role in finding the optimal sequence of tests and treatments to optimize clinical outcomes in individual patients. As we capture increasing amounts of data, we will eventually create reinforcement learning models to find optimal sequences of actions throughout an entire episode of sepsis.

There are countless possibilities to use AI to advance the clinical care of patients who suffer from sepsis. Many machine learning models can potentially aid in the early detection of sepsis, optimize the diagnostic work-up, and recommend treatment strategies. However, we are still in the early stages of adopting these tools into routine clinical practice. At the moment, few studies have shown robust and clinically meaningful benefits from using AI tools. Researchers must first overcome obstacles such as a continuous clinical evaluation of these tools, limited explainability, and the lack of medical AI training. Further research on the barriers to implementing machine learning tools in clinical practice is much needed to aid the maturation of this research field. The road to medical AI products that deliver value for patients and the healthcare community is still long and challenging but presents exciting opportunities to improve routine practice.

REFERENCES

[1] Wartman SA, Donald Combs C. Medical education must move from the information age to the age of artificial intelligence. Acad Med 2018;93:1107—9. https://doi.org/10.1097/ACM.0000000000002044.

[2] Healthcare Data Growth: An Exponential Problem n.d. https://www.nextech.com/blog/healthcare-data-growth-an-exponential-problem (accessed May 7, 2021).

[3] Schinkel M, Paranjape K, Nannan Panday RS, Skyttberg N, Nanayakkara PWB. Clinical applications of artificial intelligence in sepsis: a narrative review. Comput Biol Med 2019;115. https://doi.org/10.1016/j.compbiomed.2019.103488.

[4] Vigilante K, Escaravage S, McConnell M. Big data and the intelligence community—lessons for health care. N Engl J Med 2019;380:1888—90. https://doi.org/10.1056/nejmp1815418.

[5] Benjamens S, Dhunnoo P, Meskó B. The state of artificial intelligence-based FDA-approved medical devices and algorithms: an online database. Npj Digit Med 2020;3:1—8. https://doi.org/10.1038/s41746-020-00324-0.

[6] Singer M, Deutschman CS, Seymour CW, Shankar-Hari M, Annane D, Bauer M, et al. The third international consensus definitions for sepsis and septic shock (Sepsis-3). JAMA 2016;315:801. https://doi.org/10.1001/jama.2016.0287.

[7] Ohno-Machado L, Nadkarni P, Johnson K. Natural language processing: algorithms and tools to extract computable information from EHRs and from the biomedical literature. J Am Med Inf Assoc 2013;20:805. https://doi.org/10.1136/amiajnl-2013-002214.

[8] Panch T, Szolovits P, Atun R. Artificial intelligence, machine learning and health systems. J Glob Health 2018;8. https://doi.org/10.7189/jogh.08.020303.

[9] Komorowski M, Celi LA, Badawi O, Gordon AC, Faisal AA. The Artificial Intelligence Clinician learns optimal treatment strategies for sepsis in intensive care. Nat Med 2018;24:1716—20.

[10] Rhodes A, Evans LE, Alhazzani W, Levy MM, Antonelli M, Ferrer R, et al. Surviving sepsis campaign. Crit Care Med

2017;45:486—552. https://doi.org/10.1097/CCM.0000 000000002255.

[11] Fleuren LM, Klausch TLT, Zwager CL, Schoonmade LJ, Guo T, Roggeveen LF, et al. Machine learning for the prediction of sepsis: a systematic review and meta-analysis of diagnostic test accuracy. Intensive Care Med 2020;46:383—400. https://doi.org/10.1007/s00134-019-05872-y.

[12] Delahanty RJ, Alvarez J, Flynn LM, Sherwin RL, Jones SS. Development and evaluation of a machine learning model for the early identification of patients at risk for sepsis. Ann Emerg Med 2019;73(4):334—44.

[13] Desautels T, Calvert J, Hoffman J, Jay M, Kerem Y, Shieh L, et al. Prediction of sepsis in the intensive care unit with minimal electronic health record data: a machine learning approach. JMIR Med Informatics 2016;4:e28.

[14] Mao Q, Jay M, Hoffman JL, Calvert J, Barton C, Shimabukuro D, et al. Multicentre validation of a sepsis prediction algorithm using only vital sign data in the emergency department, general ward and ICU. BMJ Open 2018;8:e017833.

[15] Nemati S, Holder A, Razmi F, Stanley MD, Clifford GD, Buchman TG. An interpretable machine learning model for accurate prediction of sepsis in the ICU. Crit Care Med 2018;46:547—53.

[16] Taneja I, Reddy B, Damhorst G, Dave Zhao S, Hassan U, Price Z, et al. Combining biomarkers with EMR data to identify patients in different phases of sepsis. Sci Rep 2017;7:10800.

[17] Saqib M, Sha Y, Wang MD. Early prediction of sepsis in EMR records using traditional ML techniques and deep learning LSTM networks. Conf Proc. Annu Int Conf IEEE Eng Med Biol Soc IEEE Eng Med Biol Soc Annu Conf 2018;2018:4038—41.

[18] Shashikumar SP, Stanley MD, Sadiq I, Li Q, Holder A, Clifford GD, et al. Early sepsis detection in critical care patients using multiscale blood pressure and heart rate dynamics. J Electrocardiol 2017;50:739—43.

[19] MIMIC-IV v1.0 n.d. https://physionet.org/content/mimiciv/1.0/(accessed June 8, 2021).

[20] Pollard TJ, Johnson AEW, Raffa JD, Celi LA, Mark RG, Badawi O. The eICU collaborative research database, a freely available multi-center database for critical care research. Sci Data 2018;5:1—13. https://doi.org/10.1038/sdata.2018.178.

[21] van de Sande D, van Genderen ME, Huiskens J, Gommers D, van Bommel J. Moving from bytes to bedside: a systematic review on the use of artificial intelligence in the intensive care unit. Intensive Care Med 2021:1—11. https://doi.org/10.1007/s00134-021-06446-7.

[22] Schinkel M, Virk HS, Nanayakkara PWB, van der Poll T, Wiersinga WJ. What sepsis researchers can learn from COVID-19. Am J Respir Crit Care Med 2021;203:125—7. https://doi.org/10.1164/rccm.202010-4023LE.

[23] Stanski NL, Wong HR. Prognostic and predictive enrichment in sepsis. Nat Rev Nephrol 2020;16:20—31. https://doi.org/10.1038/s41581-019-0199-3.

[24] Scicluna BP, van Vught LA, Zwinderman AH, Wiewel MA, Davenport EE, Burnham KL, et al. Classification of patients with sepsis according to blood genomic endotype: a prospective cohort study. Lancet Respir Med 2017;5:816—26.

[25] Davenport EE, Burnham KL, Radhakrishnan J, Humburg P, Hutton P, Mills TC, et al. Genomic landscape of the individual host response and outcomes in sepsis: a prospective cohort study. Lancet Respir Med 2016;4:259—71. https://doi.org/10.1016/S2213-2600(16)00046-1.

[26] Seymour CW, Kennedy JN, Wang S, Chang C-CH, Elliott CF, Xu Z, et al. Derivation, validation, and potential treatment implications of novel clinical phenotypes for sepsis. JAMA 2019;321:2003. https://doi.org/10.1001/jama.2019.5791.

[27] Van Der Poll T, Van De Veerdonk FL, Scicluna BP, Netea MG. The immunopathology of sepsis and potential therapeutic targets. Nat Rev Immunol 2017;17:407—20. https://doi.org/10.1038/nri.2017.36.

[28] Schinkel M, Paranjape K, Kundert J, Nannan Panday RS, Alam N, Nanayakkara PWB. Towards understanding the effective use of antibiotics for sepsis. Chest 2021;0. https://doi.org/10.1016/j.chest.2021.04.038.

[29] Sweeney TE, Liesenfeld O, May L. Diagnosis of bacterial sepsis: why are tests for bacteremia not sufficient? Expert Rev Mol Diagn 2019;19:959—62. https://doi.org/10.1080/14737159.2019.1660644.

[30] Coburn B, Morris AM, Tomlinson G, Detsky AS. Does this adult patient with suspected bacteremia require blood cultures? JAMA, J Am Med Assoc 2012;308:502—11. https://doi.org/10.1001/jama.2012.8262.

[31] Eliakim-Raz N, Bates DW, Leibovici L. Predicting bacteraemia in validated models-a systematic review. Clin Microbiol Infect 2015;21:295—301. https://doi.org/10.1016/j.cmi.2015.01.023.

[32] Shapiro NI, Wolfe RE, Wright SB, Moore R, Bates DW. Who needs a blood culture? A prospectively derived and validated prediction rule. J Emerg Med 2008;35:255—64. https://doi.org/10.1016/j.jemermed.2008.04.001.

[33] Van Steenkiste T, Ruyssinck J, De Baets L, Decruyenaere J, De Turck F, Ongenae F, et al. Accurate prediction of blood culture outcome in the intensive care unit using long short-term memory neural networks. Artif Intell Med 2019;97:38—43. https://doi.org/10.1016/j.artmed.2018.10.008.

[34] Roimi M, Neuberger A, Shrot A, Paul M, Geffen Y, Bar-Lavie Y. Early diagnosis of bloodstream infections in the intensive care unit using machine-learning algorithms. Intensive Care Med 2020;46:454—62. https://doi.org/10.1007/s00134-019-05876-8.

[35] Yelin I, Snitser O, Novich G, Katz R, Tal O, Parizade M, et al. Personal clinical history predicts antibiotic resistance of urinary tract infections. Nat Med 2019;25:1143—52. https://doi.org/10.1038/s41591-019-0503-6.

[36] Alam N, Oskam E, Stassen PM, Exter P van, van de Ven PM, Haak HR, et al. Prehospital antibiotics in the ambulance for sepsis: a multicentre, open label, randomised trial. Lancet Respir Med 2018;6:40—50. https://doi.org/10.1016/S2213-2600(17)30469-1.

[37] Rivers E, Nguyen B, Havstad S, Ressler J, Muzzin A, Knoblich B, et al. Early goal-directed therapy in the

treatment of severe sepsis and septic shock. N Engl J Med 2001;345:1368—77. https://doi.org/10.1056/NEJMoa0 10307.

[38] Peine A, Hallawa A, Bickenbach J, Dartmann G, Fazlic LB, Schmeink A, et al. Development and validation of a reinforcement learning algorithm to dynamically optimize mechanical ventilation in critical care. Npj Digit Med 2021;4. https://doi.org/10.1038/s41746-021-00388-6.

[39] Quinten VM, van Meurs M, Ligtenberg JJ, Ter Maaten JC. Prehospital antibiotics for sepsis: beyond mortality? Lancet Respir Med 2018;6:e8. https://doi.org/10.1016/S2213-2600(18)30061-4.

[40] Dybowski R, Weller P, Chang R, Gant V. Prediction of outcome in critically ill patients using artificial neural network synthesised by genetic algorithm. Lancet 1996; 347:1146—50. https://doi.org/10.1016/S0140-6736(96)90609-1.

[41] Knaus W, Draper EA, Wagner DP, Zimmerman JE. Apache II: a severity of disease classification systemvol. 13; 1985. https://doi.org/10.1097/00003465-198603000-00013.

[42] Moons KGM, Wolff RF, Riley RD, Penny, Whiting F, Westwood M, et al. PROBAST: a tool to assess risk of bias and applicability of prediction model studies: explanation and elaboration annals of internal medicine research and reporting methods. Ann Intern Med 2019; 170:1—33. https://doi.org/10.7326/M18-1377.

[43] Kelly CJ, Karthikesalingam A, Suleyman M, Corrado G, King D. Key challenges for delivering clinical impact with artificial intelligence. BMC Med 2019;17. https://doi.org/10.1186/s12916-019-1426-2.

[44] Wong A, Otles E, Donnelly JP, Krumm A, McCullough J, DeTroyer-Cooley O, et al. External validation of a widely implemented proprietary sepsis prediction model in hospitalized patients. JAMA Intern Med 2021;181(8):1065—70. https://doi.org/10.1001/jamainternmed.2021.2626.

[45] Van Calster B, Wynants L, Timmerman D, Steyerberg EW, Collins GS. Predictive analytics in health care: how can we know it works? J Am Med Inf Assoc 2019;26: 1651—4. https://doi.org/10.1093/jamia/ocz130.

[46] Davis SE, Greevy RA, Fonnesbeck C, Lasko TA, Walsh CG, Matheny ME. A nonparametric updating method to correct clinical prediction model drift. J Am Med Inf Assoc 2019;26: 1448—57. https://doi.org/10.1093/jamia/ocz127.

[47] "Deep Learning: The Most Advanced Artificial Intelligence" - Chris Brandt | Mount Sinai - New York n.d. https://www.mountsinai.org/about/newsroom/2017/university-herald-deep-learning-the-most-advanced-artificial-intelligence-chris-brandt (accessed June 28, 2021).

[48] Paranjape K, Schinkel M, Panday RN, Car J, Nanayakkara P. Introducing artificial intelligence training in medical education. JMIR Med Educ 2019;5. https://doi.org/10.2196/16048.

[49] Paranjape K, Schinkel M, Hammer RD, Schouten B, Nannan Panday RS, Elbers PWG, et al. The value of artificial intelligence in laboratory medicine. Am J Clin Pathol 2020;155(6):823—31. https://doi.org/10.1093/ajcp/aqaa170.

[50] Demerle K, Angus DC, Seymour CW. Precision medicine for COVID-19: phenotype Anarchy or promise realized? JAMA, J Am Med Assoc 2021;325:2041—2. https://doi.org/10.1001/jama.2021.5248.

Index

'*Note:* Page numbers followed by "t" indicate tables.'

Printed and bound by CPI Group (UK) Ltd, Croydon, CR0 4YY

08/05/2025

01864765-0001